# Advances in Fertility and Reproductive Medicine

# Advances in Fertility and Reproductive Medicine

Proceedings of the 18th World Congress on Fertility and Sterility held in Montréal, Canada between 23 and 28 May 2004.

*Editors:*

**Salim Daya, M.D.**
Professor
Departments of Obstetrics & Gynecology and
Clinical Epidemiology & Biostatistics
McMaster University
Hamilton, Ontario, Canada

**Robert F. Harrison**
Professor
RCSI Department of Obstetrics and Gynaecology and
Human Assisted Reproduction Unit
Rotunda Hospital, Dublin
Ireland

**Roger D. Kempers, M.D.**
President, IFFS
Professor, Obstetrics and Gynecology, Emeritus
Mayo Medical School and May Clinic
Rochester, MN
USA

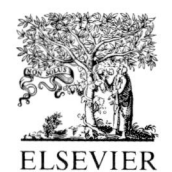

ELSEVIER

**2004**

| | | | |
|---|---|---|---|
| ELSEVIER B.V. | ELSEVIER Inc. | ELSEVIER Ltd | ELSEVIER Ltd |
| Sara Burgerhartstraat 25 | 525 B Street, Suite 1900 | The Boulevard, Langford Lane | 84 Theobalds Road |
| P.O. Box 211, 1000 AE Amsterdam | San Diego, CA 92101-4495 | Kidlington, Oxford OX5 1GB | London WC1X 8RR |
| The Netherlands | USA | UK | UK |

© 2004 Elsevier B.V. All rights reserved.

This work is protected under copyright by Elsevier, and the following terms and conditions apply to its use:

Photocopying
Single photocopies of single chapters may be made for personal use as allowed by national copyright laws. Permission of the Publisher and payment of a fee is required for all other photocopying, including multiple or systematic copying, copying for advertising or promotional purposes, resale, and all forms of document delivery. Special rates are available for educational institutions that wish to make photocopies for non-profit educational classroom use.

Permissions may be sought directly from Elsevier's Rights Department in Philadelphia, PA, USA: phone (+1) 215 238 7869, fax (+1) 215 238 2239, e-mail healthpermissions@elsevier.com. Requests may also be completed on-line via the Elsevier homepage (http://www.elsevier.com/locate/permissions).

In the USA, users may clear permissions and make payments through the Copyright Clearance Center, Inc., 222 Rosewood Drive, Danvers, MA 01923, USA; phone: (+1) (978) 7508400, fax: (+1) (978) 7504744, and in the UK through the Copyright Licensing Agency Rapid Clearance Service (CLARCS), 90 Tottenham Court Road, London W1P 0LP, UK; phone: (+44) 207 631 5555; fax: (+44) 207 631 5500. Other countries may have a local reprographic rights agency for payments.

Derivative Works
Tables of contents may be reproduced for internal circulation, but permission of Elsevier is required for external resale or distribution of such material.
Permission of the Publisher is required for all other derivative works, including compilations and translations.

Electronic Storage or Usage
Permission of the Publisher is required to store or use electronically any material contained in this work, including any chapter or part of a chapter.

Except as outlined above, no part of this work may be reproduced, stored in a retrieval system or transmitted in any form or by any means, electronic, mechanical, photocopying, recording or otherwise, without prior written permission of the Publisher. Address permissions requests to: Elsevier Rights Department, at the fax and e-mail addresses noted above.

Notice
No responsibility is assumed by the Publisher for any injury and/or damage to persons or property as a matter of products liability, negligence or otherwise, or from any use or operation of any methods, products, instructions or ideas contained in the material herein. Because of rapid advances in the medical sciences, in particular, independent verification of diagnoses and drug dosages should be made.

First edition 2004

Library of Congress Cataloging in Publication Data
A catalog record is available from the Library of Congress.

British Library Cataloguing in Publication Data
A catalogue record is available from the British Library.

International Congress Series No. 1266
ISBN: 0-444-51545-3
ISSN: 0531-5131

∞ The paper used in this publication meets the requirements of ANSI/NISO Z39.48-1992 (Permanence of Paper).
Printed in The Netherlands.

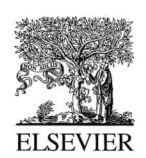

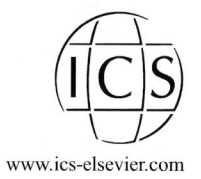

# Preface

On the occasion of its 50th anniversary, the Canadian Fertility and Andrology Society, on behalf of the International Federation of Fertility Societies (IFFS), is pleased to host the 18th World Congress on Fertility and Sterility in Montreal, Quebec, Canada. The Scientific Committee of the IFFS has worked hard to organize an outstanding scientific programme that focuses on advances in the rapidly growing field of reproductive medicine and science. Our understanding of mechanisms of disease has expanded exponentially with developments in molecular and cellular biology. Similarly, new innovations in assisted reproductive technologies have opened up numerous options for treatment of infertility and improved our understanding of the processes involved in gamete interaction and implantation. The increased focus on evidence-based practice has led to critical review of existing evidence in the areas of therapy, diagnostic assessment, causation and prognosis and has provided the framework for conducting clinical studies and therapeutic trials that have high validity. Implementation of the findings from these studies has improved clinical decision making and our understanding of disorders in reproduction. Advances in reproduction bring with them many ethical challenges that require debate and formulation of health policies. Furthermore, the long-term effects of our therapeutic strategies need to be addressed through careful and comprehensive outcome evaluation surveillance methods.

A major feature of these World Congresses, which are held every 3 years, is to provide the most current scientific information to the delegates. To accomplish this objective, we have brought together a group of recognized authorities, who, by being at the forefront of research in their specific fields in reproductive medicine and science, can share their knowledge with the participants. The manuscripts derived from these presentations have been compiled into this book of the Proceedings of the 18th World Congress in Fertility and Sterility. They include Plenary topics, which are the keynote lectures of the congress, and Trilogy lectures, a format which involves three topics grouped in thematic manner to integrate contemporary research and clinical information.

The editors wish to thank all of the contributing authors for agreeing to submit their work and for the quality and timeliness of their manuscripts which have allowed us to produce this comprehensive text on a wide range of topics in reproductive medicine and science. It will serve as a very useful resource to researchers and health care practitioners dedicated to improving the understanding and management of disorders in reproduction.

Salim Daya
Robert F. Harrison
Roger D. Kempers

0531-5131/ © 2004 Published by Elsevier B.V.
doi:10.1016/j.ics.2004.02.088

# Contents

**Preface** v

**Plenary** 1

Treating menopause in the 21st century—where do we go from here?
*I. Schiff* 3

New developments in the evaluation and management of male infertility
*R.I. McLachlan* 10

Transcultural issues in gender selection
*G.I. Serour* 21

Is human fertility declining?
*T.K. Jensen, A.N. Andersen, N.E. Skakkebæk* 32

Human embryonic stem cells—potential applications for regenerative medicine
*B. Reubinoff* 45

**Trilogy** 55

*Evidence-based infertility*

Evidence-based infertility: evaluation of the female partner
*J.A. Collins* 57

*Management of menstrual disorders*

Medical management of menstrual disorders
*J.S. Tapanainen* 63

Mirena
*S.L. Yu* 69

Menorrhagia: the role of endometrial ablation
*M.C. Sowter* 72

## Advances in contraception and sterilization

Adolescent contraception
D. Apter, R. Cacciatore, E. Hermanson — 81

## Evidence-based reproductive surgery

Evidence-based reproductive surgery: endometriosis
J.L.H. Evers — 90

Evidence-based reproductive surgery: tubal infertility
H. Dechaud, L. Reyftmann, J. Faidherbe, S. Hamamah, B. Hedon — 96

Future directions and development in reproductive surgery
T. Falcone — 107

## Optimizing outcome in assisted reproduction

Embryo transfer—a critique of the factors involved in optimizing pregnancy success
H.N. Sallam — 111

Optimizing outcome in assisted reproduction reducing multiple pregnancy
D.L. Healy, S. Breheny, V. MacLachlan, L. Rombauts, G. Kovacs — 119

Endocrine disrupters and ovarian function
W.G. Foster, M.S. Neal, E.V. YoungLai — 126

## Health in menopause

Menopause-related definitions
W.H. Utian — 133

Critique of the evidence from large trials of hormone replacement therapy
H. Rozenbaum — 139

Health in the menopause: advances in management
S.O. Skouby — 151

## Current developments in assisted reproduction

Embryo selection and health
A. Veiga, G. Arroyo, P.N. Barri — 156

In vitro maturation of human ova
A.L. Mikkelsen — 160

## Basic science in assisted reproduction

Basic science issues in assisted reproduction: gamete interaction
S. Brugo Olmedo   167

Apoptosis in testicular germ cells
D. Royere, F. Guérif, V. Laurent-Cadoret, M.-T. Hochereau de Reviers   170

Implantation and uterine receptivity
J.A. Horcajadas, F. Domínguez, J. Martín, A. Pellicer, C. Simón   177

## Fibroids

Fibroids: basic science and etiology
S. Fujii, A. Suzuki, N. Matsumura, T. Kanamori, H. Shime, K. Fukuhara, K. Takakura, M. Kariya   183

Fibroids: effect on infertility and assisted reproduction
C.M. Farquhar   191

Treatment options for uterine myoma
R. Al-Fadhli, T. Tulandi   197

## Controversies in treatment of male infertility

Guidelines in the treatment of male infertility
S. Irvine   202

Intrauterine insemination for idiopathic male subfertility
B.J. Cohlen   208

Leukocytospermia
R. Menkveld   218

## Polycystic ovarian syndrome

Polycystic ovary syndrome—diagnosis and etiology
R.J. Norman, T. Hickey, L. Moran, J. Boyle, J. Wang, M. Davies   225

Do women with polycystic ovary syndrome have an increased risk of cardiovascular disease: review of the evidence
E.O. Talbott, J.V. Zborowski, M.Y. Boudreaux   233

### Endocrine aspects of ovarian function

Ovarian bone morphogenetic proteins in female reproduction
S. Shimasaki, R.K. Moore, G.F. Erickson, F. Otsuka ......... 241

Clinical use of cytokines in ovulation induction
H. Okamura, T. Ohba, H. Katabuchi, N. Tanaka, A. Takasaki ......... 248

### Psychosocial aspect of infertility

Solo mothers: quality of parenting and child development
S. Golombok ......... 256

Exit counseling
L. Hammer Burns ......... 264

Psychosocial aspects of infertility: sexual dysfunction
A.M. Braverman ......... 270

### Infection in reproduction

Sexually transmitted chlamydial infections and subfertility
J. Paavonen ......... 277

Tuberculosis in assisted reproduction and infertility
T. Gurgan, A. Demirol ......... 287

### Ethical challenges in reproductive medicine

Ethical challenges in reproductive medicine: posthumous reproduction
G. Bahadur ......... 295

Sperm and oocyte donation: gamete donor issues
Y. Englert, E. Serena, R. Philippe, D. Fabienne, L. Chantal, D. Anne ......... 303

Saviour siblings: using preimplantation genetic diagnosis for tissue typing
G. Pennings ......... 311

### Evidence-based management of recurrent miscarriage

Evidence-based management of recurrent miscarriage: optimal diagnostic protocol
S. Daya ......... 318

Medical management of recurrent miscarriage—evidence-based approach
H.J.A. Carp ......... 328

Evidence-based management of recurrent miscarriage. Surgical management
P. Acién, M. Acién                                                                                                        335

## Paediatric outcome following infertility management

Paediatric outcome following infertility management/genetic outcome
M. Bonduelle                                                                                                              343

Parenting and child psychosocial development after infertility management
F. Gibson, C. McMahon                                                                                                     351

The long-term paediatric outcomes of assisted reproductive therapies
A.G. Sutcliffe                                                                                                            359

## Molecular reproduction

An introduction to genomics in reproduction
G.C. Weston                                                                                                               367

Mass spectrometry-based proteomics
B.L. Hood, T.D. Veenstra, T.P. Conrads                                                                                    375

## New developments in imaging and endoscopy

Office operative endoscopy in infertility
H.C. Verhoeven                                                                                                            381

Ultrasound imaging in human reproduction: what is new?
S. Kupesic                                                                                                                393

Pelvic MR imaging in infertility and recurrent pregnancy loss
C. Reinhold                                                                                                               401

**Author index**                                                                                                          409

**Keyword index**                                                                                                         411

**Plenary**

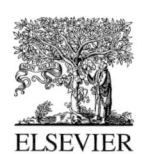

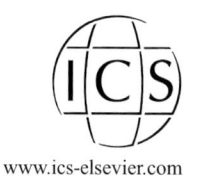

# Treating menopause in the 21st century—where do we go from here?

Isaac Schiff*

*Department of Obstetrics and Gynecology, Massachusetts General Hospital, 55 Fruit Street, Boston, MA 02114, USA*

**Abstract.** *Introduction*: The history of estrogen replacement therapy has changed dramatically during the past 40 years or so. At first it was thought that estrogens represented the fountain of youth but in the 1970s it was shown that unopposed estrogens could result in endometrial cancer. With the utilization of progestins, this particular risk disappeared. In the 1980s and 1990s, numerous observational trials found that estrogens could prevent chronic diseases such as heart disease, osteoporosis, colon cancer and even dementia. However, when prospective randomized trials were carried out in the late 1990s and published in the early 21st century, this potential benefit disappeared. And in fact we learned more about the risks of estrogen and breast cancer. When one identifies the major medical risks for not taking estrogen replacement therapy, it appears to be the development of osteoporosis. If a woman desires or requires treatment to prevent or treat osteoporosis there are other medications such as bisphosphonates or selective estrogen receptor modulators (SERMs) which are available and they may have a better benefit/risk profile. Treatment of symptoms such as vaginal atrophy can be carried out successfully with the use of vaginal estrogen tablets or a vaginal ring which is associated with minimal systemic absorption. As for the treatment of vasomotor flushes when estrogens are contraindicated one can consider the use of selective serotonin reuptake inhibitors (SSRIs). Complementary medicines such as phytoestrogens have had disappointing results. Although estrogens have received a lot of negative publicity, health care providers should continue to prescribe them because they do provide a lot of benefit predominantly symptomatic to patients. As long as the patients are fully aware of the risks, then it is reasonable to prescribe them for the appropriate patient. © 2004 Elsevier B.V. All rights reserved.

*Keywords:* Estrogen; Breast cancer; Heart disease

---

I will give the perspective and the history of estrogens and heart disease. If we go back to the 1960s and the influence of books like *Feminine Forever* it was thought that estrogens were a panacea. The theory goes that women rarely get heart attacks until they pass through menopause, that is when their ovaries stop producing estrogens. This lack of estrogens may

* Tel.: +1-11-617-726-3001; fax: +1-11-617-726-7548.
E-mail address: ISCHIFF@partners.org (I. Schiff).

increase the risks for heart disease. With the powerful influence of male physicians the obvious conclusion and thinking was to use estrogen replacement therapy to prevent recurrent heart attacks in men. The first good study of estrogens on heart disease was actually done in men in 1963 and women had to wait 35 years later to learn the effects on them. The study in men was called the Coronary Drug Project. It was an excellent study where estrogens or placebo were prescribed to men who already had a coronary insult. After 18 months the code had to be broken because one group was getting many more events. As you could anticipate, knowing what we now know, the group of men treated with the high-dose estrogens have more pulmonary emboli and more heart attacks. Of course, we appreciate that the dose of estrogen utilized was much too high. The thinking then was that if a little bit is good, a lot must be fabulous. Nevertheless, we learned in the early 1960s that estrogens did not prevent recurrent cardiac events.

It was then followed by an evaluation of men with prostate cancer who were treated with estrogens. This was in the 1960s and of course predates the treatment of GnRh agonists. As you could see, there are these men with prostate cancer receiving DES and an equal number receiving placebo. The life expectancy is the same with both groups. The difference is that men who receive the DES die of vascular disease such as pulmonary emboli or myocardial infarcts. While the men who receive the placebo die of prostate cancer. Thus, if you use estrogens for prostate cancer, you do not prolong life but you may improve on the quality of it. This was the final nail in the coffin of the use of estrogens for men.

In the early 1970s we started to see heart attacks in young women where this was never seen before. Of course, these were women who were on the birth control pill. Again in the early 1970s the dose of estrogen in the pill was probably as much as five times our current level. When the dose was reduced and we learned to not prescribe the pill to cigarette smokers the risk was reduced. But if someone were speaking to you in the mid-1970s they would be telling you that estrogens cause heart disease. We then move along to the 1980s where a number of retrospective, observational studies suggested that estrogens prevent heart disease. So we came full circle during those 20 years. It was almost like a broken clock which is right twice a day suggesting that in the 1960s estrogens were great; in the 1970s they were not and in the 1980s they were wonderful again. And a whole series of biological studies were carried out which helped confirm that estrogens were beneficial from the fact that hormones improve the HDL and LDL ratios to estrogens serving as coronary artery vasodilators.

This prompted with the best of intentions the effort by the pharmaceutical houses to obtain the indication for estrogens as a preventive for heart disease. The FDA initially was receptive but then decided not to do so and this called for a prospective randomized clinical trial. This was the beginning of the Women's Health Initiative (WHI).

As one can learn by the 1990s, very distinguished researchers were convinced that estrogens might indeed prevent heart disease. The problem was, of course, that these were all observational trials and may not have been able to take into account the healthy user effect. You cannot minimize this as many obstetrician–gynecologists and internists would avoid using estrogens for their patients whom they thought were at risk for heart disease especially based on the data from the 1970s. This would not be unreasonable given the fact that above all else we would not like to do anything that could potentially be harmful. But as one can appreciate, some drugs are never as bad as we think they are and some drugs are not as good as we think they are and emotion gets carried up in the day. Let us evaluate the HERS trial.

The HERS trial sought to prove that estrogens prevent recurrence of heart disease in women already afflicted with it. This was of course similar to the Coronary Drug Project done in men. It is randomized, prospective and the patients received both estrogen and progestin or placebo. The major findings were if you look at the 5-year endpoint, that there was no difference. What was equally interesting was that at the end of the first 2 years or so, the group that received estrogens and progestins actually had an increased risk. Then as you went out to the third and fourth year, the placebo group caught up. The investigators—and here is where emotion took over—were so convinced that if allowed to proceed for another 3–4 years, that indeed there would be many more events in the placebo group and the benefit of estrogens would be vindicated. I heard the investigators and with all due respect, some of them were so caught up emotionally that when they would present the data, instead of doing it in an objective, scientific fashion, they would conclude that estrogens were probably beneficial. (The investigators wished to carry out the study for another 3 years.) Now if you were a patient who was presented with the information and supposing the study turned out to be most positive, how would that play? Would your doctor tell you to take this drug because at the end of 8 years, your risk for heart disease would be reduced? However, there might be one little problem. If you took the medication in the first 2–3 years, your events might actually be increased, but I guess if you made it past the first 2–3 years, you would be golden. The only reason for continuing the study for another 3 years was to answer the question for women who were already on hormones, to tell them that if they were on it for 2–3 years, then probably their risk for heart disease would not be increased. The possibility that the investigators considered was that hormone replacement therapy (HRT) was like the birth control pill. With the pill, women who develop phlebitis usually get it in the first year or two. It is probably more related to genetic risk for phlebitis and that the first year or two of the pill weans out those patients. On the other hand, keep in mind that when using hormone replacement therapy, it is a much older population whose risks for most diseases go up with age. HERS II showed us no benefit when continued for 2 to 3 more years.

Now let us leave HERS II [5,7] and go on to the Women's Health Initiative [4,6,8,9,11,12,14]. The study is a very powerful one and I have the deepest respect for the people who designed it and carried it out. But since I have been asked to provide my personal perspective, I will proceed. Over the past 20 years, we learned that estrogens do indeed prevent heart disease from retrospective trials. To repeat, the pharmaceutical industry wished to get the permission for estrogens to prevent heart disease as an indication. That is perfectly reasonable. The NIH and I guess the FDA realized that we would need to have prospective data to show this. Now all the retrospective data showing estrogens prevent heart disease come from either estrogens used in unopposed fashion and the predominant estrogen in the United States is Premarin .625 or Premarin and Provera in cyclic fashion. None of the data that suggest that estrogens prevent heart disease comes from the continuous–combined formulation. The NIH and we have to congratulate them for this, decided to study estrogens as to whether or not they prevent heart disease.

The obvious question is why are the data so divergent with respect to heart disease trials and the observational studies, but the data with respect to breast cancer and colon cancer are consistent. What are the issues involved? One of the thoughts was that observational studies have as a confounding factor—the healthy user effect. Thus, the healthiest patients were using estrogens. But stroke which is related to healthy user is increased in both observational and the Women's Health Initiative study. Similarly, the same findings exist with pulmonary emboli. If one is speaking of socioeconomic features, the Nurses Health Study even adjusted for the education of the husbands assuming that all the nurses had similar educational experience. Thus, it is unlikely related to this bias.

## 1. Compliance bias

Because people who take placebo in trials focused on heart disease have a lower risk for it, it is thought that the hormone users in observational studies are more compliant. This may seem rational but it did not turn out to have the same effect on stroke. Thus, a compliance basis could only be a partial explanation.

## 2. Incomplete capture of early clinical events

Many of the observational studies would not capture information in women who initiated hormones and had a myocardial infarct within the first 2-year period. For example the investigators asked about hormone utilization only once every 2 years in the Nurses Health Study. Thus if an event occurred at 6 months, and the person stopped medications— at the end of 2 years that person would be considered a non-user of estrogens. The obvious question is why would this not show up for stroke? It is because the risk occurred later on than year 1 and year 2.

The above features are potential explanations and there may also be a biologic difference. The first one may be related to the hormone regimen, which I have already mentioned, namely that observational studies dealt with cyclic estrogens and progestins and intervention dealt with continuous–combined. The populations were different in the observational studies such as the Nurses Health Study, the BMI was 24.3 and in the WHI it was 28.5. The coronary benefits of hormones may be related to women with a lower body mass index. In addition, women in the observational studies tend to take them because they are symptomatic while in the control trials those women may be excluded. Women who are very symptomatic are less likely to sign up for them.

Women in observational studies tend to be younger and it may be related to the fact that they have less coronary artery disease. Thus, estrogens in the latter stage may destabilize a plaque due to the increase of matrix metalloproteinase which will destabilize a plaque. In the younger women who do not have atherosclerosis and start estrogen, this effect may not be seen.

Another question is why was the randomized trial terminated so early? In response to this, the WHI was designed prior to the findings of the PEPI or HERS trial and it was to test the hypothesis that estrogen plus progestin would reduce the risks of heart disease. As the study went along, findings were not consistent with the initial informed consent document. In fact, the Data Safety Monitoring Board (DSMB) required the WHI hormone program participants be given written information after year 2 indicating the presence of adverse effects. When the breast cancer rates were found to be increased, in the context of increasing risks for heart disease, stroke and pulmonary emboli, the primary hypothesis of preventive benefits of hormones was disproven. Thus, the decision was made to stop May 31, 2002.

Other complaints with this study included that women with significant symptoms were excluded and this would remove younger women. But this has already been dealt with. Another complaint is that in year 5 the placebo group had a dramatic decline in heart disease which may have led to statistical significance. Could this have been related to the placebo group getting different kinds of treatment from estrogen at that point. Another criticism included the fact that it was intention-to-treat analysis and thus there were high drop-out rates in both the treated and placebo group. If anything, this would dampen the effect of the HRT and it more likely mimics what women in general do, that as about 80% stop hormones after a few years.

Although this lecture concentrated a great deal on heart disease which was an endpoint in the WHI, it suggested that at best there is no beneficial effect and it may even be harmful. But let us keep in mind that breast cancer is the major concern of postmenopausal women in their 50s and this will affect the decision.

As I must repeat, breast cancer is by far the biggest concern our patients have [10]. The anxiety prior to a mammogram is palpable. All one has to do is tell a patient that the mammogram is abnormal and this sets into motion a whole series of crises and then if the diagnosis turns out to be cancer, who would be so cruel or cold or callus to tell the patient that they are going to live a lot longer because it is not a lethal type of cancer. In order to understand estrogens and breast cancer, let us develop it historically.

In August of 1989, the study from Sweden first suggested warning clouds that women on estrogen replacement therapy had an increased risk for breast cancer after 7–8 years of use. This study was problematic in that the estrogen used was not the one available in the United States. Nevertheless, it received wide press coverage. One of the other troubling features of the study was that in the very same month in the *American Journal of Epidemiology* which few of us in this room subscribe to, it was demonstrated that the women who started estrogens had a longer life expectancy if they develop breast cancer than the women with breast cancer who never took estrogens. This implied that it was a different type of breast cancer that was caused by estrogens. Then in the early 1990s, the Nurses Health Study again brought up the concern of long-term use of estrogens leading to an increased risk. The long-term use was more than 5 years and I reassured patients who took it for less than that time. Unfortunately, the Women's Health Initiative removed that safety free zone [2]. The risk was given in percentages in the popular press which may have been more inflammatory to patients and thus I reduced it to absolute numbers. For example, a woman aged 55–59 not on estrogens, out of 1200 women 3 would develop breast cancer in the next 12 months. This is a type of epidemic. On the other hand, those who used estrogens for more than 5 years, 4 out of 1200 would develop breast cancer. Some women when given this information said that when you go from 3 to 4, it is not that much, and they felt better on estrogens. Others said 3–4 is unacceptable and they knew they would be the fourth person and they stopped. The risk is 33%. Some studies suggested a risk; others did not find the risk, but the Women's Health Initiative came down on the side of risks. Whether it is a different type of breast cancer is not really known yet some observers have pointed out that the estrogens could not have caused it because it takes over 5 years and maybe as long as 10 years until fully formed cancer develops. My answer to that would be if it is a different type of breast cancer and thus lethal, why could it not have a shorter time period to develop. Thus, with current available information, we now have learned from the Women's Health Initiative that if anything estrogens do not prevent heart disease and may increase it; and estrogens again might increase the risk for breast cancer. And there are other concerns about the WHI.

## 3. Specific estrogen receptor modulators

Tamoxifen was utilized as a primary prevention trial to prevent breast cancer and was shown to be quite effective in the U.S. study. Tamoxifen was given to women at high risk for breast cancer and therefore low risk for osteoporosis. Raloxifene was studied in women at low risk for breast cancer and high risk for osteoporosis [1,3,13]. Both produce a reduction in risk. This may turn out to be the most common reason why raloxifene is used in the future. But I would also ask you to pay attention to the fact that raloxifene appeared to reduce the risks of breast cancer in women whose baseline endogenous estradiol level was highest. Again, it points out some biologic explanation for the association between estrogens and the risk for breast cancer.

This paper has not dealt with the effects of estrogens on Alzheimer's disease. This would be a potential benefit of the Women's Health Initiative that would change our thinking at this time and may certainly change the balance in favor. The data on Alzheimer's disease from retrospective studies appear to be positive but the randomized trials thus far need to be shown. With respect to colon cancer, our methodology of preventing it relies on colonoscopy and other diagnostic studies. As for hot flashes and vaginal dryness, estrogens are the best medication we have available.

Where do we go from here? Estrogens are not to be used to prevent heart disease. Even studies other than the WHI, which are prospective and using the patch, have not found it to be of benefit. Estrogens are certainly effective for prevention of osteoporosis but we ought to consider other medications that may have a better benefit risk profile for the patient. The safety window of 5 years has been violated by the WHI suggesting the risk for breast cancer may come even sooner. I realize that there are problems with the study but there are enough randomized trials with and retrospective data to at least make us concerned that estrogens can increase the breast cancer risk and that alone may be adequate reason why many of our patients refuse estrogens. On the other hand, some patients feel a lot better on estrogens and we have to find objective ways to measure this. Until the WHI data are evaluated, I would point out that we have to assume that estrogens have this positive effect for some women and that is adequate reason to take it. In fact, if some women feel better and want to take it long term, I would certainly prescribe it as long as they are well aware of the risks. I would not feel guilty about them doing so. As for colon cancer that is not an indication for estrogens. If one is concerned about colon cancer, one ought to do colonoscopy or the diagnostic technologies that are available to us. There are no good data to suggest how it is best to wean patients but if they are very symptomatic with hot flashes, it ought to be done slowly over time. Certainly if women have vaginal dryness or problems with sexuality one can consider using estrogen vaginal tablets or the ring which appears to have less absorption systemically than oral or transdermal. These answers are not for the women who undergo premature menopause as the data are predominantly in women over age 50. Thus the ultimate decision as to whether or not to take hormones does rely on the patient but it is also the physician who helps steer her toward what is in her best interests. It is not that the physician is relinquishing his or her responsibility but it is a joint decision which takes into account the patient's medical history, her physical exam and her feelings about taking hormones.

## References

[1] J.A. Cauley, et al., Continued breast cancer risk in postmenopausal women treated with raloxifene: 4-year results from the MORE trial. Multiple outcomes of raloxifene evaluation, Breast Cancer Res. Treat. 65 (2001) 125.
[2] R.T. Chlebowski, T. Rowan, et al., Influence of estrogen plus progestin on breast cancer and mammography in healthy postmenopausal women. The women's health initiative randomized trial, JAMA 289 (24) (2003) 3243.
[3] G.C. Davies, et al., Adverse events reported by postmenopausal women in controlled trials with raloxifene, Obstet. Gynecol. 93 (1999) 558.
[4] S.W. Fletcher, G.A. Colditz, Failure of estrogen plus progestin therapy for prevention, JAMA 288 (2002) 366.
[5] D. Grady, et al., HERS Research Group, Cardiovascular disease outcomes during 6.8 years of hormone therapy. Heart and estrogen/progestin replacement study follow-up (HERS II), JAMA 288 (2002) 49.
[6] H. Hodis, et al., Hormone therapy and the progression of coronary-artery atherosclerosis in postmenopausal women, N. Engl. J. Med. 349 (2003) 6535.
[7] S. Hulley, et al., for the HERS Research Group, Noncardiovascular disease outcomes during 6.8 years of hormone therapy. Heart and estrogen/progestin replacement study. Follow-up (HERS II), JAMA 288 (2002) 58.
[8] International Position Paper on Women's Health and Menopause—A Comprehensive Approach, National Institutes of Health, #02-3284, July 2002.
[9] J. Manson, et-al., Estrogen plus progestin and the risk of coronary heart disease N. Engl. J. Med. 349 2003: 6, 523.
[10] Million Women Study Collaborators, Breast cancer and hormone-replacement therapy in the Million Women Study, Lancet 362 (2003) 419–427.
[11] D. Petitti, Hormone replacement therapy for prevention. More evidence, more pessimism, JAMA 288 (2002) 99.
[12] S. Shumaker, et al., Estrogen plus progestin and the incidence of dementia and mild cognitive impairment in postmenopausal women. The women's health initiative memory study: a randomized controlled trial, JAMA 289 (2003) 2651.
[13] W. Utian, et al., Case Western Reserve University, Medical College of Georgia, Lilly Research Laboratories, Effect of Raloxifene HCl (60 mg/day) in postmenopausal women with pre-existing vasomotor symptoms, Annual Meeting of the North American Menopause Society, Menopause 8 (2001) 467.
[14] Writing Group for the Women's Health Initiative Investigators, Risks and benefits of estrogen plus progestin in healthy postmenopausal women. Principal results from the Women's Health Initiative randomized controlled trial, JAMA 288 (2002) 321.

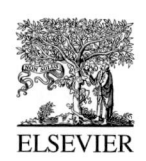

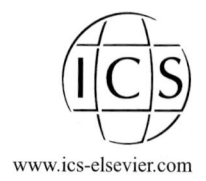

# New developments in the evaluation and management of male infertility

Robert I. McLachlan*

*Prince Henry's Institute of Medical Research, Department of Obstetrics and Gynecology and Monash IVF, Monash University, PO Box 5152, Clayton, Melbourne, Victoria, 3168, Australia*

**Abstract.** A male factor exists in 30% of infertile unions. New options, particularly ICSI, have revolutionized its management but should not create an environment wherein the evaluation of the male focuses only on ART outcomes. All men require a thorough assessment for reversible causes of infertility, comorbidities and sexual/relationship difficulties consequent upon this diagnosis. Endocrine, genetic and histological evaluations play key roles in diagnosis and must be viewed critically. Increasingly, genetic defects are being described in otherwise healthy men with 'idiopathic' spermatogenic failure, including karyotypic anomalies, Y chromosomal deletions and potentially in X-linked and autosomal genes. This new knowledge has major implications for clinical practice and the health of offspring. The background rate of natural fertility in subfertile men means that treatments should be assessed in placebo-controlled RCTs: such evidence is lacking for many common treatments. In obstructive azoospermia, the decision to use surgical correction as opposed to sperm retrieval and ICSI is affected by the surgical access and skill, female cofactors and site-specific cost-effectiveness considerations. The use of testicular sperm in nonobstructive azoospermia requires discussion of the realistic prospects for live births, and its safety for the man and his offspring. © 2004 Elsevier B.V. All rights reserved.

*Keywords:* Spermatogenesis; Testis; Semen; Gonadotropins; In vitro fertilization

## 1. Introduction

A male factor is recognised in at least 30% of infertile unions, and new therapeutic options, such as ICSI, have revolutionized the management of severe male infertility. These successes have led to a reciprocal decline in donor insemination as couples prefer to use their own gametes, although there is some uncertainty about its safety for offspring [1].

However, our ability to establish pregnancy using single sperm should not create an 'ART outcome only' approach wherein the evaluation and management of male focuses simply on the acquisition and use of sperm in the most 'cost-effective' manner. A complete and systematic evaluation of the male partner may identify conditions that are readily treatable to restore natural fertility, or that are associated with significant health risks for

---

Tel.: +61-3-95943561; fax: +61-3-95943558.

*E-mail address:* rob.mclachlan@phimr.monash.edu.au (R.I. McLachlan).

0531-5131/ © 2004 Elsevier B.V. All rights reserved.
doi:10.1016/j.ics.2004.01.107

the man or his offspring. There is also a need to consider, on an individual basis, the extent and type of information to be provided and to identify sexual or relationship difficulties consequent upon this diagnosis.

Recent progress in understanding the genetics of spermatogenesis and of male infertility provides hope for future specific diagnoses and foreshadows the development of treatments of 'idiopathic' spermatogenic failure, the commonest cause of male infertility. In the meantime, ART/ICSI provides a valuable 'bypass', rather than treatment, of disordered spermatogenesis.

The ever increasing range of diagnostic tests and treatment options require continued review of clinical practice and in the monitoring of short- and long-term outcomes for infertile men and their offspring. Fertility clinics have a responsibility to contribute to this process through active research programs or by contribution of data to appropriate organisations. Ongoing surveillance of health matters revealed during ART assessment requires the engagement of the man's primary care physician.

In this paper, a brief review and commentary will be given on the causes, investigations and management of the major types of male infertility with some perspectives on current deficiencies and future opportunities to improve care.

## 2. Clinical evaluation and causes of male infertility

The clinical history focuses on detecting the conditions listed in Fig. 1, including the assessment of pubertal development, prior cryptorchidism, genitourinary infection and symptoms of testosterone deficiency. A thorough medical history and examination with emphasis on the degree of virilization and genital examination (especially testis size/consistency, vas and epididymides, varicocele) are mandatory. The use of a proforma

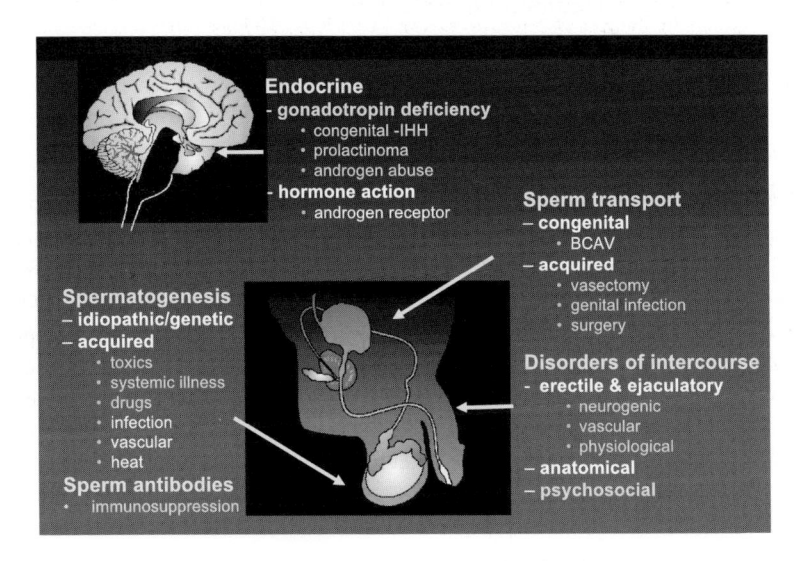

Fig. 1. Five common etiological groupings in male infertility. Those for which effective medical/surgery treatments are available are shown in *blue* on the web.

provides a basis for categorization of subjects for monitoring of outcomes and for research purposes.

Of the five common etiological groupings in male infertility, *endocrine deficiency* is the least common cause (~1%), yet specific therapies (gonadotropins, cabergoline) frequently restore both fertility and testosterone secretion. Androgen abuse reversibly suppresses FSH/LH and spermatogenesis. *Sperm transport*: bilateral congenital absence of the vas (BCAV) is characterized by the inability to palpate normal calibre vasa and low-volume acidic semen due to associated absence of the seminal vesicles. Surgery may be effective in the settings of vasectomy, ejaculatory duct obstruction (e.g., due to prostatic cysts) but rarely for epididymal lesions. *Disorders of intercourse* are a heterogeneous group including erectile dysfunction of any cause and retrograde ejaculation or 'functional' defects in transport resulting from diabetic neuropathy, retroperitoneal lymph node dissection or spinal cord injury in which setting medical approaches (e.g., electro-ejaculation and AIH) may be effective. Immunosuppression for sperm autoimmunity is an effective alternative to ICSI in some settings.

Over 60% of the cases are due to *spermatogenic disorders*. In some cases, it may be possible to reduce or withdraw spermatogenic toxins or to offer cryopreservation. Unfortunately, the majority of men with poor semen quality suffer from 'idiopathic' spermatogenic failure, but increasingly, genetic explanations are being provided. A false sense of diagnostic precision is given by such purely descriptive terms that may also imply a common causation. Abnormalities seen on routine semen analyses may only be the 'tip of the iceberg' such that functional sperm defects will escape diagnosis. One good example is the impairment of acrosome reactivity following binding to isolated zona in vitro that have been suggested to be present in 25% of normospermic men with 'idiopathic infertility' [2].

## 3. Assessment of comorbidities in infertile men

A number of conditions are more prevalent in infertile men which demand specific considerations including the following.

### 3.1. Testicular cancer

The rate of this cancer varies between regions but is increasing worldwide with infertility per se associated with a twofold increase risk of testis cancer [3], but there is a much greater risk with the history of cryptorchidism (particularly if bilateral) that may persist despite surgical correction [4]. Evaluation by testicular examination, and, generally, also ultrasonography, is required for all men with spermatogenic failure. Furthermore, when testis biopsy is performed for diagnostic reasons or for testicular sperm extraction (TESE) for ICSI, histological evaluation of a portion of the sample to exclude cancer or carcinoma in situ (CIS) is essential. CIS is managed by orchidectomy or local radiotherapy, but if unrecognised, and thus untreated, progresses to invasive cancer in 50% of patients within 5 years [5].

### 3.2. Hypoandrogenism

Hypoandrogenism is more common in men presenting with infertility. Men with Klinefelter's syndrome escape diagnosis lifelong in more than 50% of cases [6], but the opportunity to make the diagnosis occurs when they present to fertility clinics when the opportunity must be taken to assist these men through: (i) counselling the couple about the condition, (ii) achieving full masculinization with testosterone replacement, (iii) managing gynecomastia and other health issues more prevalent in these men (osteoporosis, thyroid dysfunction, rarely lymphoma and breast cancer) and (iv) realistically presenting fertility options through testicular sperm extraction/ICSI or donor insemination. Men with spermatogenic failure (idiopathic or following testicular damage or chemotherapy) uncommonly have clinical testosterone deficiency. More often, they have a mildly raised LH combined with a low-normal serum T representing 'compensated Leydig cell failure'. Evidence for benefit from androgen therapy is marginal in this setting [7]; clinical judgment, bone density and repeat testing direct treatment including long-term review by their primary care physician. In these settings of primary testicular failure, T replacement will reduce FSH/LH levels, thereby impairing residual spermatogenesis (if any) and reduce the prospects of successful TESE. Thus, without compelling reason, T treatment should be delayed until after TESE attempt.

### 3.3. Cystic fibrosis gene-related problems

The presence of unilateral or bilateral congenital absence of the vas requires evaluation for associated renal tract anomalies or variable degrees of sinopulmonary disease [8].

### 3.4. Psychosexual difficulties

These are common following the recognition of male infertility (especially spermatogenic failure) with feelings of guilt and a sense of loss and reduced masculinity, resulting in erectile and/or relationship problems. These concerns must be brought out in discussion as it may have short-term (e.g., during ART treatments) and long-term consequences (relationship break up) if left unresolved.

## 4. Laboratory evaluation

### 4.1. Assay methods

Assay methods are often chosen by laboratories for convenience and cost, and report reference ranges that have not been derived from age-appropriate healthy fertile men. As a result, FSH upper limits may be set very high (thereby missing spermatogenic failure), while for testosterone, dubious methods (e.g., automated direct free T) and variable reference ranges confuse the diagnosis of hypoandrogenism. Inhibin B provides some added accuracy in establishing testicular failure but has not found a clear place in practice [9]. Endocrine profiles are similar in severely infertile men with or without Yq deletions [10].

### 4.2. Semen analysis

The value of semen analysis is highly dependent on the quality of laboratory. WHO methodologies for manual analysis of at least two analyses (due to the inherent variability of sperm parameters) several weeks apart remains the best approach. Computer-assisted semen analysis systems are widely promoted and may appear cost efficient from a laboratory perspective. But debris in semen (requiring DNA staining for confident identification of sperm) and a lack of sensitivity at low sperm concentrations (the patients of most interest) limit their routine use in fertility laboratories. Low/variable semen volume requires examination of postorgasmic urine for the presence of sperm indicating retrograde ejaculation.

Independent predictors of in vivo and in vitro fertilizing ability include sperm velocity and morphology using the strict criteria: a progressive reduction in fertilization rates from 60% to 20% as abnormal morphology increases from less than 70% to more than 95% [11]. Manual morphology assessment is difficult to standardise between laboratories: computerised morphology holds promise in this area for predicting fertilizing ability.

*4.3. Morphological and functional basis for defective sperm structure*

Chemes and Rawe [12] recently pointed out the need to consider the morphological and functional basis for defective sperm structure, and the impact of this knowledge on the use of ART and genetic counselling. For example, primary cilial dyskinesia is associated with sinopulmonary disease and a wide range of defects in sperm flagellar elements (such as the dynein arms, microtubules and radial spokes) are only apparent on EM while dysplasia of the fibrous sheath is readily apparent as short, thick sperm tails. Both conditions may be amenable to ICSI unlike immotility due to necrospermia from which they must be distinguished. Defects in the relationship between the sperm head and neck are very important as they may result in acephalic sperm or in dysfunction of the proximal sperm centriole that impairs sperm aster formation, normal syngamy and cleavage. Agenesis (often termed globozoospermia) or hypoplasia of the acrosome profoundly impairs fertility and may not be resolved through ICSI, perhaps due to defects in oocyte activation. Functional defects may also exist such as a failure of the zona pellucida-induced acrosome reaction that appears to be a common cause of 'idiopathic' male infertility [2]. A great deal remains to be learnt about the genetic defects and their implications for ART offspring.

## 5. Genetic evaluation

Genetic defects causally related to STF are increasingly being identified. The rapid application of this knowledge to the clinic is an important challenge as it will satisfy the man's legitimate desire to understand the reason for his problem, as well as having implications for the prospects for a normal pregnancy and offspring, and for directing treatment, e.g., success of TESE. A formal relationship with a genetic counselling service is an essential part of modern practice. Current clinical considerations include the following.

*5.1. Karyotypic anomalies*

Karyotypic anomalies are well recognised in otherwise well men with STF with sex chromosome aneuploidy and autosomal translocations being seen in 13.7% in azoospermic men and 4.6% of oligospermic men [13]. These anomalies appear causally linked to spermatogenic failure, perhaps through impairment of chromosomal segregation during meiosis. Routine karyotypic analysis is widely recommended for ICSI candidates with sperm concentrations less than 10 million/ml. However, there remains an increased prevalence of aneuploidy in ejaculated or testicular sperm despite a normal peripheral karyotype, the risk appearing to rise with serum FSH and decline sperm concentration [14,15]. This probably underscores the higher rate of apparently de novo abnormalities in ICSI offspring [16].

### 5.2. Yq microdeletions

Yq microdeletions are found in 3–8% of men with spermatogenic failure and sperm concentrations less than 5 million/ml: the absence of other apparent phenotypic expressions speaks to the remarkable specialization of this region of the genome. Deletions arise in three regions of the long arm termed AZFa, AZFb and AZFc that contain testis-specific genes and others that are expressed in other tissues or which have homologues on X or autosomes. Of particular note are deleted in azoospermia (DAZ) and RNA binding motif (RBMY) genes that encode RNA binding proteins that have been causally linked to defects in spermatogenesis and exist as multiple copies. Complete sequencing of the Y chromosome has revealed there are only 27 distinct protein-coding genes present on the male-specific region of the Y chromosome. Deletions arise de novo by homologous recombination events between long stretches of highly repetitive sequences that represent palindromes.

Repping et al. [17] studied the mechanism of AZFb and AZFb+AZFc deletions by localising and sequencing the deletion junctions: homologous recombination explained seven out of the nine deletions implicating other factors aside from homology in some cases. Interestingly, massive deletion events extend between AZF regions; for example, AZFb deletions extend from palindrome P5 to the proximal arm of palindrome P1 within AZFc (6.2 Mb, 32 genes/transcripts), and deletions of AZFb+AZFc extend from P5 to the distal arm of P1, sparing distal AZFc (7.7 Mb, 42 genes/transcripts).

A more common Yq deletion (termed gr/gr, [18]) is present in 1% of the general population and results in a reduced copy number of several spermatogenic gene family members but is compatible with natural fertility (and thus, transmission). The gr/gr deletion appears to be a risk factor for infertility; that is, other factors (environmental, genetic) appear to be needed for the expression of infertility. Thus, the concept is emerging that male infertility will be a complex genetic trait rather than a 'single gene' disorder.

Deletions of the AZFc region occur in the majority of Yq deletions (80%). When involving only the AZFc region, men are usually severely oligozoospermic or azoospermic (in which case, testicular sperm for ICSI are often found). Variable histological patterns are seen with the same deletion strongly implying the involvement of other genetic or environmental factors in its pathogenesis. Deletions AZFa and AZFb extending to AZFc, are associated with severe damage to spermatogenesis and the absence of sperm at open biopsy [19, 20]. Vertical transmission of Yq deletions via ICSI has been consistently shown, and Y deletion testing is routine in ICSI candidates with a sperm concentration less than 5 million/ml.

### 5.3. Androgen receptor gene

Specific mutations in the androgen receptor gene rarely cause abnormal spermatogenesis and infertility without affecting genital development [21]. Most of the attention has been paid to expansions of the CAG repeat (polyglutamine tract) in exon 1 being associated with diminished receptor activity and oligospermia; however, this is not always found. The reason for this discrepancy is unclear, and, at this time, routine assessment of CAG length in the clinic is not indicated.

### 5.4. Cystic fibrosis transmembrane receptor (CFTR) gene

About 85% of BCAV men are heterozygotes or compound heterozygotes for cystic fibrosis transmembrane receptor (CFTR) mutations [8]. Furthermore, the presence of the 5T allelic variant in intron 8–9 is heavily overrepresented in BCAV compared with normal men and results in decreased CFTR mRNA that, when combined with a single mutation in the CFTR gene allele, results in BCAV.

## 6. Testicular histology

This evaluation is indicated to differentiate azoospermia due to spermatogenic failure vs. obstruction, and in the evaluation of spermatogenic defects when considering testicular sperm extraction in nonobstructive azoospermia. Care should be taken to appropriately fix the sample in Bouin's fluid and to use a classification that relates to clinical outcomes (e.g., success of TESE) and for understanding the pathogenesis of spermatogenic failure: (i) normal; (ii) hypospermatogenesis (hypoSG, all germ cell forms present in some or all tubules but in mildly, moderately or severely reduced numbers); (iii) germ cell arrest in which development ceases at a particular stage in every tubule; (iv) Sertoli cell-only syndrome (SCOS, or germ cell aplasia) in which every tubule lacks germ cells; (v) hyalinization—the cellular elements have disappeared leaving only thickened tubule walls; (vi) immature testis which has not been exposed to gonadotropic stimulation (prepubertal appearance). Biopsies frequently show heterogeneity, but from a practical viewpoint, the existence of hypoSG in some tubules results in this being the summary diagnosis while the use of contradictory terms such as 'partial SCOS' should be avoided.

However, histological classification is only descriptive and there are many mechanisms for the SCOS phenotype (genetic, toxins, radiation, etc.). Germ cell arrest (usually at the primary spermatocytes stage) often feature normal testicular volumes and FSH levels but has the poorest outlook for TESE suggesting a genetically based uniform failure of meiosis. On the other hand, hypoSG carries good prospects for sperm retrieval.

## 7. Management options

The outcome of treatment for spermatogenic failure may be described in terms of semen quality (and by implication fertility) but, given the background rate of natural fertility in subfertile men, is best determined by placebo-controlled RCTs assessing life table prospects of successful pregnancy [22]. Such evidence is lacking for some commonly used treatments; systematic literature reviews have found several empirical therapies to be of no or questionable fertility benefit, e.g., despite innumerable 'single arm' studies showing improvement in semen quality with varicocele ligation. Review of controlled RCT data does not reveal consistent improvements in fertility [23]. Many empirical therapies have been convincingly shown to be ineffective such as androgen rebound, mesterolone and antibiotic therapy in absence of demonstrable infection. Other treatments have been proposed but their benefits remain unsubstantiated such as treatment with FSH [24, 25], aromatase inhibitors [26], clomiphene/tamoxiphen [27,28] and vitamin/zinc supplementation [29]. Patients should be informed of the limited data showing improved conception rates and given an honest account of comparative ART outcomes.

Treatments for other conditions are classified in Table 1 according to the level of evidence that they improve fertility outcomes (natural and/or ART associated). For some treatments, RCT evidence may be found, but for others, the conclusion about effectiveness is implicit (e.g., reduced chemotherapy-induced azoospermia with new regimens) or self-evident (e.g., sperm retrieval/ICSI in BCAV). Intrauterine insemination for male factor infertility provides improvements in pregnancy rates in the absence of correctable ovulatory disturbance or without the use of FSH to achieve superovulation [30] but is not listed in the table.

Surgical treatments for obstructive azoospermia are increasingly being replaced with sperm retrieval/ICSI. The decision to undertake vasectomy reversal vs. ICSI is impacted by medical factors (obstructive interval, type of vasectomy, female age and fertility status), the availability of skilled surgical care and cost-effectiveness considerations that vary between

Table 1
Treatments for male infertility based on the level of evidence of effectiveness

*Approaches to protect/preserve fertility*
Mumps vaccination
Less gonadotoxic cancer treatments
Sperm cryopreservation (pre chemo-, vasectomy)
Early surgical correction of cryptorchidism?

*Evidence-based treatments to restore/initiate fertility*

| | |
|---|---|
| Endocrine | GnRH deficiency (congenital/acquired) with gonadotropins |
| | Hyperprolactinemia–prolactinoma treatment with cabergoline |
| | Relief of gonadotropin suppression |
| |   Cessation of opiates, androgen abuse |
| |   Treatment of systemic disease |
| Obstructive | Surgical repair, e.g., vasectomy reversal, ejaculatory duct obstruction. |
| Seminiferous tubule failure | Withdrawal of toxins—salazopyrine |
| Sperm autoimmunity | Immunosuppressive glucocorticoid treatment |
| Disorders of intercourse | Sexual counselling, electroejaculation |
| | Treatment of erectile dysfunction |

*Assisted reproductive treatments*
Obstructive azoospermia—ICSI
  Vas/epididymal: epididymal/testicular needle aspiration
  Nonsurgically remediable lesions at bladder base
Aspermia—IVF/ICSI
  Ejaculatory duct obstruction—surgical vs. ICSI
  Diabetes, spinal cord injury—alternative to electroejaculation
Spermatogenic failure
  Conventional IVF—mild–moderate semen defects
  ICSI—Severe oligospermia+/or motility+/or morphology
  Nonobstructive azoospermia–testicular sperm retrieval
Sperm antibodies—ICSI

centre/countries. Needle aspiration from the epididymis or testis is not without risk but appears well tolerated. Ejaculatory duct obstruction may be surgically remediable, but in many centres, ICSI is a viable alternative as it is for the recovery of viable sperm (as an alternative to electroejaculation) in a range of settings including ejaculatory disorders related to spinal cord injury or diabetes.

Men with nonobstructive azoospermia who are candidates for TESE are more likely to have borderline androgen deficiency preoperatively, and, as testis biopsy carries a small but important risk of testicular devascularization and atrophy [31], the possibility of lifelong hypoandrogenism must be discussed preoperatively. Microdissection of tubules may reduce the risk of hematoma and loss of testicular mass [31]. The risk of occult cancer/CIS dictates the need for formal histological assessment of a portion of the sample. Long-term studies of androgen levels and cancer in this group would be useful: one study at 18 months postbiopsy did not show a reduction in testis volume or serum testosterone [32]. Around half the nonmosaic men with Klinefelters obtain sperm for ICSI [33,34], but of 38 children born so far, only one 47XXY offspring has been reported. The success of TESE procedures does not appear lower with a past history of cryptorchidism [35]. The poorest outlook is seen in men with uniform germ cell arrest at the primary spermatocyte stage; those with extensive Yq deletions have a very poor outlook.

## 8. Conclusion

The infertile man requires full clinical assessment. ART/ICSI provides a valuable 'bypass' for the couple's problem of infertility but better understanding of the genetics of spermatogenesis provides hope for future specific diagnoses and genuine treatments of 'idiopathic' spermatogenic failure. In the meantime, the clinician is challenged to keep up with the increasing array of diagnostic tests and treatment options and to monitor the short- and long-term outcomes for infertile men and their offspring.

## Acknowledgements

The National Health and Medical Research Council of Australia is acknowledged for the support of RMcL through Fellowship Grant #169020 and Program Grant #241000.

## References

[1] E.R. Maher, M. Afnan, C.L. Barratt, Epigenetic risks related to assisted reproductive technologies: epigenetics, imprinting, ART and icebergs? Hum. Reprod. 18 (2003) 2508–2511.
[2] D.Y. Liu, et al., Frequency of disordered zona pellucida (ZP)-induced acrosome reaction in infertile men with normal semen analysis and normal spermatozoa–ZP binding, Hum. Reprod. 16 (2001) 1185–1190.
[3] H. Moller, N.E. Skakkebaek, Risk of testicular cancer in subfertile men: case–control study, BMJ 318 (1999) 559–562.
[4] J.M. Hutson, Cryptorchidism and hypospadias, in: R. McLachlan, L. DeGroot (Eds.), Male Reproductive Endocrinology, Chapter 19, http://www.ENDOTEXT.org.
[5] E. Niels, et al., Testicular cancer pathogenesis, diagnosis and endocrine aspects, in R. McLachlan, L. DeGroot (Eds.), Male Reproductive Endocrinology, Chapter 13, http://www.ENDOTEXT.org.
[6] A. Bojesen, S. Juul, C.H. Gravholt, Prenatal and postnatal prevalence of Klinefelter syndrome: a national registry study, J. Clin. Endocrinol. Metab. 88 (2003) 622–626.
[7] S.J. Howell, et al., Randomized placebo-controlled trial of testosterone replacement in men with mild Leydig cell insufficiency following cytotoxic chemotherapy, Clin. Endocrinol. (Oxf.) 55 (2001) 315–324.

[8] T. Dork, et al., Distinct spectrum of CFTR gene mutations in congenital absence of vas deferens, Hum. Genet. 100 (1997) 365–377.
[9] F.H. Pierik, et al., Serum inhibin B as a marker of spermatogenesis, J. Clin. Endocrinol. Metab. 83 (1998) 3110–3114.
[10] P.A. Tomasi, et al., The pituitary–testicular axis in Klinefelter's syndrome and in oligo–azoospermic patients with and without deletions of the Y chromosome long arm, Clin. Endocrinol. (Oxf.) 59 (2003) 214–222.
[11] G. Baker, Clinical management of male infertility in: R. McLachlan, L. DeGroot (Eds.), Male Reproductive Endocrinology, Chapter 7, http://www.ENDOTEXT.org.
[12] H.E. Chemes, V.Y. Rawe, Sperm pathology: a step beyond descriptive morphology. Origin, characterization and fertility potential of abnormal sperm phenotypes in infertile men, Hum. Reprod. Updat. 9 (2003) 405–428.
[13] E. Van Assche, et al., Cytogenetics of infertile men, Hum. Reprod. 11 (Suppl 4) (1996) 1–24.
[14] A.E. Calogero, et al., Aneuploidy rate in spermatozoa of selected men with abnormal semen parameters, Hum. Reprod. 16 (2001) 1172–1179.
[15] J. Levron, et al., Sperm chromosome abnormalities in men with severe male factor infertility who are undergoing in vitro fertilization with intracytoplasmic sperm injection, Fertil. Steril. 76 (2001) 479–484.
[16] M. Bonduelle, et al., Prenatal testing in ICSI pregnancies: incidence of chromosomal anomalies in 1586 karyotypes and relation to sperm parameters, Hum. Reprod. 17 (2002) 2600–2614.
[17] S. Repping, et al., Recombination between palindromes P5 and P1 on the human Y chromosome causes massive deletions and spermatogenic failure, Am. J. Hum. Genet. 71 (2002) 906–922.
[18] S. Repping, et al., Polymorphism for a 1.6-Mb deletion of the human Y chromosome persists through balance between recurrent mutation and haploid selection, Nat. Genet. 35 (2003) 247–251.
[19] C. Kamp, et al., High deletion frequency of the complete AZFa sequence in men with Sertoli-cell-only syndrome, Mol. Hum. Reprod. 7 (2001) 987–994.
[20] C.V. Hopps, et al., Detection of sperm in men with Y chromosome microdeletions of the AZFa, AZFb and AZFc regions, Hum. Reprod. 10 (2003) 1660–1665.
[21] R. Ochsenkuhn, D.M. DeKretser, The contributions of deficient androgen action in spermatogenic disorders, Int. J. Androl. 26 (2003) 195–201.
[22] H.W. Baker, Medical treatment for idiopathic male infertility: is it curative or palliative? Baillière's Clin. Obstet. Gynaecol. 11 (1997) 673–689.
[23] J.L. Evers, J.A. Collins, Assessment of efficacy of varicocele repair for male subfertility: a systematic review, Lancet 361 (2003) 1849–1852.
[24] A. Kamischke, et al., Recombinant human follicle stimulating hormone for treatment of male idiopathic infertility: a randomized, double-blind, placebo-controlled, clinical trial, Hum. Reprod. 13 (1998) 596–603.
[25] C. Foresta, et al., Use of recombinant human follicle-stimulating hormone in the treatment of male factor infertility, Fertil. Steril. 77 (2002) 238–244.
[26] J.D. Raman, P.N. Schlegel, Aromatase inhibitors for male infertility, J. Urol. 167 (2002) 624–629.
[27] World Health Organization, A double-blind trial of clomiphene citrate for the treatment of idiopathic male infertility, Int. J. Androl. 15 (1992) 299–307.
[28] D.A. Adamopoulos, et al., Effectiveness of combined tamoxifen citrate and testosterone undecanoate treatment in men with idiopathic oligozoospermia, Fertil. Steril. 80 (2003) 914–920.
[29] W.Y. Wong, et al., Effects of folic acid and zinc sulfate on male factor subfertility: a double-blind, randomized, placebo-controlled trial, Fertil. Steril. 77 (2002) 491–498.
[30] E.G. Hughes, The effectiveness of ovulation induction and intrauterine insemination in the treatment of persistent infertility: a meta-analysis, Hum. Reprod. 12 (1997) 1865–1872.
[31] L.M. Su, et al., Testicular sperm extraction with intracytoplasmic sperm injection for nonobstructive azoospermia: testicular histology can predict success of sperm retrieval, J. Urol. 161 (1999) 112–116.
[32] T. Schill, et al., Clinical and endocrine follow-up of patients after testicular sperm extraction, Fertil. Steril. 79 (2003) 281–286.
[33] S. Friedler, et al., Outcome of ICSI using fresh and cryopreserved–thawed testicular spermatozoa in patients with nonmosaic Klinefelter's syndrome, Hum. Reprod. 16 (2001) 2616–2620.

[34] G.D. Palermo, et al., Births after intracytoplasmic injection of sperm obtained by testicular extraction from men with nonmosaic Klinefelter's syndrome, N. Engl. J. Med. 338 (1998) 588–590.
[35] J.D. Raman, P.N. Schlegel, Testicular sperm extraction with intracytoplasmic sperm injection is successful for the treatment of nonobstructive azoospermia associated with cryptorchidism, J. Urol. 170 (2003) 1287–1290.

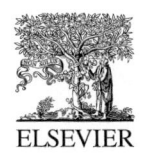

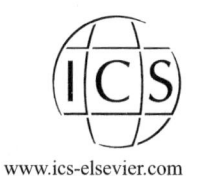

# Transcultural issues in gender selection

G.I. Serour*

*Department of Obstetrics and Gynecology and the International Islamic Center for Population Studies and Research, Al-Azhar University, 40 Talaat Harb Street, City Center, Cairo 00202, Egypt*

**Abstract.** *Introduction*: Gender selection is the term currently used when the couple tries to dictate the sex of the baby to be born. The sex of the baby may be chosen before fertilization or at conception by preimplantation genetic diagnosis (PGD). Gender selection may be performed for medical or social indications. The latter had created an intense legal and ethical debate all over the world. Gender selection is becoming increasingly advertised and practiced around the world. The paper discusses gender selection in different cultures, procreative autonomy of women, and legal and ethical issues in gender selection. *Material*: The desire for gender selection is a reflection of culture, tradition, religion, civilization, education, and available technologies in the community. Gender selection and preference as they had been practiced in different cultures are discussed. Legal issues surrounding gender selection and attempts to criminalize its practice in some countries are analysed. Different ethical issues in gender selection such as whether it reinforces male preference, interferes with nature, is sexist, or conflicts with procreative autonomy of women are discussed. The possible positive and negative effects of gender selection are explored. The statements of different international organizations on the issue of gender selection are reviewed. The controversial issue of whether indications for gender selection justify creation of embryos and how to deal with these embryos are discussed. *Results*: The review of literature has revealed the pressing need for concerned international organizations as IFFS to issue their guidelines on this important issue. Soon, gender selection may become available on the counter, and we shall then be faced with the outcome of its bizarre use. *Conclusion*: Gender bias must be tackled at more fundamental and comprehensive social, economic, political, and legal levels worldwide. Till we achieve these long-term goals, gender selection may not be unethical in some particular instances to overcome some societal customs, and to meet procreative autonomy of some couples. Practices of gender selection intended to promote gender discrimination are unacceptable independent of cultural, religious, political and societal demands. © 2004 Published by Elsevier B.V.

*Keywords:* Transcultural; Gender; Gender selection; Ethics-legal

---

Gender selection is the term currently used when the woman with or without her partner tries to dictate the sex of the baby to be born. It is now possible to attempt to choose the sex of the baby before fertilization by separating the X- and Y-chromosome-bearing sperms based on the 2.8% difference in their DNA content using the microsort sperm

---

* Tel.: +20-202-5755869, Cellular: +20-122116039; fax: +20-202-5754271.
 *E-mail address:* giserour@thewayout.net (G.I. Serour).

0531-5131/ © 2004 Published by Elsevier B.V.
doi:10.1016/j.ics.2004.02.008

separation technique or by preimplantation genetic diagnosis (PGD). The indications for gender selection are broadly divided into medical and social [1]. The paper discusses the practice of gender selection in different cultures, procreative autonomy, and legal and ethical issues in gender selection in the light of available modern technology.

## 1. Gender selection in different cultures

The desire for gender selection is a reflection of culture, tradition, religion, civilization, education, and available medical technologies in a given society or community, all of which may influence the morality and the mentality of the people living in these societies and communities. Ancient Egyptians believed that women of certain complexion were destined to have boys. Early Greeks believed that tying off the left testicle would produce boys because the male-determining sperms were derived from the right testicle. The Babylonian Talmud advises couples on means to favour the birth of either a male or a female child. The Hebrew Talmud suggested that placing the marriage bed in a North–South direction favoured the conception of boys. When the woman emits her semen before the man, the child will be a boy; otherwise, it will be a girl. Sons are important for religious reasons. In Judaism, it is the son who says the kaddish for a dead father. [2] Arabs more than 1400 years ago, before Islam, used to practice infanticide for gender selection. The Holy Quran described this act and condemned it [3]. The Shi'its and some Sunnis would allow gender selection for social indications while some Sunnis would not.

In China, the practice of female infanticide was mentioned in the historical records. Sons are important for religious reasons [1]. In the traditional family genogram in the ancestral halls, only the names of sons and grandsons and not daughters are put onto the list. The traditional cultural norm in old China was to unilaterally divorce women who cannot bear a son. The issue of gender preference was complicated by the introduction of the one child policy. Couples in urban areas are usually allowed to have one child. In rural areas, couples whose first child is a girl may have a second child, but only after a specific time period [4]. Chinese women may want to get rid of a female fetus so that they may try again for a male child. This practice is leading to a serious imbalance in sex ratio in China. In some provinces in China, the sex ratio was more than 120 boys for every 100 girls [1].

In India, having more than one daughter is a curse, whereas any number of sons is welcomed. Sons are important economically and provide support for aging parents. Until recently, daughters did not have a right to inherit any part of the ancestral or other property of the parents. Further, at the time of marriage, among a vast majority of Hindus, the prospective husband and his parents generally demand substantial dowries: This practice substantially continues, even though the country's law now prohibits it. Therefore, a girl child becomes a financial burden on the parents. India is, in fact, today known for the large number of dowry deaths where the young bride either kills herself or is killed by her in-laws for refusing to ask her parents, after the marriage, for more money, in addition to what was initially agreed upon as the dowry to be paid by the girl's family. In some communities in India, although few, female infanticide at birth is a common practice [5]. Under the above circumstances, there is an extreme desire on the part of a vast majority of Indian couples to use modern technology to ensure the birth of only a male child particularly with national policy emphasis on small families [6]. The proportion of females to males had dropped from 935:1000 in 1981 to 927:1000 in 1991. In certain communities in the northern states of Bihar and Rajasthan, the ratio has plummeted to 600:1000, one of the lowest in the world [1]. In the age group of 0–6 years, sex ratio was 927 females to 1000 males. It was 820 females per 1000 males in Harayana, while Punjab has 793 females per 1000 males [7]. In Korea, a similar situation exists, which created an imbalance in the sex ratio. For the fourth child in Korea, there were two males born for every female [8].

In Canada, a national survey of preferences regarding the sex of children showed that a large majority of Canadians do not prefer children of one sex or the other [9]. The Royal Commission found that preferences were generally seen as unimportant, almost trivial. The survey showed that virtually all prospective parents want, and feel strongly about having, at least one child of each sex. Another study on sex preference in Canada showed that neither boys nor girls are preferred as first-born children by women and their husbands/partners. The attitudinal measure showed that sons are preferred as first-born children among parents with a sex preference. However, the greater percentage of zero-parity women have no sex preference for their first-born child [1]. Gender selection for nonmedical reasons has been practiced in the United States for decades. In Australia, requests for gender selection are not common.

In Europe, Aristole advised sexual intercourse in Northern wind to get a boy and in Southern wind to get a girl. In Germany, a father was advised to take an axe to bed with him if he wanted to conceive a boy. Millot, the obstetrician of Queen Marie Antoinette of France (1820), wrote: "it is the last movement of the woman that determines the sex of the child: it is the side on which she lies at ejaculation time that drives to sex of the child: always a boy when she is on the right side and always a girl on the left side" [10]. In France, women desiring a boy were provided, a diet rich in potassium and sodium and poor in magnesium and calcium concentration [11]. A London clinic revealed that in 902 couples in Europe, gender selection is based more on ethical individual concern than a social need. Europeans expressed they would have had a baby regardless of whether sex selection was possible or not [12].

In Japan, the head of a family was always the man. He governed everything in the family, and the first son held the right to succeed almost all the family property under legal protection. This structure mandated a boy as at least one of their children. The increasing average longevities of men and women in Japan affected their preference for female offspring suspecting that they would be better taken care of by daughters rather than sons later in life [13].

## 2. Procreative autonomy

The procreative autonomy is the right of the person to freely choose his/her reproductive performance including his/her reproductive potentials. Though procreative autonomy is basically a personal decision, yet some would argue that it is not merely so. Reproduction itself is a process that does not involve solely the person who makes the choice. It also involves the other partner, the baby to be born, the family, the society, and the world at large [14]. On receiving new technologies in human reproduction, we have to demonstrate a tolerance of innovation and respect for individual autonomy.

Dworkin [15] defined a right of procreative autonomy as "a right [of people] to control their own role in procreation unless the state has a compelling reason for denying them that control. The decision not to implant in vitro created embryos is within the unfettered discretion of any woman. While she is entitled to refuse to implant any embryos, the decision to select between embryos is constrained by morality. She should not choose between them in ways which might constitute unfair discrimination. Choosing between embryos would only constitute unfair discrimination, if the reasons for preferring some embryos to others focused on features which there would be no legitimate reasons to prefer [16]. If couples use contraceptive technology to prevent conception of both boys and girls, why cannot couples use their procreative autonomy to prevent birth of one sex or the other?

## 3. Legal issues in gender selection

Female infanticide, a practice that was prevalent in the past in many societies, has not been completely abolished. It has been brought forward at an earlier stage of conception as figures from China, India, and Korea have shown. This is the basis for measures taken to ban and even criminalize gender selection in many parts of the world [1,17].

In Canada, Bill C-13, first introduced in May 2003, proposes to make it a crime for any person who, for the purpose of creating a human being, knowingly: performs any procedure or provides, prescribes, or administers anything that would ensure or increase the probability that an embryo will be of a particular sex, or that would identify the sex of an in vitro embryo, except to prevent, diagnose or treat a sex-linked disorder or disease (Clause 5 (1) (e) [18]). In the USA, the law requiring a model program for certification of ART centers specifically states that in developing the model certification program, " the secretary [of Health and Human Services] may not establish any regulation, standard or requirement which has the effect of exercising supervision or control over the practice of medicine and ART programs" [19]. Thus, existing regulations allow private ART clinics to create and destroy embryos and to operate pretty much on their own [20].

In Australia, gender selection employing artificial insemination or IVF is banned explicitly in Victoria, Australia, by section 50 of the Infertility Treatment Act 1995. In South Australia, section 13 of the Reproductive Technology Act 1988 requires that artificial fertilization only be used for the treatment of infertility. Both acts provide exceptions to avoid the risk of transmission of a genetic defect [1].

In India, gender selection was banned by a law issued in 1994 [21]. The Indian Medical Association and the Medical Council of India have ordered doctors to stop providing sex determination services and participation in any selective abortion of female fetuses.

In Japan, clinical application of PGD is restricted exclusively to medical indications with the consent from the couple and the respective families after consulting the genetic counselor and/or physicians specialized in human genetics and submitting their written consent [22,23].

In Spain, the law which dates back to 1988 clearly expressed that the sex cannot be preselected. No mention of the methods or reasons is included. In Article 20, it indicates that sex selection or genetic manipulation for nontherapeutic or unauthorised therapeutic purposes is prohibited [24].

In the UK, the HFEA banned authorised IVF centers from performing PGD for gender selection for non therapeutic indications. However, it does not prohibit gender selection offered in intrauterine insemination clinics using the sperm separation technique.

To ban gender selection and assume that such choice is sexist is unjust and oppressive. It is even more so if laws introducing criminal penalties on such a choice are introduced as it is proposed in Canada [18]. In societies where gender selection is apparently sexist, the ethics of legal prohibition warrant attention. Experience in India has shown that implementation of legislation to ban gender selection was not successful. Legislation in ART takes long time and may hinder developments in this rapidly advancing field [22,25]. It may be better for the ordinance to lay down broad principles and regulatory framework [26], if necessary.

## 4. Ethical issues

As much as the use of gender selection technologies for prevention of diseases is welcomed and encouraged, its use for social indications had created a great deal of ethical debate. Recommendations may change as science and technology change, as understanding of processes deepens and as society's mores change [27]. Gleicher and Karande [28] emphasized that there is no difference in the ethical issues associated with prefertilization gender selection or PGD. It must be emphasized that these ethical arguments do not necessarily lead to a self-determined conclusion; rather, they expose considerations that require or warrant attention, balance, and prioritizations. There are a number of questions and arguments to be made in this context.

Is gender selection unnatural? The whole practice of medicine is unnatural (people naturally fall ill and die prematurely), if we were to accept an ethic which required us not to interfere with what was natural, there would be little for medical practitioners and medical scientists to do. The principle that it is better to do something good than to do nothing good should be emphasized. It must be better to make good use of something than to allow it to be wasted. It must surely be more ethical to help some people than to help no one [16]. Almost two million babies were already born using IVF and ICSI since they were introduced. Is this unnatural? Or is it a natural scientific development which the scientific body accepted, developed, and celebrated? New reproductive techniques and technologies have always triggered fears of unnatural, harmful outcomes, social disruption, and destruction of conventional families. In human reproduction, any change in custom or practice in this emotionally charged area has always elicited a response from established custom and law of horrified negation at first, then negation without horror, then slow and gradual curiosity, study, evaluation, and finally a very slow but steady acceptance.

Does gender selection reinforce male preference and attribute to society's gender stereotyping? Jewish, Christian, and Islamic teaching show that it is highly significant to children that they be accepted by their parents as a divine gift to be loved for what they uniquely are and not merely because they conform to the parents' hopes or expectations. At present, society is becoming more aware of the immense injustice and harm inflicted on women by cultural structures and patterns that constantly tell a girl, "You should have been a boy". It is argued that gender selection for nonmedical reasons will reinforce this male preference pattern, lead to a serious distortion of the sex ratio, identify gender as a reason to value one person over another, or contribute to society's gender stereotyping.

Gender selection at least will tell the child, "You are loved because you conform to your parents' preferences". This seems an injustice to the child and further reinforces the cultural message that children exist primarily to fulfil the needs of the parents rather than for their own sake. Such implication is already built into many cultural structures and we have an ethical responsibility to fight against it. Choosing the sex of children seems incompatible with the attitude of virtually unconditional acceptance that developmental psychologists have found to be essential to successful parenting [29]. But until we change these societal attitudes, which is likely to take a long time to achieve, are we not protecting the children of the unwanted sex, by gender selection, from being exposed to this conditional acceptance, improper remarks, and discriminative treatment of their parents? While gender selection in the West is unlikely to disturb the sex ratio [30], more openly available gender selection would further distort the sex ratio in Asia. There were 100 million women missing in 1990 as a result of various forms of discrimination [31].

Is gender selection sexist? Many feminists view any efforts to plan the sex of future children as epitomising sexism [32]. The stereotypical concept that pro-male sexism is inherent in sex selection, rooted in perceptions of pervasive devaluation of girl children, may be contradicted in particular countries, such as Canada, by empirical studies [9]. There may be preference in some families for a first born child to be male, but this preference, if offensive to equal priority and opportunity between the sexes, can be addressed by permitting gender selection only for second or subsequent children, rather than by absolute prohibition [17]. Gender selection may be allowed under these conditions for purposes of family balancing in countries in which no demonstrable pro-male sex bias exists among prospective parents. This appears to be ethically neutral and tolerable [33]. Support of such tolerance lies in respect for prospective parents' autonomy and avoiding harm of compelling a woman's repeat pregnancies to achieve family balance of both sexes in the family. Gender selection based on sex is clearly sexual, but not necessarily sexist. The intention of a couple who have a child of one sex to have another child of the other sex is a sexual but not a sexist preference. Feminist ethics demand that the effects of any decision on women's lives be a feature of moral discussion and decision making and focuses on the need to develop a moral analysis that fits the actual world in which we live [34]. Until societies overcome and eliminate their son-preference, the prohibition of gender selection would burden and endanger women's health and lives. Women will go through successive unwanted pregnancies or ART trials, with all their implications and risks until they conceive a boy [35]. The risks are even more increased in developing countries, where gender preference is more likely to prevail as compared with the developed countries [36].

Is gender selection of the first child or of one sex ethical? The greatest social harm of gender selection arises when the gender of the first child is chosen or gender selection is used to produce one sex only in the family. Selection for first children will overwhelmingly favour males, particularly if one child family population policies apply. This has been the experience with the use of technology of gender selection in India, China, Jordan [37], and Saudi Arabia (Samir Abbas, personal communication). This would be considered as unethical and sexist, and involves tremendous social harm.

Does gender selection justify creating embryos? The question arises whether the desire for gender variety in children, even if not sexist, is a strong enough reason to justify creating and discarding embryos. No one has yet marshalled evidence showing that the need or desire for gender variety in children is substantial and important, or whether many parents would refrain from having another child if PGD for gender variety was not possible. If that case is made, then PGD for gender variety might be acceptable as well [38]. Donation of embryos of the undesired sex to infertile couples, in cultures that allow this practice, is one alternative. Also, they may be cryopreserved for transfer to the couple in the future, or donated for research. The ethics committee of the American Society of Reproductive Medicine (ASRM) indicated that PGD for gender selection generally "should be discouraged" for couples not going through IVF, and "not encouraged" for couples who were [39]. The chair of the ethics committee found that PGD for gender balancing would be acceptable [40]. However, the full committee later concluded that it had not yet received enough evidence that the need for gender variety was so important in families that it justified creating and discarding embryos for that purpose [38]. In the future, if such evidence was forthcoming, then PGD for gender variety might also be acceptable. Given the legitimacy of wanting to raise children of both genders, reasonable persons might find that this need outweighs the symbolic costs of creating and discarding embryos for that purpose [41].

Does prohibition of gender selection conflict with procreative autonomy and liberty of women? If we admit that individuals enjoy procreative liberty and that serious reasons must be provided if a limitation on reproductive freedom is to be justified, one cannot accept that gender selection for non-medical reasons is ethically inappropriate and ought to be discouraged. Universal prohibition of gender selection for social reasons would itself risk prejudice to women in societies, where births remain central to women's well-being. Family balancing was considered acceptable, for instance where a wife had borne three or four daughters, and it was in her and her family's best interests that another pregnancy should be her last. Employing gender selection to ensure the birth of a son might then be approved, to satisfy a sense of family obligation and to save the women from increasingly risk-laden pregnancies [42]. Gender selection should be offered only after proper counselling of the couple with the reproductive medicine physician, geneticist, social scientist, and psychiatrist [1]. Most feminists agree that women must gain full control over their own reproductive lives if they are to free themselves from male dominance [34]. Is gender selection not one of these reproductive choices of women?

Does gender selection have a negative effect on children to be born, family, and society? Gender selection might have a negative psychological impact on children themselves. Children who are sex selected could feel subtly harmed, controlled, or invidiously different from other children not so conceived. If a daughter knows that she was "planned-to-be-second", she may "suffer a loss of confidence or self-esteem". Even if a daughter is first-born, she may be damaged if she learns that whereas she was not sex selected, her younger brother was. Also, there is the possibility that a given method of gender selection may fail, with the child of the unwanted sex experiencing parental rejection or developing feelings of inadequacy. Whether gender selection is performed or not depends upon parental needs served and balancing it against harm posed to embryos, children, and society. When gender selection service becomes available, who will make the decision? Is it the potential mother? Or her partner or both? Or is it the family? This may create unnecessary conflict in the family and bring more suppression of the female partner. The availability of gender selection may open the door widely for those who are sexist to achieve their goals, particularly in Eastern countries such as what happened in India. More seriously, the availability of the service may encourage those with tendencies towards gender preferences, who never practiced it in the past, to demand it once the service becomes available. This will attribute to increased gender stereotyping in both Western and Eastern societies. Moreover, in countries with limited health resources, gender selection may cause misallocation of these resources.

Does gender selection have any benefits or positive effects? A direct effect of the availability of techniques of gender selection might some day reduce the incidence and prevalence of female feticide/infanticide [43]. Whether the imbalance of sex ratio which resulted from gender selection in some countries has any advantage is very questionable. Though this may be ominous for the present generation of children, it provides possible attitudinal changes in the future reversing female vulnerability and the force of male dominance. This may lead to a higher value of the rarer gender, interbreeding of different populations and reduce population growth. Gender selection may even save public funds by preventing the birth and the cost of unwanted repeated pregnancies.The size and make up of families could become a matter of choice rather than chance for couples favouring this approach. Exercising the right to choose family planning and/or balancing would have a positive effect on the quality of life of the parents and children delivered unto them [44].

## 5. Gender selection and international organizations

The World Health Organization indicated in 1998, "The use of prenatal diagnosis for paternity testing, except in cases of rape or incest, or for gender selection, apart from sex-linked disorders, is not acceptable" [45]. The WHO statement did not refer to prefertilization or preimplantation gender selection. The American College of Obstetricians and Gynaecologists accepts, as ethically permissible, the practice of gender selection to prevent sex-linked genetic disorders. The College opposes meeting requests for gender selection for personal and family reasons, due to the concern that such requests may ultimately support sexist practices [46]. The Ethics Committee of the ASRM concluded that PGD for sex selection for non-medical reasons should be discouraged because it poses a risk of unwarranted gender bias, social harm, and results in the diversion of medical resources from genuine medical need [39]. However, in its recent review on preconception gender selection for non-medical reasons the committee recognised the serious ethical concerns that such a practice raises and counsels against its widespread use. It concludes that sex selection aimed at increasing gender variety in families may not so greatly increase the risk of harm to children, women, or society so that its use should be prohibited or condemned as unethical in all cases [47]. The FIGO Ethics Committee recognised that the use of pre-conceptional sex selection to avoid sex-linked genetic disorders is an indication that is completely justifiable on medical grounds. It can be justified on social grounds in certain cases for the objective of allowing children of the two sexes to enjoy the love and care of parents. However, it must not conflict with other social values where it is practised, and it should never be used as a tool for sex discrimination against either sex particularly the female [48]. The ESHRE Task Force on Ethics and Law in 2001 stated, regarding the ethical concerns related to the technique of PGD..."we are aware of the risks of abuse for non-medical reasons. Information and consent of the couple, public transparency and the respect of professional guidelines will limit abuse" [49]. In a more recent statement, the committee has not been able to reach a unanimous decision. Two positions can be distinguished: those opposed to every application of sex selection for non-medical reasons and those who accept sex selection for family balancing [50]. The Vatican instruction states that, "procedures such as sex preselection cannot be justified, for whatever medical or social indications, on grounds of possible beneficial consequences for humanity" [51].

## 6. Conclusion

With the rapid progress in technology, gender selection scarcely used today, may tomorrow become available on the counter. The medical profession will then be confronted with implications of its unregulated use. Tight regulations should reassure people that gender selection will not lead to designer babies and deal with problems associated with it as record keeping, handling of embryos, sex discrimination, and public funds use [1,52–56].

The following are proposed recommendations:

1. Sex bias must be tackled at more fundamental and comprehensive social, economic, political and legal levels worldwide. Until we achieve these long-term goals, gender selection may not be unethical in some particular instances. Gender selection intended to maintain and promote gender discrimination is unacceptable, independently of cultural, religious, political economical, or social demands.
2. When technology is used for non medical indications tight regulations should be implemented.
3. Prohibitions are unnecessary and oppressive when there is no sex bias.
4. Gender selection should only be offered after proper informative and implicative counselling.
5. Healthy embryos of the unwanted sex, created by PGD for gender selection, may be donated to infertile couples, research, or transferred to the genetic mother.
6. Centers providing gender selection must keep a balanced sex ratio within the center and within every year.
7. When health resources are limited, the service may be provided in private sectors. A mechanism has to be found to enable the needy to have access to this service.
8. The conscious of the couple and the physician is the decisive factor in gender selection.

## References

[1] G.I. Serour, Family and sex selection, in: D.L. Healy, et al. (Eds.), Reproductive Medicine in the Twenty-First Century. Proceedings of the 17th World Congress on Fertility and Sterility, Melbourne, Australia, The Parthenon Publishing Group, Boca Raton, London, New York, Washington, D.C., 2002, pp. 97–106.
[2] J.G. Schenker, Gender selection: cultural and religious perspectives, Journal of Assisted Reproduction and Genetics 19 (9) (2002) 400–410.
[3] Holy Quran, Sura Al-Takwir 8–9.
[4] C.L.W. Chan, et al., Gender selection in China, its meanings and implications, Journal of Assisted Reproduction and Genetics 19 (9) (2002) 426–430.
[5] P.M. Bhargava, Ethical issues in modern biological technologies, Reproductive Biomedicine Online 7 (3) (2003) 276–285.

[6] A. Malpani, A. Malpani, D. Modi, Preimplantation sex selection for family balancing in India, Human Reproduction 17 (2002) 11–12.
[7] Registrar General of India, Provisional Population totals, Census of India 2001 (New Delhi: Office of the Registrar General India, 2001. Available at http://www.censusindia.net/resultsmain).
[8] Z. Yi, et al., Causes and implications of the recent increase in the reported sex ratio at birth in China, Population and Development Review 19 (1993) 282–302.
[9] Royal Commission on New Reproductive Technologies, Proceed with care: final report of the Royal Commission (Ottawa: Minister of Government Services Canada, 1993, 889).
[10] J.A. Millot, m'art de procréer les sexes à volonté, 4 edn., Vers. 1820.
[11] Stoolkowski et Emmeriche: Influence de la nutrition minerale de la vache sur la repartition des sexes dans la descendance, Annales d'Endocrinologie 32 (1971) 3.
[12] J. Cohen, Gender selection: is there a European view? Journal of Assisted Reproduction and Genetics 19 (9) (2002) 417–419.
[13] T. Mori, H. Watanabe, Ethical considerations on Indications for gender selection in Japan, Journal of Assisted Reproduction and Genetics 19 (9) (2002) 420–425.
[14] G.I. Serour, Reproductive choice: a Muslim perspective, in: J. Harris, S. Holm (Eds.), The Future of Human Reproduction. Ethics, Choice, and Regulation, Clarendon Press, Oxford, 2000, pp. 191–202.
[15] R. Dworkin, Life's Dominion, Harper Collins, London, 1993, p. 148.
[16] J. Harris, Rights and reproductive choice, in: J. Harris, S. Holm (Eds.), The Future of Human Reproduction. Ethics, Choice and Regulation, Clarendon Press, Oxford, 2000, pp. 5–37.
[17] B. Dickens, Can sex selection be ethically tolerated? Editorial, Journal of Medical Ethics 28 (6) (2002) 335–336.
[18] The proposed Assisted Human Reproduction Act, section (5) (1) (e).
[19] USC 42 §§ 263a-2 (i) (1), 2003 and USC 42 §§ 263a-2 (i) (2), 2003.
[20] D.P. Wolf, An opinion on regulating the assisted reproductive technologies, Journal of Assisted Reproduction and Genetics 20 (7) (2003) 290–292.
[21] The Pre-natal Diagnostic Techniques (Regulation and Prevention of Misuse) Act, 1994. Indian Parliament Act No. 57 of 1994.
[22] N. Takeshita, et al., Regulating assisted reproductive technologies in Japan, Journal of Assisted Reproductive and Genetics 20 (7) (2003) 260–264.
[23] Executive Board of Japan Society of Obstetrics and Gynaecology, Guidelines on preimplantation genetic diagnosis, Nippon Sanka Fujinka Gakkai Zasshi, (2000) 52 (Announcement to society members).
[24] M. Boada, A. Veiga, P.N. Barri, Spanish regulations on assisted reproduction techniques, Journal of Assisted Reproduction and Genetics 20 (7) (2003) 271–275.
[25] J. Montagut, Y. Mmenezo, How to legislate in human reproduction: the French experience, Journal of Assisted Reproduction and Genetics 20 (7) (2003) 287–289.
[26] E.H.Y. Ng, et al., Regulating reproductive technology in Hong Kong, Journal of Assisted Reproduction and Genetics 20 (7) (2003) 281–286.
[27] M.M. Cadieux, Sex preselection and full disclosure, Fertility and Sterility 8 (2) (2003) 469.
[28] N. Gleicher, V. Karande, Gender selection for non medical indications, Fertility and Sterility 78 (3) (2002) 460–462.
[29] President's Commission for the Study of Ethical Problems in Medicine and Biomedical and Behavioral Research, Screening and Counseling for Genetic Conditions, U.S. Government Printing Office, Washington, DC, 1983, pp. 56–59.
[30] J.L. Simpson, S.A. Carson, The reproductive option of sex selection, Human Reproduction 14 (1999) 870–872.
[31] A. Sen, More Than 100 Million Women are Missing, Rev. Books, NY, 1990, p. 61.
[32] S.M. Wolf (Ed.), Feminism and Bioethics: Beyond Reproduction, Oxford Univ. Press, New York, 1996, p. 336.
[33] G. Pennings, Ethics of sex selection for family balancing as a morally acceptable application of sex selection, Human Reproduction II (1996) 2339–2345.
[34] S. Sherwin, No Longer Patient: Feminist Ethics and Health Care, Temple Univ. Press, Philadelphia, 1992, pp. 102–103.

[35] G.I. Serour, et al., Complications of assisted reproduction techniques: a review, Assisted Reproduction 9 (1999) 214–232.
[36] M.F. Fathalla, The girl child, International Journal of Gynecology and Obstetrics 70 (1) (2000) 7–12.
[37] Z. Kilani, L. Haj Hassan, Sex selection and preimplantation genetic diagnosis at the Farah Hospital, Reproductive Biomedicine Online 4 (1) (2001) 68–70.
[38] J.A. Robertson, Sex selection for gender variety by preimplantation genetic diagnosis, Fertility and Sterility 78 (2002) 463.
[39] J.A. The Ethics Committee of the American Society of Reproductive Medicine, Sex selection and preimplantation genetic diagnosis, Fertility and Sterility 72 (4) (1999) 595–5980.
[40] G. Kolata, in: Society Approves Embryo Selection, vol. 26, The New York Times, 2001 Sept. 26, p. A14.
[41] J.A. Robertson, Extending preimplantation genetic diagnosis: medical and non-medical uses, Journal of Medical Ethics 29 (2003) 213–216.
[42] G.I. Serour, B.M. Dickens, Assisted reproduction developments in the Islamic world, International Journal of Gynecology and Obstetrics, Ethical and Legal Column 74 (2001) 187–193.
[43] N. Pandiyan, Embryo sex selection: a social comment on the article by Malpani and Malpani, Reproductive Biomedicine Online 4 (1) (2001) 9–10.
[44] D.L. Hill, M.W. Surrey, H.C. Danzer, Is gender selection an appropriate use of medical resources? Journal of Assisted Reproduction and Genetics 19 (9) (2002) 438–439.
[45] World Health Organization, Proposed International Guidelines on Ethical Issues in Medical Genetics and Genetic services, WHO, Geneva, 1998.
[46] American College of Obstetricians and Gynecologists (ACOG), Committee on Ethics. Sex Selection Committee opinion No. 177, November 1996 in ACOG Ethics in Obstetrics and Gynecology (Washington, DC: ACOG, 2002), 85-8, repr. In Int. J. Gynecol. Obstet. 56 (1997) 199–202.
[47] Ethics Committee of the American Society for Reproductive Medicine, Preconception gender selection for nonmedical reasons, Fertility and Sterility 75 (5) (2001) 861–864.
[48] FIGO Committee for the Ethical aspects of human reproduction and Women's health, Sex selection, FIGO Recommendations on Ethical Issues in Obstetrics and Gynecology, FIGO, London, 2003, pp. 9–10.
[49] ESHRE Task Force on Ethics and Law, The moral status of the pre-implantation embryo, Human Reproduction 16 (2001) 1046–1048.
[50] The ESHRE Ethics Task Force, F. Shenfield, et al., Task force 5: preimplantation genetic diagnosis, Human Reproduction 18 (3) (2003) 649–651.
[51] Congregation for the doctrine of the faith, Instruction on respect for human life in its origin and on the dignity of procreation, 1. 6. p. 20.
[52] F.A. Flinter, Preimplantation genetic diagnosis: needs to be tightly regulated editorial, BMJ 322 (2001) 1008–1009.
[53] J. Egozcue, Preimplantation social sexing: a problem of proportionality and decision making, Journal of Assisted Reproduction and Genetics 19 (9) (2002) 440–442.
[54] M. Meseguer, et al., Gender selection: ethical, scientific, legal and practical issues, Journal of Assisted Reproduction and Genetics 19 (9) (2002) 443–446.
[55] A.C. Katayama, US ART practitioners soon to begin their forced march into a regulated future, Journal of Assisted Reproduction and Genetics 20 (7) (2003) 265–270.
[56] R.J. Cooke, B.M. Dickens, M.F. Fathalla (Eds.), Sex Selection—Abortion in Reproductive Health and Human Rights, vol. 12, Clarendon Press, Oxford, 2003, pp. 363–371.

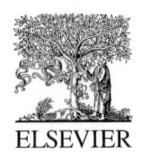

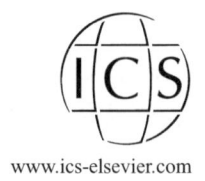

#  Is human fertility declining?

Tina Kold Jensen[a,b,*], Anders Nyboe Andersen[b], Niels Erik Skakkebæk[c]

[a] *Department of Environmental Medicine, University of Southern Denmark, Institute of Public Health, Winsloewsparken 17, 5000 Odense C, Denmark*
[b] *The Fertility Clinic, Rigshospitalet, Denmark*
[c] *University Department of Growth and Reproduction, Rigshospitalet, Denmark*

**Abstract.** During the past decades, we have witnessed a remarkable decline in fertility rates (number of births per 1000 women of reproductive age) in the industrialized world. It seems beyond doubt that the enormous social changes of our societies play the major role in this decline, but we argue that reduced fecundity (the ability to conceive) in the population may be a contributing factor. The time taken to conceive (Time To Pregnancy, TTP) has proven a valuable tool in measuring fecundity of a couple, but few studies have attempted to study trends in TTP. Another proposed marker is the spontaneous dizygotic twinning rate, which has declined until the 80s where the use of ovulation-inducing agents introduced increase. Fecundity may be affected both by female and male factors. Semen quality may have deteriorated considerably during the past 50 years and large geographical differences exist. Not many studies among unselected men from the general population exist, but when studying semen quality in an unselected population of young Danish men we found an alarmingly low semen quality. In addition, other biological markers of male fecundity may have changed in prevalence—hypospadias, cryptorchidism and testicular cancer. Changes in ovarian function (biological female factors) may also contribute to a change in the fecundity, although the literature in this field is sparser. We lack information on the roles of modern lifestyle and food contaminants (including endocrine disrupters) on reproductive function in males, as well as in females. It is therefore important that we, even though it is time consuming and costly, continue to monitor semen quality and begin to monitor fecundity, including trends in waiting time to pregnancy.
© 2004 Published by Elsevier B.V.

*Keywords:* Fertility; Fecundity; Time trends; Male factors; Female factors; Semen quality

## 1. Introduction

Demographers define fertility as the number of births per 1000 women of reproductive age. It has declined tremendously in the industrialised world [1,2] during the last decades. The number of children per women is less than two in many Western countries, including

\* Corresponding author. Department of Environmental Medicine, University of Southern Denmark, Institute of Public Health, Winsloewsparken 17, 5000 Odense C, Denmark. Tel.: +4565503077; fax: +4565911458.
*E-mail address:* tkjensen@health.sdu.dk (T.K. Jensen).

0531-5131/ © 2004 Published by Elsevier B.V.
doi:10.1016/j.ics.2004.01.113

several European countries and Japan [3], and is too low to sustain the population at the current level (Fig. 1). Major changes in the social structure of modern society are beyond doubt mainly to blame for this decline. Women educate and work outside their home and they benefit from more effective contraception to delay childbearing. In most European countries the average age at the birth of the first child is increasing, and in Denmark it is currently 29 years for women.

Demographic fertility is, however, not a very sensitive measure of the biological fertility, the ability to conceive (fecundity). Some couples may never have their desired number of children and some may take longer to conceive than planned. It is important to consider the possibility that decreased fecundity may contribute to the decreasing fertility rate [4]. Indeed, infertility treatment has become an increasing part of the health care system. In Denmark in 1999, 3.2% of all children were born after the use of assisted reproductive technology (ART) using IVF or ICSI [5]. In addition, an established 1.3% of all children are born after artificial insemination with donor or husband semen. Furthermore, most recent data from the Danish Fertility Society have shown that the number of pregnancies after ART has increased by 19% from 1997 to 1999. The number of pregnancies after ART in Denmark in 2002 was 7.5% of all pregnancies and 6.4% of all births are after some form of ART. Furthermore, 37.4% of all ART treatments are ICSI treatments. This could be due to an increase in the number of infertile couples, but could also be caused by more couples seeking treatment and even better success rates.

It seems important to study time trends in biological fecundity, defined as the probability of a couple to conceive in a menstrual cycle. The development of the use of the time taken to conceive (Time To Pregnancy, TTP) has proven a valuable tool in this research [6,7]. Another proposed marker of couple fecundity is the spontaneous dizygotic twinning rate, as it reflects not only the frequency of double ovulations but also the probability of fertilization and the survival of the zygotes [8].

Fecundity is a measure of the ability *of a couple* to conceive. It may, therefore, be affected both by female and male factors. Several studies have shown that sperm

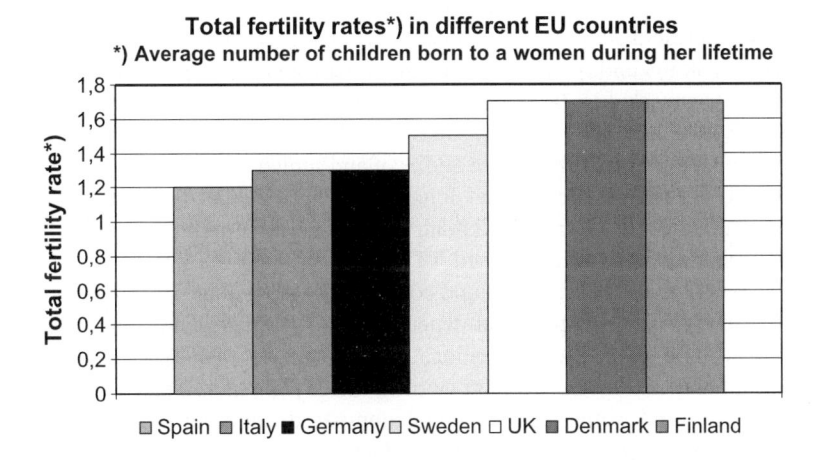

Fig. 1. The average number of children per women in different European countries.

concentration and morphology is correlated to the time to pregnancy of a couple [9–12]. Semen quality may have deteriorated considerably during the past 50 years and large geographical differences exist [13]. In addition, other biological markers of male fecundity may have changed in prevalence—hypospadias, cryptorchidism and testicular cancer [14]. But, changes in ovarian function (biological female factors) may also contribute to a change in the fecundity, although the literature in this field is sparser.

This article will review and discuss trends in biological fecundity and discuss the contribution of male and female biological factors. The contribution of social factors is not a main focus.

## 2. Time to pregnancy (TTP)

Fecundity can be measured by the use of the time taken to conceive (Time To Pregnancy, TTP). TTP has been proven to be a valuable tool to measure fecundity since it is easy to obtain information about and well recalled [15,16]. Little is known about the true prevalence and time trends in TTP because population—based data are generally not available. Some population studies have reported no decline in fecundity with calendar time [17,18]. In Britain, a cross-sectional study showed significantly increasing fecundity over calendar time, after adjustment for truncation bias [19]. Two transient dips in fertility were observed. A Swedish study among 400,000 women found a decrease in subfecundity (TTP>1 year) from 1983 to 1993, which followed a birth cohort pattern [20]. The analysis did not take into account truncation bias at both ends of the study period, which occurs when a calendar time cut off date is imposed (e.g. when data were collected), after which pregnancies are no longer included. This bias has the effect of artificially overestimating fecundity in the most recent category [21].

Some studies have reported spatial variation in TTP. A study comparing TTP among English and Finnish couples from previously performed studies found that Finnish couples tended to have a shorter TTP than English couples [22]. However, the populations and the TTP questions were not directly comparable and no control for known confounders could be performed. In a joint European study, the longest TTP was found in France followed by East Germany, northern Italy, West Germany, Denmark, Sweden and southern Italy. The highest risk of subfecundity (TTP>12 months) was found in Poland, northern Italy, Germany and Denmark [23,24]. A highly structured and validated questionnaire was developed and used in all of the study areas. In a joint European study among pregnant couples from Finland, Denmark, France and Scotland semen samples, as well as TTP data, were collected. French couples waited longer to conceive than the rest, but the study included only 200 couples from each country and had a low participation rate [25].

Numerous studies have dichotomised TTP and examined the percentages of couples with TTP above 12 months, the subfecund couples. The percentage of subfecundity varies from 3 to 28 in different countries, but depends on the sampling and study design. Some studies have been conducted in occupational settings among potentially exposed women [27]; some studies were among pregnant women, thereby not including couples who never conceived [28,29]; and, some were by population-based sampling [26,30]. Furthermore, information about the potential confounding factors were often not complete and not accounted for: parental age, caffeine and alcohol intake and smoking, timing of sexual intercourse, recent use of oral contraceptives and occupational exposures. In addition, numerous biases may operate when analysing TTP; recall bias, infertility treatment bias, truncation bias, behavioural bias, planning bias. They have all previously been discussed [7,31,32].

## 3. Dizygotic twin rate

Lazar has suggested [8] that a dizygotic twinning (DZ) rate may be used as a marker of fecundity. The change of a woman carrying DZ twins to term depends on several factors: (1) the occurrence of double ovulations, (2) coitus in the fertile period, (3) fertilisation of both ova and (4) both embryos carried to term [8,33,34]. If any of these steps were affected, a changed trend in the twinning rate would result. A decline in sperm count may reduce the chance of both ova being fertilised, whereas the use of ovulation-inducing agents may increase the risk of double ovulations.

A decline in the DZ twinning rate has been observed in many developed countries from the 1960s to the 1980s, for example, in Italy [35], Holland [36], UK [37], New Zealand [33], Australia [38], Japan [39] and Hong Kong [40]. Conflicting reports from the USA show that either the DZ rates fell until 1970 and then rose, or declined from the 1940s to 1964 and then were stable until the late 1970s when it increased. This lack of decline in 1970s USA is in contrast to Canada, where the rates declined from 1951 to 1977, and is probably caused by the earlier introduction of ovulation-inducing agents in USA. A Danish study found [41] that the age and parity-adjusted total twinning rate decreased from 1931 to 1977, and since the monozygotic rate was almost constant; the decline was mainly caused by a decline in the spontaneous DZ twin rate. Few data for undeveloped countries exist but a decline in the DZ twin rate has been observed in India and South Africa, whereas the twinning rates have been stable in Bangladesh. The cause for the decline is mainly unknown, but the decline in semen quality has been suggested to be responsible [33,34].

There are, however, large geographical difference in the DZ twin rates across countries and it is affected by heritability, race, maternal age and parity, season, war periods and ovulation-inducing agents. From around the 80s an increase in the DZ twinning rate occurred in many countries [42]. This is believed to be mainly caused by the increased use of ovulation-inducing agents. However, this iatrogenic-induced increase may mask a serious and continuing decline in the true (spontaneous) DZ twinning rate, and we are completely unaware of a recent trend in the DZ twinning rates.

In contrast, the monozogotic (MZ) twin rate has been constant and it is generally believed to be a random, embryological event, which is not subject to environmental or genetic influences and is independent of maternal age, parity and race. The observed rate, in fact, has remained relatively stable in many countries, including Denmark, Italy, Israel, UK, Holland and Japan. Tong and Short [43] has, therefore, suggested that the DZ:MZ rate can be used as a measure of trends in DZ twins.

## 4. Male factors

Male reproductive health has been a focus in recent years after the meta-analysis by Carlsen et al. in 1992 [13], which reported a significant decline in sperm concentration of almost 50% in average sperm concentration from 1940 to 1990. Semen quality can be determined from the following semen variables: semen volume (ml), sperm concentration (mill/ml), percentage of motile sperms, percentage of sperms with normal morphology and the calculated total sperm count (concentration×volume, mill), and is by far the most important male factor for fecundity. A study indicated that men with sperm counts below 40 mill/ml had reduced fecundity [10]. Since most of the published literature to date has focused on sperm concentration, and since there is large variability among technicians when counting morphology and motility, the following will focus on sperm concentration [44].

The limitations of any meta-analysis are that often information about important confounders, like period of abstinence, is not available and cannot be taken into account. Likewise, differences in semen analysis techniques in different laboratories may affect the findings. This would, however, create imprecise estimates of semen concentration, but it is not very likely that this would explain this large decline in semen concentration. In a more extensive reanalysis of the data from the meta-analysis [13], Swan et al. [45] took into account the period of abstinence, age, proven fertility, method of analysis and aim of the individual study and confirmed a significant mean sperm concentration decline of 1.5% per year in the USA between 1938 and 1988 and of 3.1% per year in Europe between 1971 and 1990.

Following the meta-analysis [46] various laboratories analysed their own data. Many longitudinal retrospective trends in semen characteristics of more or less homogeneous groups of men recruited in a single centre during a long period of time have been published. Many men were recruited from infertility clinics [47–51]. It is impossible to draw any conclusion from these studies since the availability of infertility services and the behaviour of infertile couples has changed during the last 30 years. Some of the men were partners of women with tubal disease and may, therefore, be selected because they had a good semen quality in order to be included in in-vitro fertilization. In addition, some studies of potential semen donors who had fathered a child [52–55] or were young students [56–58] have been performed. It is, however, difficult to determine selection processes that recruit men for semen donors and these may have changed over time.

Many factors have to be taken into account when analysing sperm concentration, since it varies greatly among individuals [46]. There is a tenfold difference between the 10th and the 90th percentile of the distribution of sperm concentration in fertile men [59]. Furthermore, many population characteristics may influence semen quality: sexual activity and period of abstinence, occupation, age, medication and diseases, nutrition, smoking habits, stress and season at delivery of the sample. In addition, the mode of semen collection and analysis is very important as there is large intra- and inter-technician variability. Furthermore, the participation rates in semen quality studies do not exceed 50%. Self-volunteers are often better educated people or men with doubts about their own fertility and, consequently, eager to participate to get information on their own health status. It is, therefore, important to obtain information about their motivation for participation and about non-participants so that the selection process can be described. It is preferable to study men from the general population, recruited with the same procedures and from whom information about the above factors is present and semen analysis is standardized.

Few studies have investigated men from the general population [60–64]. A worldwide study among partners of pregnant women was undertaken. In this study, semen quality among 1082 fertile men from four European cities (Copenhagen, Denmark; Paris, France; Edinburgh, Scotland; and Turku, Finland) were compared [65]. The lowest sperm concentrations and total counts were detected for Danish men, followed by French and Scottish men; Finnish men had the highest sperm counts. A study using the same inclusion criteria has been undertaken in four centres in the US among 512 partners of pregnant women [66]. Sperm concentration and motile sperms were significantly lower in Columbia (Missouri), than in big cities including New York, Minnesota and Los Angeles.

Partners of pregnant women are selected with respect to their fertility and are, therefore, likely to have a better semen quality than the general male population, since they have been able to conceive. Very few studies of unselected men from the general population have been conducted, as they are very costly and time-consuming. Nevertheless, they are extremely important if semen quality among men from the general population should be monitored. Recently, a joint European study tried to overcome these problems by approaching all young men who are required to have a compulsory physical examination to determine their fitness for military service in some countries. Their semen quality and reproductive hormone profile were investigated [67]. Similar inclusion criteria, questionnaires and quality control for the semen analysis were used in each country. Among 968 young men, the Finnish and Estonian men had higher sperm concentration than the Norwegian and Danish men, and an east–west gradient in the Nordic-Baltic area, paralleling the incidences of testicular cancer, was found [68]. The participation rate was around 20%, but we believe that these men are representative for 18–20-year-old men from the general population. Firstly, their age and educational status did not differ from non-participants; secondly they had no prior knowledge of their fertility and were, therefore, not inclined to participate because of suspected fertility problems. And thirdly, we enrolled 179 Danish military conscripts from whom only a blood sample was drawn. The participation rate in this cohort was 79% and their reproductive serum hormones did not differ from that of the conscripts who also delivered a semen sample [69]. In Denmark the semen quality among these young men from the general population was alarmingly low [69]; 21% had sperm counts below 20 mill/ml (lower WHO limit) and 43% below 40 mill/ml [69] (a study indicated that men with sperm counts below 40 mill/ml had reduced fecundity [10]). A large number of these men may, therefore, be expected to experience fertility problems in the future. In addition, evidence is emerging that semen quality is lower among younger cohorts. A meta-analysis of semen quality of normal Danish men suggested a birth cohort-related decline in semen quality [70], and the trend seems to continue as the younger cohorts born around 1980 had the lowest sperm counts of all cohorts examined (Fig. 2) [69]. This means that the average young man has a lower fecundity than the average older man. This might be reflected in the fertility rates. In this respect, the fertility rates of teenagers are particularly interesting as they to a large extent reflect unplanned pregnancies caused by lack of contraceptive use or contraceptive failure. Fertility rates among Danish teenagers are showing a subtle, but constant, fall. Similar findings have been observed in many countries. The decline in birth rates among female teenagers is not counterbalanced by an increase in the rate of induced abortion in Denmark (which has been legal since 1973). Both abortion rates and the total pregnancy rate (number of abortions and births per 1000 in the relevant population) have been decreasing among teenagers [4]. Although most social scientists will argue that this decline is caused

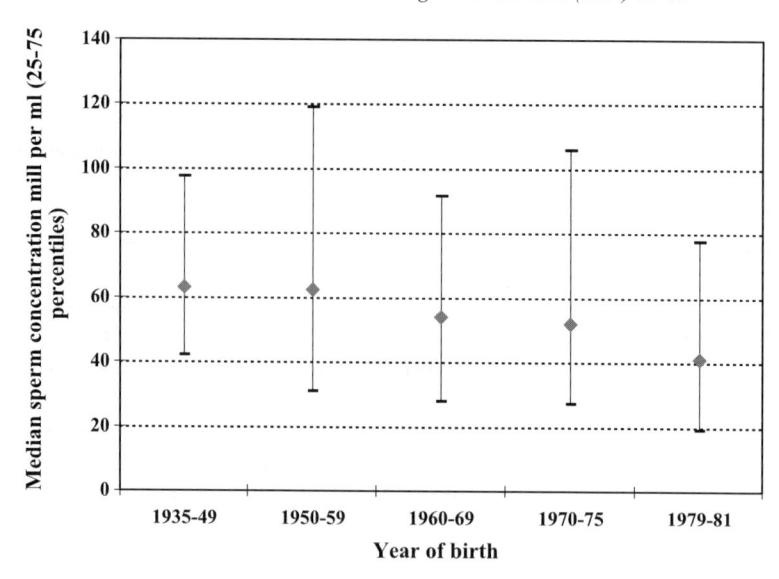

Fig. 2. Median sperm concentration and 25–75th percentiles according to year of birth from 10 Danish studies of men born between 1935 and 1975 (reconstructed from 70) and 708 men from the general Danish population born from 1979 to 1981 [69].

by changes in social factors and use of more effective contraception (including the introduction of the morning after pill), it is not well documented and the fall may not be attributed to social factors alone. A recent study showed that the use of contraception and education levels among Danish teenagers during the past 10 years has been largely unchanged [71]. Neither is it likely that diminished sexual activity is the cause [71]. It therefore seems particularly important to follow the younger cohorts to see whether their future fertility rates will be affected.

## 5. Testicular dysgenesis syndrome (TDS)

The importance of declining semen quality lies partly in its possible link with other problems of male reproductive organs, such as a widespread rise in the incidence of testicular cancer [68], which follows a birth cohort pattern [72]. Interestingly, a similar east–west gradient is observed; the age-standardised incidence of testicular cancer is substantially lower in Finland and the Baltic countries than in the rest of Scandinavia [68]. The precursor of testicular cancer, the carcinoma in situ germ cell, is probably of foetal origin and tends to occur in testes harbouring other histologic abnormalities [14]. Furthermore, men with testicular cancer have been found to have lower fertility than normal men even before the cancer develops [73]. This suggests that the underlying defect arises in early life and is related to infertility. An increase in hypospadias and cryptorchidism has also been observed in some geographical areas [74,75]. It is interesting that male infertility, testis cancer, hypospadias and undescending testis all are risk factors for each other. A hypothesis has suggested the existence of a pathogenetic link, the testicular dysgenesis syndrome (TDS) [14] (Fig. 3). TDS may be a result of genetic, as well as

## Testicular Dysgenesis Syndrome

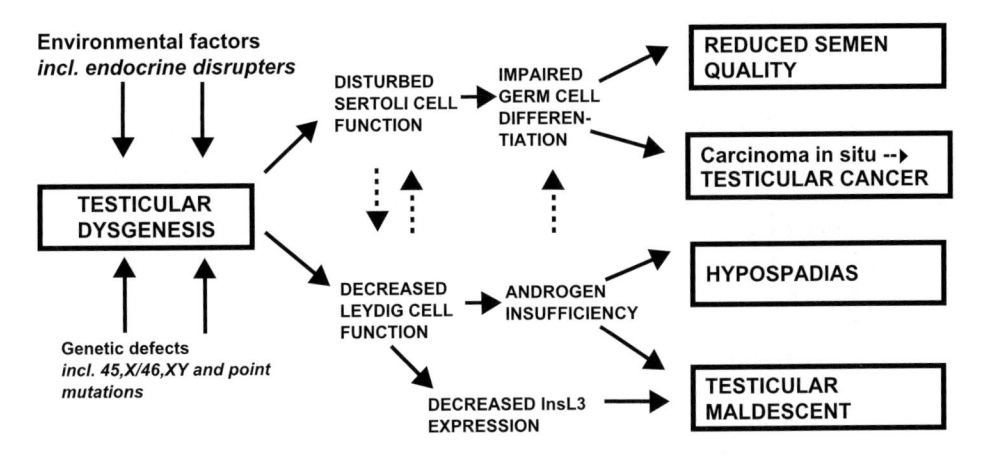

Fig. 3. Testicular Dysgenesis Syndrome (TDS).

environmental factors, causing poor testicular development. Endocrine disruption due to environmental agents with estrogenic [76] and/or anti-androgenic [77] effects have been suggested to be responsible for these parallel changes. The syndrome most often causes impaired spermatogenesis and, only in rare cases, the full range of its signs, including genital malformations and testicular cancer.

## 6. Female factors

In contrast to male factors where semen quality is a measurable marker for testicular function, it is more difficult to study trends in female factors. Anovulation, following ovarian dysfunction in younger women, is common. Premature ovarian failure is defined as secondary amenorrhea and elevated gonadotrophins before the age of 40. Its incidence is unknown, but it is suggested to affect 1–3% of all women and 5% have menopause between the age of 40 and 44 years [78,79].

Polycystic ovarian syndrome (PCOS) is a common and complex endocrine disorder, but little is known about its aetiology [80]. It is a form of ovarian dysfunction defined by multiple cysts in the ovaries, anovulation, hirsutism, infertility and obesity. Some women only have multiple cysts in the ovaries (PCO). In infertile populations of women, the prevalence has been found to be up to 44% and 10–20% of young normal women have been found to have PCOS, which has made some gynaecologists believe that the incidence is increasing [81]. Ultrasound is, however, now routinely used in gynaecologic practice, therefore making the diagnosis easier. Furthermore, no prevalence in an unselected group of women has been reported. It is, therefore, not possible to draw conclusions about trends in PCOS.

Historic studies indicate an age-related decrease in biological fertility both in developed and undeveloped countries [82,83]. Decline in the number of eggs and the rate of spontaneous abortions increase. In a group of women not using birth control (Hutterite women), fecundity decreased already from the age of 25 years [84] and studies among infertile women have found decreases from 31 years [85,86]. Likewise, more studies have reported lower fecundity with older age among women from the general population [87–89]. Since women postpone childbirth, this may be a contributing factor to the reported decline in fecundity and a confounder that needs to be accounted for.

## 7. The role of lifestyle for male and female fecundity

The lifestyles of individuals in the western world have changed tremendously during the past decades. The percentages of smokers first increased and are now decreasing in many countries. Likewise, more alcohol is consumed and an increase in the average body mass index, resulting in an increased prevalence towards obesity, is another major health problem [90].

Smoking has been related to reduced fecundity among women and a meta-analysis suggested that it reduces the chance of conceiving in a menstrual cycle by up to 30% [91]. In a meta-analysis smoking has also been found to reduce semen quality [92]. In addition, some studies have found that women exposed to smoking in utero take longer to conceive [93,94] but one study was not able to confirm this [95]. Likewise, semen quality has been reported to be reduced among men exposed to smoking in utero in two independent studies [96,97].

Obesity has previously been related to reduced female fertility with prolonged waiting time to pregnancy among women with a body mass index (BMI) above 25 $kg/m^2$ [98]. There are, however, to our knowledge no studies investigating the relationship between BMI and male fertility and semen quality.

Thus, it is beyond doubt that lifestyle factors may contribute to changes in fecundity. Recent studies suggest that fetal exposure is also important for reproduction in later life. This makes it even more difficult to obtain solid information about lifestyle effects on fecundity.

## 8. Conclusion

Should we be concerned about the current situation with fertility rates far below population replacement levels in many Western countries? Probably. Not so much because of what we know, as what we do not know, e.g. (1) We do not know when the current decreasing trends in fertility rates will end; (2) Although we assume that the decreasing trends in fertility rates are due to social factors (and therefore reversible), we do not actually have good scientific evidence for this assumption; (3) We do not know why so many couples show up in fertility clinics due to poor semen quality of the male partner; and, (4) We lack information on the roles of modern lifestyle and food contaminants (including endocrine disrupters) on reproductive function in males as well as in females. It is, therefore, important that we, even though it is time consuming and costly, continue to monitor semen quality and begin to monitor fecundity, including trends in waiting time to pregnancy.

## Acknowledgements

This study was supported by the European Union (contract No QLK4-1999-01422/BMH4-CT96-0314), Danish Environmental Agency, Danish Research Council (Grant no. 9700883), Super post-doc from Danish MRC paid TKJs salary (Grant no. SV1736).

## References

[1] R.B. Kaufmann, et al., The decline in US teen prenancy rates, 1990–1995, Pediatrics 102 (1998) 1141–1147.
[2] D. Pearce, G. Cantisani, A. Laihonon, Changes in fertility and family sizes in Europe, Popul. Trends, (95) (1999 Spring) 33–40.
[3] W. Lutz, B.C. O'Neill, S. Scherbov, Demographics. Europe's population at a turning point, Science 299 (5615) (2003) 1991–1992.
[4] T.K. Jensen, et al., Poor semen quality may contribute to recent decline in fertility rates, Hum. Reprod. 17 (2002) 1437–1440.
[5] K.G. Nygren, A.N. Andersen, Assisted reproductive technology in Europe, 1999. Results generated from European registers by ESHRE. European Society of Human Reproduction and Embryology, Hum. Reprod. 17 (2002) 3260–3274.
[6] D.D. Baird, A.J. Wilcox, C.R. Weinberg, Use of time to pregnancy to study environmental exposures, Am. J. Epidemiol. 124 (1986) 470–480.
[7] M. Joffe, Asclepios projekt. Time to pregnancy: a measure of reproductive function in either sex, Occup. Environ. Med. 54 (1997) 289–294.
[8] P. Lazar, D. Hemon, C. Berger, Twinning rate and reporductive failures, in: W.E. Nance (Ed.), Twin Research: Biology and Epidemiology, Alan R. Liss, New York, 1977, pp. 125–132.
[9] B.C. Dunphy, L.M. Neal, I.D. Cooke, The clinical value of conventional semen analysis, Fertil. Steril. 51 (1989) 324–329.
[10] J.P. Bonde, et al., The relation between semen quality and fertility. A population based study of 430 first-pregnancy planners, Lancet 352 (1998) 1172–1177.
[11] E. Bostofte, J. Serup, H. Rebbe, Relation between sperm count and semen volume, and pregnancies obtained during a twenty-year follow-up period, Int. J. Androl. 5 (1982) 267–275.
[12] R. Slama, et al., Time to pregnancy and semen parameters: a cross-sectional study among fertile couples from four European cities, Hum. Reprod. 17 (2) (2002) 503–515.
[13] E. Carlsen, et al., Evidence for decreasing quality of semen during past 50 years, Br. Med. J. 305 (1992) 609–613.
[14] N.E. Skakkebaek, et al., Germ cell cancer and disorders of spermatogenesis: an environmental connection? (Review) (61 refs), APMIS 106 (1998) 3–11 (Discussion 12).
[15] M. Joffe, et al., Long-term recall of time-to-pregnancy, Fertil. Steril. 60 (1993) 99–104.
[16] G.A. Zielhuis, M.E.J.L. Hulscher, E.I.M. Florack, Validity and reliability of a questionnaire on fecundability, Int. J. Epidemiol. 21 (1992) 1151–1156.
[17] W.D. Mosher, Reproductive impairments in the United States, 1965–1982, Demography 22 (1985) 415–430.
[18] A. Templeton, C. Fraser, B. Thompson, The epidemiology of infertility in Aberdeen, Br. Med. J. 301 (1990) 148–152.
[19] M. Joffe, Time trends in biological fertility in Britain, Lancet 355 (2000) 1961–1965.
[20] O. Akre, et al., Human fertility does not decline: evidence from Sweden, Fertil. Steril. 71 (1999) 1066–1069.
[21] T.K. Jensen, et al., Selection bias in determining the age dependence of waiting time to pregnancy, Am. J. Epidemiol. 152 (6) (2000) 565–572.
[22] M. Joffe, Decreased fertility in Britain compared with Finland, Lancet 347 (1996) 1519–1522.
[23] S. Juul, W. Karmaus, J. Olsen, The European infertility and subfecundity study group. Regional differences in waiting time to pregnancy: pregnancy-based surveys from Denmark, France, Germany, Italy and Sweden, Fertil. Steril. 14 (1999) 1250–1254.
[24] W. Karmaus, S. Juul, European infertility and subfecundity group. Infertility and subfecundity in population-based samples from Denmark, Germany, Italy, Poland and Spain, Eur. J. Public Health 9 (1999) 229–235.
[25] T.K. Jensen, et al., Regional differences in waiting time to pregnancy among fertile couples from four European cities, Hum. Reprod. 16 (12) (2001) 2697–2704.
[26] J.P. Bonde, et al., A follow-up study of environmental and biologic determinants of fertility among 430 Danish first-pregnancy planners: design and methods, Reprod. Toxicol. 12 (1998) 19–27.

[27] P. Thonneau, et al., Incidence and main causes of infertility in a resident population (1 850 000) of three French regions (1988–1989), Hum. Reprod. 6 (1991) 811–816.
[28] T.K. Jensen, et al., Fecundability in relation to body mass and menstrual cycle patterns, Epidemiology 10 (1999) 422–428.
[29] D.D. Baird, A.J. Wilcox, Cigarette smoking associated with delayed conception, JAMA 253 (1985) 2979–2983.
[30] A. Wilcox, C.R. Weinberg, D.D. Baird, Caffeinated beverages and decreased fertility, Lancet ii (1988) 1453–1455.
[31] M. Joffe, Invited commentary: the potential for monitoring of fecundity and the remaining challenges, Am. J. Epidemiol. 157 (2) (2003) 89–93.
[32] C.R. Weinberg, D.D. Baird, A.J. Wilcox, Sources of bias in studies of time to pregnancy, Stat. Med. 13 (1994) 671–681.
[33] W.H. James, Recent secular trends in dizygotic twinning rates in Europe, J. Biosoc. Sci. 18 (4) (1986) 497–504.
[34] W.H. James, Secular trends in monitors of reproductive hazard, Hum. Reprod. 12 (3) (1997) 417–421.
[35] F. Parazzini, et al., Trends in multiple births in Italy: 1955–1983, Br. J. Obstet. Gynaecol. 98 (6) (1991) 535–539.
[36] J.F. Orlebeke, et al., Changes in the DZ unlike/like sex ratio in The Netherlands, Acta Genet. Med. Gemellol. (Roma.) 40 (3–4) (1991) 319–323.
[37] M. Murphy, K. Hey, Twinning rates, Lancet 349 (9062) (1997) 1398–1399.
[38] J.D. Doherty, P.A. Lancaster, The secular trend of twinning in Australia, 1853–1982, Acta Genet. Med. Gemellol. (Roma.) 35 (1–2) (1986) 61–76.
[39] Y. Imaizumi, Twinning rates in Japan, 1951–1990, Acta Genet. Med. Gemellol. (Roma.) 41 (2–3) (1992) 165–175.
[40] S. Tong, D. Caddy, R.V. Short, Use of dizygotic to monozygotic twinning ratio as a measure of fertility, Lancet 349 (9055) (1997) 843–845.
[41] P. Rachootin, J. Olsen, Secular changes in the twinning rate in Denmark, Scand. J. Soc. Med. 8 (1980) 89–94.
[42] Y. Imaizumi, A comparative study of twinning and triplet rates in 17 countries, 1972–1996, Acta Genet. Med. Gemellol. 47 (1998) 101–114.
[43] S. Tong, R.V. Short, Dizygotic twinning as a measure of human fertility, Hum. Reprod. 13 (1) (1998) 95–98.
[44] N. Jørgensen, et al., Semen analysis performed by different laboratory teams: an intervariation study, Int. J. Androl. 20 (1997) 201–208.
[45] S.H. Swan, E.P. Elkin, L. Fenster, Have sperm densities declined? A reanalyses of global trend data, Environ. Health Perspect. 105 (1997) 1228–1232.
[46] P. Jouannet, et al., Semen quality and male reproductive health: the controversy about human sperm concentration decline, APMIS 109 (2001) 333–344.
[47] J. de Mouzon, et al., Declining sperm count. Semen quality has declined among men born in France since 1950, Br. Med. J. 313 (7048) (1996) 43–45.
[48] F. Menchini-Fabris, et al., Declining sperm counts in Italy during the past 20 years, Andrologia 28 (6) (1996) 304.
[49] E.V. Younglai, J.A. Collins, W.G. Foster, Canadian semen quality: an analysis of sperm density among eleven academic fertility centers, Fertil. Steril. 70 (1) (1998) 76–80.
[50] I. Tortolero, et al., Semen analysis in men from Merida, Venezuela, over a 15-year period, Arch. Androl. 42 (1) (1999) 29–34.
[51] M. Almagor, et al., Changes in semen quality in Jerusalem between 1990 and 2000: a cross-sectional and longitudinal study, Arch. Androl. 49 (2) (2003) 139–144.
[52] J. Auger, et al., Decline in semen quality among fertile men in Paris during the past 20 years, N. Engl. J. Med. 332 (1995) 281–285.
[53] L. Bujan, et al., Time series analysis of sperm concentration in fertile men in Toulouse, France between 1977 and 1992, Br. Med. J. 312 (1996) 471–472.
[54] E. Vicari, et al., Sperm characteristics in fertile men and healthy men of the south–east Sicily from year 1982 to 1999, Arch. Ital. Urol. Androl. 75 (1) (2003) 28–34.

[55] D.J. Handelsman, Sperm output of healthy men in Australia: magnitude of bias due to self-selected volunteers, Hum. Reprod. 12 (12) (1997) 2701–2705.
[56] K. Van Waeleghem, et al., Deterioration of sperm quality in young healthy Belgian men, Hum. Reprod. 11 (1996) 325–329.
[57] J. Gyllenborg, et al., Secular and seasonal changes in semen quality among young Danish men: a statistical analysis of semen samples from 1927 donor candidates during 1977–1995, Int. J. Androl. 22 (1) (1999) 28–36.
[58] M.F. Costello, et al., No decline in semen quality among potential sperm donors in Sydney, Australia, between 1983 and 2001, J. Assist. Reprod. Genet. 19 (6) (2002) 284–290.
[59] P. Jouannet, et al., Study of a group of 484 fertile men: Part I. Distribution of semen characteristics, Int. J. Androl. 4 (4) (1981) 440–449.
[60] S. Irvine, et al., Evidence of deteriorating semen quality in the United Kingdom: birth cohort study in 577 men in Scotland over 11 years, Br. Med. J. 312 (1996) 467–471.
[61] P. Bilotta, R. Guglielmo, M. Steffe, Analysis of decline in seminal fluid in the Italian population during the past 15 years, Minerva Ginecol. 51 (6) (1999) 223–231.
[62] C.A. Paulsen, N.G. Berman, C. Wang, Data from men in greater Seattle area reveals no downward trend in semen quality: futher evidence that deterioration of semen quality is not geographically uniform, Fertil. Steril. 65 (1996) 1015–1020.
[63] A. Benshushan, et al., Is there really a decrease in sperm parameters among healthy young men? A survey of sperm donations during 15 years, J. Assist. Reprod. Genet. 14 (6) (1997) 347–353.
[64] H. Fisch, et al., Semen analyses in 1,283 men from the United States over a 25-year period: no decline in quality, Fertil. Steril. 65 (1996) 1009–1014.
[65] N. Jorgensen, et al., Regional differences in semen quality in Europe, Hum. Reprod. 16 (5) (2001) 1012–1019.
[66] S.H. Swan, et al., Geographic differences in semen quality of fertile U S. males, Environ. Health Perspect. 111 (4) (2003) 414–420.
[67] N. Jorgensen, et al., East–West gradient in semen quality in the Nordic-Baltic area: a study of men from the general population in Denmark, Norway, Estonia and Finland, Hum. Reprod. 17 (8) (2002) 2199–2208.
[68] H.-O. Adami, et al., Testicular cancer in nine Northern European countries, Int. J. Cancer 59 (1994) 33–38.
[69] A.G. Andersen, et al., High frequency of sub-optimal semen quality in an unselected population of young men, Hum. Reprod. 15 (2000) 366–372.
[70] J.P. Bonde, et al., Year of birth and sperm count in 10 Danish occupational studies, Scand. J. Work Environ. & Health 24 (1998) 407–413.
[71] Frederiksberg Kommunes Sundhedsafdeling. Young 1999, a sexual profile (In Danish). Frederiksberg, Copenhagen: Forebyggelsessekretariatet; 1999.
[72] R. Bergström, et al., Increase in testicular cancer incidence in six European countries: a birth cohort phenomenon, J. Natl. Cancer Inst. 88 (1996) 727–733.
[73] H. Moeller, N.E. Skakkebaek, Risk of testicular cancer in subfertile men: case control study, Br. Med. J. 318 (1999) 559–562.
[74] M.B. Jackson, John Radcliffe Hospital Cryptorchidism Research Group, The epidemiology of cryptorchidism, Horm. Res. 30 (1988) 153–156.
[75] H. Dolk, Rise in prevalence of hypospadias, Lancet 351 (1998) 770.
[76] R.M. Sharpe, N.E. Skakkebæk, Are oestrogens involved in falling sperm counts and disorders of the male reproductive tract? Lancet 341 (1993) 1392–1395.
[77] W.R. Kelce, et al., Persistent DDT metabolite, p,p'DDE is a potent androgen receptor antagonist, Nature 375 (1995) 581–585.
[78] N. Santoro, Mechanisms of premature ovarian failure, Ann. Endocrinol. 64 (2003) 87–92.
[79] J.L. Luborsky, et al., Premature menopause in a multiethnic population study of the menopause transistion, Hum. Reprod. 18 (2003) 199–206.
[80] K. Lakhani, et al., Polycyctic ovaries, Brit. J. Radiol. 75 (2002) 9–16.
[81] E. Kousta, et al., The prevalence of polycyctic ovaries in women with infertility, Hum. Reprod. 14 (1999) 2720–2723.

[82] W.C. Robinson, Regional variation in the age-specific natural fertility curve, J. Biosoc. Sci. 19 (1987) 57–64.
[83] G.P. Mineau, J. Trussell, A specification of marital fertility by parents' age, age at marriage and marital duration, Demography 19 (1982) 335–350.
[84] U. Larsen, J.W. Vaupel, Hutterite fecundability by age and parity: strategies for frailty modeling of event histories, Demography 30 (1993) 81–102.
[85] B.M. van Noord-Zaadstra, et al., Delaying childbearing: effect of age on fecundity and outcome of pregnancy, Br. Med. J. 302 (1991) 1361–1365.
[86] S. Friedmann, Artificial donor insemination with frozen human semen, Fertil. Steril. 28 (1977) 1230–1233.
[87] G. Howe, et al., Effects of age, cigarette smoking, and other factors on fertility: findings in a large prospective study, Br. Med. J. 290 (1985) 1697–1700.
[88] Fedération CECOS, D. Schwartz, M.J. Mayaux, Female fecundity as a function of age, N. Engl. J. Med. 306 (1982) 404–406.
[89] J. Olsen, Subfecundity according to the age of the mother and the father, Dan. Med. Bull. 37 (1990) 281–282.
[90] A.H. Mokdad, et al., The continuing epidemics of obesity and diabetes in the United States, JAMA. J. Am. Med. Assoc. 286 (10) (2001) 1195–1200.
[91] C. Augood, K. Duckitt, A.A. Templeton, Smoking and female infertility: a systematic review and meta-analysis, Hum. Reprod. 13 (1998) 1532–1539.
[92] M.F. Vine, et al., Cigarette smoking and sperm density: a meta-analysis, Fertil. Steril. 61 (1994) 35–43.
[93] T.K. Jensen, et al., Adult and prenatal exposure to tobacco smoke as risk indicators of fertility among 430 Danish couples, Am. J. Epidemiol. 148 (1998) 992–997.
[94] C.R. Weinberg, A.J. Wilcox, D.D. Baird, Reduced fecundability in women with prenatal exposure to cigarette smoking, Am. J. Epidemiol. 129 (1989) 1072–1078.
[95] D.D. Baird, A.J. Wilcox, Future fertility after prenatal exposure to cigarette smoke, Fertil. Steril. 46 (1986) 368–372.
[96] T.K. Jensen, et al., Association of in utero exposure to maternal smoking with reduced semen quality and testis size in adulthood: A cross-sectional study of 1,770 young men from the general population in five European countries, Am. J. Epidemiol. 159 (2004) 49–58.
[97] L. Storgaard, et al., Does smoking during pregnancy affect sons sperm counts? Epidemiology 14 (2003) 278–286.
[98] B.M. Zaadstra, et al., Fat and female fecundity: prospective study of effect of body fat distribution on conception rates, Br. Med. J. 306 (1993) 484–487.

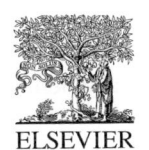

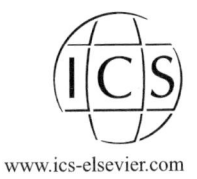

# Human embryonic stem cells—potential applications for regenerative medicine

Benjamin Reubinoff*

*Department of Obstetrics and Gynecology and the Goldyn Savad Institute of Gene Therapy, The Hadassah Embryonic Stem Cell Research Center, Hadassah University Hospital, Jerusalem 91120, Israel*

**Abstract.** Human embryonic stem (hES) cells attract profound scientific and public attention due to their far-reaching potential applications in regenerative medicine. Given the capability of hES cells to proliferate extensively in culture and their pluripotent potential, hES cells may serve as a renewable unlimited source of cells for transplantation therapy. In addition, genetically manipulated, transplanted hES cells may serve as vectors that carry and express genes in target organs in the course of gene therapy. While hES cells show great promise, bulk cultures of standardized cells suitable for clinical trials should be developed, and additional research is required to control the growth and differentiation of the cells and to overcome the risk of tumor formation and graft rejection. The recent development of humanized, feeder-free culture systems, methods to genetically modify the cells, and strategies to derive highly enriched populations of differentiated cells of a specific type are encouraging. It is anticipated that these achievements will set the stage for further developments that may eventually allow the exploitation of the great potential of hES cells for cell and gene therapy. © 2004 Published by Elsevier B.V.

*Keywords:* Human embryonic stem cells; Transplantation

## 1. Introduction

The derivation of embryonic stem (ES) cell lines from human blastocysts [1,2] establishes a new avenue for the treatment of human diseases. Given the self-renewal potential of human ES (hES) cells, combined with their capability to differentiate into any cell type, these cells can potentially provide an unlimited source of cells for transplantation therapy. Transplanted hES cell-derived progeny may restore tissue function in a wide range of human diseases, which are associated with loss of cells or cellular dysfunction. In addition, hES cells may serve as an unlimited donor source of various types of cells in the construction of tissues by tissue engineering. Lastly, hES cells may be also invaluable for gene therapy, as genetically modified transplanted cells may transmit and express specific genes in target organs.

---

* Tel.: +972-51-874659; fax: +972-2-6430982.
 *E-mail address:* reubinof@md2.huji.ac.il (B. Reubinoff).

0531-5131/ © 2004 Published by Elsevier B.V.
doi:10.1016/j.ics.2004.02.002

While the promise of hES cells for regenerative medicine is tremendous, additional developments are required to exploit their potential clinical value. Limitations of currently used culture systems should be overcome, and standardized pathogen-free cells that will be suitable for clinical trials should be developed. Pure cultures of differentiated functional cells of a specific type are required for transplantation, and issues such as the possible induction of immune rejection by transplanted hES cells should be addressed. Potential hazards, such as the formation of teratoma tumors, or differentiated cells from a nondesired lineage should be vigorously evaluated. Here, we will review the reported progress in resolving some of these issues and discuss the obstacles that need to be further addressed to allow hES cell therapy.

## 2. Human ES cells eligible for clinical use

The existing hES cell lines are not ideal for clinical use. The majority of the cell lines reported worldwide to date were derived from mouse fibroblast feeder layers. The direct contact with the mouse feeders renders these lines xenotransplantation products. In addition, the screening of embryo donors and reagents was not compliant with the requirements of regulatory authorities, and the cells have been exposed to materials derived from animal species.

Extensive testing for human adventitious agents and animal-derived pathogens may be attempted to overcome these limitations and to obtain regulatory approval to use existing cell lines for human transplantation.

An alternative approach would be to derive new hES cell lines using a nonanimal culture system fully compliant with regulations for the production of therapeutic products. It has been demonstrated that the use of mouse feeders may be replaced by propagation of the hES cells on extracellular matrices in the presence of a mouse embryonic, fibroblast-conditioned medium [3]. While this system avoids direct contact between mouse feeders and hES cells, the risk of cross-transfer of animal pathogens from the animal-conditioned medium to the hES cells is not avoided. The capability of human feeders, combined with animal-free reagents to support the derivation and propagation of hES cell lines, was demonstrated [4,5]. Furthermore, as shown in a recent publication, a combination of growth factors and matrices could replace the need for feeders [6]. In conclusion, it appears that current technology allows the development of hES cells eligible for clinical use. The development of these cells is required to exploit the remarkable therapeutic potential of hES cells.

## 3. Bulk cultures of undifferentiated, standardized hES cells

The culture systems that are currently used to propagate hES cells have limitations. The cultures most commonly have some level of background differentiation. While the cytokine leukemia inhibitory factor (LIF) can replace the requirement of a feeder layer and support the derivation and propagation of mouse ES cell lines [7], it cannot support undifferentiated proliferation of hES cells in the absence of feeders [1,2]. Although the combination of LIF, basic fibroblast growth factor, and transforming growth factor β1 can support undifferentiated proliferation of hES cells on fibronectin [6], very little is known about the regulatory pathways that govern the undifferentiated proliferation of hES cells, and uncovering these pathways is a major challenge for the future. Manipulation of these pathways may improve the growth of hES cells in the absence of feeders and may facilitate the growth of pure bulk cultures of undifferentiated cells. Standardized, pure populations of undifferentiated hES cells on a large scale are needed as a platform for the development of more specialized, differentiated cells for transplantation.

## 4. Purified preparations of differentiated cells from ES cells

Human ES cells spontaneously differentiate into a variety of somatic cells representing all three embryonic germ layers when cultured for prolonged periods without replenishment of feeders, or when they are cultured in suspension within aggregates, termed embryoid bodies (EBs) [1,2,8]. However, a mixture of differentiated cells of multiple types is generated following spontaneous differentiation, while pure populations of differentiated cells of one type are required for transplantation therapy.

To establish pure preparations of differentiated progeny of a specific cell type, further study of the regulatory pathways that govern the differentiation of hES cells is required. The potential of growth and differentiation-inducing factors to direct the differentiation of hES cells towards specific cell types has been demonstrated [9–11]. However, while these results are encouraging, growth factors most commonly could enhance the differentiation toward specific lineages but could not direct differentiation exclusively to one cell type [9].

Differentiation towards a specific lineage may be enhanced by coculture with various cell types. For example, bone marrow-derived stromal cells can induce hematopoietic differentiation of hES cells [12], and visceral–endoderm-like cells enhance their differentiation into cardiomyocytes [13]. However, the major drawback of coculture systems is that they do not direct differentiation exclusively into one cell type. In addition, coculture systems raise complex regulatory compliance issues, in particular when cells from an animal source are used.

An alternative approach to generate pure or highly enriched populations of differentiated cells could rely on the selection of specific cells from a mixed population of differentiated cells. Selection may be based on morphology [14], biophysical properties, such as density [15], and on the expression of lineage-specific cell surface markers [16,17]. Alternatively, lineage-specific promoter constructs driving selectable markers may be used for genetic selection [18]. Selective culture conditions favouring growth, adhesion, and differentiation into cells of a desired lineage and repressing other cell types is an additional approach. Lastly, differentiation into a specific cell type may be enhanced by forced expression of key transcription factors in the developmental pathway of a desired lineage [19,20].

Given the current limitations in directing the differentiation of hES cells into one cell type by exogenous signals, it appears that combining the various strategies detailed above may prove most effective for the establishment of pure or highly enriched cultures of differentiated cells.

Indeed, highly enriched (>90%) cultures of neural progenitors (NPs) were successfully developed from hES cells by methods that combined the various approaches. Spontaneous differentiation was initially induced by the formation of EBs or high-density cultures. This step was followed by the combination of NP-selection and culture under selective conditions that are known to promote the proliferation of NPs [14,16,21]. Human ES cell-derived NPs can differentiate in culture to various types of mature neurons [14,16,21], which can respond to neurotransmitters and fire action potentials [16]. They also give rise to astrocytes and, occasionally, also into oligodendroglia progenitors [14,16,21]. Following transplantation into the neonatal mouse brain ventricles, the NPs participate in host brain development [14,21].

Various protocols for the development of enriched cultures of other cell types were also reported. Percoll gradient separation was used to enrich (70%) EB-derived differentiated cells for cardiomyocytes [15]. Treatment with DMSO, followed by sodium butyrate, induces differentiation into cultures enriched for hepatocyte-like cells [10]. Lastly, cultures enriched for (78%) putative endothelial cells were isolated from EB-derived, differentiated hES cells by immunosorting of PCAM1-expressing cells. The sorted PCAM1+ cells displayed characteristics of vessel endothelial cells in vitro, formed tube-like structures when cultured on Matrigel, and created microvessels following transplantation into SCID mice [17].

These results are encouraging because they demonstrate that enriched cultures of both committed progenitors and differentiated cells may be obtained from hES cells in vitro. However, it should be noted that the cultures that are developed following these approaches are, at best, highly enriched and are not pure. Further purification may be required to allow the use of such differentiated cell preparations for therapeutic applications. Moreover, additional studies are required to demonstrate that the differentiated cells that are derived in vitro are functional and have properties similar to those of their in vivo counterparts.

## 5. Embryonic stem cell-derived functional graft

The function of grafts following transplantation of hES cell-derived progeny has not been reported as yet. However, stable functional grafts have been obtained following the transplantation of mouse ES cell-derived, differentiated progeny from various lineages.

The curative potential of mouse ES cell-derived neural progeny was demonstrated after transplantation into animal models of neural diseases. Early studies demonstrated that mouse ES cells can differentiate into oligodendrocytes capable of remyelinating axons in host brain and spinal cord [22–24]. Mild neurological improvement was demonstrated after transplantation of ES cell-derived neural progeny to the injured rat spine [23]. These observations lay the foundation for the hope that human axonal remyelination by hES cell-derived oligodendrocytes will be feasible, offering a new avenue to treat neurological disabilities associated with spinal cord injuries, MS, and other demyelination disorders.

Transplantation of a low dose of undifferentiated mouse ES cells into the midbrain of Parkinsonian rats resulted in a gradual and sustained neurological improvement. However, transplantation of undifferentiated ES cells was associated with the formation of teratoma tumors [25]. Engraftment of ES cell-derived, differentiated neural progeny committed to a midbrain fate resulted in significant functional improvement in animal models of Parkinson's disease [19,26]. Teratoma tumor formation was not observed [19]. The grafted cells were found to have electrophysiological properties similar to those of midbrain DA neurons [19].

The potential of ES cell-derived, hematopoietic precursors to restore hematopoiesis after transplantation to irradiated mice has been demonstrated [27,28]. In addition, insulin-producing cells have been recently derived from ES cells. After transplantation to animal models of diabetes, the cells integrated and could secrete insulin. However, circulating insulin levels were elevated to subnormal levels, and the correction of the diabetic state was either partial and/or short term [18,20,29,30].

Given these encouraging results in the mouse ES cell system, it appears that it will also be possible to establish functional grafts from hES cells. Nevertheless, extensive research is still required to adapt methods from the mouse to the hES cell system, and/or to develop novel efficient methods to direct the differentiation of hES cells towards functional progeny. Other issues that need to be addressed include: the best mode of cell delivery, the stage of development in which the cells should be at the time of transplantation, the optimal number of cells that should be engrafted, and the means to assure their survival in light of possible immune rejection.

## 6. Strategies to overcome potential immune rejection

It is possible that transplantation of hES cells will activate an immune rejection response. However, at present, the immunogenicity of hES cells and its correlation with differentiation is unclear. A single study has recently demonstrated very low expression levels of MHC class I proteins that increased to moderate levels following in vitro or in vivo differentiation of hES cells. MHC class II antigens were not expressed by undifferentiated or differentiated cells [31]. Therefore, in contrast to transplanted solid organs, which harbor MHC class II-expressing APCs, homogenous, nonimmune cell populations differentiated from ES cells are expected not to express MHC class II antigens, and, as a result, may provoke host rejection to a lesser degree [32]. Further research is required to characterize the cellular and humeral immune response to engrafted hES cells.

In the case that transplanted hES cells will induce an immunologic rejection response in the recipient, a few strategies other than immunosuppressive therapy have been suggested. One approach may be to increase HLA matching between the transplanted hES cells and the recipients by the establishment of banks with a large number of hES cell lines with a variety of MHC phenotypes.

A potential alternative strategy may be the establishment of a "universal" donor ES cell line by "knocking out" [33] the expression of MHC genes [32,34]. Such a cell line will not induce rejection or will induce just minor immune responses. It should be noted that this approach would not prevent non-MHC-mediated rejection. Genetic modification of hES cells could also be used to suppress the host immune response by the repression or induction of expression of genes encoding for immune-regulating molecules [32,34]. At this stage, the effectiveness of these approaches has never been experimentally proven.

An alternative approach to overcoming possible rejection may be the induction of specific lifelong transplantation tolerance. It has been shown in animal models that engraftment of allogeneic hematopoietic progenitors may induce lifelong hematolymphoid chimerism and immune tolerance to other grafts from the same donor [35]. There are also indications in humans that this approach may be effective. Typically, the reported cases involved a kidney transplanted due to renal failure, complicating the transplantation of allogeneic hematopoietic progenitors [36]. This approach may be implemented with hES cells by transplanting hES cell-derived, hematopietic stem cells and creating lifelong hematolymphoid chimerism in the recipient and tolerance to engrafted, differentiated cells from the same parental hES cell line.

Lastly, potential graft rejection may be prevented by the approach of therapeutic cloning, where human ES cells are derived from an embryo that was cloned from the patient's own tissues and are then used for autologus transplantation [37]. The feasibility of therapeutic cloning has been demonstrated in the mouse model [38]. Pluripotent ES cell lines have been successfully derived from cloned embryos [38]. Their capability to give rise to mature, functioning dopaminergic neurons was demonstrated both in vitro and in vivo. After transplantation, they corrected behavioral deficits in Parkinsonian mice [26]. A complete demonstration of the concept of therapeutic cloning, in combination with gene therapy, was recently reported [28]. Cloned embryos were developed from nuclei donated by an immune-deficient mouse strain. ES cells were derived from these cloned embryos and, following the repair of the genetic defect, were directed to differentiate into hematopoietic progenitors that successfully reconstituted a healthy hematopietic system following autologous transplantation. Immune rejection of the graft or graft-versus-host reaction were not observed. While the origin of mitochondrial DNA of cloned embryos is the enucleated oocyte, it appears from this and other studies [39] that autologous, engrafted cells containing foreign mitochondrial DNA will not be rejected by the host.

The process of "therapeutic cloning" should be clearly distinguished from "reproductive cloning," where a cloned duplicate organism of the nucleus donor is created. Reproductive cloning is inefficient and is associated with a high rate of gestational or neonatal developmental failures and numerous offspring abnormalities [37,40]. These adverse outcomes are probably related to epigenetic errors during the rapid nuclear reprogramming of the donor nucleus [37,41,42]. At present, reproductive cloning is considered unsafe and is also morally unaccepted by most people [41].

The poor outcome of reproductive cloning raises concerns whether similar reprogramming-related adverse outcomes will also occur in ES cells originating from cloned embryos. It appears that the derivation of ES cells from cloned embryos is more efficient than the generation of cloned offspring [37]. This may be related to the nature of the process of derivation of ES cells, which possibly allows for the selection only of normally reprogrammed cells [37]. Further studies are required to evaluate possible deleterious epigenetic abnormalities within ES cells that will be generated from reprogrammed adult somatic cells.

There are additional substantial limitations to the performance of therapeutic cloning. Somatic cell nuclear transfer is costly, technically complex, and its yield is not high. It is questionable whether it will be practical to generate a specific cell line per patient. In addition, restricted oocyte availability may limit the widespread use of therapeutic cloning. Recently, the potential of mouse ES cells to differentiate into oocyte-like cells was reported [43]. The ES cell-derived, oogonia-like cells could complete meiosis and generate embryo-like structures following parthenogeneic activation [43]. Although these cells are not completely identical to gonadal oocytes, their cytoplasm might have the same potential to induce reprogramming of somatic nuclei. Given the unlimited proliferation capacity of ES cells, these oocyte-like cells may potentially serve as large-scale alternatives to gonadal oocytes for therapeutic cloning. It still remains to be seen whether it will be possible to derive these oocyte-like cells from hES cells and whether they will indeed support reprogramming.

## 7. Potential complications of hES cell transplantation

The major hazards of hES cell transplantation therapy are the potential formation of teratoma tumors or the development of tissues other than the desired one. When undifferentiated ES cells are transplanted, they give rise to teratoma tumors [1,2]. These tumors may develop if the transplanted preparation of ES cell-derived, differentiated progeny will include relatively undifferentiated cells [25]. In principle, transplanting pure populations of fully committed cells from the desired lineage may prevent both the formation of teratoma tumors and nondesired tissues.

Additional safety measures may be used to protect recipients of hES cells from potential tumor formation. These may include the transplantation of genetically modified ES cell lines in which the expression of the transgene will destroy all undifferentiated cells. An alternative approach may be to modify the ES cells so that they will be amenable to destruction upon the administration of a specific drug. The feasibility of this approach was recently demonstrated with genetically modified hES cells [44].

There is limited data regarding the safety of transplanting hES cell-derived progeny. Two recent publications reported the transplantation of hES cell-derived, highly enriched cultures of neural progenitors into the brain ventricles of newborn mice [14,21]. Teratoma formation, or the formation of nonneural tissues, was not observed in the recipient animals [14,21]. Yet, intraventricular clusters composed of mature and immature neuroepithelial cells were reported in one of these publications [14]. Long-term studies are required to determine the safety of hES cell-derived progeny transplantation and to rule out potential hazards such as tumor formation or the development of cells from other lineages.

## 8. Conclusions

The recent development of hES cell lines establishes a new avenue for the potential treatment of diseases. Human ES cells may serve as an unlimited source of cells for transplantation and gene therapy. Current data indicates that hES cells may be cultured without the support of feeders, may be genetically modified, and that highly enriched cultures of lineage-specific progenitors may be derived from them. Furthermore, studies in the mouse model demonstrate the potential of transplanted, genetically modified ES cells to generate functional grafts and to correct genetic defects. ES cells offer novel approaches, such as therapeutic cloning, to overcome potential immune rejection after transplantation. These results set the stage for further developments that may eventually allow the exploitation of hES cells for transplantation and gene therapy. Nevertheless, new cell lines eligible for clinical use, improved control of the growth and differentiation of hES cells, analysis of their therapeutic effect in animal models of disease, and rigorous evaluation of safety are all required to allow the utilization of hES cells for cell and gene therapy.

## References

[1] J.A. Thomson, et al., Embryonic stem cell lines derived from human blastocysts, Science 282 (1998) 1145–1147.
[2] B.E. Reubinoff, et al., Embryonic stem cell lines from human blastocysts: somatic differentiation in vitro, Nat. Biotechnol. 18 (2000) 399–404.
[3] C. Xu, et al., Feeder-free growth of undifferentiated human embryonic stem cells, Nat. Biotechnol. 19 (2001) 971–974.
[4] M. Richards, et al., Human feeders support prolonged undifferentiated growth of human inner cell masses and embryonic stem cells, Nat. Biotechnol. 20 (2002) 933–936.
[5] M. Amit, et al., Human feeder layers for human embryonic stem cells, Biol. Reprod. 68 (2003) 2150–2156.

[6] M. Amit, et al., Feeder and serum-free culture of human embryonic stem cells, Biol. Reprod. (2003).
[7] J. Nichols, E.P. Evans, A.G. Smith, Establishment of germ-line-competent embryonic stem (ES) cells using differentiation inhibiting activity, Development 110 (1990) 1341–1348.
[8] J. Itskovitz-Eldor, et al., Differentiation of human embryonic stem cells into embryoid bodies compromising the three embryonic germ layers, Mol. Med. 6 (2000) 88–95.
[9] M. Schuldiner, et al., From the cover: effects of eight growth factors on the differentiation of cells derived from human embryonic stem cells, PNAS 97 (2000) 11307–11312.
[10] L. Rambhatla, et al., Generation of hepatocyte-like cells from human embryonic stem cells, Cell Transplant 12 (2003) 1–11.
[11] R.H. Xu, et al., BMP4 initiates human embryonic stem cell differentiation to trophoblast, Nat. Biotechnol. 20 (2002) 1261–1264.
[12] D.S. Kaufman, et al., Hematopoietic colony-forming cells derived from human embryonic stem cells, Proc. Natl. Acad. Sci. U. S. A. 98 (2001) 10716–10721.
[13] C. Mummery, et al., Differentiation of human embryonic stem cells to cardiomyocytes: role of coculture with visceral endoderm-like cells, Circulation 107 (2003) 2733–2740.
[14] B.E. Reubinoff, et al., Neural progenitors from human embryonic stem cells, Nat. Biotechnol. 19 (2001) 1134–1140.
[15] C. Xu, et al., Characterization and enrichment of cardiomyocytes derived from human embryonic stem cells, Circ. Res. 91 (2002) 501–508.
[16] M.K. Carpenter, et al., Enrichment of neurons and neural precursors from human embryonic stem cells, Exp. Neurol. 172 (2001) 383–397.
[17] S. Levenberg, et al., Endothelial cells derived from human embryonic stem cells, Proc. Natl. Acad. Sci. U. S. A. 99 (2002) 4391–4396.
[18] B. Soria, et al., Insulin-secreting cells derived from embryonic stem cells normalize glycemia in streptozotocin-induced diabetic mice, Diabetes 49 (2000) 157–162.
[19] J.H. Kim, et al., Dopamine neurons derived from embryonic stem cells function in an animal model of Parkinson's disease, Nature 418 (2002) 50–56.
[20] P. Blyszczuk, et al., Expression of Pax4 in embryonic stem cells promotes differentiation of nestin-positive progenitor and insulin-producing cells, Proc. Natl. Acad. Sci. U. S. A. 100 (2003) 998–1003.
[21] S.C. Zhang, et al., In vitro differentiation of transplantable neural precursors from human embryonic stem cells, Nat. Biotechnol. 19 (2001) 1129–1133.
[22] O. Brustle, et al., Embryonic stem cell-derived glial precursors: a source of myelinating transplants, Science 285 (1999) 754–756.
[23] J.W. McDonald, et al., Transplanted embryonic stem cells survive, differentiate and promote recovery in injured rat spinal cord, Nat. Med. 5 (1999) 1410–1412.
[24] S. Liu, et al., Embryonic stem cells differentiate into oligodendrocytes and myelinate in culture and after spinal cord transplantation, PNAS 97 (2000) 6126–6131.
[25] L.M. Bjorklund, et al., From the cover: embryonic stem cells develop into functional dopaminergic neurons after transplantation in a Parkinson rat model, PNAS 99 (2002) 2344–2349.
[26] T. Barberi, et al., Neural subtype specification of fertilization and nuclear transfer embryonic stem cells and application in Parkinsonian mice, Nat. Biotechnol. 21 (2003) 1200–1207.
[27] M. Kyba, R.C. Perlingeiro, G.Q. Daley, HoxB4 confers definitive lymphoid–myeloid engraftment potential on embryonic stem cell and yolk sac hematopoietic progenitors, Cell 109 (2002) 29–37.
[28] W.M. Rideout III, et al., Correction of a genetic defect by nuclear transplantation and combined cell and gene therapy, Cell 109 (2002) 17–27.
[29] Y. Hori, et al., Growth inhibitors promote differentiation of insulin-producing tissue from embryonic stem cells, Proc. Natl. Acad. Sci. U. S. A. 99 (2002) 16105–16110.
[30] N. Lumelsky, et al., Differentiation of embryonic stem cells to insulin-secreting structures similar to pancreatic islets, Science 292 (2001) 1389–1394.
[31] M. Drukker, et al., Characterization of the expression of MHC proteins in human embryonic stem cells, Proc. Natl. Acad. Sci. U. S. A. 99 (2002) 9864–9869.
[32] J.S. Odorico, D.S. Kaufman, J.A. Thomson, Multilineage differentiation from human embryonic stem cell lines, Stem Cells 19 (2001) 193–204.

[33] T.P. Zwaka, J.A. Thomson, Homologous recombination in human embryonic stem cells, Nat. Biotechnol. 21 (2003) 319–321.
[34] D.S. Kaufman, J.A. Thomson, Human ES cells—haematopoiesis and transplantation strategies, J. Anat. 200 (2002) 243–248.
[35] I.L. Weissman, Translating stem and progenitor cell biology to the clinic: barriers and opportunities, Science 287 (2000) 1442–1446.
[36] T.R. Spitzer, et al., Combined histocompatibility leukocyte antigen-matched donor bone marrow and renal transplantation for multiple myeloma with end stage renal disease: the induction of allograft tolerance through mixed lymphohematopoietic chimerism, Transplantation 68 (1999) 480–484.
[37] K. Hochedlinger, R. Jaenisch, Nuclear transplantation, embryonic stem cells, and the potential for cell therapy, N. Engl. J. Med. 349 (2003) 275–286.
[38] T. Wakayama, et al., Differentiation of embryonic stem cell lines generated from adult somatic cells by nuclear transfer, Science 292 (2001) 740–743.
[39] R.P. Lanza, et al., Generation of histocompatible tissues using nuclear transplantation, Nat. Biotechnol. 20 (2002) 689–696.
[40] K. Eggan, et al., Hybrid vigor, fetal overgrowth, and viability of mice derived by nuclear cloning and tetraploid embryo complementation, Proc. Natl. Acad. Sci. U. S. A. 98 (2001) 6209–6214.
[41] R. Jaenisch, I. Wilmut, Developmental biology. Don't clone humans! Science 291 (2001) 2552.
[42] W.M. Rideout III, K. Eggan, R. Jaenisch, Nuclear cloning and epigenetic reprogramming of the genome, Science 293 (2001) 1093–1098.
[43] K. Hubner, et al., Derivation of oocytes from mouse embryonic stem cells, Science 300 (2003) 1251–1256.
[44] M. Schuldiner, J. Itskovitz-Eldor, N. Benvenisty, Selective ablation of human embryonic stem cells expressing a "suicide" gene, Stem Cells 21 (2003) 257–265.

# Trilogy

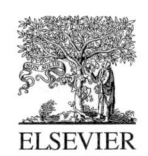

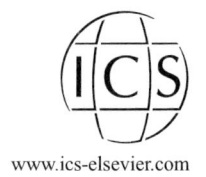

# Evidence-based infertility: evaluation of the female partner

John A. Collins*

*Department of Obstetrics and Gynaecology, McMaster University, Hamilton, Canada*
*Department of Obstetrics and Gynaecology, Dalhousie University, Halifax, Canada*

**Abstract.** Infertility, involving at least 1 year of attempted conception without success, affects 10,000 couples per million populations. Evaluation of a couple is generally indicated after a year, by which time most normal couples attempting conception would have been successful. The principles of evidence-based medicine indicate that the diagnostic tests should correlate with the outcome of interest to couples, that is live birth. In the female partner, these tests are assessment of ovulation by cycle history or mid-luteal progesterone and of tubal pathology by *Chlamydia* antibody testing, tubal patency tests or laparoscopy. The chief female categories of infertility are ovulation disorders (25%), tubal disease (15%) and endometriosis (10%). Male infertility is the primary diagnosis in approximately 25% of cases and contributes to a further 15% to 25% of the remaining cases. The infertility remains unexplained in at least 20% of cases because numerous reproductive defects are undetectable with current methods. Undetectable deficiencies in oocyte or sperm quality and tubal function may contribute to fertilization failure and diminished embryo quality. Even high quality embryos may undergo implantation failure by means that are poorly understood. Research is needed to improve awareness of potential fertility defects before and after fertilization and possible errors in embryonic development. © 2004 Published by Elsevier B.V.

*Keywords:* Infertility; Anovulation; Tubal disease; Endometriosis; Unexplained infertility

## 1. Introduction

Infertility, which affects approximately 10,000 couples per million populations in developed countries, is one of the most prevalent chronic health disorders involving young adults [1]. Defined as 1 year of attempted conception without success, infertility is clinically distinct from the inability to carry a pregnancy, or recurrent, spontaneous pregnancy loss. The chief female categories of infertility are ovulation disorders (25%), tubal disease (15%) and endometriosis (10%). Male infertility is the primary diagnosis in approximately 25% of cases and contributes to a further 15–25% of the remaining cases. The infertility remains unexplained in approximately 20% of cases, because numerous reproductive defects cannot be detected with current diagnostic methods.

---

* 400 Maders Cove Road, RR # 1, Mahone Bay NS, Canada B3J 2E0. Tel.: +1-902-624-6178; fax: 1-902-624-0115.
*E-mail address:* collinsj@auracom.com (J.A. Collins).

Clinical evaluation of a couple having regular, unprotected intercourse is generally indicated after a year or more, because by that time 85% of normal couples attempting conception would have been successful. Earlier assessment is indicated in some circumstances, such as the presence of amenorrhea or when the female partner is more than 35 years of age. The diagnostic assessment should begin with history, physical examination and pre-conceptional counselling, and it is usually most appropriate to have both partners involved in the initial workup. The current focus of diagnostic testing is on the use of a limited panel of specific investigations that correlate with the likelihood of live birth, rather than a broad range of screening tests. Typical couples will require semen analysis, serum progesterone in the mid-luteal phase and an assessment of tubal pathology. Laparoscopy may be indicated initially when there is a high probability of tubal disease or endometriosis. Elevation of basal FSH estimation is indicated in women with a potentially poor ovarian response and a diminished likelihood of conception.

The diagnosis and treatment of female infertility illustrate how evidence from medical care research should be considered, together with the personal preferences of couples and non-medical issues such as cost and convenience, when making clinical decisions.

## 2. Assessment of ovulation

### 2.1. Initial assessment

Ideally, the aim of testing is to evaluate whether there is regular release of an oocyte capable of being fertilized, but clinical testing to detect ovulation is a poor guide to oocyte quality. A detailed history will disclose ovulatory dysfunction in the form of amenorrhea, oligomenorrhea, dysfunctional uterine bleeding or the presence of lactation with or without cycle abnormalities. The prevalence of amenorrhea is approximately 3% in the population and also among infertile couples [2,3]. If the history reveals contributing factors, such as thyroid disease, hyperandrogenism, pituitary tumor, eating disorder, extremes of weight loss or exercise, hyperprolactinemia or obesity, these disorders should be rectified. The specific cause of ovulatory dysfunction may remain unknown, especially in oligo-ovulation.

### 2.2. Preliminary laboratory evaluation

Laboratory evaluation may not be needed in patients with short-term amenorrhea or oligomenorrhea prior to initiation of a short course of therapy. In other patients, mid-luteal serum progesterone provides presumptive evidence of ovulation [4]. Mid-luteal progesterone levels greater than 10.0 ng/ml (30 nM/l) are compatible with the 10th percentile of progesterone concentration in cycles of conception, but any level greater than 5.0 ng/ml (15 nM/l) is sufficient to reflect luteinization. In women over 35 years of age, or those with a history of ovarian surgery, FSH estimation on cycle day 3 is indicated to rule out a poor ovarian response and a diminished likelihood of conception.

### 2.3. Further testing

Further testing depends on which of four broad categories of ovulation disorders may be suspected from the initial assessment: hyperprolactinemic anovulation, hypergonadotrophic anovulation, hypogonadotrophic anovulation and normogonadotrophic anovulation. Normogonadotrophic anovulation, including polycystic ovary syndrome, is the most frequent and also the most challenging to treat.

### 2.3.1. Hyperprolactinemic anovulation

Prolactin and thyroid-stimulating hormone should be evaluated in women with ovulatory disturbances and lactation. When repeated prolactin concentrations are higher than normal, and primary hypothyroidism has been ruled out, pituitary magnetic resonance imaging is indicated to rule out microadenoma, empty sella syndrome or a macroadenoma. Even mildly elevated prolactin levels may be a sign of another organic central nervous system lesion, such as congenital aqueductal stenosis, non-functioning adenomas or conditions, which cause pituitary stalk irritability. Because the association between pituitary tumor and level of prolactin is not robust [5], MRI should not be restricted to specific threshold levels, but should be done whenever prolactin levels are above normal.

### 2.3.2. Hypergonadotrophic anovulation

This category is referred to as WHO Type III anovulation. If the FSH value is elevated in a woman with oligo-amenorrhea, the unlikely possibility of a random ovulatory peak should be excluded by ensuring that two values are obtained approximately 10 days apart. In some cases, FSH concentrations initially fluctuate in a high range and then rise to the menopausal range. In women under 30 with premature ovarian failure, a karyotype should be obtained to rule out mosaic XY cell lines and other sex chromosome abnormalities, such as translocation or short arm deletion. Elevated FSH levels and premature ovarian failure are more common in women who are carriers of the premutation of Fragile X syndrome [6].

### 2.3.3. Hypogonadotrophic anovulation

This category is referred to as WHO Type I anovulation. Weight loss, malnutrition and excessive exercise contribute to hypogonadotrophic anovulation, and counseling may be useful. Estimations of thyroxine-stimulating hormone and prolactin levels are indicated. The duration of the amenorrhea and the clinical condition are better indications of endogenous estrogen production than estradiol estimation, progesterone challenge testing or cervical mucus assessment. When stress, weight loss and excessive exercise are unlikely to cause the amenorrhea, magnetic resonance imaging may be indicated to rule out organic disease.

### 2.3.4. Normogonadotrophic anovulation

This category is referred to as WHO Type II anovulation. Investigations should include testosterone and sex hormone-binding globulin estimation (SHBG), as well as ovarian ultrasound. In a study which evaluated numerous clinical and endocrine variables, there were three significant predictors of success with induction of ovulation: lower free androgen index, lower BMI and a history of oligomenorrhea rather than amenorrhea [7]. Polycystic ovary syndrome (PCOS) is the most common component of this category and the criteria for this diagnosis involves any two of the following: cycle abnormality, androgen excess and ovarian ultrasound abnormality. Thus, PCOS involves women with bleeding intervals greater than 35 days, evidence of elevated androgen (hirsutism or elevated free androgen index (FAI): >4.5 [FAI=testosterone×100/SHBG]) or polycystic ovary morphology on ultrasound (ovarian volume>10 ml and/or follicle number>12/ovary in at least one ovary).

## 2.4. Other tests

Basal temperature records, endometrial biopsies and clomiphene citrate challenge tests are no longer recommended as routine investigations of the infertile couple. Keeping a basal temperature record is unnecessary in women with regular menstrual cycles and can be a distracting duty. Endometrial biopsy is a painful test, which has been superseded for confirmation of ovulation by mid-luteal progesterone assessment. The test is not accurate in evaluating an out-of-phase endometrium, and in any case, luteal phase defect is more common among fertile women [8,9]. The clomiphene challenge test provides no more accuracy in the assessment of ovarian reserve than basal FSH. Finally, luteinized, unruptured follicles, which are more common in women taking non-steroidal, anti-inflammatory agents, usually are not repetitive and this is unlikely to be a cause of infertility [10].

## 3. Assessment of tubal function

Available tests of tubal function describe tubal patency and appearance but fail to assess tubal functions, including the transport and sustenance of sperm and oocyte before fertilization and of the embryo after fertilization. The tubal abnormality that is most likely to cause infertility is impaired function or closure as a long-term consequence of infection, which may have been asymptomatic. Typically, infertile women have a 15% pre-test likelihood of tubal obstruction.

## 3.1. Screening tests

Serological testing for *Chlamydia trachomatis* antibody is a useful, initial screening test because a negative test result greatly reduces the likelihood that distal tubal pathology will be found at laparoscopy [11]. Hysterosalpingography (HSG) is also a screening test, because while it can demonstrate proximal and distal tubal occlusion, peritubal pathology cannot be visualized. Also, in some cases, cornual occlusion may result from myometrial spasm and require further evaluation. A more recent screening test is hystero-contrast-sonography (HyCoSy) in which contrast enhancement enables tubal visualisation by ultrasound. Predictive values with respect to blinded laparoscopy findings were similar with HSG and HyCoSy. Pain and patient preferences were also similar for both tests [12].

## 3.2. Laparoscopy

Laparoscopy is regarded as the reference test for the assessment of tubal and pelvic pathology because the test of patency by dye transit can be observed, and the procedure offers direct visualization of the peritoneal surfaces in the pelvis. Laparoscopy is not an ideal reference standard, however, for two reasons. First, the results are distant from the gold standard for the outcome of infertility, which is birth of a healthy child. Second, occasionally technical problems during the laparoscopy procedure may cause failure of the dye to transit the tube or interfere with pelvic visualization. Nevertheless, the laparoscopic procedure can demonstrate tubal patency and document proximal or distal tubal occlusive disease, peritubular adhesions and endometriosis.

*3.3. Test properties*

The 15% pre-test likelihood of tubal obstruction is reduced to approximately 8% if the *Chlamydia* antibody test is normal and to 5% if the HSG or HyCoSy result is normal. An abnormal result in any screening test is less reliable and warrants laparoscopy.

*3.4. Clinical approach*

In clinical practice, laparoscopy is indicated as the primary procedure whenever the history or physical examination suggest there is a higher than average likelihood of tubal or peritoneal disease. In patients at lower risk, *Chlamydia* antibody testing can serve to delay the need for invasive testing, but when conception has not occurred within a few months, a visual assessment by HSG or HyCoSy is indicated.

## 4. Endometriosis

The diagnosis of endometriosis cannot be made without visualization of the disease by laparoscopy. Endometriosis is found in 5–10% of women with infertility. Since laparoscopic ablation of endometriosis may improve fertility, should early laparoscopic assessment be offered to all infertile female partners? Two randomized clinical trials have evaluated the effectiveness of laparoscopic ablation with respect to ongoing pregnancy or live birth, with significant [13] and insignificant [14] results. The trials are clinically homogeneous and when the data are combined there is no significant statistical heterogeneity. The overall pregnancy rates were 27% and 18% in the treated (laparoscopy ablation) and control (laparoscopy only) groups, respectively. The absolute treatment difference is 8.7%, yielding a number needed to treat (NNT) rounded up to 12 (95% CI 6, 112).

Thus, the combined evidence indicates that among patients with endometriosis, for every 12 ablations during laparoscopy there will be a single additional birth during a year of follow-up, compared with diagnostic laparoscopy only. Only a fraction of patients considering laparoscopy, however, will be found to have endometriosis. If endometriosis were diagnosed in 20% of the infertility laparoscopy procedures in a given clinical practice, the preoperative number needed to treat would be 12 divided by 20%, which is 60. This treatment effect is not large enough to be a factor in the decision about when to have a laparoscopy during the investigation of infertility.

## 5. Conclusions

Although experience with in vitro fertilization, intracytoplasmic sperm injection and other research efforts have expanded knowledge of reproductive mechanisms, the diagnostic process has evolved more by discarding old tests than by finding useful new ones. The most useful tests correlate directly with the likelihood of conception and these are semen analysis, assessment of tubal disease and ovulation detection. Other tests are less useful because the results are not correlated with pregnancy. These tests include sperm penetration assay in the zona-free hamster oocyte, post-coital tests, sperm penetration into cervical mucus, sperm antibody tests and endometrial biopsy.

For example, the post-coital test only mirrors semen analysis findings, is difficult to schedule, adds no information on cervical function and fails to discriminate between couples with a good and bad prognosis. The test does not contribute to choice of treatment or increase conception rates [15].

To improve treatment results in female infertility will require research to discover as-yet-unknown causes of infertility that coexist with recognized diagnoses. Unknown causes may include post-fertilization defects that cannot possibly respond to the pre-fertilization interventions that now comprise many of the available treatments.

## References

[1] E.H. Stephen, A. Chandra, Updated projections of infertility in the United States: 1995 to 2025, Fertil. Steril. 70 (1998) 30–34.
[2] F. Pettersson, H. Fries, S.J. Nillius, Epidemiology of secondary amenorrhea: I. Incidence and prevalence rates, Am. J. Obstet. Gynecol. 117 (1973) 80–86.
[3] J.A. Collins, E.A. Burrows, A.R. Willan, The prognosis for live birth among untreated infertile couples, Fertil. Steril. 64 (1995) 22–28.
[4] The ESHRE Capri Workshop Group, Guidelines to the prevalence, diagnosis, treatment and management of infertility, 1996, Hum. Reprod. 11 (1996) 1775–1807.
[5] P. Touraine, et al., Long-term follow-up of 246 hyperprolactinemic patients, Acta Obstet. Gynecol. Scand. 80 (2001) 162–168.
[6] D.J. Allingham-Hawkins, et al., Fragile X premutation is a significant risk factor for premature ovarian failure: the International Collaborative POF in Fragile X study—preliminary data, Am. J. Med. Genet 83 (1999) 322–325.
[7] B. Imani, et al., Predictors of patients remaining anovulatory during clomiphene citrate induction of ovulation in normogonadotropic oligo-amenorrheic infertility, J. Clin. Endocrinol. Metab. 83 (1998) 2361–2365.
[8] J. Balasch, et al., The usefulness of endometrial biopsy for luteal phase evaluation in infertility, Hum. Reprod. 7 (1992) 973–977.
[9] The Reproductive Medicine Network, The endometrial biopsy as a diagnostic tool in the evaluation of the infertile patient, Fertil. Steril. 78 (2002) S2.
[10] The ESHRE Capri Workshop Group, Physiopathological determinants of human infertility, Hum. Reprod. Updat. 8 (2002) 435–447.
[11] J.A. Land, et al., Performance of five serological *Chlamydia* antibody tests in subfertile women, Hum. Reprod. 18 (2003) 2621–2627.
[12] A.B. Dijkman, et al., Can hysterosalpingocontrast-sonography replace hysterosalpingography in the assessment of tubal subfertility? Eur. J. Radiol. 35 (2000) 44–48.
[13] S. Marcoux, R. Maheux, S. Berube and The Canadian Collaborative Group on Endometriosis, Laparoscopic surgery in infertile women with minimal or mild endometriosis, N. Engl. J. Med. 337 (1997) 217–222.
[14] F. Parazzini and Gruppo Italiano per lo Studio dell'Endometriosi, Ablation of lesions or no treatment in minimal-mild endometriosis in infertile women: a randomized trial, Hum. Reprod. 14 (1999) 1332–1334.
[15] S.G. Oei, et al., Effectiveness of the postcoital test: randomised controlled trial, BMJ 317 (7157) (1998) 502.

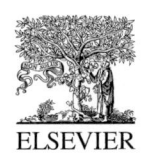

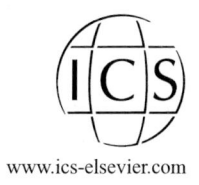

# Medical management of menstrual disorders

## Juha S. Tapanainen*

*Department of Obstetrics and Gynecology, University of Oulu, P.O. Box 5000, FIN-90014 Oulu, Finland*

**Abstract.** A vast majority of women experience menstrual disorders some time in their life. Complaints of excessive menstrual loss, in particular, have a substantial impact on gynecological services. It is estimated that 5% of women consult their physician with menstrual problems each year, and up to 30% of reproductive age women suffer from menorrhagia. Menorrhagia is defined as blood loss of more than 80 ml per cycle, but already lower amounts may result in iron-deficient anemia. Before starting the medication for heavy menstrual bleeding, the possible organic cause should be assessed, and the age, pregnancy desires, general health and patient preference should be considered. The combined oral contraceptive pills (COCPs), prostaglandin inhibitors and tranexamic acid are still recommended as the first line of therapy for menorrhagia, especially in nulliparous women. All of these also have the added advantage of relieving dysmenorrhea. Other drugs, such as danazol and gonadotropin-releasing hormone agonists (GnRHa), reduce menstrual blood loss effectively, but due to side effects, their use is limited to special cases. Luteal progestins are widely used for the treatment of heavy menstrual bleeding, but women with regular ovulatory cycles suffering from menorrhagia do not benefit from the treatment. © 2004 Published by Elsevier B.V.

*Keywords:* Menstrual disorder; Menorrhagia; Prostaglandin inhibitor; Tranexamic acid; Contraceptive pill

## 1. Introduction

Menstruation normally starts between the ages of 11 and 13 years, and stops between 45 and 50 years of age. The average blood loss per period is between 30 and 40 ml. The most common menstrual disorders are dysfunctional uterine bleeding, premenstrual syndrome (PMS) and dysmenorrhea. A vast majority of women suffer from these symptoms during their reproductive life span, but dysfunctional uterine bleeding occurs most commonly during adolescence and in premenopause when the cycles are or become anovulatory. The patterns of abnormal uterine bleeding include menorrhagia, polymenorrhea, oligoamenorrhea and metrorrhagia. Menorrhagia means excessive menstrual bleeding; in polymenorrhea, bleeding episodes occur in less than 21 days; oligomenorrhea means scanty menstruation or long menstrual periods over 35 days; and metrorrhagia means irregular bleeding at any time between menstrual periods.

---

* Tel.: +358-8-3153172; fax: +358-8-3154310.
 *E-mail address:* juha.tapanainen@oulu.fi (J.S. Tapanainen).

0531-5131/ © 2004 Published by Elsevier B.V.
doi:10.1016/j.ics.2004.01.106

Table 1
Medical treatment of menorrhagia

| |
|---|
| Prostaglandin synthetase inhibitors |
| Drugs affecting coagulation system |
|   Tranexamic acid |
|   Ethamsylate |
| Combined oral contraceptive pills |
|   Standard-cycle pills |
|   Trimonthly-cycle pills |
| Progestins |
| Other |
|   Danazol |
|   GnRH agonists |

This chapter will concentrate on the medical treatment of excessive menstrual bleeding (Table 1), and other menstrual disorders will be touched only briefly. The use of the levonorgestril intrauterine system for the treatment of menorrhagia will be discussed in chapter XX.

## 2. Menorrhagia

Menorrhagia is defined as blood loss of 60–80 ml per cycle [1,2]. Women with regular but heavy or long-lasting menstrual bleeding are more likely to have ovulatory cycles, while menorrhagia with intermenstrual bleeding or spotting is often associated with unovulatory cycles and may result in hyperplasia due to the unopposed, continuous estrogen effect. The prevalence of endometrial hyperplasia in cases of normal weight women under 45 years of age is 2.3%, but it is already 8% in women over 45 [3]. Eighty percent of women with menorrhagia have no anatomical pathology, such as uterine fibroids, polyps or adenomyosis, and over one-third of the women undergoing hysterectomy for heavy bleeding have their normal uteri removed [4,5].

## 3. Menstrual disorders in adolescence

The maturation of the hypothalamic–pituitary–ovarian axis takes place during the first 2 years after menarche, but in 20% of adolescents anovulatory cycles, last up to 5 years [6]. Adolescent females suffering from menstrual disorders are concerned about their personal image, and, therefore, early treatment is very important. The treatment strategies depend on the etiology of the pathologic causes of anovulation. The most important are polycystic ovary syndrome (PCOS), hypothalamic dysfunction associated with exercise and eating disorders, and endocrinopathies. Coagulation disorders are a common cause of menorrhagia in teenagers. These include thrombocytopenia, idiopathic thrombocytogenic purpura, platelet dysfunction and von Willebrandt disease [7]. Because coagulopathies are found in 10–30% of adolescents with excessive menstrual bleeding [8,9], they have to be excluded before starting the medical treatment of other causes of menorrhagia. The adolescent who is heavily bleeding (juvenile metropathy) needs immediate hormonal intervention. She should take oral contraceptives containing 30–35 μg ethinyl estradiol four times a day for 2 days; thereafter, the dose should be reduced over 3 days to 1 tablet a day. If necessary, a contraceptive pill containing 50 μg ethinyl estradiol should be used. After 5 days of acute treatment, the patient should start a new 21- or 28-pill pack and continue the therapy for several months [6,10]. The most common problems related to menstruation in adolescence are dysmenorrhea and irregular or heavy bleeding, and they can often be treated successfully with nonsteroidal anti-inflammatory drug (NSAIDs) and/or oral contraceptive pills.

## 4. Medical management of menorrhagia

### 4.1. Prostaglandin synthetase inhibitors

The rationale in using NSAIDs was based on their ability to decrease endometrial prostaglandin levels, which are elevated in menorrhagia [11]. NSAIDs decrease menstrual blood loss by 20–50% [12]. The NSAIDs used most often include acetylsalicylic acid, diclofenac, ibuprofen, indomethacin, mefenamic acid and meclofenamic acid. Mefenamic acid is the most commonly studied of these drugs, but data comparing different NSAIDs in the treatment of menorrhagia are limited. Nevertheless, it is widely accepted that the clinical efficacy of different NSAIDs is similar. Based on the Cochrane Review by Lethaby et al. [13], they are more effective than placebo but less effective than tranexamic acid or danazol [14]. Compared with other treatments, like luteal progestin, ethamsylate, oral contraceptive pills or the levonorgestril intrauterine system, no differences were observed but most studies were underpowered [13]. Moreover, small, nonrandomized cohort studies have shown that the levonorgestril intrauterine system used for contraceptive purposes decreases menstrual bleeding after 12 months by more than 90% [15,16]. Randomized trials have shown that its effectiveness in the treatment of menorrhagia is similar [17,18]. To obtain optimal effect, the treatment with NSAIDs should be started a few days before menstruation, on the first day of menses at the latest, and should be continued until cessation of bleeding. Furthermore, the dosage should be high enough based on the recommendations of the manufacturer.

### 4.2. Drugs affecting coagulation system

Plasminogen activators cause fibrinolysis, and their tissue concentrations increase in the endometrium of women with heavy menstrual bleeding. Tranexamic acid, a plasminogen activator inhibitor, has been used for the treatment of menorrhagia for a long time. The other drug, ethamsylate, reduces capillary bleeding by affecting platelet function and has also been in clinical use for a number of years. There are several studies on the effect of tranexamic acid in menorrhea but only one comparing tranexamic acid with ethamsylate. In this study by Bonnar [19,20], tranexamic acid (1 g four times daily for cycle days 1–5) was significantly more effective. No significant differences were found in the subjective assessment by the study subjects, although there was a trend in favour of tranexamic acid. Moreover, in the Cochrane Review by Lethaby et al. [20], tranexamic acid was also found to be more effective in reducing heavy menstrual bleeding than placebo, NSAIDs and luteal phase progestin. It reduced menstrual blood flow by 25–50%. Tranexamic acid had no more adverse events than placebo, and long-term studies have failed to demonstrate any increase in the risk of thrombosis. There are no studies comparing tranexamic acid with contraceptive pills and the levonorgestril intrauterine system.

### 4.3. Combined oral contraceptive pill

Combined oral contraceptive pills (COCPs) have been used for years for the treatment of menorrhagia. Their efficacy was first recognized by women using pills only for contraception, and later on, this observation was confirmed objectively in several trials [12]. The reduction of menstrual bleeding by oral contraceptives is probably a result of induced atrophy in the endometrium. Besides contraception, COCPs have several beneficial effects, such as good cycle control and antiandrogenic effects, which make them acceptable for long-term therapy. Although there are a large number of studies on the effect of COCPs on menorrhagia, there is only one randomized, controlled trial comparing the efficacy of COCP, mefenamic acid, naproxen and danazol [21,22]. The crossover trial was small, consisting of 45 patients, and there were no significant differences in menstrual blood loss between the treatments. The overall blood loss reduced 43% in the COCP group. Trimonthly-cycle oral contraceptive therapy has been used to postpone withdrawal bleeding and reduce the frequency of menstruation. Typically, it consists of 84 days of estrogen–progestin, followed by a pill-free interval of 7 days, and reduces the yearly number of withdrawal bleeding episodes from 12 to 4 [23–25]. The contraceptive effectiveness and the side effect profile [26] of extended COCP regimens are similar to those of standard COCP. Thus, this therapy will offer a good alternative for women suffering from menorrhagia, at least, later in reproductive age.

### 4.4. Progestins

The use of progestin in the anovulatory patient to coordinate menstrual cycle is effective when given cyclically in the luteal phase (c.d. 15–24), but a patient with regular menstrual cycle and menorrhagia do not benefit from the treatment [12]. However, progestin therapy for 21 days of the cycle [27,28], or injectable long-acting progestins [29], reduce menstrual blood flow by inducing endometrial atrophy. Progestin therapy administered from cycle days 5 to 26 may be beneficial for some patients, but due to side effects such as mood changes, nausea, headache, tiredness and atherogenic changes in lipid profile, it is limited for the short-term use [28]. In the Cochrane Review [28], cyclical progestin administered during the luteal phase was found to be less effective when compared with tranexamic acid, danazol or the levonorgestril intrauterine system. The subdermal contraceptive implant system (Norplant) somewhat reduces menstrual blood loss when used for contraceptive purposes [30], but for the treatment of excessive menstrual bleeding, it is not effective enough. Thus, oral or subdermal progestins are not the first line therapy for menorrhagia, but the 21 days' treatment may be useful for some women with anovulatory irregular cycles and intermenstrual bleeding associated with excessive menstrual bleeding.

### 4.5. Other medical treatments

Danazol is a synthetic androgen derived from testosterone. It has both antiestrogenic and antiprogestogenic activity. It reduces estrogen levels and thereby causes endometrial atrophy and amenorrhea in some women [31]. In the Cochrane Review by Beaumont et al. [14], despite wide confidence intervals, danazol (100–200 mg daily) was found to be more effective in reducing menstrual blood flow than placebo, progestins, NSAIDs and oral contraceptive pills, but it has more side effects than NSAIDs and progestins. The commonly reported side effects were acne, weight gain, headache, nausea and tiredness [14]. There are no randomized trials comparing danazol with tranexamic acid or the levonorgestril intrauterine system. Thus, danazol is effective for the treatment of severe menorrhagia, but due to its side effect profile and the need for continuing treatment, its use is limited to special cases.

Gonadotropin-releasing hormone agonists (GnRHa) are an alternative for the treatment of heavy menstrual bleeding. By downregulating pituitary gonadotropin secretion, they cause a hypoestrogenic state and endometrial atrophy. GnRHas are very effective in reducing menstrual blood loss [32], but long-term treatment is not possible due to hypoestrogenic symptoms and bone loss.

## 5. Conclusions

Before starting medication for heavy menstrual bleeding, the possible organic cause should be excluded. There are several drugs available for the medical treatment of menorrhagia, but only a few of them are effective enough and meet patient acceptability. Traditional drugs, NSAIDs and tranexamic acid are still useful, safe and can be used long-term. The dosage has to be high enough and the medication should be started at the latest on the first day of menstruation. For young women and especially for those requiring contraception, combined oral contraceptive pills are often the drug of choice and, in the case of dysmenorrhea, can be combined with NSAIDs. Trimonthly-cycle oral contraceptive therapy may offer a useful alternative for women suffering from menorrhagia. Cyclical progestins are not effective enough for menorrhagia unless given monthly for 21 days. Danazol and GnRHas reduce menstrual blood loss significantly but cannot be recommended for first-line therapy or long-term use because of their side effects.

## References

[1] L. Hallberg, et al., Menstrual blood loss and iron deficiency, Acta Med. Scand. 180 (1966) 639–650.
[2] B.J. Cohen, Y. Gibor, Anemia and menstrual blood loss, Obstet. Gynecol. Surv. 35 (1980) 597–618.
[3] C.M. Farquhar, et al., An evaluation of risk factors for endometrial hyperplasia in premenopausal women with abnormal menstrual bleeding, Am. J. Obstet. Gynecol. 181 (1999) 525–529.
[4] A. Clarke, et al., Indications for and outcome of total abdominal hysterectomy for benign disease: a prospective cohort study, Br. J. Obstet. Gynaecol. 102 (1995) 611–620.
[5] D. Gath, P. Cooper, A. Day, Hysterectomy and psychiatric disorder: I. Levels of psychiatric morbidity before and after hysterectomy, Br. J. Psychiatry 140 (1982) 335–350.
[6] E.H. Qiunt, Y.R. Smith, Abnormal uterine bleeding in adolescents, J. Midwifery Women's Health 48 (2003) 186–191.
[7] J.A. Bevan, et al., Bleeding disorders: a common cause of menorrhagia in adolescents, J. Pediatr. 138 (2001) 856–861.
[8] Y.R. Smith, E.H. Quint, R.B. Hertzberg, Menorrhagia in adolescents requiring hospitalization, J. Pediatr. Adolesc. Gynecol. 11 (1998) 13–15.
[9] C. Duflos-Cohade, M. Amandruz, E. Thibaud, Pubertal metrorrhagia, J. Pediatr. Adolesc. Gynecol. 9 (1996) 16–20.
[10] G.B. Slap, Menstrual disorders in adolescence, Bailliére's Best Pract. Res., Clin. Obstet. Gynaecol. 17 (2003) 75–92.

[11] S.K. Smith, et al., Prostaglandin synthesis in the endometrium of women with ovular dysfunctional uterine bleeding, Br. J. Obstet. Gynaecol. 88 (1981) 434–442.
[12] G.A. Irvine, I.T. Cameron, Medical management of dysfunctional uterine bleeding, Bailliére's Best Pract. Res., Clin. Obstet. Gynaecol. 13 (1999) 189–202.
[13] A. Lethaby, C. Augood, K. Duckitt, Nonsteroidal anti-inflammatory drugs for heavy menstrual bleeding (Cochrane Review), The Cochrane Library, Issue, vol. 4, Wiley, Chichester, UK, 2003.
[14] H. Beaumont, et al., Danazol for heavy menstrual bleeding (Cochrane Review), The Cochrane Library, Issue, vol. 4, Wiley, Chichester, UK, 2003.
[15] J.K. Andersson, G. Rybo, Levonorgestrel-releasing intrauterine device in the treatment of menorrhagia, Br. J. Obstet. Gynaecol 97 (1990) 690–694.
[16] T. Luukkainen, J. Toivonen, Levonorgestrel-releasing IUD as a method of contraception with therapeutic properties, Contraception 52 (1995) 269–276.
[17] I. Milsom, et al., A comparison of flurbiprofen, tranexamic acid, and a levonorgestrel-releasing intrauterine contraceptive device in the treatment of idiopathic menorrhagia, Am. J. Obstet. Gynecol. 164 (1991) 879–883.
[18] R. Hurskainen, et al., Quality of life and cost-effectiveness of levonorgestrel-releasing intrauterine system versus hysterectomy for treatment of menorrhagia: a randomised trial, Lancet 357 (2001) 273–277.
[19] J. Bonnar, B.L. Sheppard, Treatment of menorrhagia during menstruation: randomised controlled trial of ethamsylate, mefenamic acid, and tranexamic acid, Br. Med. J. 313 (1996) 579–582.
[20] A. Lethaby, C. Farquhar, I. Cooke, Antifibrinolytics for heavy menstrual bleeding (Cochrane Review), The Cochrane Library, Issue, vol. 4, Wiley, Chichester, UK, 2003.
[21] I.S. Fraser, et al., Blood and total fluid content of menstrual discharge, Obstet. Gynecol. 65 (1985) 194–198.
[22] V. Iyer, C. Farquhar, R. Jepson, Oral contraceptive pills for heavy menstrual bleeding (Cochrane Review), The Cochrane Library, Issue, vol. 4, Wiley, Chichester, UK, 2003.
[23] N.B. Loudon, et al., Acceptability of an oral contraceptive that reduces the frequency of menstruation: the tri-cycle pill regimen, Br. Med. J. 2 (1977) 487–490.
[24] P.J. Sulak, et al., Extending the duration of active oral contraceptive pills to manage hormone withdrawal symptoms, Obstet. Gynecol. 89 (1997) 179–183.
[25] J.B. Braunstein, et al., Economics of reducing menstruation with trimonthly-cycle oral contraceptive therapy: comparison with standard-cycle regimens, Obstet. Gynecol. 102 (2003) 699–708.
[26] L. Miller, J.P. Hughes, Continuous combination oral contraceptive pills to eliminate withdrawal bleeding: a randomized trial, Obstet. Gynecol. 101 (2003) 653–661.
[27] G.A. Irvine, et al., Randomised comparative trial of the levonorgestrel intrauterine system and norethisterone for treatment of idiopathic menorrhagia, Br. J. Obstet. Gynaecol. 105 (1998) 592–598.
[28] A. Lethaby, G. Irvine, I. Cameron, Cyclical progestogens for heavy menstrual bleeding (Cochrane Review), The Cochrane Library, Issue, vol. 4, Wiley, Chichester, UK, 2003.
[29] I.S. Fraser, Bleeding arising from the use of exogenous steroids, Bailliére's Best Pract. Res., Clin. Obstet. Gynaecol. 13 (1999) 203–222.
[30] C.G. Nilsson, P. Holma, Menstrual blood loss with contraceptive subdermal levonorgestrel implants, Fertil. Steril. 35 (1981) 304–306.
[31] T.H. Chimbira, et al., Reduction of menstrual blood loss by danazol in unexplained menorrhagia: lack of effect of placebo, Br. J. Obstet. Gynaecol. 87 (1980) 1152–1158.
[32] R.W. Shaw, H.M. Fraser, Use of a superactive luteinizing hormone releasing hormone (LHRH) agonist in the treatment of menorrhagia, Br. J. Obstet. Gynaecol. 91 (1984) 913–916.

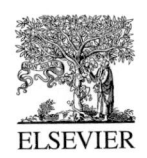

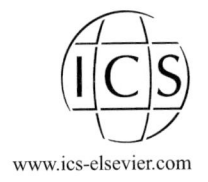

# Mirena

## Su Ling Yu[*]

*Department of Obstetrics and Gynecology, Singapore General Hospital, Outram Road, Singapore 169608, Singapore*

**Abstract.** Mirena is a levonorgestrel-releasing intrauterine system (LNG-IUS). It comprises a T-shaped plastic frame with a cylinder of the synthetic progestogen levonorgestrel that permits the slow and controlled release over 24 h of 20 µg levonorgesterel into the uterus. It was first approved in Finland in 1990 and approved by the FDA in 2001. Contraceptive effect is due to suppression of levonorgestrel on the endometrium, prevents sperm from reaching the egg. A cumulative pregnancy rate of 0.0–0.5 has been reported, which equals that of tubal ligation. Besides providing highly effective contraception, there are noncontraceptive benefits with Mirena. Noncontraceptive benefits include reduction in heavy menstrual bleeding, reduced growth of uterine fibroids, reduction in dysmenorrhoea and some benefits in the suppression of endometriosis. It is most suitable for older women of reproductive age when it can improve anovulatory dysfunctional bleeding. It can also act as the progestogen in hormone replacement therapy for postmenopausal women. Randomised studies of Mirena have been done comparing it with norethisterone, transcervical resection of the endometrium, endometrial ablation as well as hysterectomy. Irregular, breakthrough bleeding is the most common side effect and the most common reason for discontinuation. This occurs up to 6 months after use of Mirena. Other concerns include infection, ovarian cysts and ectopic pregnancy. The continuation rate for MIRENA was reported to be 0.65 at 5 years in Finnish women. Gross cumulative rates at 5 years per 100 women were for expulsion 5.9, removal for bleeding problems 16.7, removal for pain 4.3 and removal for pelvic inflammatory disease 1.2 in a UK study. © 2004 Published by Elsevier B.V.

*Keywords:* Mirena; LNG-IUS; Progestogen; Levonorgestrel; Contraceptive; Heavy menstrual bleeding

## 1. What is mirena?

Mirena is a levonorgestrel-releasing intrauterine system (LNG-IUS). It comprises a T-shaped plastic frame with a cylinder of the synthetic progestogen levonorgestrel that permits the slow and controlled release over 24 h of 20 µg levonorgestrel into the uterus [1]. It was first approved in Finland in 1990 and by the FDA in 2001. Mirena is used as a parenteral hormonal contraceptive method and lasts for 5 years.

---

[*] Tel.: +65-63214651; fax: +65-62253464.
 *E-mail address:* gogysl@sgh.com.sg (S.L. Yu).

0531-5131/ © 2004 Published by Elsevier B.V.
doi:10.1016/j.ics.2004.01.103

## 2. How does it work?

Mirena is inserted into the uterine cavity using its own inserter, differently inserted compared with the usual intrauterine contraceptive device. Ovulation is usually not inhibited. Its main effect is a local progestogenic effect on the endometrium and cervical mucus. Features of atrophy and extensive decidualisation are seen within a month of insertion of Mirena. Studies have shown suppression of estrogen, progesterone and androgen receptors of the endometrium. The progestogenic effects on the endometrium were observed to return to normal within 3 months of removal of the device with a complete return to previous fertility [2].

The contraceptive effect is due to suppression of levonorgestrel on the endometrium preventing sperm from reaching the egg. Cumulative pregnancy rates of 0.0–0.5 have been reported [3]. This equals that of tubal ligation.

## 3. What are the noncontraceptive benefits?

Besides providing highly effective contraception, there are noncontraceptive benefits with Mirena. Noncontraceptive benefits include reduction in heavy menstrual bleeding, reduced growth of uterine fibroids, reduction in dysmenorrhoea and suppression of endometriosis. It is most suitable for older women of reproductive age when it can improve anovulatory dysfunctional bleeding. It can also act as the progestogen in hormone replacement therapy for postmenopausal women.

Much has been reported on the great reduction of menstrual blood, of up to 80% in women with menorrhagia, after insertion of Mirena. Up to 66% of women have reported oligomenorrhea to amenorrhea up to 12 months. This method of treatment of menorrhagia has compared favourably with nonsteroidal, antiinflammatory drugs, tranexamic acid as well as progestogen treatments.

Randomised studies of Mirena on women with menorrhagia have been done comparing Mirena with medical treatment, transcervical resection of the endometrium, endometrial ablation as well as hysterectomy [4]. The quality of life measurement appears to be similar at one year with the Mirena treatment compared with hysterectomy [5].

Grigorieva et al. [6] reported a reduction of fibroid volume in a study involving 67 women with at least one fibroid using the Mirena for at least 1 year.

Small studies have shown that the use of Mirena had resolved endometrial hyperplasia and reduced the severity of dysmenorrhoea as compared with the copper IUD, and reduced the stage of endometriosis [7–9].

The future role of Mirena may be in the protection of the endometrium, in place of oral progestrogen, in hormone replacement therapy. A nonrandomised study showed good protection of the endometrium in 5 years of treatment with Mirena and oral estrogen or the estradiol patch [10].

## 4. What are the side effects?

Irregular breakthrough bleeding is the most common side effect and the most common reason for discontinuation. This occurs in up to 53% of women after 3 months of using Mirena [11]. This could be due to extensive decidualisation, downregulation of endometrial hormonal receptors, disturbed angiogenesis, as well as local inflammatory factors [12].

Other concerns include premenstrual syndrome, infection, ovarian cysts and ectopic pregnancy.

The continuation rate for Mirena was reported to be 0.65 at 5 years in Finnish women. Gross cumulative rates at 5 years per 100 women were expulsion 5.9, removal for bleeding problems 16.7, removal for pain 4.3 and removal for pelvic inflammatory disease 1.2 in a UK study [13,14].

## 5. Conclusion

Despite the problem of unscheduled bleeding, Mirena still plays an important role for older women with heavy periods who also want contraception. More studies should be done on its role in improving such conditions as endometriosis, fibroids and endometrial hyperplasia.

## References

[1] C.C. Nilsson, P. Lahteenmaki, T. Luukkainen, Patterns of ovulation and bleeding with a low levonorgestrel-releasing intrauterine device, Contraception 21 (1980) 155–164.
[2] K. Andersson, I. Batar, G. Rybo, Return to fertility after removal of a levonorgestrel-releasing intrauterine device and Nava-T, Contraception 46 (1992) 575–584.
[3] T. Luukkainen, et al., Effective contraception with the levonorgestrel-releasing intrauterine device: 12 month report of a European multicenter study, Contraception 35 (1987) 169–179.
[4] J. Majoribanks, C. Farquhar, A. Lethaby, Surgery versus medical therapy for heavy menstrual bleeding (Cochrane Review), The Cochrane Library, Update Software, Oxford, 2003, p. 2.
[5] R. Hurskainen, et al., Quality of life and cost-effectiveness of levonorgestrel-releasing intrauterine system versus hysterectomy for treatment of menorrhagia: a randomised trial, Lancet 357 (2001) 273–277.
[6] V. Grigorieva, et al., Use of a levonorgestrel-releasing intrauterine system to treat bleeding related to uterine leiomyomas, Fertil. Steril. 79 (2003) 1194–1198.
[7] A. Perino, et al., Treatment of endometrial hyperplasia with levonorgestrel-releasing intrauterine devices, Acta Eur. Fertil. 18 (1987) 137–144.
[8] I. Sivin, J. Stern, Health during prolonged use of levonorgestrel 20 micrograms/d and the copper TCu 380AG intrauterine contraceptive devices: a multicentre study. International Committee for Contraception Research (ICCR), Fertil. Steril. 61 (1994) 70–71.
[9] L. Fedele, et al., Use of a levonorgestrel-releasing intrauterine device in the treatment of rectovaginal endometriosis, Fertil. Steril. 75 (2001) 485–488.
[10] E. Varila, T. Wahlstrom, I. Rausomo, A 5-year follow-up study on the use of a levonorgestrel-releasing intrauterine system in women receiving hormone replacement therapy, Fertil. Steril. 76 (2001) 969–973.
[11] G.A. Irvine, et al., Randomised comparative trial of levonorgestrel-releasing intrauterine system and norethisterone for the treatment of idiopathic menorrhagia, Br. J. Obstet. Gynaecol. 105 (1998) 592–598.
[12] C. Hilary, Endometrial effects of progestogens, Gynaecol. Forum. 8 (3) (2003) 6–10.
[13] T. Backman, et al., Sixty thousand woman-years of experience on the levonorgestrel intrauterine system: an epidemiological survey in Finland, Eur. J. Contracept. Reprod. Health Care Suppl. 1 (2001) 23–26.
[14] M. Cox, J. Tripp, S. Balcksell, Clinical performance of the levonorgestrel intrauterine system in routine use by the UK Family Planning and Reproductive Health Research Network: 5-year report, J. Fam. Plan. Reprod. Health Care 28 (2) (2002) 73–77.

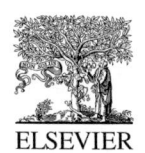

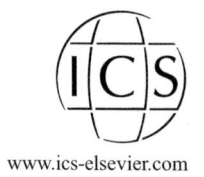

# Menorrhagia: the role of endometrial ablation

## Martin C. Sowter*

*Obstetrics and Gynaecology, National Women's Hospital, Claude Road, Epsom, 1001 Auckland, New Zealand*

**Abstract.** Menorrhagia has an enormous impact on many women's lives and, until the early 1990s, the only treatments widely available were relatively ineffective oral therapies and hysterectomy. Since then, women seeking treatment for menorrhagia have also been able to choose from a much wider range of treatments, including endometrial resection or ablation and the levonorgestrel-releasing intra-uterine device. Hysteroscopic resection/ablation has been extensively studied and compared with other medical and surgical treatments in well-conducted randomised trials. Long-term follow-up and safety data are also available. More recently, a potentially bewildering number of new surgical therapies have also become available, for which in some cases much less information is available. These treatments have been developed with the aim of providing a quick, safe way of destroying the endometrium, without requiring the surgical skills or general anaesthesia needed for hysteroscopic ablation/resection. However, as experience is gained with the use of progestogen-releasing devices for the treatment of menorrhagia, some question whether there is much role for endometrial ablation in any form. This review considers each currently available technology individually, assesses the role of endometrial ablation in the treatment of menorrhagia, and suggests what characteristics are required of the ideal ablation device. © 2004 Published by Elsevier B.V.

*Keywords:* Menorrhagia; Endometrial ablation; Levonorgestrel intrauterine system; Hysterectomy

## 1. Introduction

Menorrhagia has an enormous impact on many women's lives and, until the early 1990s, the only treatments widely available were relatively ineffective oral therapies and hysterectomy. However, for the last decade, women seeking treatment for menorrhagia have also been able to choose from a much wider range of therapies, including a potentially bewildering number of new surgical therapies that aim to permanently remove or destroy the endometrium. This review considers each currently available technology individually, assesses the role of endometrial ablation in the treatment of menorrhagia, and suggests what characteristics are required of the ideal ablation device.

---

*Abbreviations:* FEAT, first generation ablation therapy; SEAT, second generation ablation therapy.
* Tel.: +64-9-638-9909; fax:+64-9-631-1101.
*E-mail address:* martinsowter@xtra.co.nz (M.C. Sowter).

## 2. First-generation ablation therapy (FEAT)

Three techniques for the hysteroscopic removal or ablation of the endometrium have been described: Nd-YAG laser ablation [1], trans-cervical resection of the endometrium (TCRE) [2] and rollerball ablation [3]. All three techniques are referred to as first-generation ablation therapies (FEAT) and data from observational studies [4-6] and randomised trials [7] suggest that there is no difference in clinical outcomes among the three techniques.

FEAT have been compared in randomised trials with recommended [8] first-line medical treatments, and satisfaction rates, post-treatment haemoglobin concentrations, pain scores and quality of life measures are better after FEAT [9]. Randomised trials comparing endometrial resection with the levonorgestrel-releasing intra-uterine device (LNG-IUS) show slightly higher amenorrhoea rates and reduced blood loss following resection [10,11]. When compared with hysterectomy, operating time, hospital stay and direct costs are less after FEAT [12-14]. However, patient satisfaction rates are slightly, but significantly, higher after hysterectomy [15]. Within 5 years of treatment, up to 15% of women will have a second ablation treatment and 10-25% will have a hysterectomy [16-19].

Reported complications from FEAT include uterine perforation, haemorrhage, pelvic sepsis and fluid overload syndromes [20]. The UK-based MISTLETOE audit, which reported on 10,686 procedures, included two deaths and an overall complication rate ranging from 2.1% for laser ablation to 6.4% for loop resection [20].

FEAT have been described as the most thoroughly evaluated new surgical treatment of recent times [21]. Long-term outcome data show that many women can avoid any further surgical intervention following treatment using a FEAT technique. However, a significant level of operator skill and training is required to produce reliable results safely. FEAT also require general anaesthesia, expose the patient to the risk of fluid overload and can be time-consuming. The rapid development of a range of so-called second generation (SEAT) or global ablation therapies that can be used by a gynaecologist with no operative hysteroscopic skills make it likely that FEAT will, in future, be only infrequently used.

## 3. Second generation ablation therapy (SEAT)

In the last decade, a number of second generation devices have been developed with the aim of making the efficacy and safety of endometrial ablation less operator-dependent and also to permit the use of this treatment in a clinic, rather than an operating theatre setting. Each treatment modality is reviewed briefly below.

### 3.1. Balloon systems

These devices use an inflatable balloon on the end of a disposable probe, which is inserted into the uterine cavity and through which heated fluid is then circulated. Balloon inflation pressure ensures close contact between the heat source and endometrium and also produces a degree of endometrial ischaemia, reducing the cooling effect of uterine blood flow. Some devices have a heating element and thermistor within the intra-uterine balloon and no mechanism for circulating the fluid within the balloon (ThermaChoice™, Gynecare, Menlo Park, CA, USA [22]). Others heat saline or glycine within a separate unit and circulate it through the intra-uterine balloon (CavaTerm™, Wallsten Medical, Morges,

Switzerland [23]; Menotreat™, ATOS Medical, Hörby, Sweden [24]) or have an umpellar within the balloon to circulate fluid (ThermaChoice II™, Gynecare). Treatment times are 8 min for Thermachoice, 11 min for Menotreat and 15 min for Cavaterm. The devices require dilation of the cervix to between 5 mm (Thermachoice) and 8 mm (Cavaterm). Most recently, a new balloon ablation system, Thermablate (MDMI Technologies, Richmond, B.C., Canada) has been described [25]. In this system, a biocompatible liquid contained within a disposable catheter-balloon unit is heated to an initial temperature of 173 °C and forced into an intra-uterine balloon through a series of pressurisation and depressurisation cycles over a treatment period of only 2 min.

Randomised trials have compared these devices with FEAT [26–28], with each other [29] and with the levonorgestrel-releasing intra-uterine device [30]. These studies suggest that there is little difference between individual balloon devices and between SEAT and FEAT in effectiveness, even over 3 years of follow-up. Studies comparing balloon therapies with the LNG-IUS are small, but suggest either no difference in post-operative blood loss and health-related quality of life indices, or some small benefits in favour of balloon ablation [30,31].

### 3.2. Intrauterine laser devices

A device using diffused laser energy from an intra-uterine array of three 830-nm diode laser fibres has been developed (ELITT™, Sharplan Laser, Needham, MA, USA) [32]. Two lateral fibres and a single central fibre on a disposable handset are introduced into the uterus and the cavity is illuminated for a treatment time of 7 min. Rates of amenorrhoea of up to 70% at 12 months have been reported [32,33], but larger studies and randomised comparisons with other treatments are awaited.

### 3.3. Multi-electrode radio-frequency ablation

The Vestablate™ (Valleylab, Boulder, USA) [34] system uses radiofrequency thermal energy applied globally within the uterine cavity to desiccate the endometrium. It consists of a polymer balloon covered with 12 monopolar electrodes inflated within the uterine cavity to bring the electrodes into contact with the endometrium for a treatment time of 4–7 min. Non-randomised clinical studies suggest that similar amenorrhoea and success rates to FEAT can be expected [35,36].

### 3.4. Bipolar impedance controlled ablation

Novasure (Novasure, Palo Alto, CA, USA) [37] uses bipolar electrosurgical energy to ablate the endometrium. The device consists of a conductive metallic wire mesh over a triangular frame that is expanded within the uterus. Prior to activation, intra-uterine pressure is measured by the injection of carbon dioxide gas to check for cavity perforation and a vacuum is then produced to ensure close contact with the endometrium [38]. Tissue impedance is measured during a treatment time of about 90 s and the device is switched off when endometrial desiccation has occurred. Randomised trials have shown Novasure to be as effective as rollerball ablation at 12 months [39] and associated with lower intra-operative pain, lower post-operative analgesia requirement [40] and a higher amenorrhoea rate than balloon ablation systems [41].

## 3.5. Hot saline instillation systems

Fluid infused through the cervix at pressures below 70 mm Hg will not spill into the peritoneal cavity [42] and this principle is utilised by hydrothermal ablation devices. In the Hydrotherm Ablator™ (BEI Medical systems, Boston Scientific, Teterboro, NJ, USA [43,44]), 0.9% saline is infused through the inflow channel of a standard 3-mm hysteroscope covered by a 7.8-mm disposable insulating sheath at a pressure of 50 mm Hg. Treatment time is 10 min at an intra-uterine temperature of 90 °C. A multicentre randomised trial comparing the HydroTherm Ablator with rollerball ablation reported similar amenorrhoea rates and improvements in quality of life scores at 12 months [44]. Another device (EnAbl system™, Innerdyne Medical, Sunnyvale, CA, USA [45]) has also been described that repeatedly instills and aspirates saline over 15 min at a pressure of 30 mm Hg through an intra-uterine catheter with a heater, monitoring thermocouple and collapsible cage contained within its tip. Both devices switch off if fluid is lost from the uterine cavity.

## 3.6. Microwave energy

Electromagnetic energy can be used to ablate the uterine cavity (Microwave Endometrial Ablation (MEA™), Microsulis, Portsmouth, UK) [46]. A 9-mm-diameter reusable probe using a microwave frequency of 9.2 GHz, produces heat penetration at its tip to a depth of 6 mm within the uterus. Temperature is indicated on a graphical display and the operator ensures that the probe tip remains within a therapeutic temperature band (75–85 °C) as the probe is moved slowly across the uterine cavity and gradually withdrawn over a typical treatment time of 3 min. Uniquely for a SEAT device, the control unit records treatment profiles for all patients each probe is used for, potentially facilitating the collection of audit data. Randomised trials comparing MEA with endometrial resection [47], its use with local and general anaesthesia [48] and long-term follow-up data on large enough numbers of patients to produce meaningful safety data [49] are available. Amenorrhoea rate of 40% at 12 months and very similar retreatment rates at 3 years to FEAT devices [46,47] have been reported.

## 3.7. Cryo-ablation therapy

A number of gas mixtures and devices have been developed over the last 35 years for endometrial cryoablation [50,51], but it has been difficult to find a gas mixture with a temperature–pressure relationship that permits the use of an applicator small enough to be inserted into the uterine cavity. Recently, an effective device has become commercially available. Her-Choice™ Uterine Cryoablation Therapy™ (Cryogen, San Diego, CA, USA) consists of a cryoprobe and 5 mm diameter disposable sheath with a tip surface temperature of −100 °C that is inserted into the uterus for two freeze–thaw cycles over a total treatment time of about 10 min [52]. Trans-abdominal ultrasound is used to monitor the expansion of the hyperechoic edge of the "ice-ball" of treated tissue. A multicentre randomised trial has shown cryoablation to be similarly effective to rollerball ablation [52,53].

## 3.8. Chemical cautery of the endometrium

Demonstrating that all medical treatments will be re-invented regularly, the transcervical application of trichloroacetic acid (TCA) to the endometrium to chemically cauterise the endometrium has very recently been reported [54], many years after the use of other chemical agents, such as formalin and quinacrine, were suggested [55]. In this clinical study, 95% TCA was applied directly to the endometrium using a cotton-swab applicator on three occasions 1 week apart in 90 women. Over 80% reported a satisfactory reduction in menstrual loss at 6 months.

*3.9. Photodynamic therapy*

The application of 5-aminolevulinic acid (ALA), a photosensitising drug, to the endometrial surface and subsequent light activation via a trans-cervical catheter can be used to produce reactive oxygen intermediates that induce cellular necrosis [56,57]. Early clinical studies of a commercial prototype with a balloon catheter used to keep the ALA within the uterus for 4–6 h prior to the insertion of a reflecting balloon light-diffuser have recently been reported (Medlight, Lausanne, Switzerland) [58].

## 4. Which SEAT to use?

In most developed countries, gynaecologists will have a choice of three or more SEAT devices, but many will work in a setting where they or their hospital can purchase only one type of SEAT. Some devices have only short-term follow-up data available, but most SEAT devices appear to produce similar results: 20–50% of women experience complete amenorrhoea 12 months post-operatively and 80–90% report a reduction in menstrual loss. Individual small trials may show one SEAT to be more effective in producing amenorrhoea than another, but patient satisfaction rates seem to be remarkably very similar for all devices.

Most commercially available SEAT devices have been used successfully with only local anesthesia or sedation [59,60]. What little comparative data of intra-operative and post-operative discomfort that are available suggest that some techniques, such as bipolar impedance controlled ablation and cryo-ablation, may be inherently less painful than other SEAT devices. Some treatments are undeniably faster than others and require varying degrees of cervical dilatation, which will affect how confident clinicians will feel about using each SEAT outside an operating theatre. Versatility is another important consideration and the ability to treat women with a uterus distorted by fibroids is an important advantage that will allow some therapies, such as microwave ablation and hot-saline instillation, to be used to treat a wider range of women than others. Treatment costs are an important consideration, although in an increasingly crowded market, costs per treatment are likely to become very similar for each device. Perhaps the most important consideration is patient safety. Most SEAT devices require the blind insertion of a potent energy source into the uterine cavity and have been developed with the aim of enabling gynecologists with limited hysteroscopic skills to offer ablation therapy. Serious complications associated with uterine perforation will inevitably happen and some devices have attempted to provide ways of recognizing this occurrence before SEAT activation. With appropriate training, individual clinicians should be able to expect a low risk of complications with all currently available devices, but larger follow-up studies and the continued meticulous reporting and analysis of serious complications are needed to rule out the possibility that some devices are less safe than others. A final consideration will be whether the companies producing these devices are able to provide long-term support and product availability: some early SEAT devices have already been withdrawn [61] and it is unlikely that all or even a majority of the devices described above will be commercially available in 5 years' time.

## 5. Will the levonorgestrel intrauterine system replace ablation?

Two important disadvantages of endometrial ablation are its lack of reliable contraceptive effect and the permanent damage it causes to the endometrium, making future pregnancy hazardous [62]. The LNG-IUS (Mirena™ Schering, Berlin, Germany) is not only long-acting, completely reversible and at least as effective a contraceptive as female sterilisation [63,64], it also has a profound effect on menstrual blood loss. With 6–12 months of use, a mean reduction in menstrual blood loss of 70–90% has been reported [65]. Continuance rates for the LNG-IUS when used for menorrhagia are high, but up to 25% of women will request removal because of side effects [65]. A significant minority of women using the LNG-IUS are dissatisfied with an unpredictable and irregular bleeding pattern [65]. Meta-analysis of trials comparing the LNG-IUS with FEAT show that the LNG-IUS is associated with a smaller reduction in blood loss and a lower amenorrhoea rate, although satisfaction rates are very similar [66]. Trials comparing the LNG-IUS with SEAT devices are starting to appear [30,31], but long-term comparisons are not yet available. These studies suggest that ablation leads to less unscheduled bleeding, a higher amenorrhoea rate and fewer subsequent side effects. However, its ease of insertion, contraceptive efficacy and reversibility make the LNG-IUS a very attractive alternative to endometrial ablation, even if it proves to be less effective than SEAT.

These data suggest that, for women who need an effective outpatient treatment for their menorrhagia, the LNG-IUS may be their first choice. For women uncertain about their future fertility plans, it could be their only choice. However, what data are available do not show endometrial ablation to be any less effective than the LNG-IUS. The apparent lack of post-treatment side effects with SEAT devices means that they should not be reserved for women who have found the LNG-IUS unacceptable. It seems entirely reasonable to offer women with a completed family endometrial ablation as an alternative to the levonorgestrel-releasing intra-uterine system.

## 6. Where to from here?

Endometrial ablation has a firmly established and well-evaluated role in the treatment of menorrhagia. Early studies have favourably compared the efficacy, safety and cost of first-generation techniques with hysterectomy. Interestingly, contemporaneous nationally collected data in the UK and the USA suggest that their use has had no impact on hysterectomy rates [67,68] and it has been estimated that, in the late 1990s, fewer than 20,000 endometrial ablations were undertaken annually in the USA, compared with 700,000 hysterectomies [69]. It is possible that this imbalance will change: second-generation devices now mean that it should be possible for all gynaecologists treating women with menorrhagia to offer an effective day-case or outpatient surgical alternative to hysterectomy. It is also possible that these treatments will merely lower the threshold for surgical intervention and, indeed, endometrial ablation increasingly appears to be an alternative to the levonorgestrel-releasing intra-uterine system, rather than hysterectomy [70]. It is unlikely that one ablation device will prove to be substantially more effective than any other, but all have the potential to cause serious harm: individual gynaecologists or clinics will need to decide which device(s) they should purchase and ensure that the operators are appropriately trained in their use. Professional bodies will need to ensure that robust training programmes are available and mechanisms for the collection of reliable safety and long-term outcome data exist.

## Acknowledgements

The author has never received any financial or non-financial gift, grant or aid from any of the companies that have developed or market the devices described in this article.

## References

[1] M.H. Goldrath, T.A. Fuller, S. Segal, Laser photovaporisation of the endometrium for the treatment of menorrhagia, Am. J. Obstet. Gynecol. 140 (1981) 14–19.
[2] A.H. DeCherney, M.P. Diamond, G. Lavy, Endometrial ablation for intractable uterine bleeding: hysteroscopic resection, Obstet. Gynecol. 70 (1987) 668–670.
[3] T.G. Vancaillie, Electrocoagulation of the endometrium with the ball-end resectoscope, Obstet. Gynecol. 74 (1989) 425–427.
[4] H. O'Connor, A. Magos, Endometrial resection for the treatment of menorrhagia, New Engl. J. Med. 335 (1996) 151–156.
[5] G. Phillips, P.F. Chein, R. Garry, Risk of hysterectomy after 1000 consecutive laser ablations, Br. J. Obstet. Gynaecol. 105 (1998) 897–903.
[6] W.R. Meyer, et al., Thermal balloon and rollerball ablation to treat menorrhagia: a multicentre comparison, Obstet. Gynecol. 92 (1998) 98–103.
[7] S. Bhattacharya, et al., A pragmatic randomised comparison of transcervical resection of the endometrium with endometrial laser ablation for the treatment of menorrhagia, Br. J. Obstet. Gynaecol. 104 (1997) 601–607.
[8] Royal College of Obstetricians and Gynaecologists, Guidelines: the initial management of menorrhagia, RCOG, London, 1999.
[9] K.G. Cooper, D.E. Parkin, A.M. Garrat, A.M. Grant, Two year follow up of women randomised to medical management or transcervical resection of the endometrium for heavy menstrual loss: clinical and quality of life outcomes, Br. J. Obstet. Gynaecol. 106 (1997) 258–265.
[10] P.G. Crosignani, P. Vercellini, P. Mosconi, Levonorgestrel-releasing intrauterine device versus hysteroscopic endometrial resection in the treatment of dysfunctional uterine bleeding, Obstet. Gynecol. 90 (1997) 257–263.
[11] O. Istre, B. Trolle, Treatment of menorrhagia with the levonorgestrel intrauterine system versus endometrial resection, Fertil. Steril. 76 (2001) 304–309.
[12] N. Dwyer, J. Hutton, G.M. Stirrat, Randomised controlled trial comparing endometrial resection with abdominal hysterectomy for treatment of menorrhagia, Br. J. Obstet. Gynaecol. 100 (1993) 237–243.
[13] H. O'Connor, et al., Medical research council randomised trial comparing endometrial resection with abdominal hysterectomy for treatment of menorrhagia, Br. Med. J. 349 (1997) 897–901.
[14] Aberdeen Endometrial Ablation Trials Group, A randomised trial of endometrial ablation versus hysterectomy for the treatment of dysfunctional uterine bleeding: outcomes at four years, Br. J. Obstet. Gynaecol. 106 (1999) 360–366.
[15] M.J. Schulper, et al., Randomised trial comparing hysterectomy and transcervical endometrial resection: effect on health related quality of life and costs two years after surgery, Br. J. Obstet. Gynaecol. 103 (1996) 142–149.
[16] V.H. Boujida, et al., Five-year follow-up of endometrial ablation: endometrial coagulation versus endometrial resection, Obstet. Gynecol. 99 (2002) 988–992.
[17] R. Comino, R. Torrejon, I. Sanchez-Ortega, Long-term results of endometrial ablation-resection, J. Am. Assoc. Gynecol. Laparosc. 9 (2002) 268–271.
[18] M. Shankar, N.J. Naftalin, N. Taub, The long-term effectiveness of endometrial laser ablation: a survival analysis, Eur. J. Obstet., Gynecol. Reprod. Biol. 108 (2002) 75–79.

[19] S.C. Nicholson, et al., Endometrial resection in Oxford: the first 500 cases—a five year follow up, J. Obstet. Gynaecol. 15 (1995) 38–43.
[20] C. Overton, J. Hargreaves, M. Maresh, A national survey of the complications of endometrial destruction for menstrual disorders: the MISTLETOE study, Br. J. Obstet. Gynaecol. 104 (1997) 1351–1359.
[21] R. Garry, Endometrial ablation and resection: validation of a new surgical concept, Br. J. Obstet. Gynaecol. 104 (1997).
[22] R.S. Neuwirth, et al., The endometrial ablator: a new instrument, Obstet. Gynecol. 83 (1994) 792–796.
[23] J.A. Hawe, et al., Cavaterm thermal balloon ablation for the treatment of menorrhagia, Br. J. Obstet. Gynaecol. 106 (1999) 1143–1148.
[24] W.R. Meyer, et al., Thermal balloon and rollerball ablation to treat menorrhagia: a multicenter comparison, Obstet. Gynecol. 92 (1998) 98–103.
[25] P.S. Mangeshikar, A. Kapur, D.B. Yackel, Endometrial ablation with a new thermal balloon system, J. Am. Assoc. Gynecol. Laparosc. 10 (2003) 27–32.
[26] F.D. Loffer, Three-year comparison of thermal balloon and rollerball ablation in the treatment of menorrhagia, J. Am. Assoc. Gynecol. Laparosc. 8 (2001) 48–54.
[27] J. Hawe, et al., A randomised controlled trial comparing the Cavaterm endometrial ablation system with the Nd: YAG laser for the treatment of dysfunctional uterine bleeding, Br. J. Obstet. Gynaecol. 110 (2003) 350–357.
[28] W.R. Meyer, et al., Thermal balloon and rollerball ablation to treat menorrhagia: a multicentre comparison, Obstet. Gynecol. 92 (1998) 98–103.
[29] K.K. Vihko, R. Raitala, E. Taina, Endometrial thermoablation for the treatment of menorrhagia: comparison of two methods in outpatient setting, Acta Obstet. Gynecol. Scand. 82 (2003) 269–274.
[30] M. Soysal, S. Soysal, S. Ozer, A randomized controlled trial of levonorgestrel releasing IUD and thermal balloon ablation in the treatment of menorrhagia, Zentralb. Gynakol. (2002) 213–219.
[31] J. Barrington, A. Arunkalaivanan, M. Abdel-Fattah, Comparison between the levonorgestrel intrauterine system (LNG-IUS) and thermal balloon ablation in the Treatment of menorrhagia, Eur. J. Obstet., Gynecol., Reprod. Biol. 108 (2003) 72–74.
[32] J. Donnez, et al., Endometrial laser intrauterine thermotherapy: the first series of 100 patients observed for 1 year, Fertil. Steril. 74 (2000) 791–796.
[33] K. Jones, et al., Endometrial laser intrauterine thermotherapy for the treatment of dysfunctional uterine bleeding: the first British experience, Br. J. Obstet. Gynaecol. 108 (2001) 749–753.
[34] R. Sonderstrom, P. Brooks, S. Corson, Endometrial ablation using a distensible multielectrode balloon, J. Am. Assoc. Gynecol. Laparosc. 3 (1996) 403–407.
[35] S.L. Corson, et al., One-year results of the Vesta system for endometrial ablation, J. Am. Assoc. Gynecol. Laparosc. 7 (2000) 489–497.
[36] K.D. Jones, L. Spangler, C. Sutton, Endometrial ablation using a distensible multielectrode balloon: a long-term follow up report, Gynaecol. Endosc. 11 (2002) 43–45.
[37] J. Cooper, et al., A randomized, multicenter trial of safety and efficacy of the NovaSure system in the treatment of menorrhagia, J. Am. Assoc. Gynecol. Laparosc. 9 (2002) 418–428.
[38] US Food and Drug Administration Center of Devices and Radiologic Health, Summary of safety and effectiveness data: novaSure impedance controlled endometrial ablation system (2001) P010013.
[39] J. Cooper, et al., A randomized, multicenter trial of safety and efficacy of the NovaSure system in the treatment of menorrhagia, J. Am. Assoc. Gynecol. Laparosc. 9 (2002) 418–428.
[40] P. Laberge, et al., Assessment and comparison of intra-operative and post-operative pain associated with Novasure and Thermachoice endometrial ablation systems, J. Am. Assoc. Gynecol. Laparosc. 10 (2003) 223–232.
[41] J. Abbott, et al., A double-blind randomized trial comparing the Cavaterm and NovaSure endometrial ablation systems for the treatment of dysfunctional uterine bleeding, Fertil. Steril. 80 (2003) 203–208.
[42] V. Baker, G. Adamson, Threshold intrauterine perfusion pressures for intraperitoneal spill during hydrotubation and correlation with tubal adhesive disease, Fertil. Steril. 64 (1995) 1066–1069.
[43] S. Corson, A multicenter evaluation of endometrial ablation by Hydro ThermAblator and rollerball for treatment of menorrhagia, J. Am. Assoc. Gynecol. Laparosc. 8 (2001) 359–367.
[44] US Food and Drug Administration, Center of Devices and Radiologic Health. Summary of Safety and

Effectiveness Data: HydroThermAblator Endometrial Ablation System, BEI Medical Systems Company Rockville, MD: 2001. PMA 000040.
[45] H. Bustos-Lopez, et al., Endometrial Ablation with the EnAbl System, J. Am. Assoc. Gynecol. Laparosc. 3 (1996) S5.
[46] D. Hodgson, et al., Microwave endometrial ablation: development, clinical trials and outcomes at three years, Br. J. Obstet. Gynaecol. 106 (1999) 684–694.
[47] C. Bain, K. Cooper, D. Parkin, Microwave endometrial ablation versus endometrial resection: a randomised controlled trial, Obstet. Gynecol. 99 (2002) 983–987.
[48] S. Wallage, et al., A randomised trial comparing local versus general anaesthesia for microwave endometrial ablation, Br. J. Obstet. Gynaecol. 110 (2003) 779–807.
[49] D. Parkin, Microwave endometrial ablation (MEA™: a safe technique? Complication data from a prospective series of 1400 cases, Gynaecol. Endosc. 9 (2000) 385–388.
[50] W. Cahan, Cryosurgery of the uterine cavity, Am. J. Obstet. Gynecol. 99 (1967) 138–153.
[51] W. Droegemueller, B.E. Greer, E.L. Makowski, Preliminary observations of cryocoagulation of the endometrium, Am. J. Obstet. Gynecol. 107 (1970) 958–961.
[52] US Food and Drug Administration Center for Devices and Radiologic Health, Summary of Safety and Effectiveness Data: Her Option Uterine Cryoablation Therapy System, Cryogen Rockville. PMA P000032b, 2001.
[53] J. Dobak, J. Williams, Extirpated uterine endometrial cryoablation with ultrasound visualization, J. Am. Assoc. Gynecol. Laparosc. 7 (2000) 95–101.
[54] T. Kucukozkan, et al., Chemical ablation of the endometrium with trichloracetic acid, Int. J. Gynecol. Obstet. 84 (2004) 41–46.
[55] J. Schenker, W. Polishuk, Regeneration of rabbit endometrium following instillation of chemical agents, Gynecol. Invest., (1973) 1–13.
[56] P. Wyss, L.O. Svaasand, Y. Tadir, Photomedicine of the endometrium: experimental concepts, Hum. Reprod. 10 (1995) 221–226.
[57] M. Gannon, S. Brown, Photodynamic therapy and its applications in gynaecology, Br. J. Obstet. Gynaecol. 106 (1999) 1246–1254.
[58] P. Wyss, et al., Photodynamic endometrial ablation: a morphological study, Lasers Surg. Med. 32 (2003) 305–309.
[59] H. Fernandez, S. Capella, F. Audibert, Uterine balloon therapy under local anaesthesia for the treatment of menorrhagia: a pilot study, Hum. Reprod. 12 (1997) 2511–2514.
[60] L. Byrd, K. Chia, Balloon ablation: is this an outpatient procedure? J. Obstet. Gynaecol. 22 (2002) 205–208.
[61] R. Thijssen, Radiofrequency-induced endometrial ablation: an update, Br. J. Obstet. Gynaecol. 104 (1997) 608–613.
[62] T. El-Toukhy, M. Hefni, Pregnancy after hydrothermal endometrial ablation and laparoscopic sterilisation, Eur. J. Obstet., Gynecol., Reprod. Biol. 106 (2003) 222–224.
[63] T. Luukkainen, et al., Five years' experience with levonorgestrel-releasing IUDs, Contraception 33 (1986) 139–148.
[64] H. Peterson, et al., The risk of pregnancy after tubal sterilization: findings from the U.S. Collaborative Review of Sterilization, Am. J. Obstet. Gynecol. 174 (1996) 1161–1168.
[65] A. Stewart, et al., The effectiveness of the levonorgestrel-releasing intrauterine system in menorrhagia: a systematic review, Br. J. Obstet. Gynaecol. 108 (2001) 74–86.
[66] A. Lethaby, I. Cooke, M. Rees, Progesterone/progestogen releasing intrauterine systems versus either placebo or any other medication for heavy menstrual bleeding. Cochrane Database Systematic Reviews 2000, CD002126.
[67] C. Farquhar, C. Steiner, Hysterectomy rates in the United States 1990–1997, Obstet. Gynecol. 99 (2002) 229–234.
[68] S. Bridgeman, K. Dunn, Has endometrial ablation replaced hysterectomy for the treatment of dysfunctional uterine bleeding? National figures, Br. J. Obstet. Gynaecol. 106 (1999) 531–534.
[69] R. Garry, Evidence and techniques in endometrial ablation: consensus, Gynaecol. Endosc. 11 (2002) 5–17.
[70] F. Nagele, T. Rublinger, A. Magos, Why do women choose endometrial ablation rather than hysterectomy, Fertil. Steril. 69 (1998) 1063–1066.

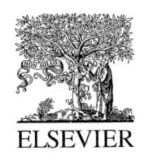

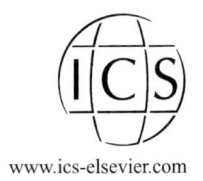

# Adolescent contraception

## Dan Apter*, Raisa Cacciatore, Elina Hermanson

*The Sexual Health Clinic, Family Federation of Finland, Kalevankatu 16, POB 849, 00101 Helsinki, Finland*

**Abstract.** Sexual health for adolescents is based on three components: recognizing sexual rights, sexuality education and counseling, and confidential, high quality services. Contraception needs to include prevention of both STIs and pregnancies. The main options for adolescents are condoms, backed up by emergency contraception, and oral contraceptives in a longer, mutually monogamous relationship. Condoms and hormonal contraception together can be well recommended for adolescents. Condom use should not be stopped before it is reasonably certain that the partner is STI-negative. Other alternatives can be considered in special cases. Improved contraceptive methods do not automatically lead to reduced numbers of adolescent abortions. The prevention of unintended adolescent pregnancies requires four elements: a desire to use protection, a good contraceptive method, ability to obtain the contraceptive method, and ability to use it. All these components are important and if one is missing, contraception will fail. In the developed countries, we have good contraceptive methods, but improvements are still needed in the other components. When adolescent sexuality is not condemned, but sexuality education and sexual health services instead are provided, it is possible to profoundly improve adolescent sexual health at comparatively small costs. Each year new groups of young people mature, requiring new efforts. © 2004 Published by Elsevier B.V.

*Keywords:* Condoms; Hormonal contraception; Sexuality education; Sexual health services; STI

## 1. Introduction

Sexual development brings along dreams and wishes of a new kind of relationship, an opportunity to intimate closeness with another person. A maturing young person is in many aspects lonely and uncertain, and thus vulnerable. She needs adult support. A growth milieu supporting the self-esteem of the young person, together with adequate and sufficient sexual education, helps her to make choices to maintain and protect her sexual health [1]. Sexual health for adolescents is based on three fundamental components: (1) recognizing sexual rights, (2) sexuality education and counseling, and (3) confidential high quality services. These components all need to be considered together. A holistic approach to contraceptive provision involves considering the individual's overall sexual and reproductive health needs. By informing adolescents of potential risks, benefits and uncertainties in

---

\* Corresponding author. Tel.: +358-9-61-62-22-26; fax: +358-9-645-017.
*E-mail address:* dan.apter@vaestoliitto.fi (D. Apter).

0531-5131/ © 2004 Published by Elsevier B.V.
doi:10.1016/j.ics.2004.01.072

language they can understand, clinicians can enable women to reach their own contraceptive choices. Access for women can be enhanced by service innovations, such as nurse prescribing. Several means of prevention need to be considered:

1. Prevention of pregnancy—use of contraceptive methods;
2. Prevention of STIs—use of condoms and avoiding risks;
3. Prevention of bad feelings/desperation—use of sense, consideration and avoiding risk taking.

## 2. Sexual behavior

National surveys conducted in Europe show differences in the transition to younger age at first intercourse. This transition first started in the Nordic countries, and followed in most other Western European countries. The mean age of women at their first intercourse decreased after the 1960s by 2 to 3 years. During the 1980s, this age remained rather stable. In some countries, a further decrease occurred in the 1990s. A similar decrease started in Central and Eastern Europe one generation later (20–30 years). Mean ages at first intercourse are 17 to 18 years for women and men in western Europe, whereas it is reported to be around 20 for women in eastern European countries, as summarized by Bajos et al. [2].

## 3. Sexuality education

Knowledge about various contraceptive methods and a desire to use protection is essential for successful contraception. Sexuality education can take place at three levels. The most general one reaching large populations is information campaigns through, for example, the mass media. These might provide information about a new contraceptive method or draw attention to a problem, but are not likely to profoundly change behavior. Adolescents obtain much information through mass media. The message should be tailored in a suitable form. An example of this was our leaflet to promote condom use among boys. A cartoon character told Business news: "Banks do not hand out millions to just anyone. Why would you? A condom makes sure you will have the exclusive right to your sperm until you want to merge it with an egg cell you consider worth the fusion." (full text in http://www.seksuaaliterveys.org/kondomikampanja/index_eng.html). Another

Table 1
National adolescent friendly clinic initiative, with key elements identified as important

(1) Management
(2) Client rights
(3) Access
(4) Environment of care
(5) Drugs, supplies, equipment
(6) Trained staff
(7) Information, education, communication
(8) Client assessment
(9) Individualized client care
(10) Continuity of care

According to Reproductive Health Research Organization, South Africa; http://www.rhru.co.za.

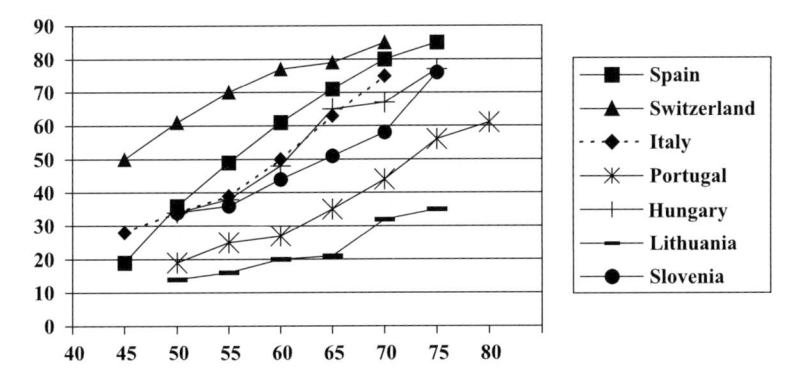

Fig. 1. Percentage use of contraception at first intercourse in relation to year of birth 1945–1980. From Ref. [2].

form is the sexuality education typically given in schools or other social situations, where a group of young persons of similar age listens to lectures, views educational material and can discuss the matters. The different developmental stages of the pupils require a lot from the teacher. Some might have reached a developmental stage already beyond the information given, and others in the group are perhaps not yet interested. For all it is important to realize that sexual issues can be discussed, including personal feelings. The third approach is counseling, which occurs in direct interpersonal relationship and is based on recognizing individual needs. Although it is time-consuming and thus expensive, counseling can be highly effective [3] as it is easy to individualize and might include very sensitive areas. It needs to be highly confident and free of oppressing judgments. The closer sexuality education programs and sexual health services work together, the better are the results.

## 4. Sexual health services

Services for adolescents can be provided in various settings, as long as certain basic principles are observed (Table 1). The needs of adolescents differ from those of adults. High quality care of adolescents calls for special clinics. The clinic should have a youth-friendly atmosphere [1], where young people can feel welcome and comfortable. Unquestionable confidentiality is important. The providers must not moralize and judge the adolescents, but treat adolescents with respect indicating that young people are important. Most important is strengthening of self-esteem, contributing to a feeling that their body and their sexuality are valuable and need to be protected. In that way adolescents learn to respect and take care of themselves and others. Services should be available at an affordable price, which preferably means free of charge. The threshold to come to the clinic should be low. The adolescents

Table 2
Recommended choices of contraception for adolescents

(1) Condom+emergency contraception
(2) Oral contraceptives+condom
(3) Oral contraceptives or other hormonal contraception

Table 3
Answers by female students in Finland to the question "What contraceptive method did you use at your most recent intercourse?" and the percentage of having had intercourse, by school grade

| Grade | Secondary school | | High school | |
| --- | --- | --- | --- | --- |
| | Grade 8 | Grade 9 | 1 | 2 |
| Age range | 14–15 | 15–16 | 16–17 | 17–18 |
| Nothing % | 21 | 17 | 10 | 8 |
| Condom % | 60 | 50 | 50 | 42 |
| OC % | 11 | 25 | 33 | 42 |
| Condom and OC % | 7 | 7 | 6 | 7 |
| Other method % | 1 | 1 | 1 | 1 |
| Percentage of all having had intercourse | 17 | 33 | 41 | 57 |

From the School Health Study in 2002, http://www.stakes.fi/kouluterveys.

should be able to drop in or get an appointment without having to wait long. In many respects, school health care may provide an easy-access service, which can fulfill the requirements for high standard adolescent care.

## 5. Use of contraception among adolescents

Contraceptive prevalence and method used varies markedly [4]. With increasing availability, the percentages that have used some contraception at first intercourse have increased (Fig. 1).

Using a condom is the most common first contraceptive method. With increasing age and entering a more stable relationship, adolescents switch to hormonal methods, mainly the combined oral contraceptives (COC). Double contraception, condom for protection against STIs and COC for better protection against pregnancies, is recommended (Table 2), but except in the Netherlands, is not largely used. The contraceptive method used during the most recent intercourse is given in Table 3 for Finland and Table 4 for some other European countries.

The figures for abortion generally show an inverse correlation to contraceptive use. Where reliable modern methods are widely used, the need for abortion is low. In Russia, the majority of pregnancies end in abortion [5], which remains the primary method of birth control.

Table 4
Contraceptive use (%) among adolescents in some European countries[a]

| Country | Armenia | Czech. Rep. | Romania | Slovenia | Netherlands | Spain | Hungary |
| --- | --- | --- | --- | --- | --- | --- | --- |
| Year | 2000 | 1997 | 1999 | 1994 | 1993 | 1995 | 1992–1993 |
| Age | 15–19 | 15–19 | 15–19 | 15–19 | 18–19 | 18–19 | 18–19 |
| Pill | 2.1 | 40.7 | 8.2 | 27.1 | 88.0 | 44.4 | 48.1 |
| IUD | 2.8 | 5.5 | 1.0 | 0.0 | 0.0 | 7.6 | 3.7 |
| Condom | 2.6 | 0.0 | 1.9 | 8.0 | 0.0 | 12.1 | 11.1 |
| Withdrawal | 7.5 | 3.5 | 31.1 | 20.3 | | 21.6 | 11.1 |
| Other method | 10.5 | 3.8 | 4.2 | 0.0 | | 0.0 | 0.0 |
| No contraceptive method used | 74.5 | | | 8.1 | 7.0 | 7.1 | 3.7 |

[a] Sources: FFS, CDC and DHS surveys as summarized in Ref. [2].

## 6. Various contraceptive methods

The adolescent chooses to use the method she is most comfortable with, that suits her particular life situation at the moment, and that she knows well based on sufficient counseling.

### 6.1. Condom

Condoms are a well-suited contraception for adolescents, because they prevent pregnancies and diminish the risks of STIs and cervical cytology changes. Young people know these benefits, but are still not using condoms regularly. Many circumstances influence condom use, like the price, difficulties in buying them, unplanned sexual experiences, alcohol and drug using and the willingness to take risks. The use of a condom may inconveniently interrupt the sexual act, because the placement of it on a penis must occur after erection has taken place, but before intercourse begins. Street survival strategies, including sexual activity for money and drug use, put street youths in situations at considerable risk for HIV-infection [6]. Use of the female condom has remained rather limited in most countries.

### 6.2. Emergency contraception

Emergency contraception, or postcoital contraception, is a method used after intercourse to prevent the beginning of a pregnancy, thus it is not related to abortion. Levonorgestrel only (1.5 mg) is replacing the Yuzpe method of a high-dose of ethinylestradiol (200 µg) combined with levonorgestrel (1 mg), as it has less side effects and higher efficacy [7]. A recent WHO study [8] showed that the two levonorgestrel tablets could be taken together as a single dose making the use easier. Increasing the interval from intercourse to emergency contraception use lowers the efficacy [9], as it should be taken as soon as possible, and after 72 h its efficacy is questionable. There are no contraindications to levonorgestrel emergency contraception, and it is now available without prescription in most European countries. According to statistics in Finland, removing the need of prescription for emergency contraception increased its use and decreased the number of abortions among 15–19-year-old girls by 10% within 6 months (Apter, manuscript in preparation).

Emergency contraception is a good addition to condom use since if the condom breaks, there is still a further possibility to prevent pregnancy. However, the preventive efficacy of emergency contraception should not be overestimated, it is much lower than the regularly used COC.

### 6.3. Combined oral contraception

COC is widely used in adolescence. It is useful in a stable relationship. However, this can mean anything between 1 week to 1 year, and condom use should not be stopped before it is reasonably certain that the partner is STI-negative. Condoms and COC together can be well recommended for adolescents.

What should a clinician assess before prescribing COC? The Faculty of Family Planning and Reproductive Health Care Guidance [10] provided evidence-based recommendations and good practice points for clinicians advising women considering their *first prescription* of COC.

Clinical history taking and examination allows an assessment of medical eligibility for COC use. In this context, the clinical history should include medical, sexual (to assess risk of STI), family and drug history, as well as details of reproductive health and previous contraceptive use. With this information, clinicians can advise women appropriately on their contraceptive options, taking account of both medical and social factors. It should be noted that breast examination, pelvic and genital examination, cervical cytology screening and routine laboratory tests do not contribute substantially to COC safety, and are therefore not recommended routinely before starting COC. Particularly, fear of the pelvic examination might reduce the likelihood of young adolescents seeking services. Blood pressure measurement is essential and mandatory in all women prior to COC use. Women with a BP measurement consistently over 140 mm Hg systolic and/or 90 mm Hg diastolic should be advised against the use of the COC. Ideally, the risk of STI should be assessed and opportunistic Chlamydia testing offered when appropriate. For females with a family history of venous thromboembolism in a first degree relative under the age of 45 years, who, having considered other contraceptive methods, still wish to use COC, a thrombophilia screen should be performed.

COC can be used from menarche onwards unless there are medical or other contraindications. Contraindications are basically the same for adolescents as for adults [11]. Women with a body mass index above 30 should be counseled regarding an increased risk for thromboembolism. Focal migraine is associated with risks of COC use that outweigh the benefits. Epilepsy medication and other liver enzyme-inducing drugs are not very uncommon, and reduce the efficacy of hormonal contraception.

There are several noncontraceptive benefits for adolescents using COC. They often have irregular cycles, and with COC the bleedings come regularly. A randomized, double-blind, placebo-controlled trial showed a significant reduction in dysmenorrhea with COC [12]. The amount of bleeding usually decreases. Acne, a common condition in adolescence, significantly improves with COC (summarized in Ref. [10]). Some get help for PMS-like symptoms [13].

*6.4. New routes*

New ways of administering combined estrogen–progestin preparations are now available. The contraceptive vaginal ring is a good alternative for those who have difficulties in taking tablets daily, as it remains 3 weeks in place in the vagina. It has particularly good bleeding control [14], and in our practice has worked well for adolescents. The dermal patch is another new alternative, which is changed weekly.

*6.5. Progestin only contraception*

The progestin only pill needs to be taken more accurately than COC, and is frequently associated with poor bleeding control [15]. Therefore, its use is limited to contraindications/problems with other methods.

Adolescents have extensively used implants. First, the Norplant six implant system, and later Jadelle with two and Implanon with one implant. Contraceptive efficacy is excellent, but bleeding control very variable. About a third are amenorrheic, which can be seen as an additional benefit.

The progestin-releasing IUD, such as Mirena, is most efficient in reducing the amount of bleeding and menstrual pain. In adolescents whose uterine size approaches that of adults, it can be well inserted. With appropriate counseling, the amenorrheic effect is seen as an important benefit.

Hormonal injections are commonly used in some countries, but not much in Europe. Using Medroxyprogesterone every 3 months has been related to a tendency of weight increase and some concerns of bone mineral [16,17].

### 6.6. Intrauterine device

The ideal IUD user is a woman who has at least one child and who has a normal menstrual period (not painful and not abundant). The risk of pelvic inflammatory disease is the most important problem in young women. It is important to preserve the fertility of young women, who may change partners frequently. Thus, the IUD is not the contraceptive method of choice for adolescents [18]. The progestin-releasing IUD can be used to treat abundant bleeding, and it offers some protection against pelvic inflammatory disease.

### 6.7. Diaphragms and spermicides

Diaphragms, cervical caps, spermicides, sponges and vaginal condoms are not the first choice for adolescents because they often are uncomfortable and difficult to use, so the application is not consistent and correct [19]. They might also increase the incidence of vaginitis, because the removal may be delayed after intercourse and postcoital hygiene is variable. Contraceptive efficacy is rather low [15], but for special situations these methods need to be available.

### 6.8. Periodic abstinence and withdrawal

Adolescents often have very irregular menstrual cycles making rhythm methods unreliable, and it is difficult also for adults to have systematical abstinence. For very young adolescents, it is reasonable to encourage abstinence, and to emphasize the emotional aspects of a relationship and the desirability of sometimes saying "no" [20].

Withdrawal is a widely used method among adolescents, but it mainly prevents sexual pleasure.

## 7. Is it possible to affect adolescent sexual health?

The level of sexual health of young people is relatively good in the Nordic countries in international comparisons. Indicators of this are the relatively low numbers of unintended pregnancies, abortions and sexually transmitted diseases. Today's condition has evolved over a long span of time. Sixty years ago the situation in Finland was quite different: illegal abortions and STIs were common, sex education was nonexistent and attitudes towards sexuality and contraception were negative. The overall development in society—gender equality, equal education opportunities for boys and girls, development of the health care system, positive attitude changes of the state and Church—have all made it possible to reach the present situation through extended provision of sufficient and reliable sexuality education, confidential services and a wide selection of contraceptive methods.

However, continuous efforts are needed. In the 1990s, due to economical depression and other structural changes in Finland, preventive services for adolescents were severely cut together with reductions in sexuality education. This was followed by increases in adolescent abortions and chlamydia infections.

A recent example of increasing resources for adolescent sexual health followed by a profound decrease in the number of unintended pregnancies and adolescent abortion is Slovenia. Internationally, much remains to be done. In KwaZulu-Natal Province of South Africa, the incidence of HIV, unintended pregnancies and sexual violence against adolescent girls are very high, but the political leadership is still confused. In USA, the level of teenage deliveries and abortions remain high. The US administration, which has blocked payments to the United Nations Population Fund, has tried to make its "abstinence-only" sex education part of international policy, with harmful results.

The Nordic experience shows that with persistent and committed actions many problems can be prevented and solved. It requires political commitment.

## 8. Conclusions

For adolescents, contraception always needs to include the prevention of STIs, as well as pregnancies. Also, the prevention of early sexual activity, i.e. before psychological maturation, is important. Counseling should include all areas of risk taking behavior: alcohol and drug use, smoking, traveling alone, and situations easily leading to abuse. It is important to teach self-respect and responsibility. The contraceptive choice should be individualized, considering all circumstances. The main options for adolescents are condoms, backed up by emergency contraception and oral contraceptive pills in a longer, mutually monogamous relationship. Other alternatives can be considered in special cases.

Improved contraceptive methods do not automatically lead to reduced numbers of adolescent abortions. The prevention of unintended adolescent pregnancies requires four elements: a desire to use protection, a good contraceptive method, ability to obtain the contraceptive method, and ability to use it. All these components are important, and if one is missing, contraception will fail. In developed countries, we have good contraceptive methods, but improvements are still needed in all the other components. Motivation to take care of oneself and others' growths is based on many interactions, and to that we could all contribute as parents, teachers and health care providers.

When adolescent sexuality is not condemned, but sexuality education and sexual health services instead are provided, it is possible to profoundly improve adolescent sexual health with comparatively small costs; but each year new groups of young people mature, requiring new efforts. Education, counseling and services are all needed. If the resources are cut too much or not given, negative effects are soon evident.

## References

[1] P. McIntyre (Ed.), Adolescent Friendly Health Services—An Agenda for Change, WHO, Geneva, 2002.
[2] N. Bajos, A. Guillaume, O. Kontula, Reproductive health behaviour of young Europeans, Population Studies, No. 42, vol. 1, Council of Europe Publishing, Strasbourg, 2003.

[3] B.T. Johnson, M.P. Carey, K.L. Marsh, K.D. Levin, L.A.J. Scott-Sheldon, Interventions to reduce sexual risk for the human immunodeficiency virus in adolescents, 1985–2000: a research synthesis, Arch. Pediatr. Adolesc. Med. 157 (2003) 381–388.
[4] UNFPA, State of the World Population, Making 1 Billion Count: Investing in Adolescents' Health and Rights, United Nations Population Fund, New York, 2003, www.unfpa.org.
[5] World Health Organization, Regional Office for Europe, Copenhagen, From abortion to contraception. Conference report, 1990.
[6] G.C. Luna, Street youth: adaptation and survival in the AIDS decade, J. Adolesc. Health 12 (1991) 511–514.
[7] WHO Task Force on Postovulatory Methods of Fertility Regulation, Randomized controlled trial of levonorgestrel versus the Yuzpe regimen of combined oral contraceptives for emergency contraception, Lancet 352 (1998) 428–433.
[8] H. von Hertzen, G. Piaggio, J. Ding, et al, Low dose mifepristone and two regimens of levonorgestrel for emergency contraception: a WHO multicentre randomised trial, Lancet 360 (2002) 1803–1810.
[9] G. Piaggio, H. von Hertzen, D.A. Grimes, P.F.A. Van Look, Timing of emergency contraception with levonorgestrel or the Yuzpe regimen, Lancet 353 (1999) 721–722.
[10] Faculty of Family Planning C.E.U. Reproductive Health Care, FFPRHC Guidance: first prescription of combined oral contraception, J. Fam. Plan. Reprod. Health Care 29 (2003) 209–222.
[11] World Health Organization, Medical Eligibility Criteria for Contraceptive Use, WHO, Geneva, 2000.
[12] S. Hendrix, N. Alexander, Primary dysmenorrhea treatment with a desogestrel-containing low dose oral contraceptive, Contraception 66 (2002) 393–399.
[13] D. Apter, A. Borsos, W. Baumgartner, et al, Effect of an oral contraceptive containing drospirenone and ethinylestradiol on general well-being and fluid-related symptoms, Eur. J. Contracpt. Reprod. Health Care 8 (2003) 37–51.
[14] T.O. Dieben, F.J. Roumen, D. Apter, Efficacy, cycle control, and user acceptability of a novel combined contraceptive vaginal ring, Obstet. Gynecol. 100 (2002) 585–593.
[15] R.A. Hatcher, W. Rinehart, R. Blackburn, J.S. Geller, J.D. Shelton, The Essentials of Contraceptive Technology, Population Information Program, Baltimore, 2003.
[16] C. Westhoff, Bone mineral density and DMPA, J. Reprod. Med. 47 (2002) 795–799.
[17] D. Scholes, A.Z. LaCroix, L.E. Ichikawa, W.E. Barlow, S.M. Ott, Injectable hormone contraception and bone density: results from a prospective study, Epidemiology 13 (2002) 581–587.
[18] R. Cacciatore, D. Apter, Alternative contraceptive choices for the adolescent, Fertil. Control Rev. 2 (1993) 7–10.
[19] R. Hatcher, D. Warner, New condoms for men and women, diaphragms, cervical caps, and spermicides: overcoming barriers to barriers and spermicides, Curr. Opin. Obstet. Gynecol. 4 (1992) 513–521.
[20] C. Donovan, Adolescent sexuality: better, more accessible sex education is needed, Br. Med. J. 300 (1990) 1026–1027.

ized controlled trials (RCTs). Six trials have been published with respect to medical treatment; two reported surgical treatment. The overall pregnancy rate in the (untreated) controls of all eight RCTs together was 28% [95% confidence interval (CI), 24–33%]. This rate does not differ significantly from the one reported by Taylor and Collins in their review of 20 studies of 2026 couples with essentially unexplained subfertility of 33% (95% CI, 31–35%). Two RCTs studied the effect on pregnancy rates of surgical resection or ablation of the endometriosis lesions. Neither study allowed for estimating the effect of ablation of lesions on pregnancy chances since, in both studies, apart from ablation of the lesions, lysis of adhesions was also performed. The larger of the two studies did show an overall benefit from surgical removal of the endometriotic implants; the smaller one did not. We conclude that surgery for minimal or mild endometriosis might modestly enhance fecundity in women with otherwise unexplained subfertility, but it cannot be excluded that this improvement is due to removal of adhesions rather than implants. © 2004 Published by Elsevier B.V.

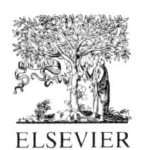

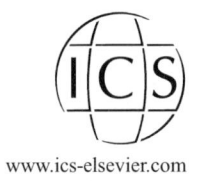

# Evidence-based reproductive surgery: endometriosis

Johannes L.H. Evers*

*Deparment of Obstetrics and Gynaecology, Research Institute GROW, Maastricht University and Academisch Ziekenhuis Maastricht, P. Debyelaan 25, PO Box 5800, Maastricht 6202 AZ, The Netherlands*

**Abstract.** In order to answer the question as to whether surgical removal of implants should be performed at all, one should first address the question as to whether endometriosis per se affects fertility. For this, one could study spontaneous pregnancy rates in untreated control subjects in randomized controlled trials (RCTs). Six trials have been published with respect to medical treatment; two reported surgical treatment. The overall pregnancy rate in the (untreated) controls of all eight RCTs together was 28% [95% confidence interval (CI), 24–33%]. This rate does not differ significantly from the one reported by Taylor and Collins in their review of 20 studies of 2026 couples with essentially unexplained subfertility of 33% (95% CI, 31–35%). Two RCTs studied the effect on pregnancy rates of surgical resection or ablation of the endometriosis lesions. Neither study allowed for estimating the effect of ablation of lesions on pregnancy chances since, in both studies, apart from ablation of the lesions, lysis of adhesions was also performed. The larger of the two studies did show an overall benefit from surgical removal of the endometriotic implants; the smaller one did not. We conclude that surgery for minimal or mild endometriosis might modestly enhance fecundity in women with otherwise unexplained subfertility, but it cannot be excluded that this improvement is due to removal of adhesions rather than implants. © 2004 Published by Elsevier B.V.

*Keywords:* Endometriosis; Surgery; Pregnancy rate; Unexplained subfertility

## 1. Introduction

Whether or not endometriosis affects female fertility has been a subject of ongoing debate for many years now. Both believers and nonbelievers appear to be able to find enough reliable data in the scientific literature to corroborate their respective claims. The problem is compounded by the fact that endometriosis is not a singular finding in all women. Many women are found to have, apart from endometriosis, secondary disorders such as pelvic adhesions and endometriomas.

In order to answer the question as to whether endometriosis per se affects fertility, one would have to study fertility in untreated women with endometriosis only, and with otherwise unexplained subfertility. Such women can be found in the control groups of randomized controlled trials (RCTs) of subfertile women with minimal and mild endometriosis.

---

* Tel.: +31-43-3876764; fax: +31-43-3874765.
*E-mail address:* jev@sgyn.azm.nl (J.L.H. Evers).

0531-5131/ © 2004 Published by Elsevier B.V.
doi:10.1016/j.ics.2004.01.009

## 2. The search for evidence

The fact that we live in the age of evidence-based medicine will not have escaped anyone. Quality assurance and technology assessment are the focus of both political as well as medical attention. Whereas authority-driven medicine has served an important role for ages, patients nowadays request and deserve that we do not impose unfounded diagnostic tests and treatments on them, but provide evidence of their proven efficacy, their potential harm, and their eventual shortcomings. Unfortunately, hard evidence is rare in reproductive medicine. Many of the diagnostic procedures we perform are not based on sound scientific evidence; many treatments lack objective evaluation. In endometriosis, many uncertainties come together: we do not understand the disease, we fail to appreciate its relationship— if any—with impaired fertility, we disagree on the means to make a firm diagnosis, and the disease so far escapes rational treatment.

Endometriosis-associated impairment of fertility has been a heavily disputed issue among clinicians. The advent of clinical epidemiology, and later of evidence-based medicine, has introduced many question marks in our discourse of the causes and consequences of the disease. Clinical epidemiology has long relied on (modifications of) Koch's postulates for addressing causality. Wheeler and Malinak [1] have looked at these postulates with regard to endometriosis-associated subfertility. They concluded that no sound evidence exists from experiments in humans for the putative relationship between endometriosis and subfertility; that there is no strong statistical association — if any—between endometriosis and subfertility, except for the more complex cases with adhesions and endometriomas; that the association is not consistent from study to study; that the temporal relationship between the two is not correct (endometriosis preceding subfertility complaints in some women and vice versa in others); that there does not exist a dose–response relationship; that the association is not specific; and that the situation in subfertile women with endometriosis does not show a clear analogy to proven causal relations in other fields of medicine. They concluded that they could only confirm that the association between clinically recognized endometriosis and decreased fertility may make some epidemiological, and perhaps some biological, sense [1]. From applying Koch's postulates to the endometriosis literature, they deduced that, in a clinical and epidemiological sense, there is insufficient scientific evidence for endometriosis and impaired fertility to be causally related.

When considering fertility in women with endometriosis, two clinical questions predominate: Do women with endometriosis suffer from impairment of fertility, and, if so, does treatment improve their pregnancy chances? In other words, does endometriosis affect fertility, and does treatment restore fertility?

### 2.1. Does endometriosis affect fertility?

Whether endometriosis decreases fertility is a question that can best be studied in a prospective, observational cohort study of two groups of couples without any fertility-impairing factors—one group with and one without documented endometriosis (and endometriosis only)—with all other factors (age, sexual activity, and socio-economic class) being equal (i.e., to compare—from the very moment they wish to start a family—the spontaneous pregnancy rate in proven, normal young couples with that in proven, normal young couples of whom the female partner has endometriosis as the only abnormal finding). Since it would require a laparoscopy to be performed on perfectly healthy young women even before they started attempting to achieve a pregnancy, a study like this one will, obviously, never be performed.

This option being an illusion, several less robust trial designs remain. One is to compare the spontaneous pregnancy rate in couples with unexplained subfertility after a complete fertility work-up to that in couples with unexplained subfertility except for the finding of endometriosis from laparoscopy, with the ages and durations of subfertility being equal in both groups. One way to assess the spontaneous pregnancy rate in women with endometriosis is to study nontreated control subjects participating in randomised, controlled trials. There have been eight studies reported from which figures such as these can be derived [2–9]. Together, they involved 387 control participants, who achieved a crude spontaneous pregnancy rate of 30% [95% confidence interval (CI), 26–35%]. This rate does not differ significantly from the combined, spontaneous pregnancy rate of 33% (95% CI, 31–35%) from 20 studies involving 2026 couples with unexplained subfertility, as reported by Taylor and Collins [10] in a review of the literature.

Studying the results of therapeutic donor insemination in women whose male partners have azoospermia offers an alternate way to address the issue. Three studies may offer insights [11–13]. The crude spontaneous pregnancy rates in women with endometriosis during 12 months of follow-up ranged from a low figure of 29% in a few women (2/7) in one study [12] to a "normal" conception rate of 17/21 (81%) in another [13], as compared with 51% in women without endometriosis [12]. Overall, pregnancies occurred in 38/59 cases (64%) and 46/91 controls (51%) (i.e., if anything, a more favourable outcome occurred in cases than in controls).

## 2.2. Does treatment restore fertility?

Five RCTs have shown that medical treatment does not improve pregnancy chances in subfertile women with endometriosis [2,3,5–7] (Table 1). The issue of surgical treatment, however, is more delicate. No RCT has been published so far reporting spontaneous pregnancy rates following surgical treatment of endometriosis (and endometriosis only) in women with subfertility. Two studies have been published (one from Canada involving 341 women and one from Italy involving 101 women) reporting surgical removal of endometriosis and adhesions in subfertile women with mild or minimal endometriosis [8,9] (Table 2). Both studies have been criticized because, after surgery, the participants

Table 1
Odds ratios (OR) for pregnancy in five randomised, controlled trials of medical treatment of minimal and mild endometriosis

| Trial | Cases | Cases pregnant | Controls | Controls pregnant | OR | 95% CI |
| --- | --- | --- | --- | --- | --- | --- |
| Thomas and Cooke [7] | 20 | 5 | 17 | 4 | 1.1 | 0.2–6.7 |
| Bayer et al. [2] | 37 | 13 | 36 | 17 | 0.6 | 0.2–1.7 |
| Telimaa et al. [5] | 18 | 6 | 14 | 6 | 0.7 | 0.1–3.6 |
| Telimaa [6] | 17 | 7 | 14 | 6 | 0.9 | 0.2–4.9 |
| Fedele et al. [3] | 35 | 17 | 36 | 17 | 1.1 | 0.4–3.0 |
| Common OR | 127 | 48 | 117 | 50 | 0.8 | 0.5–1.4 |

Table 2
OR for pregnancy in two randomised, controlled trials of surgical treatment of minimal and mild endometriosis, as adapted by Crosignani and Vercellini [14]

| Trial | Cases | Cases pregnant | Controls | Controls pregnant | OR | 95% CI |
|---|---|---|---|---|---|---|
| Marcoux et al. [8] | 172 | 63 | 169 | 37 | 2.1 | 1.2–3.4 |
| Gruppo Italiano per lo Studio dell'Endometriosi [9] | 54 | 12 | 47 | 13 | 0.7 | 0.3–2.0 |
| Common OR | 226 | 75 | 216 | 50 | 1.6 | 1.0–2.6 |

were informed about whether the procedure was or was not performed in their respective case; it cannot be excluded that this knowledge might have affected the outcome.

The Canadian study is, by far, the largest published RCT on any treatment of endometriosis in subfertile women to date [8]. The trial offers evidence that surgical treatment of minimal and mild endometriosis improves the pregnancy chances in a woman with subfertility, although it does not restore fertility to the level one would expect in such women, and most definitely not to normal. During the 36 weeks of follow-up, conception occurred in 50 (29%) of the 172 women randomised to have surgery and in 29 (17%) of the 169 women randomised not to undergo treatment. The (36-week) pregnancy rate of 17% in the untreated participants from this surgical RCT compares unfavourably with the combined (6-month) pregnancy rate of 28% in the untreated participants from the five medical RCTs mentioned above. Since there is no reason to presume that being an untreated control subject in a medical RCT provides for better pregnancy chances than being an untreated control subject in a surgical RCT, it is not yet possible to draw firm conclusions from the finding of the Canadian study.

The Italian study included 101 participants [9]. During the 12 months of follow-up, conception occurred in 12 (22%) of the 54 women randomised to have surgery and in 13 (28%) of the 47 women randomised to no treatment. The (1-year) pregnancy rate of 28% in the untreated participants from this surgical RCT is similar to the combined pregnancy rate of 28% in the untreated participants from the five medical RCTs mentioned above, although the latter result was obtained after only 6 months of follow-up.

In a letter to the editor, Crosignani and Vercellini [14] pointed out the differences between the Canadian and Italian studies. They stipulated that the Canadian study reported only pregnancies that had reached >20 weeks of gestation, whereas the Italian study reported any pregnancies. They proceeded to give comparable data for the Canadian and Italian studies [i.e., all pregnancies (63/172 in the surgery group versus 37/169 in the no-surgery group in the Canadian study and 12/54 and 13/47, respectively, in the Italian study) or only pregnancies >20 weeks (50/172 and 29/169 in the Canadian trial, and 10/54 and 10/47 in the Italian trial)] (Table 2). It is unfortunate that neither of the trials allows for calculation of the pregnancy rate following surgical removal of endometriosis lesions only (i.e., in those women who did not have or did not need lysis of adhesions performed), since this figure would give the only clear answer to the question of whether removal of lesions, as such, will improve a woman's subsequent pregnancy chances. In the Canadian study, 284 women did not have adhesions. In these women, the destruction of implants also increased the 36-week cumulative probability of a pregnancy that lasts beyond 20 weeks (cumulative incidence ratio, 1.6; 95% CI, 1.1–2.5; $p<0.05$). If one bases calculations on the absolute treatment effect of achieving any pregnancy in both studies combined (10%), the number needed to treat (NNT) would be 10, indicating that, in order to achieve one additional pregnancy, 10 women would have to have their minimal or mild endometriosis lesions removed via laparoscopy. Crosignani and Vercellini [14] pointed out that, considering that one cannot identify women with minimal or mild endometriosis before surgery and that the proportion of women undergoing laparoscopy for unexplained subfertility may not be more than 50%, the NNT at least doubles. Also, if endometriosis occurs in 50% of women with unexplained subfertility, the NNT would double again. One would, therefore, have to perform between 20 and 40 diagnostic laparoscopies and remove all visible endometriotic implants (and perform complete adhesiolysis) to achieve one additional pregnancy. The ESHRE Capri Workshop on the optimal use of infertility diagnostic tests and treatments concluded that randomised, controlled trials demonstrated only a "modest efficacy of endometriosis ablation in increasing the pregnancy rate in infertile women" [15].

## 3. Discussion

From the present review, it seems, therefore, reasonable to conclude that there exists no, or only very, limited evidence today to support the contention that endometriosis per se causes subfertility, that there is no support for the contention that medical treatment of minimal and mild endometriosis improves pregnancy chances in subfertile couples, and, finally, that there is statistical evidence for a slight beneficial effect of surgical removal of the lesions, but the clinical relevance of this finding is limited and the effect may be short-lived. The same holds true for occult disease. No evidence exists to support the contention that medical treatment of occult endometriosis improves pregnancy chances in subfertile couples. Although statistical evidence does exist for a slight beneficial effect of surgical removal of minimal and mild lesions, the clinical relevance of less severe forms of endometriosis (i.e., occult disease) is undefined. Occult disease can (and should not) be removed. Medical treatment will render minimal and mild disease only temporarily invisible, allowing the lesions to reemerge with time. Surgical treatment can remove visible lesions but will leave behind dozens, if not hundreds, of invisible (occult) ones, which, after removal of the visible lesions, may develop into minimal endometriosis and proceed from there.

## 4. Conclusion

One can conclude that resection or ablation of minimal and mild endometriosis appears to only modestly enhance fecundity in women with otherwise unexplained subfertility. There is still a need for properly conducted, prospective trials of resection or ablation of minimal and mild endometriosis lesions in women with otherwise unexplained subfertility without adhesions.

## References

[1] J.M. Wheeler, L.R. Malinak, Does mild endometriosis cause infertility? Semin. Reprod. Endocrinol. 6 (1988) 239–251.

[2] S.R. Bayer, M.M. Seibel, D.S. Saffan, M.J. Berger, M.L. Taymor, Efficacy of danazol treatment for minimal endometriosis in infertile women: a prospective, randomised study, J. Reprod. Med. 33 (1988) 179–183.
[3] L. Fedele, F. Parazzini, E. Radici, Buserelin acetate versus expectant management in the treatment of infertility associated with minimal or mild endometriosis: a randomized clinical trial, Am. J. Obstet. Gynecol. 166 (1992) 1345–1350.
[4] C.E. Overton, P.C. Lindsay, B. Johal, A randomized, double-blind, placebo-controlled study of luteal phase dydrogesterone (Duphaston) in women with minimal to mild endometriosis, Fertil. Steril. 62 (1994) 701–707.
[5] S. Telimaa, L. Ronnberg, A. Kauppila, Placebo-controlled comparison of danazol and high-dose medroxyprogesterone acetate in the treatment of endometriosis after conservative surgery, Gynecol. Endocrinol. 1 (1987) 363–371.
[6] S. Telimaa, Danazol and medroxyprogesterone acetate inefficacious in the treatment of infertility in endometriosis, Fertil. Steril. 50 (1988) 872–875.
[7] E.J. Thomas, I.D. Cooke, Successful treatment of asymptomatic endometriosis: does it benefit infertile women? Br. Med. J. 294 (1987) 1117–1119.
[8] S. Marcoux, R. Maheux, S. Berube, and the Canadian Collaborative Group on Endometriosis, Laparoscopic surgery in infertile women with minimal or mild endometriosis, N. Engl. J. Med. 337 (1997) 217–222.
[9] Gruppo Italiano per lo Studio dell'Endometriosi, Ablation of lesions or no treatment in minimal–mild endometriosis in infertile women: a randomized trial, Hum. Reprod. 14 (1999) 1332–1334.
[10] P.J. Taylor, J.A. Collins, Unexplained Infertility, Oxford Medical Publications, Oxford, 1992.
[11] J.A. Portuondo, A.D. Echanojauregui, C. Herran, I. Alijarte, Early conception in patients with untreated mild endometriosis, Fertil. Steril. 39 (1983) 22–25.
[12] R.P.S. Jansen, Minimal endometriosis and reduced fecundability: prospective evidence from an artificial insemination by donor program, Fertil. Steril. 46 (1986) 141–143.
[13] F.J. Rodriguez-Escudero, J.L. Neyro, B. Corcostegui, J.A. Benito, Does minimal endometriosis reduce fecundity? Fertil. Steril. 50 (1988) 522–524.
[14] P.G. Crosignani, P. Vercellini, Evidence may change with more trials: concepts to be kept in mind, Hum. Reprod. 15 (2000) 2448.
[15] P.G. Crosignani, B.L. Rubin, Optimal use of infertility diagnostic tests and treatments. The ESHRE Capri Workshop Group, Hum. Reprod. 15 (2000) 23–32.

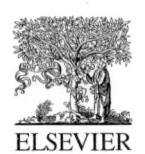

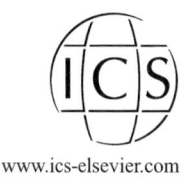

# Evidence-based reproductive surgery: tubal infertility

Herve Dechaud[*], Lionel Reyftmann, Jacques Faidherbe, Samir Hamamah, Bernard Hedon

*Department of Obstetrics and Gynecology, Reproductive Medicine, CHU Arnaud De Villeneuve, 371 avenue Doyen Gasto, Giraud, 34295 Montpellier Cedex 5, France*

**Abstract.** The goal for any infertile couple is to explore all reasonable attempts to achieve pregnancy. The couple with infertility resulting from tubal disease has two therapeutic options to achieve this goal: reconstructive tubal surgery and in vitro fertilization. However, the increasing demand for new techniques of assisted reproduction has called into question the value of the more established methods of treatment for tubal infertility. There are some causes of tubal infertility for which surgery has virtually no chance of success. For these situations, in vitro fertilization is clearly the only therapeutic option. For other situations, the decision-making process requires detailed discussion on the effectiveness, adverse effects and cost of the procedures. Endoscopic evaluation of the tubal mucosa is essential for the selective application of tubal surgery. The available evidence shows that tubal surgery can be as, or more, effective as in vitro fertilization for cases of filmy adhesions, mild distal tubal occlusion and proximal obstruction. It may, however, be reasonable to discuss in vitro fertilization with any couple without pregnancy 12 months after tubal surgery. In women with moderate to severe distal tubal disease, the diminishing success rates from surgery suggest that in vitro fertilization should be considered as the first line of treatment. In the case of unsuccessful reconstructive surgery, or if a hydrosalpinx is irreparably damaged, a salpingectomy prior to in vitro fertilization has to be considered. Tubal surgery has indisputable benefits for the patient if infertility is cured by the intervention. A successful tubal repair gives the patient the possibility of conceiving more than once without further treatment. It also gives the couple the psychological advantage of being able to conceive spontaneously. Probably the most pragmatic viewpoint is to consider reproductive surgery and in vitro fertilization as complementary options that are directed towards increasing the overall probability of achieving a pregnancy in the most efficient manner. © 2004 Published by Elsevier B.V.

*Keywords:* Hydrosalpinx; Proximal tubal occlusion; Tubal reversal of sterilization; Tubal surgery; Laparoscopy

## 1. Introduction

The highest level of evidence in therapy studies requires at least one high-quality systematic review or two high-quality randomized, controlled trials. Besides the best

---

[*] Corresponding author. Tel.: +33-4-67336536; fax: +33-4-67336468.
*E-mail address:* h-dechaud@chu-montpellier.fr (H. Dechaud).

0531-5131/ © 2004 Published by Elsevier B.V.
doi:10.1016/j.ics.2004.01.117

available scientific knowledge, evidence-based medicine relies also on clinical judgment, practical skills and the patient's individual situation and desire.

The goal for any infertile couple is to explore all reasonable attempts to achieve pregnancy. The couple with infertility resulting from tubal disease has two therapeutic options to achieve this goal: reconstructive tubal surgery and in vitro fertilization. However, the increasing demand for new techniques of assisted reproduction has called into question the value of the more established methods of treatment for tubal infertility. In fact, the question is to know if tubal surgery is obsolete today or not. If not, what is the place for tubal surgery as compared with in vitro fertilization procedures? Probably the most pragmatic viewpoint is to consider reproductive surgery and in vitro fertilization as complementary options that are directed towards increasing the overall probability of achieving a pregnancy in the most efficient manner.

## 2. Evidence-based medicine and tubal surgery

The true benefits of surgery are difficult to assess adequately because of the selectivity of cases and reporting and the lack of controlled studies. However, not all tubal damage is suitable for surgery, and tubal surgery should only be performed by gynecologists who have had appropriate training in microsurgery and laparoscopy and who operate a steady volume of patients to maintain a high level of skill [1–4]. Moreover, it is now known that better results can be obtained by appropriate selection of cases based on the severity and location of the tubal pathology [5].

There are some causes of tubal infertility for which surgery has virtually no chance of success. These include bilateral salpingectomy, bilateral multisite tubal obstruction and complete tubal obstruction by dense pelvic adhesions. For these situations, in vitro fertilization is clearly the only therapeutic option. For other situations, the decision-making process requires detailed discussion on the effectiveness, adverse effects and cost of the procedures.

### 2.1. Hydrosalpinx

Distal tubal obstruction with various degrees of dilatation and mucosal damage continues to be a common cause of infertility. Infertility caused by hydrosalpinges may be overcome by two different treatment methods: surgical distal tubal repair or in vitro fertilization. Preoperative investigations are crucial to determine patients suitable for surgical repair or for in vitro fertilization, with or without salpingectomy [6]. To achieve this aim, pelvic laparoscopy and tubal endoscopy (salpingoscopy or falloposcopy) are useful [7–9].

#### 2.1.1. Salpingostomy

The objective of salpingostomy is to create a new ostium with a well-everted fimbrial or ampullar mucosa. Salpingostomy was previously performed through laparotomy and microsurgical techniques, which have been replaced by laparoscopy to a large extent today. The outcome, in terms of pregnancies, is directly correlated to the tubal mucosal status. Only patients with preserved mucosa within their hydrosalpinges have a fair pregnancy chance subsequent to reconstructive surgery [10].

No randomized, controlled trial compared distal tubal surgery by laparotomy and by laparoscopy. Table 1 summarized the main series concerning laparotomy and laparoscopy for treating distal pathology of the tubes.

In conclusion, operative laparoscopy seems to be an effective treatment for hydrosalpinx in terms of pregnancy outcome. However, a metaanalysis of four studies comparing laparoscopic versus open microsurgical salpingostomy shows a significant decrease of total (odds ratio, 0.49 [0.31–0.76]) and intrauterine (0.59 [0.37–0.96]) pregnancy rates after laparoscopic salpingostomy versus open microsurgical salpingostomy [20].

Two randomized, controlled trials investigated the use of the CO2 laser at infertility surgery. There was no significant difference in pregnancy outcome after salpingostomy [20]. Three randomized studies compared the results of salpingostomy, with and without prosthesis, to maintain tubal patency. There was no significant difference in pregnancy rates.

No randomized, controlled trial compared distal tubal surgery and in vitro fertilization.

### 2.1.2. Salpingectomy

Tubal pathologies lead to a lower embryo implantation rate than other forms of infertility [21]. This finding seems to be associated with the severity of the tubal disease [22]. Distal tubal occlusion with a hydrosalpinx is particularly associated with a problem of embryo implantation, as well as with a lower clinical pregnancy rate [23]. Some investigators have suggested that this defect of implantation can be improved by bilateral salpingectomy [24–26].

Three randomized, controlled trials were included in a Cochrane review in order to determine if salpingectomy could be useful for patients with hydrosalpinx before undergoing in vitro fertilization [27]. Surgical treatment of hydrosalpinges versus nonsurgical management increased the odds of live birth plus ongoing viable pregnancy (OR 2.13, 95% CI 1.24–3.65) and of pregnancy (OR 1.75, 95% CI 1.07–2.86). No significant differences were seen in the odds of ectopic pregnancy (OR 0.42, 95% CI 0.08–2.14), miscarriage per pregnancy (OR 0.49, 95% CI 0.16–1.52), treatment complications (OR 5.8, 95% CI 0.35–96.79) or implantation per embryo transferred (OR 1.34, 95% CI 0.87–2.05). The reviewer's conclusions were that the metaanalysis of randomized trials does show a statistically significant benefit of laparoscopic salpingectomy for hydrosalpinges prior to in vitro fertilization. A number needed to treat calculation suggests that between seven and eight women would need to have a salpingectomy prior to in vitro fertilization to gain one additional live birth.

Table 1
Outcome of salpingostomy

| Microsurgical | | | Laparoscopical | | |
|---|---|---|---|---|---|
| Reference | n | Pregnancy rate (%) | Reference | n | Pregnancy rate (%) |
| Strandell et al. [11] | 109 | 36 | Dubuisson et al. [16] | 81 | 37 |
| Winston and Margara [12] | 323 | 43 | Canis et al. [17] | 87 | 40 |
| Singhal et al. [13] | 97 | 40 | Donnez et al. [18] | 25 | 20 |
| Schlaff et al. [14] | 95 | 27 | Taylor et al. [6] | 139 | 24.5 |
| Donnez and Casanas-Roux [15] | 83 | 38 | Milingos et al. [19] | 61 | 20.5 |

There is a degree of subjectivity in the selection of patients for tubal surgery. Depending on the degree of expertise in techniques, the same patient might be operated on in a given institution, but not in another. This bias in the selection of patients is a hindrance to the completion and significance of multicentric studies. This is possibly also the reason for the difficulty in carrying out this type of work.

Despite the number of studies on the impact of tubal pathology—particularly hydrosalpinx—on embryo implantation, the pathophysiology remains unclear. A hydrosalpinx forms after the destruction of the fimbria and, consequently, by accumulation of diverse tubal secretions. Given the continuity of the hydrosalpinx with the uterine cavity, these secretions may flow into the uterus and disrupt the process of embryo implantation [28]. The resulting dysfunction in endometrial receptivity may be caused by several phenomena [29]. The cause may be mechanical, but it seems more likely to be an inadequate chemical composition of the hydrosalpinx liquid [30]. Another hypothesis is that a hydrosalpinx causes an inflammatory endometrial reaction that prevents further endometrial and/or embryo development. This inflammatory reaction can be quantified in the endometrium by an excess of macrophages in patients with tubal sterility [31]. Several studies showed that patients with hydrosalpinx expressed fewer endometrial integrins in comparison with control subjects [32,33]. A bilateral salpingectomy reestablished the expression of these integrins, and thus indicated the deleterious effect of a hydrosalpinx on the endometrium. The authors hypothesized that this diagnostic tool can screen for a subgroup of patients with hydrosalpinx for whom salpingectomy would be beneficial.

However, conclusions of this debate might be qualified in order to avoid many unnecessary salpingectomies [34]. Actually, the group of hydrosalpinges suitable for randomized salpingectomy was previously described by hysterosalpingography or diagnostic laparoscopy. If these hydrosalpinges are enlarged enough to be visible on ultrasound, they're probably thin-walled hydrosalpinges. In this restricted group of hydrosalpinges (in opposition to thick-walled hydrosalpinges), the results of surgical salpingostomy, reported in the literature, are usually good. The reason is that the prognosis of these hydrosalpinges is not based on the size of the hydrosalpinx itself, but on the quality of the remaining tubal mucosa after opening the tube. Thus, the diagnosis of enlarged hydrosalpinx by ultrasound is not sufficient to perform salpingectomy before an in vitro fertilization procedure [35]. In order to improve the likelihood of pregnancy for each patient, physicians have to carefully discriminate which hydrosalpinx has to be removed or is suitable for surgical repair [36]. The enlargement of the hydrosalpinx could probably be a bad prognosis but above all, an excellent indication of tubal endoscopy. The appraisal of the tubal mucosa must remain the most important parameter, especially in the group of thin-walled hydrosalpinges without salpingitis isthmica nodosa associated.

The best moment to remove the fallopian tubes needs to be established so that each patient has the maximal possibility of becoming pregnant in optimal conditions. The efficacy of salpingectomy to treat cases of severe and irreversible tubal pathology before or during in vitro fertilization attempts remains a subject of debate. However, salpingectomy as a specific response to repeated embryo nonimplantation improves the pregnancy rate per transfer [37]. This surgical act also reduces the number of in vitro fertilization attempts needed to obtain pregnancy. The reduction in the number of attempts needed to obtain pregnancy has both economic and psychological impact, neither of which is negligible. This needs to be taken into consideration in the evaluation of indications for salpingectomy in this group of patients.

No randomized, controlled trial tested the efficacy of the other surgical procedures for treating hydrosalpinges prior to in vitro fertilization. In the literature, several procedures were described: transvaginal needle aspiration of the hydrosalpinx before the ovarian stimulation or at the time of oocyte retrieval; proximal tubal occlusion to prevent uterine spill of hydrosalpinx contents; salpingostomy in selected cases of hydrosalpinges; and the use of antibiotics. All of these procedures have to be evaluated in a prospective, well-designed trial [38,39].

## 2.2. Patent phimosis

Fimbrial phimosis is a partial obstruction of the distal end of a fallopian tube. This is due to the presence of peritoneal adhesive bands surrounding the terminal end of the tube. The treatment of this condition is fimbrioplasty. Nevertheless, evaluation of the results of fimbrioplasty is complicated by the fact that most authors did not distinguish between complete obstruction of the fimbrial end of the tube and phimosis and did not distinguish fimbrioplasty and salpingostomy [40,41].

No randomized, controlled trial compared fimbrioplasty by laparotomy (microsurgical) or by laparoscopy. Similarly, no randomized, controlled study investigated the role of fimbrioplasty compared with in vitro fertilization. Despite the difficulties of diagnosis, the different surgical procedures described to treat phimosis (and associated pathologies such as adhesions) and the extremely variable durations of follow-up, few authors report results of fimbrioplasty in terms of pregnancy rate (Table 2).

Because no prospective data are available comparing results of microsurgery with the laparoscopic approach, it is almost impossible to indicate the most suitable procedure. If with both approaches similar pregnancy rates are obtained, laparoscopic surgery is the preferred method because of the decreased invasiveness.

Results of fimbrioplasty depend on mucosal appearance and degree of peritubal adhesions [16,47]. The ability of salpingoscopy or falloposcopy to provide better patient selection should be further evaluated in case of fimbrial pathologies [7,8].

## 2.3. Proximal tubal occlusion

Nonfilling of tubes at the time of hysterosalpingography results from either tubal occlusion or tubal obstruction. The pathophysiology is complex because different

Table 2
Outcome of fimbrioplasty

| Microsurgical | | | Laparoscopical | | |
|---|---|---|---|---|---|
| Reference | N | Pregnancy rate (%) | Reference | n | Pregnancy rate (%) |
| Donnez and Casanas-Roux [15] | 132 | 61 | Dubuisson et al. [43] | 31 | 35 |
| Lavy et al. [42] | 134 | 60 | Saleh and Dlugi [44] | 88 | 39.8 |
| | | | Kasia et al. [45] | 108 | 36 |
| | | | Audebert et al. [40] | 35 | 74.3 |
| | | | Schmidt et al. [46] | 66 | 28.8 |

etiologies could be identified for this condition [48]. Salpingitis isthmica nodosa occur primarily around the intramural and proximal isthmic endosalpinx. Lesions grow over time and eventually obliterate the tubal lumen. Polyps usually present as well-defined, small lesions that project into the tubal lumen. They rarely lead to complete blockage. Endometriosis is a known cause of proximal tubal blockage, involving the intramural oviduct. Tubal proximal obstruction is a time-limited process that may be reversible, such as tubal spasm or plugging by amorphous material.

The treatment of proximal tubal occlusion may be performed by two techniques: surgical treatment or radiographic treatment (selective salpingography, transcervical catheterization under fluoroscopic guidance, and transcervical balloon tuboplasty). No randomized, controlled trial compared surgical and radiographic procedures to treat proximal occlusion. Proximal tubal surgery needs magnification, good visualization of abnormal changes, tissue care, delicate hemostasis and precise anastomosis. The main reason for this is that the lumen of the isthmic–interstitial segment is 0.1–0.4 mm in diameter. Microsurgical tubocornual anastomosis is the gold standard to treat proximal blockage. No prospective study compared surgery by laparotomy and by laparoscopy. The hysteroscopic transcervical tubal catheterization is the other method described to treat proximal occlusion. An operative hysteroscope is inserted into the uterus and the tubal ostia are visualized. Once proximal blockage is confirmed, the uterine ostial access catheter is introduced and the tip of the guide wire is placed at the tubal ostia, and pressure is applied until patency is achieved.

In 1999, Honore et al. [49] made a metaanalysis comparing the results of the surgical and radiographic method. Two distinct groups were identified within the radiographic group through heterogeneity analysis: a "low" success group and a "high" success group. Recognizing that this may reflect unidentified confounders (patient selection), each group was considered separately (Table 3).

This metaanalysis suggests that radiographic therapies for proximal blockage produce live birth rates that are lower than those obtained with microsurgery. However, it is difficult to draw firm conclusions about the effectiveness of these methods because coexisting tubal pathology was not always described [50].

No randomized, controlled trial compared surgical treatment of proximal blockage and in vitro fertilization. Complementary use of microsurgery and in vitro fertilization improves the prognosis for selected patients with pathological proximal tubal blockage [51].

## 2.4. Tubal sterilization

More than 1% of sterilized women seek restoration of fertility. The very large number of tubal sterilizations performed each year has created a significant demand for reversal.

Table 3
Comparison of relative effectiveness of treatments of proximal tubal occlusion

| Technique | Number of patients | % of ongoing pregnancies | Relative risk | CI | p |
|---|---|---|---|---|---|
| Microsurgery versus | 175 | 47.4 | | | |
| Radiographic "low" success | 46 | 8.7 | 6.8 | 2.5–18.3 | 0 |
| Radiographic "high" success | 163 | 28.8 | 1.6 | 1.1–2.4 | 0.0005 |
| Hysteroscopic surgery | 45 | 48.9 | 0.9 | 0.6–1.6 | NS |

Microsurgical tubotubal anastomosis has yielded excellent results in such instances, and the reported viable pregnancy rates vary between 55% and 78% [52]. Recent improvements in laparoscopic instrumentation allow tubal anastomosis to be performed by laparoscopy [53]. In the largest series by laparoscopy, the pregnancy rate was 82.8% [54]. The laparoscopic approach has several advantages over laparotomy, but the surgeon should have expertise in both microsurgical tubal anatomosis and laparoscopic suturing [55].

No randomized, controlled trial compared tubal anastomosis for reversal by laparotomy and by laparoscopy. The results seem to be similar with the two methods. Prognostic factors of reversal of tubal sterilization are widely described in the literature, but there is no consensus about them except for the age of the woman at the time of surgery [56–58]. The learning curve is considerable and the technique may not be attainable by all surgeons, despite their best efforts. Reproductive surgeons will become experts in microendoscopy and laparoscopic microsurgery and will operate a large enough volume to maintain and develop this expertise.

Tubal anastomosis may be performed by two techniques: the one-stitch technique and the microsurgical anastomosis performed in two layers. No comparative study compared the efficiency of these two techniques.

In order to increase the results of microsurgery by laparoscopy, robotic assistance was tested for reversal of sterilization. A few studies were reported and conclusions are that robotic assistance increases operative time without an appreciable improvement in patient recovery or clinical outcomes [59].

No prospective study compared tubal surgery for reversal and in vitro fertilization. The patient should know the options available to her and the factors that affect the pregnancy rate. In the near future, it will be very important to perform randomized, controlled trials in order to answer this question. Microsurgery offers good results in terms of pregnancy and avoids the risks of in vitro fertilization, especially multiple pregnancies.

## 2.5. Peritubal adhesions

Pelvic adhesions are implicated in the etiology of up to 20% of infertility cases and are frequently associated with tubal damage. The major determinant of success in surgical correction of tubal infertility is the severity of damage suffered by the tube and adnexal adhesions. When periadnexal adhesions are the sole lesion, subsequent infertility is dependent upon the severity and extent of these adhesions. One of the difficulties in infertility related to adhesions is to find the best scoring system analyzing the implication of adhesions and its treatment on subsequent fertility [60]. Several scoring systems were described in the literature [61].

One nonrandomized study compared open adhesiolysis versus no treatment and found significantly more pregnancies in the treatment group compared with the control group [62].

One study compared laparoscopic versus open microsurgical adhesiolysis [63]. Pregnancy rates did not differ significantly between the techniques. There was a nonsignificant increase in terms of intrauterine pregnancy rate and a nonsignificant reduction in ectopic pregnancy rates. Unfortunately, no prospective, randomized data are available comparing microsurgery with endoscopic surgery. In 1995, Filippini et al. [64] analyzed the literature and compared 12 studies of laparoscopic salpingo-ovariolysis (923 patients) and 13 studies of salpingo-ovariolysis by laparotomy (600 patients). Rates of intrauterine pregnancies were 46.5% versus 54.8%, respectively. Similarly, the ectopic pregnancy rates were 6.4% and 4.1%, respectively. The results of laparoscopic treatment are similar to those obtained by microsurgery.

One prospective and randomized study evaluated the chance of adhesion formation after laparoscopic salpingo-ovariolysis and determined the efficacy of early second-look laparoscopy [65]. The conclusions are that the chance of moderate and severe adhesion reformation after laparoscopic salpingo-ovariolysis was 40.2%. The chance of pregnancy did not increase compared with patients who did not undergo second-look laparoscopy. The odds of pregnancy, live birth, ectopic pregnancy and miscarriage were not significantly different with postoperative hydrotubation versus no hydrotubation or with second-look laparoscopy and adhesiolysis versus no second-look laparoscopy [66]. No prospective, randomized study demonstrated the efficacy of transvaginal hydrolaparoscopy for adhesiolysis [67].

Numerous studies investigated liquid or agents for preventing adhesions after surgery for subfertility. A Cochrane review concluded that none of the pharmacological or liquid agents investigated in a randomized, controlled fashion was shown to improve postoperative pregnancy rates [68]. There was some evidence that steroids reduced the incidence and severity of postoperative adhesion formation. Dextran appeared neither to reduce the incidence or severity of adhesions.

No randomized, controlled trial compared surgical adhesiolysis and in vitro fertilization.

## 3. Conclusion

The available evidence shows that tubal surgery can be as, or more, effective than in vitro fertilization for cases of filmy adhesions, mild distal tubal occlusion and proximal obstruction. It may, however, be reasonable to discuss in vitro fertilization with any couple without pregnancy 12 months after tubal surgery. In women with moderate to severe distal tubal disease, the diminishing success rates from surgery suggest that in vitro fertilization should be considered as the first line of treatment. In the case of unsuccessful reconstructive surgery or if a hydrosalpinx is irreparably damaged, a salpingectomy prior to in vitro fertilization has to be considered. Endoscopic evaluation of tubal mucosa is essential for the selective application of tubal surgery. Most reproductive surgical studies lack control groups and the choice of procedure and surgical technique is variable and unrandomized [69].

Although no randomized, prospective trials exist to compare laparotomy and laparoscopic procedures, the laparoscopic approach offers the advantages associated with this mode of access, which include the avoidance of laparotomy incisions, the possibility to perform the procedure during the initial diagnostic laparoscopy, an ambulatory basis, a reduction of postoperative discomfort during the recovery period, decreased health care costs, and a more effective reduction of peritoneal reformation [70,71].

Tubal surgery has indisputable benefits for the patient if infertility is cured by the intervention. A successful tubal repair gives the patient the possibility of conceiving more than once without further treatment. It also gives the couple the psychological advantage of being able to conceive spontaneously.

## References

[1] B.A. Goff, et al., Surgical skills assessment: a blinded examination of obstetrics and gynecology residents, Am. J. Obstet. Gynecol. 186 (2002) 613–617.
[2] A.J. Watson, et al., The results of tubal surgery in the treatment of infertility in non-specialist hospitals, Br. J. Obstet. Gynaecol. 97 (1990) 561–568.
[3] C.S. Miranda, A.R. Carvajal, Complications of operative gynecological laparoscopy, J. Soc. Laparoendosc. Surg. 7 (2003) 53–58.
[4] R. Philosophe, Avoiding complications of laparoscopic surgery, Fertil. Steril. 80 (2003) 30–39.
[5] B. Hedon, et al., Critical evaluation of the fallopian tube. Fertility and Reproductive Medicine, in: R.D. Kempers, J. Cohen, A.F. Haney (Eds.), Proceedings of the XVI World Congress on Fertility and Sterility, San Francisco, 4–9 October 1998, (1998) pp. 61–70.
[6] R.C. Taylor, J. Berkowitz, P.F. McComb, Role of laparoscopic salpingostomy in the treatment of hydrosalpinx, Fertil. Steril. 75 (2001) 594–600.
[7] R. Marana, G.F. Catalano, L. Muzii, Salpingoscopy, Curr. Opin. Obstet. Gynecol. 15 (2003) 333–336.
[8] H. Dechaud, J.P. Daures, B. Hedon, Prospective evaluation of falloposcopy, Hum. Reprod. 13 (1998) 1815–1818.
[9] G. Vasquez, W. Boeckx, I. Brosens, Prospective study of tubal mucosal lesions and infertility in hydrosalpinges, Hum. Reprod. 10 (1995) 1075–1078.
[10] G. Mage, et al., A preoperative classification to predict the intrauterine and ectopic pregnancy rates after distal tubal microsurgery, Fertil. Steril. 46 (1986) 807–810.
[11] A. Strandell, et al., Background factors and scoring systems in relation to pregnancy outcome after fertility surgery, Acta Obstet. Gynecol. Scand. 74 (1995) 281–287.
[12] R.M.L. Winston, R.A. Margara, Microsurgical salpingostomy is not an obsolete procedure, Br. J. Obstet. Gynaecol. 98 (1991) 637–642.
[13] V. Singhal, T.C. Li, I.D. Cooke, An analysis of factors influencing the outcome of 232 consecutive tubal microsurgery cases, Br. J. Obstet. Gynaecol. 98 (1991) 628–636.
[14] W.D. Schlaff, et al., Neosalpingostomy for distal tubal obstruction: prognostic factors and impact of surgical techniques, Fertil. Steril. 54 (1990) 984–990.
[15] J. Donnez, F. Casanas-Roux, Prognostic factors of fimbrial microsurgery, Fertil. Steril. 46 (1986) 200–204.
[16] J.B. Dubuisson, et al., Laparoscopic salpingostomy: fertility results according to the tubal mucosal appearance, Hum. Reprod. 9 (1994) 334–339.
[17] M. Canis, et al., Laparoscopic distal tuboplasty: report of 87 cases and a four years experience, Fertil. Steril. 56 (1991) 616–621.
[18] J. Donnez, M. Nisolle, F. Casanas-Roux, CO2 laser laparoscopy in infertile women with adnexal adhesions and women with tubal occlusion, J. Gynecol. Surg. 5 (1989) 47–53.
[19] S.D. Milingos, et al., Laparoscopic treatment of hydrosalpinx: factors affecting pregnancy rate, J. Am. Assoc. Gynecol. Laparosc. 7 (2000) 355–361.
[20] A. Watson, P. Vandekerckhove, R. Lilford, Techniques for pelvic surgery in subfertility, Cochrane Database Syst. Rev. 4 (2003) (CD000221).
[21] H. Dechaud, et al., Embryo implantation rate changes with the etiology of infertility. IFFS 1995, Contracept. Fertil. Sex. 23 (1995) 144–145.
[22] R. Wainer, et al., Does hydrosalpinx reduce the pregnancy rate after in vitro fertilization?, Fertil. Steril. 68 (1997) 1022–1026.
[23] E. Camus, et al., Pregnancy rates after in vitro fertilization in cases of tubal infertility with and without hydrosalpinx: a meta-analysis of published comparative studies, Hum. Reprod. 14 (1999) 1243–1249.
[24] A. Strandell, The influence of hydrosalpinx on IVF and embryo transfer: a review, Hum. Reprod. Updat. 6 (2000) 387–395.
[25] H. Dechaud, et al., Does previous salpingectomy improve implantation and pregnancy rates in patients with severe tubal factor infertility who are undergoing in-vitro fertilization? A pilot prospective randomized study, Fertil. Steril. 69 (1998) 1020–1025.
[26] A. Strandell, et al., Hydrosalpinx and IVF outcome: a prospective, randomized trial in Scandinavia on salpingectomy prior to IVF, Hum. Reprod. 14 (1999) 2762–2769.

[27] N.P. Johnson, W. Mak, M.C. Sowter, Surgical treatment for tubal disease in women due to undergo in vitro fertilization, Cochrane Database Syst. Rev. 3 (2003) (CD002125).
[28] O. Eytan, et al., The mechanism of hydrosalpinx in embryo implantation, Hum. Reprod. 16 (2001) 2662–2667.
[29] L.C. Ajonuma, E.H. Ng, H.C. Chan, New insights into the mechanisms underlying hydrosalpinx fluid formation and its adverse effect on IVF outcome, Hum. Reprod. Updat. 8 (2002) 255–264.
[30] A. Strandell, A. Lindhard, Why does hydrosalpinx reduce fertility? The importance of hydrosalpinx fluid, Hum. Reprod. 17 (2002) 1141–1145.
[31] H. Dechaud, et al., Evaluation of endometrial inflammation by the quantification of macrophages, T lymphocytes, and interleukin-1 and-6 in human endometrium, J. Assist. Reprod. Genet. 15 (1998) 612–618.
[32] W.R. Meyer, et al., Hydrosalpinges adversely affect markers of endometrial receptivity, Hum. Reprod. 12 (1997) 1393–1398.
[33] I. Bildirici, et al., A prospective evaluation of the effect of salpingectomy on endometrial receptivity in cases of women with communicating hydrosalpinges, Hum. Reprod. 16 (2001) 2422–2426.
[34] H. Dechaud, B. Hedon, What effect does hydrosalpinx have on assisted reproduction? The role of salpingectomy remains controversial, Hum. Reprod. 15 (2000) 234–235.
[35] H. Dechaud, Hydrosalpinges suitable for salpingectomy, Hum. Reprod. 15 (2000) 2464–2465.
[36] A. Strandell, How to treat hydrosalpinges: IVF as the treatment of choice, Reprod. Biomed. Online 4 (2002) 37–39.
[37] H. Dechaud, et al., Salpingectomy for repeated embryo non-implantation after in vitro fertilization in patients with severe tubal factor infertility, J. Assist. Reprod. Genet. 17 (2000) 200–206.
[38] N. Hammadieh, et al., The effect of hydrosalpinx on IVF outcome: a prospective, randomised controlled trial of vaginal ultrasound-guided hydrosalpinx aspiration during egg collection, Fertil. Steril. 80 (2003) 131–132.
[39] P.J. Puttemans, I.A. Brosens, Salpingectomy improves in-vitro fertilization outcome in patients with a hydrosalpinx: blind victimization of the Fallopian tube? Hum. Reprod. 11 (1996) 2079–2081.
[40] A. Audebert, J.L. Pouly, P. Von Theobald, Laparoscopic fimbrioplasty: an evaluation of 35 cases, Hum. Reprod. 13 (1998) 1496–1499.
[41] N.P. Johnson, L. Sadler, M. Merrilees, IVF and tubal pathology—not all bad news, Aust. N. Z. J. Obstet. Gynaecol. 42 (2002) 285–288.
[42] G. Lavy, M.P. Diamond, A.H. De Cherney, Ectopic pregnancy: its relationship to tubal reconstructive surgery, Fertil. Steril. 47 (1987) 543–556.
[43] J.B. Dubuisson, et al., Terminal tuboplasties by laparoscopy: 65 consecutive cases, Fertil. Steril. 54 (1990) 401–403.
[44] W.A. Saleh, A.M. Dlugi, Pregnancy outcome after laparoscopic fimbrioplasty in nonocclusive distal tubal disease, Fertil. Steril. 67 (1997) 474–480.
[45] J.M. Kasia, et al., Laparoscopic fimbrioplasty and neosalpingostomy. Experience of the Yaounde General Hospital, Cameroon (report of 194 cases), Eur. J. Obstet. Gynecol. Reprod. Biol. 73 (1997) 71–77.
[46] S. Schmidt, et al., Predicting the outcome of infertility surgery, Arch. Gynecol. Obstet. 264 (2000) 116–118.
[47] F. Audibert, et al., Therapeutic strategies in tubal infertility with distal pathology, Hum. Reprod. 6 (1991) 1439–1442.
[48] R. Woolcott, Proximal tubal occlusion: a practical approach, Hum. Reprod. 11 (1996) 1831–1833.
[49] G.M. Honore, A.E. Holden, R.S. Schenken, Pathophysiology and management of proximal tubal blockage, Fertil. Steril. 71 (1999) 785–795.
[50] R. Wiedemann, et al., Beyond recanalizing proximal tubal occlusion: the argument for further diagnosis and classification, Hum. Reprod. 11 (1996) 986–991.
[51] T. Tomazevic, et al., Microsurgery and in-vitro fertilization and embryo transfer for infertility resulting from pathological proximal tubal blockage, Hum. Reprod. 11 (1996) 2613–2617.
[52] V. Gomel, C. James, Restoration of fertility after tubal sterilization: tubo-tubal anastomosis versus in vitro fertilization, Fertil. Contracept. Sex 18 (1990) 439–443.
[53] C.H. Koh, G.M. Janik, Laparoscopic microsurgery: current and future status, Curr. Opin. Obstet. Gynecol. 11 (1999) 401–407.
[54] T.K. Yoon, H.R. Sung, H.G. Kang, Laparoscopic tubal anastomosis: fertility outcome in 202 cases, Fertil. Steril. 72 (1999) 1121–1126.

[55] A. Sammour, T. Tulandi, Laparoscopic fertility-promoting procedures of the fallopian tube and the uterus, Int. J. Fert. Women's Med. 46 (2001) 145–150.
[56] J. Trussell, E. Guilbert, A. Hedley, Sterilization failure, sterilization reversal, and pregnancy after sterilization reversal in Quebec, Obstet. Gynecol. 101 (2003) 677–684.
[57] M.M. Hanafi, Factors affecting the pregnancy rate after microsurgical reversal of tubal ligation, Fertil. Steril. 80 (2003) 434–440.
[58] S.H. Kim, et al., Microsurgical reversal tubal sterilization: a report on 1118 cases, Fertil. Steril. 68 (1997) 865–870.
[59] J.M. Goldberg, T. Falcone, Laparoscopic microsurgical tubal anastomosis with and without robotic assistance, Hum. Reprod. 18 (2003) 145–147.
[60] R. Marana, et al., Correlation between the American Fertility Society classifications of adnexal adhesions and distal tubal occlusion, salpingoscopy, and reproductive outcome in tubal surgery, Fertil. Steril. 64 (1995) 924–929.
[61] The American Fertility Society, The American Fertility Society classifications of adnexal adhesions, distal tubal occlusion, tubal occlusion secondary to tubal ligation, tubal pregnancies, Mullerian anomalies and intrauterine adhesions, Fertil. Steril. 49 (1988) 944–955.
[62] T. Tulandi, et al., Treatment dependent and treatment independent pregnancy among women with periadnexal adhesions, Am. J. Obstet. Gynecol. 48 (1990) 354–357.
[63] H. Reich, Laparoscopic treatment of extensive pelvic adhesions, including hydrosalpinges, J. Reprod. Med. 32 (1987) 736–742.
[64] F. Filippini, et al., Critical analysis of the adhesiolysis results, Ref. Gynecol. Obstet. Spec. Issue (1995) 137–141.
[65] S. Alborzi, S. Motazedian, M.E. Parsanezhad, Chance of adhesion formation after laparoscopic salpingo-ovariolysis: is there a place for second-look laparoscopy? J. Am. Assoc. Gynecol. Laparosc. 10 (2003) 172–176.
[66] N.P. Johnson, A. Watson, Postoperative procedures for improving fertility following pelvic reproductive surgery, Cochrane Database Syst. Rev. 2 (2003) (CD001897).
[67] S. Gordts, R. Campo, I. Brosens, Experience with transvaginal hydrolaparoscopy for reconstructive tubo-ovarian surgery, Reprod. Biomed. Online 4 (2002) 72–75.
[68] A. Watson, P. Vandekerckhove, R. Lilford, Liquid and fluid agents for preventing adhesions after surgery for subfertility, Cochrane Database Syst. Rev. 3 (2003) (CD001298).
[69] G.D. Adamson, V.L. Baker, Subfertility: causes, treatment and outcome, Best Pract. Res., Clin. Obstet. Gynaecol. 17 (2003) 169–185.
[70] P. Lundorff, et al., Adhesion formation after laparoscopic surgery in tubal pregnancy: a randomized trial versus laparotomy, Fertil. Steril. 55 (1991) 911–915.
[71] M. Granberg, et al., Economic evaluation of infertility treatment for tubal disease, J. Assist. Reprod. Genet. 20 (2003) 301–308.

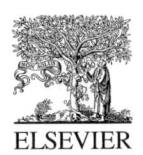

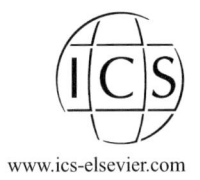

# Future directions and development in reproductive surgery

Tommaso Falcone*

*Department of Obstetrics and Gyneoclogy-A81, Cleveland Clinic Foundation, 9500 Euclid Avenue, Cleveland, OH 44195, USA*

**Abstract.** The future of surgery, and reproductive surgery in particular, will involve the use of sophisticated technology. This technology will revolutionize the operating room and the teaching of the art of surgery to the next generation. It will allow for a fully integrated operating room with capacity for robotic surgery, teleconsultation, and possibly telesurgery. Virtual reality and augmented reality will be part of an integrated operative field that the surgeon will view while performing the surgery. This same technology will be the basis of simulation programs that will teach the operative techniques to trainees. © 2004 Published by Elsevier B.V.

*Keywords:* Robotics; Virtual reality; Augmented reality

## 1. Introduction

The future of reproductive surgery, as in all surgical specialties, lies in the integration of sophisticated technology into the operating room. Traditionally, surgeons have relied on their experience with very little external input to carry out the procedure. Essentially, the operating room was an isolated experience. Surgical skill was passed on to a new generation of surgeons without any clearly defined educational methods. This situation is in contradistinction to the training of an airline pilot, in which sophisticated technology and simulation play an integral role.

In the future, the operating room team will have the ability to bring in all preoperative information on the patient, especially imaging results, into the operative field. Intra-operative teleconsultation can occur with ease. The operating surgeon will be able to obtain a consult from a colleague some distance away. The distant surgeon will be able to get the direct real time image of the operative field on his own screen, offer an opinion, and, in some circumstances, assist that surgeon from a distance. This scenario is not truly futuristic, since the technology to implement it is available today. However, the

---

* Tel.: +1-216-360-9332; fax: +1-216-445-5526.
  *E-mail address:* falcont@ccf.org (T. Falcone).

0531-5131/ © 2004 Published by Elsevier B.V.
doi:10.1016/j.ics.2004.01.084

more sophisticated visualization processes, such as augmented reality, are not yet available.

## 2. Robotic systems

Surgical robots have been available for several years [1–7]. Most surgical robots were designed to perform specific surgical procedures. In some specialties, such as neurosurgery, the robots are navigational, that is they identify a trajectory towards the lesion. The surgery is performed conventionally. There are two commercially available robotic systems that have been used for gynecologic procedures, Zeus (Computer Motion, Goleta, CA) and da Vinci (Intuitive Surgical, Mountain View, California). The first commercial application of robotics was the Automated Endoscopic System for Optimal Positioning (AESOP) device by Computer Motion to hold and position the laparoscope [2]. It provided a steady, hands-free image and the ability to move the scope by a foot pedal initially, then later by voice activation. The development of speech algorithms, which interpret speech patterns from different individuals, made the latter possible.

The world's first robot-assisted gynecologic surgical procedure was reported with the Zeus robotic system in 1999 [1]. This system has three remote-controlled robotic arms, allowing a single surgeon to manipulate the laparoscope and two laparoscopic surgical instruments simultaneously. AESOP holds the laparoscope and is directed by voice commands. The robotic arms are separate units also attached to the sides of the operating table.

The surgeon is seated at a mobile console that can be positioned anywhere in the operating room. The console consists of a video monitor and two handles that control the robotic arms holding the surgical instruments. In the original trial, the handles resembled traditional surgical instruments. The handles have been modified on the recent prototypes to solid ovals resembling large eggs that fit into the palms of the hands.

A computer controller translates the surgeon's movements of the handles to the robotic arms. There is no observed delay between the movement of the handles and the movement of the instruments. The operator's movements can be scaled according to his specifications. For example, a scaling ratio of 10:1 means that for every 1 cm the surgeon moves the handles at the console, the robotic surgical instruments would move 1 mm at the surgical site. Tremors and small, unintended hand motions that are the result of holding instruments for a prolonged period can be filtered out. Thus, the instruments may be controlled more precisely throughout the procedure.

Several interchangeable instruments have been developed for use with the robotic arms, including scissors, graspers, needle holders, and micro-unipolar cautery. The robotic device is not very bulky and is fairly quick and easy to attach to the operating table. Surgical assistants can move around the patient easily and have ready access to the abdomen and vagina.

There were significant limitations to this robotic device. It was difficult to place the robots properly around the table if the patient was in the lithotomy position. Proper port placement was less cosmetically pleasing, because the ports must be placed high on the abdomen to accommodate the length of the instruments attached to the robotic arms. The depth perception was no better than conventional laparoscopy. The haptic feedback was not sufficiently sophisticated to be of practical value. Therefore, the surgeon still had to rely on visual cues to assess the tensile strength of the tissue and sutures. This limitation led to numerous needle and suture breaks. It required many hours of training to interpret the visual cues that would prevent this from occurring.

A three-dimensional image was possible by wearing special glasses while looking at a traditional monitor. However, it was not a true 3D image and the resolution and clarity were compromised, to the point where it was easier to work from the better quality 2D image. The main drawback of the robot was the lack of articulation at the tip of the instruments. This limitation led to difficulties in placing the sutures at the precise angle, such that either undue tissue manipulation was required or the needle placement was suboptimal. The procedures included in this report were first performed in 1998. Since then, the ZEUS system has been upgraded and now has an articulation at the tip of the instruments. Computer Motion calls this articulation a Micro Wrist, which more closely follows the movements of the human wrist. Although this modification is clearly an improvement over earlier prototypes in providing additional degrees of freedom, its movements are not totally instinctive. For example, to obtain a 360° motion at the articulated instrument tip, the shaft of the instrument has to be rotated.

The other commercially available robotic system that has been used in gynecologic surgery is the da Vinci system (Intuitive surgical, Mountain View, California) [5]. The basic concept of this surgical robot is the same. The surgeon controls the movements of the robotic surgical instruments by manipulating the handles while seated at a console away from the surgical field. The da Vinci system has a dual lens 12 mm laparoscope that provides true binocular 3D vision with great clarity. The surgeon looks through a viewer on the console. The assistants observe the procedure on conventional 2D monitors.

The laparoscope is also controlled by moving the handles at the console. The most impressive part of the system is the intra-abdominal articulation of the microinstruments 2 cm from the tip. This articulation serves the same function as a human wrist. Controlling the movements of the instrument tips is intuitive and requires minimal training. The main limitation of the da Vinci device is its size. The robot tower houses the surgical arms of the robot, as well as the laparoscope holder. Once the tower is positioned in the operative field, the surgical assistants have very limited access to the abdomen and perineum. Since the system is attached to the patient, it must be disengaged prior to any changes in the position of the operating table.

A significant limitation of both robotic systems is the technical skill required to set up and maintain the robot during surgery. In spite of having a dedicated engineer from the manufacturer present throughout all of our robotic cases, technical problems occurred frequently. Furthermore, additional support was required from the manufacturer to address specific problems that arose during the surgical cases.

The use of these robots for telesurgery has captured the imagination of many surgeons. This innovation would allow a local surgeon to accomplish specialized procedures with the help of a distant expert. There are still logistical issues that need to be resolved. However, telesurgery has already been accomplished with present-day technology [8,9]. Internet bandwidth and point-to-point latency are the major technical advances that have limited this application. Cost is another issue. However, most of these problems will be resolved in the near future.

## 3. Operating room integration

Although surgical consoles were originally designed to perform a surgical procedure robotically, they will be used, in the future, for integration of information about the patient. Preoperative data, especially images, can be imported easily into the surgical field, so that the surgeon does not act by recall alone. Virtual reality is a computer model of the environment. Interaction with the artificial environment can be accomplished easily. Augmented reality is inclusion in the images of the real world images of an artificial nature. In this way, anatomic or pathologic images can be overlaid on the real-time images of the surgical field. For the moment, these are static images, but in time they will have the capacity to change as the surgery progresses. This modification will be accomplished with sensors at the effector's tips that will update the images as the surgery progresses.

## 4. Simulation

The teaching of surgical procedures needs to evolve from "training on the job" to a process that has clearly defined tasks and endpoints within the context of a standardized but changing surgical environment. Surgical simulation uses the principles of interactive, augmented or virtual reality. The surgeon trainee will be required to learn surgical procedures on simulators that assess specific tasks and give immediate feedback. The trainee proceeds through different levels until a procedure is mastered. These same principles will apply to practicing surgeons who wish to learn new surgical techniques. The era of the weekend surgical course such as with the introduction of the laparoscopic cholecystectomy is over.

## References

[1] T. Falcone, J. Goldberg, A. Garcia-Ruiz, H. Margossian, L. Stevens, Full robotic assistance for laparoscopic tubal anastomosis: a case report, J. Laparoendosc. Adv. Surg. Tech., Part A 9 (1999) 107–113.
[2] L. Mettler, M. Ibrahim, W. Jonat, One year of experience working with the aid of a robotic assistant (the voice-controlled optic holder AESOP) in gynecologic endoscopic surgery, Hum. Reprod. 13 (1998) 2748–2750.
[3] T. Falcone, J.M. Goldberg, H. Margossian, L. Stevens, Robotically assisted laparoscopic microsurgical anastomosis: a human pilot study, Fertil. Steril. 73 (2000) 1040–1042.
[4] J.M. Goldberg, T. Falcone, Laparoscopic microsurgical tubal anastomosis with and without robotic assistance, Hum. Reprod. 18 (2003) 145–147.
[5] M. Degueldre, J. Vandromme, P.T. Huong, G.B. Cadiere, Robotically assisted laparoscopic microsurgical tubal reanastomosis: a feasibility study, Fertil. Steril. 74 (2000) 1020–1023.
[6] H. Margossian, T. Falcone, Robotically assisted laparoscopic hysterectomy and adnexal surgery, J. Laparoendosc. Adv. Surg. Tech., Part A 11 (2001) 161–165.
[7] C. Diaz-Arrastia, C. Jurnalov, G. Gomez, C. Townsend, Laparoscopic hysterectomy using a computer-enhanced surgical robot, Surg. Endosc. 16 (2002) 1271–1273.
[8] J. Marescaux, J. Leroy, M. Gagner, F. Rubino, D. Mutter, M. Vix, S. Butner, M. Smith, Transatlantic robot-assisted telesurgery, Nature 413 (2001) 379–380.
[9] G. Janetschek, G. Bartsch, L.R. Kavoussi, Transcontinental interactive laparoscopic telesurgery between the United States and Europe, J. Urol. 160 (1998) 1413.

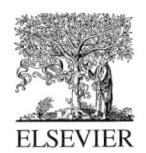

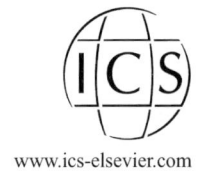

# Embryo transfer—a critique of the factors involved in optimizing pregnancy success

Hassan N. Sallam*

*Obstetrics and Gynaecology, The University of Alexandria, 22 Victor Emanuel Square, Smouha, Alexandria 21615, Egypt*
*Alexandria Fertility Centre, Alexandria, Egypt*

**Abstract.** Various modifications have been suggested to optimize embryo transfer (ET) during assisted reproduction [in vitro fertilization (IVF) and intracytoplasmic sperm injection (ICSI)]. However, not all of these modifications have been evaluated by randomized controlled trials (RCTs). The aim of this work was to evaluate these modifications by taking an evidence-based approach. Meta-analyses and RCTs have shown that the pregnancy rate is significantly increased by performing a dummy ET before the actual transfer, by ultrasound-guided ET, and by depositing the embryos 2 cm below the uterine fundus. Similarly, meta-analyses and RCTs have shown that bed rest after ET, flushing the cervical canal before ET, sexual intercourse around the time of ET, use of a fibrin sealant, use of a soft catheter as opposed to a rigid catheter, and slow withdrawal of the catheter after ET did not affect the pregnancy rate. The value of removing the cervical mucus prior to ET, performing ET with a full bladder, avoiding the use of a volsellum, and routine administration of antibiotics following ET remains to be studied by RCTs. © 2004 Published by Elsevier B.V.

*Keywords:* Embryo transfer; IVF; ICSI; Assisted reproduction; Evidence-based medicine

## 1. Introduction

Despite numerous developments in the field of assisted reproduction, the implantation rate of replaced embryos remains low. It is estimated that 85% of the embryos replaced during in vitro fertilization (IVF) or intracytoplasmic sperm injection (ICSI) fail to implant [1]. The exact cause of this low implantation rate is unknown, but may reside in the technique of embryo transfer (ET), the efficiency of endometrial receptivity, or the ability of the embryo to invade the endometrium properly. In order

---

*Abbreviations:* ET, embryo transfer; RCT, randomized controlled trial; IVF, in vitro fertilization; ICSI, intracytoplasmic sperm injection; OR, odds ratio; CI, confidence intervals.
\* Tel.: +20-3-4245750, +20-3-4279409, +20-3-4292323; fax: +20-3-4873663.
*E-mail address:* hnsallam@link.net (H.N. Sallam).

to improve implantation rates, various modifications of the ET technique have been suggested. This presentation will attempt to assess these modifications based on evidence.

## 2. Gentle and atraumatic technique

It has been claimed by some, but not all, studies that difficult ETs are associated with diminished pregnancy and implantation rates and that a gentle and atraumatic technique is necessary to achieve good results. We have also reported that changing the catheter and the presence of blood on the catheter tip during ET significantly diminish the pregnancy and implantation rates [2]. In a recent meta-analysis, we have found that difficult transfers are indeed associated with significantly diminished pregnancy [odds ratio (OR)=0.73; 95% CI (0.63–0.85)] and implantation rates [OR=0.64; 95% CI (0.52–0.77)] compared with easy transfers (Fig. 1) [3].

## 3. Performing a trial embryo transfer before the actual procedure

It has been suggested that performing a trial (mock or dummy) ET before the actual transfer increases the pregnancy and implantation rates, and various studies have been published in this respect. However, only one of these studies was a randomized controlled trial (RCT), where the authors found that the pregnancy and implantation rates were significantly higher in the dummy transfer group as compared with the no-dummy transfer group [4].

## 4. Embryo transfer under ultrasound guidance

Performing ET under ultrasound guidance was also claimed to improve pregnancy and implantation rates over the clinical touch method in some, but not all, published studies. We have conducted a meta-analysis of RCTs and found that, compared with the clinical touch method, abdominal ultrasound-guided transfer significantly increases the clinical

Review: Difficult embryo transfers
Comparison: 01 Difficult versus easy transfers
Outcome: 01 Pregnancy rate

| Study or sub-category | Difficult transfers n/N | Easy transfers n/N | OR (fixed) 95% CI | Weight % | OR (fixed) 95% CI |
|---|---|---|---|---|---|
| Leeton, 1982 | 0/28 | 34/159 | | 2.58 | 0.06 [0.00, 1.07] |
| Wood, 1985 | 28/169 | 102/659 | | 8.60 | 1.08 [0.69, 1.71] |
| Tur-Kaspa, 1998 | 30/120 | 121/734 | | 6.31 | 1.69 [1.07, 2.67] |
| Abusheikha, 1999 | 2/17 | 16/40 | | 2.08 | 0.20 [0.04, 1.00] |
| Nabi, 1999 | 16/69 | 280/1135 | | 6.10 | 0.92 [0.52, 1.64] |
| Noyes, 1999 | 30/67 | 474/847 | | 9.50 | 0.64 [0.39, 1.05] |
| Burke, 2000 | 5/15 | 53/195 | | 1.25 | 1.34 [0.44, 4.10] |
| Tomas, 2002 | 72/342 | 1355/4465 | | 37.68 | 0.61 [0.47, 0.80] |
| Sallam, 2003 | 23/149 | 142/635 | | 11.30 | 0.63 [0.39, 1.03] |
| Spandorfer, 2003 | 33/106 | 914/2157 | | 14.60 | 0.61 [0.40, 0.94] |
| Total (95% CI) | 1082 | 11026 | | 100.00 | 0.73 [0.63, 0.85] |

Total events: 239 (Difficult transfers), 3491 (Easy transfers)
Test for heterogeneity: Chi² = 25.85, df = 9 (P = 0.002), I² = 65.2%
Test for overall effect: Z = 4.00 (P < 0.0001)

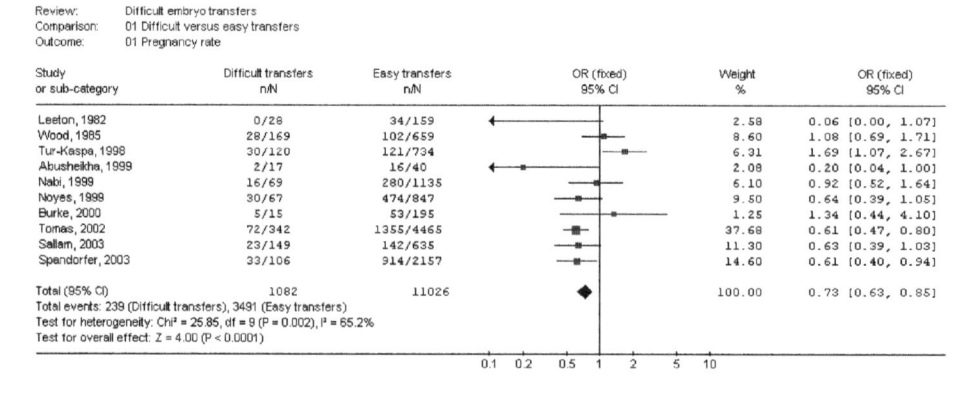

Fig. 1. A meta-analysis of controlled studies showing that difficult transfers are associated with diminished pregnancy rates in IVF and ICSI [3].

| Review: | Ultrasound guided embryo transfer |
|---|---|
| Comparison: | 01 Ultrasound versus clinical touch |
| Outcome: | 01 Clinical pregnancy rate |

| Study or sub-category | Ultrasound guided n/N | Clinical touch n/N | OR (fixed) 95% CI | Weight % | OR (fixed) 95% CI |
|---|---|---|---|---|---|
| Coroleu et al | 91/182 | 61/180 | | 17.74 | 1.95 [1.28, 2.98] |
| Tang et al | 104/400 | 90/400 | | 38.52 | 1.21 [0.88, 1.67] |
| Garcia-Velasco | 112/187 | 103/187 | | 23.89 | 1.22 [0.81, 1.84] |
| Matorras et al | 67/255 | 47/260 | | 19.85 | 1.62 [1.06, 2.46] |
| Total (95% CI) | 1024 | 1027 | | 100.00 | 1.42 [1.17, 1.73] |

Total events: 374 (Ultrasound guided), 301 (Clinical touch)
Test for heterogeneity: Chi² = 3.99, df = 3 (P = 0.26), I² = 24.8%
Test for overall effect: Z = 3.58 (P = 0.0003)

Fig. 2. A meta-analysis of RCTs showing that transabdominal ultrasound-guided embryo transfers are associated with an increased clinical pregnancy rate in IVF and ICSI [5] (with the kind permission of the editor of *Fertility and Sterility*).

pregnancy rate [OR=1.42; 95% CI (1.17–1.73)] and the ongoing pregnancy rate [OR=1.49; 95% CI (1.22–1.82)] (Figs. 2 and 3) [5].

## 5. Embryo transfer with a full bladder

It has been suggested that straightening the utero-cervical angle by performing ET with a full bladder could improve pregnancy and implantation rates [6]. We have also found that the utero-cervical angle measured by ultrasound is related to the pregnancy and implantation rates (Fig. 4) and that patients with acute utero-cervical angles (>60°) had significantly lower pregnancy rates compared with patients with no angles [OR=0.36; 95% CI (0.16–0.52)] [7]. Moulding the catheter according to the measured angle resulted in a lower incidence of difficult transfers [OR=0.25; 95% CI (0.16–0.40)], as well as higher pregnancy rates [OR=1.57; 95% CI (1.08–2.27)]. However, no RCTs have so far been published to evaluate performing ET with and without a full bladder.

## 6. Removing the cervical mucus prior to embryo transfer

In a retrospective study, Nabi et al. [8] found that embryos were significantly more likely to be retained when the ET catheter was contaminated with mucus (3.3% vs. 17.8%,

| Review: | Ultrasound guided embryo transfer |
|---|---|
| Comparison: | 01 Ultrasound versus clinical touch |
| Outcome: | 03 On-going pregnancy rate |

| Study or sub-category | Ultrasound guided n/N | Clinical touch n/N | OR (fixed) 95% CI | Weight % | OR (fixed) 95% CI |
|---|---|---|---|---|---|
| Coroleu et al | 85/182 | 52/180 | | 17.62 | 2.16 [1.40, 3.33] |
| Tang et al | 94/400 | 76/400 | | 36.75 | 1.31 [0.93, 1.84] |
| Garcia-Velasco | 100/187 | 94/187 | | 27.65 | 1.14 [0.76, 1.71] |
| Matorras et al | 57/255 | 37/260 | | 17.98 | 1.74 [1.10, 2.74] |
| Total (95% CI) | 1024 | 1027 | | 100.00 | 1.49 [1.22, 1.82] |

Total events: 336 (Ultrasound guided), 259 (Clinical touch)
Test for heterogeneity: Chi² = 5.47, df = 3 (P = 0.14), I² = 45.1%
Test for overall effect: Z = 3.89 (P < 0.0001)

Fig. 3. A meta-analysis of RCTs showing that transabdominal ultrasound-guided embryo transfers are associated with an increased, ongoing pregnancy rate in IVF and ICSI [5] (with the kind permission of the editor of *Fertility and Sterility*).

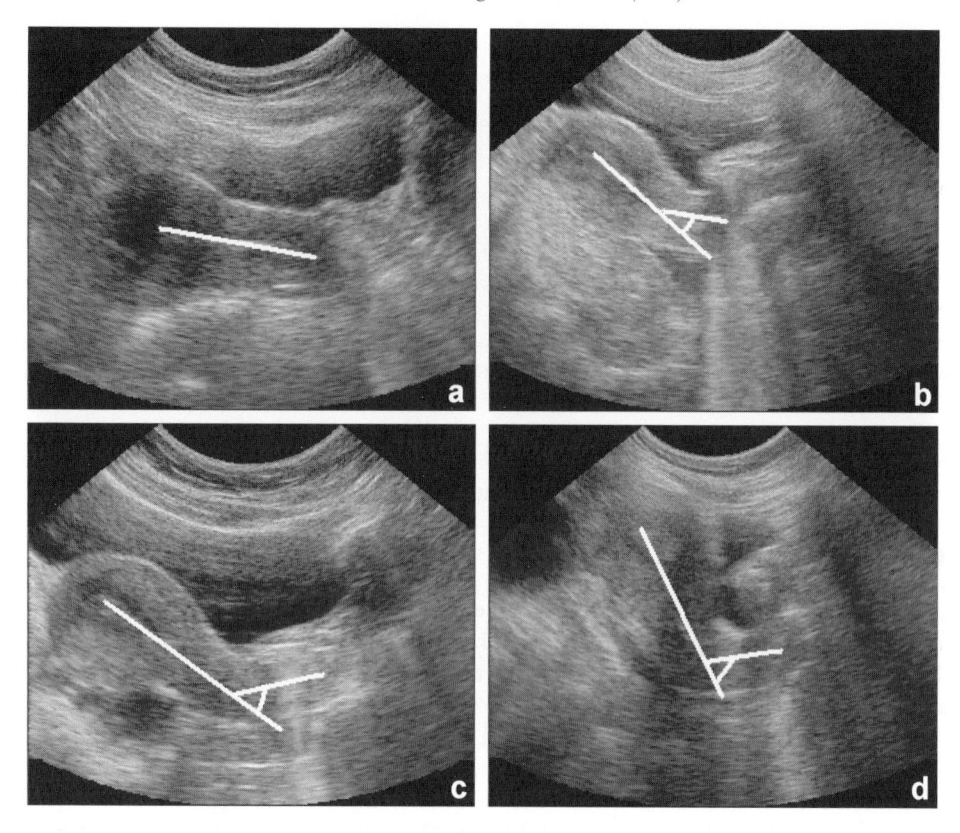

Fig. 4. Measuring the utero-cervical angle by transabdominal ultrasonography: (a) no angle, (b) small angle (<30°), (c) moderate angle (30–60°), (d) large angle (>60°) [7] (with the kind permission of the editor of *Human Reproduction*).

$p$=0.000001). Consequently, the removal of the cervical mucus prior to ET has been claimed to improve the pregnancy and implantation rates, but no randomized trials have so far been published on the routine aspiration of the mucus prior to ET.

## 7. Flushing the cervical canal with culture medium prior to embryo transfer

Vigorous flushing of the cervical canal with culture medium prior to ET has been suggested as a method to improve implantation in assisted reproduction. In 1999, MacNamee [9] reported that vigorous flushing of the cervical canal and the use of a soft catheter improved the pregnancy and implantation rates. However, in an RCT, we have found no statistically significant difference with and without flushing in pregnancy rates (25.5% and 34.5%, $p$=0.4053) or implantation rates (15.38% and 17.46%, $p$=0.7687) [10].

## 8. Avoiding the use of a tenaculum (volsellum)

The use of a tenaculum was found to stimulate uterine junctional zone contractions affecting implantation of the transferred embryos [11]. Similarly, Dorn et al. [12] found an elevation in oxytocin level when the tenaculum was applied to the cervix during ET and remained elevated until the end of the ET procedure. Whether this practice results in lower pregnancy and implantation rates remains to be shown.

## 9. The type of catheter

The relationship between the types of catheter used in ET remains unresolved. Some studies have reported better results with soft catheters. Other studies found the complete opposite and a third group reported no difference. We have recently conducted a meta-analysis of RCTs, comparing soft with rigid catheters, and found no statistically significant differences in the pregnancy rates between the two types [OR=0.98; 95% CI (0.75–1.28)] (Fig. 5) [13].

## 10. Site of embryo deposition

In an RCT, Coroleu et al. [14] reported that the implantation rate was significantly higher when the embryos were deposited 2 cm below the uterine fundus compared with when deposited 1 cm below the fundus. It has also been suggested that midfundal deposition of the embryos results in a lower incidence of ectopic pregnancies compared with deep fundal deposition, but these claims have not been substantiated in large RCTs [15].

## 11. Slow withdrawal of the embryo transfer catheter

In an RCT, Martinez et al. [16] found no statistically significant difference in pregnancy rate when the catheter was withdrawn immediately after ET compared with when it was left for 30 s in the uterus before its withdrawal. They concluded that either the waiting interval was insufficient to detect differences, or that the retention time before withdrawing the catheter is not a factor influencing pregnancy rates.

## 12. The use of a fibrin sealant

The addition of a fibrin sealant (glue) to the culture medium containing the embryos during ET was suggested in an attempt to improve pregnancy rates and a case–control

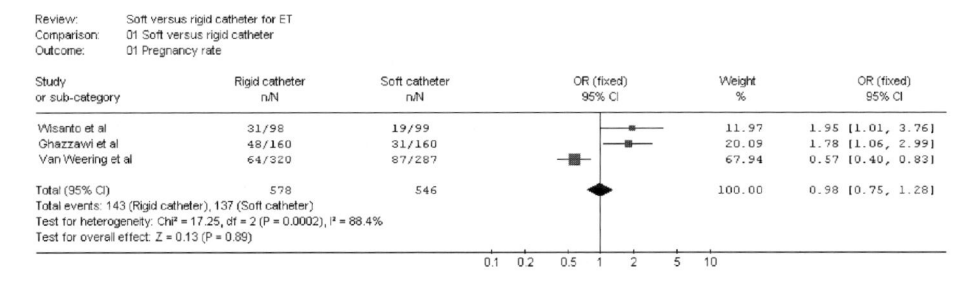

Fig. 5. A meta-analysis of RCTs showing no statistically significant difference in the clinical pregnancy rate between using soft and rigid ET catheters [13].

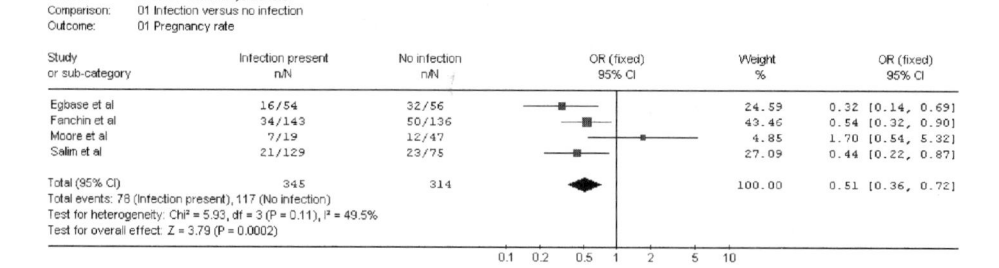

| Study or sub-category | Infection present n/N | No infection n/N | Weight % | OR (fixed) 95% CI |
|---|---|---|---|---|
| Egbase et al | 16/54 | 32/56 | 24.59 | 0.32 [0.14, 0.69] |
| Fanchin et al | 34/143 | 50/136 | 43.46 | 0.54 [0.32, 0.90] |
| Moore et al | 7/19 | 12/47 | 4.85 | 1.70 [0.54, 5.32] |
| Salim et al | 21/129 | 23/75 | 27.09 | 0.44 [0.22, 0.87] |
| Total (95% CI) | 345 | 314 | 100.00 | 0.51 [0.36, 0.72] |

Total events: 78 (Infection present), 117 (No infection)
Test for heterogeneity: Chi² = 5.93, df = 3 (P = 0.11), I² = 49.5%
Test for overall effect: Z = 3.79 (P = 0.0002)

Fig. 6. A meta-analysis of controlled studies showing that cervical infection during ET is associated with diminished pregnancy rates in IVF and ICSI [22].

study reported higher pregnancy rates [17]. However, two RCTs failed to confirm these findings [18,19].

## 13. Bed rest after embryo transfer

In 1998, Sharif et al. [20] reported that the clinical pregnancy rate in their patients who had no bed rest following ET was significantly higher than the national data (30% vs. 22.9%). These findings were confirmed in an RCT conducted by Botta and Grudzinskas [21] who found no statistically significant differences in clinical pregnancy rate between patients who had a 2-h period of bed rest following ET compared with those who had bed rest for only 20 min.

## 14. Routine administration of antibiotics following embryo transfer

Microbial infection of the cervix was found to be a cause of diminished pregnancy and implantation rates in some, but not all, published studies. We have recently conducted a meta-analysis of controlled studies and found that the clinical pregnancy [OR=0.51; 95% CI (0.36–0.72)] and implantation rates [OR=0.43; 95% CI (0.31–0.61)] were indeed diminished in the presence of cervical infection (Fig. 6) [22]. However, the effect of routine administration of antibiotics following oocyte retrieval or ET has not been studied by RCTs and is still a matter of debate.

## 15. Sexual intercourse

Sexual intercourse around the time of embryo transfer has also been suggested as a cause of low implantation rates after assisted reproduction. However, when an RCT was conducted by Tremellen et al. [23], the clinical pregnancy rate was not affected by sexual intercourse and, contrary to expectations, the implantation rate was significantly increased for patients who had sexual intercourse around the time of embryo transfer.

## 16. Conclusions

Embryo transfer remains a delicate but essential step in assisted reproduction. RCTs have shown that the pregnancy rate is significantly increased by performing a dummy ET before the actual transfer, by ultrasound-guided ET, and by depositing the embryos

2 cm below the uterine fundus. Similarly, RCTs have shown that bed rest after ET, flushing the cervical canal before ET, sexual intercourse around the time of ET, use a fibrin sealant, use of a soft catheter as opposed to a rigid catheter, and slow withdrawal of the ET catheter did not affect the pregnancy rate. The value of removing the cervical mucus prior to ET, performing ET with a full bladder, avoiding the use of a volsellum, and routine administration of antibiotics following ET remains to be studied by RCTs.

## References

[1] R.G. Edwards, Clinical approaches to increasing uterine receptivity during human implantation, Hum. Reprod. 10 (1995) 60–66.
[2] H.N. Sallam, et al., Impact of technical difficulties, choice of catheter, and the presence of blood on the success of embryo transfer—experience from a single provider, J. Assist. Reprod. Genet. 20 (2003) 135–142.
[3] H. Sallam, S. Sadek, A.F. Agameya, Does a difficult embryo transfer affect the results of IVF and ICSI? A meta-analysis of controlled studies, Fertil. Steril. 80 (2003) S127.
[4] R. Mansour, M. Aboulghar, G. Serour, Dummy embryo transfer: a technique that minimizes the problems of embryo transfer and improves the pregnancy rate in human in vitro fertilization, Fertil. Steril. 54 (1990) 678–681.
[5] H.N. Sallam, S.S. Sadek, Ultrasound-guided embryo transfer: a meta-analysis of randomized controlled trials, Fertil. Steril. 80 (2003) 1042–1046.
[6] A. Lewin, et al., The role of uterine straightening by passive bladder distension before embryo transfer in IVF cycles, J. Assist. Reprod. Genet. 14 (1997) 32–34.
[7] H.N. Sallam, et al., Ultrasound measurement of the utero-cervical angle prior to embryo transfer—a prospective controlled study, Hum. Reprod. 17 (2002) 1767–1772.
[8] A. Nabi, et al., Multiple attempts at embryo transfer: does this affect in-vitro fertilization treatment outcome? Hum. Reprod. 12 (1997) 1188–1190.
[9] P. MacNamee, Vigorous flushing the cervical canal with culture medium prior to embryo transfer, Paper presented at the World Congress of IVF, Sydney, 1999.
[10] H.N. Sallam, et al., The importance of flushing the cervical canal with culture medium prior to embryo transfer, Fertil. Steril. 3 (2000) 64–65.
[11] P. Lesny, et al., Junctional zone contractions and embryo transfer: is it safe to use a tenaculum? Hum. Reprod. 14 (1999) 2367–2370.
[12] C. Dorn, et al., Serum oxytocin concentration during embryo transfer procedure, Eur. J. Obstet. Gynecol. Reprod. Biol. 87 (1999) 77–80.
[13] H.N. Sallam, The evidence-based practice of assisted reproduction, in: J. Bonnar, W. Dunlop (Eds.), Recent Adv. Obstetr. Gynaecol. vol. 22, The Royal Society of Medicine Press, London, England, UK, 2003, pp. 95–108.
[14] B. Coroleu, et al., The influence of the depth of embryo replacement into the uterine cavity on implantation rates after IVF: a controlled, ultrasound-guided study, Hum. Reprod. 17 (2002) 341–346.
[15] A. Nazari, et al., Embryo transfer technique as a cause of ectopic pregnancy in in vitro fertilization, Fertil. Steril. 60 (1993) 919–921.
[16] F. Martinez, et al., Ultrasound-guided embryo transfer: immediate withdrawal of the catheter versus a 30 second wait, Hum. Reprod. 16 (2001) 871–874.
[17] I. Bar-Hava, et al., Fibrin glue improves pregnancy rates in women of advanced reproductive age and in patients in whom in vitro fertilization attempts repeatedly fail, Fertil. Steril. 71 (1999) 821–824.
[18] W. Feichtinger, et al., The use of fibrin sealant for embryo transfer: development and clinical studies, Hum. Reprod. 7 (1992) 890–893.
[19] Z. Ben-Rafael, et al., The use of fibrin sealant in in vitro fertilization and embryo transfer, Int. J. Fertil. Menopausal Stud. 40 (1995) 303–306.
[20] K. Sharif, et al., Is bed rest following embryo transfer necessary? Fertil. Steril. 69 (1998) 478–481.

[21] G. Botta, G. Grudzinskas, Is a prolonged bed rest following embryo transfer useful? Hum. Reprod. 12 (1997) 2489–2492.
[22] H. Sallam, S. Sadek, F. Ezzeldin, Does cervical infection affect the results of IVF and ICSI? A meta-analysis of controlled studies, Fertil. Steril. 80 (2003) S110.
[23] K.P. Tremellen, et al., The effect of intercourse on pregnancy rates during assisted human reproduction, Hum. Reprod. 15 (2000) 2653–2658.

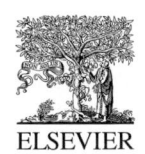

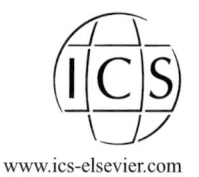

# Optimizing outcome in assisted reproduction reducing multiple pregnancy

David L. Healy[a,*], Sue Breheny[b], Vivien MacLachlan[b], Luk Rombauts[a], Gab Kovacs[a]

[a] *Department of Obstetrics and Gynaecology, Monash Medical Centre, Level 5, 246 Clayton Road, Clayton 3168, Melbourne, Victoria, Australia*
[b] *Monash IVF, Australia*

**Abstract.** *Introduction*: Optimizing outcome in assisted reproduction requires definition of a successful outcome. We suggest delivery of a single term gestation, live baby, per cycle of assisted reproduction initiated is the most relevant standard of success. We have defined this outcome as the birth emphasising a successful singleton at term (BESST). *Methods*: We have evaluated the BESST outcome in a series of patients requiring controlled ovarian hyperstimulation–intrauterine insemination (COH–IUI) as well as series of patients requiring in vitro fertilisation (IVF). *Results*: We found that our BESST outcome for COH–IUI was 6%. We also found that our BESST statistic over a large IVF program was 11%. *Conclusions*: Clinical ART is now established worldwide in both developed and developing nations. Although the science is mature, the outcome of treatment and the reporting of endpoints require emphasis if reducing multiple pregnancy and reducing damage to babies is to occur. We propose the singleton, term gestation, live birth rate of the baby per cycle begun as the BESST measure of ART success. © 2004 Published by Elsevier B.V.

*Keywords:* Assisted reproduction; Live birth rate per cycle; Single pregnancy; Success rate; Term gestation; In vitro fertilisation; Ovulation induction; Ovulation enhancement; Controlled ovarian hyperstimulation–intrauterine insemination

## 1. Introduction

Optimizing outcome in assisted reproduction requires agreement on what primary outcome will be measured. We suggest that a fundamental strategy to optimising outcome in all assisted reproductive technologies (ARTs)–ovulation induction (OI), controlled ovarian hyperstimulation–intrauterine insemination (COH–IUI) and all in vitro fertilisation (IVF) methods including intracytoplasmic sperm injection (ICSI), pivots upon methods to prevent multiple pregnancy and to emphasise a new statistic measuring outcome.

---

\* Corresponding author. Tel.: +61-03-9594-5488; fax: +61-9594-6389.
*E-mail address:* david.healy@med.monash.edu.au (D.L. Healy).

0531-5131/ © 2004 Published by Elsevier B.V.
doi:10.1016/j.ics.2004.01.079

Multiple pregnancy is the most frequent and most serious iatrogenic complication of ART [1]. It is universally recognized that multiple gestation, and its attendant prematurity, is associated with increased mortality and morbidity, both for mothers and fetuses [2-4]. Indeed, complications are so common that some have classified multiple pregnancy as a major pathology [5].

We suggest the establishment of a new definition of a successful outcome in all assisted reproductive technologies. We have called this the birth emphasising a successful singleton at term (BESST) statistic. The BESST statistic is the singleton, term gestation, live birth rate of one baby per cycle of fertility treatment initiated.

Although a seemingly simple act, the importance of setting a new BESST endpoint cannot be overstated. It will focus the philosophical change already underway—the recognition that delivery of a single healthy baby is the most appropriate endpoint. Singleton live birth rate per cycle started has been advocated, in response to the high incidence of multiples, by the European Society of Human Reproduction and Embryology [1] and by the World Health Organization [6]. If the object is a healthy baby, the specification of 'term gestation' is also justified.

IVF/ICSI programmes should express outcome as a proportion of all treatment cycles initiated. Oocyte retrieval is a significant component of assisted reproductive technology, accounting for much of the stress, financial burden, and almost all of the surgical risk [7]. Moreover, the exclusion of cycles from which oocyte retrieval is not attempted is inappropriate. Although less daunting, the cost of follicular stimulation is not insignificant; nor is the emotional burden of a cycle that is terminated prior to oocyte retrieval. Inclusion of all cycles initiated, regardless of outcome, is most appropriate because it best represents the burden of treatment endured by a couple.

There has been considerable controversy in the medical literature regarding the incidence of multiple pregnancy and multiple birth following not only IVF but also ovulation induction and various forms of ovulation enhancement. The consensus from major centers in the United States and Europe seems to be that the multiple pregnancy rates associated with ovulation induction are a damaging problem and, as highlighted by Jones and Schnorr [8], "a grave disservice to patients". The president, two past presidents and president-elect of the American Society of Reproductive Medicine have noted that triplets and higher births result in approximately 40% of instances of ovulation induction [9]. These authorities have emphasized that guidelines to avoid high-order multiple pregnancies caused by ovulation induction have not been published.

## 2. Ovulation induction

Follicle-stimulating hormone was first reported to induce ovarian follicle growth, ovulation and pregnancy in patients with hypogonadotropic hypogonadism, approximately 40 years ago. Subsequent series of anovulatory infertile patients reported results from the administration of FSH injections also for eugonadotropic hypogonadism and for polycystic ovary syndrome (PCOS) [10,11].

Studies from the United Kingdom and Australia emphasized low-dose gonadotropin treatment with small stepwise increments above a threshold dosage [12,13].

## 3. Controlled ovarian hyperstimulation and intrauterine insemination

Follicle-stimulating hormone administration to normally ovulating but infertile women rapidly followed the first report of pregnancies after IVF-ET using gonadotropin injections to induce multiple co-dominant folliculogenesis [14]. Around the same time, FSH injections also began to be administered to infertile women who were spontaneously ovulatory. These patients were not undertaking IVF treatment but were undergoing controlled ovarian hyperstimulation before IUI (COH–IUI) for the treatment of their infertility [15,16].

Widespread expansion of IVF and COH–IUI programs have subsequently occurred. Recent editorials have lamented an epidemic of multiple pregnancies arising from these assisted reproductive technologies. It appears in the USA that an individual infertile couple is at significantly greater risk of a high order multiple pregnancy from COH–IUI or ovulation induction regimens than they are from IVF [17,18].

Between January 1, 1999, and December 31, 2000, we prospectively treated 234 consecutive patients referred for COH–IUI by specialist gynecologists because of continuing infertility. Patients referred by gynecologists had already had tests of tubal patency and were not further operated upon by us by diagnostic laparoscopy and hysteroscopy to cement a diagnosis of idiopathic infertility. Five hundred and ten treatment cycles were administered. Women had regular ovulatory cycles, 23–34 days apart with mid luteal phase serum progesterone concentrations >30 nmol/l taken as confirmation of spontaneous ovulation. All patients had normal serum FSH concentrations of <10 U/l on cycle day 3 indicating adequate ovarian reserve. Women with known tubal disease, who had at least one normal looking uterine tube at laparoscopy, were eligible for this study. A semen analysis was considered abnormal by World Health Organization criteria.

The first day of menstrual bleeding was defined as Day 1 of the spontaneous cycle. Treatment commenced on Day 2 with recombinant human FSH (RhFSH; Puregon; Organon Australia; Gonal-F; Serono Australia). The typical median starting dose was 112 IU of RhFSH per day. In individual patients weighing <45 kg, the commencement dose was 75 IU of RhFSH subcutaneously daily. In individuals with a body mass index of 25–30, a daily commencement dosage of 150 IU RhFSH subcutaneously was used.

Decisions about ongoing treatment were made on the basis of vaginal ultrasound ovarian scanning and serum estradiol concentrations. The initial dose of RhFSH was maintained for ≥5 days before any increase. If there was no dominant follicle (>10 mm maximum diameter) after 5 days, the dosage was increased from 112 IU subcutaneously daily to 150 IU subcutaneously daily for a further 5 days. If a follicle equal to 10 mm maximum diameter emerged, the dose of RhFSH was maintained until that follicle reached a diameter of 14 mm and the endometrium was ≥8 mm or more in bilaminar thickness.

At that diameter, a single dose of human chorionic gonadotropin (hCG) 5000 IU, was administered intramuscularly and RhFSH was stopped. If there were more than three follicles ≥14 mm in diameter or greater, the cycle was stopped due to the risk of multiple pregnancy and/or ovarian hyperstimulation syndrome. The couple were advised to not have sexual intercourse for 3 weeks.

In the treatment cycle, patients were evaluated three times per week, Monday to Friday. If, despite ovulation, pregnancy did not occur during the first cycle of treatment, RhFSH was reintroduced at the same dosage on Day 2 of the next cycle. In women who developed more than three follicles, the treatment protocol was amended for the next cycle so that a smaller starting dose was used. In some patients, this was as low as 50 IU RhFSH subcutaneously daily. If no pregnancy had occurred despite three to four cycles of COH–IUI, the patients were reviewed and tubal status assessed by laparoscopy if not already performed within the previous 1 year.

Each patient and/or their obstetrician provided information on whether the ongoing pregnancy was single or multiple. Outcome measures included the gestation at delivery, method of delivery, birth weight, congenital abnormalities and neonatal outcome. The primary endpoint of this study was pregnancy resulting in the birth of one normal baby at term gestation. Birth rate was calculated per started cycle. A normal baby was defined as any newborn child examined by a paediatrician in which the baby was without any notifiable birth defect.

The age of the women, body mass index, duration of infertility and parity for the cohort were respectively (median and range) 33 years (23–43), 23 (18–37) and 24 months (12–90). Seventy six percent were nulliparous.

Pregnancy rate varied considerably depending on which end-point was used. The pregnancy rate was 11% per cycle commenced if +βhCG (the β subunit of human chorionic gonadotrophin) was the endpoint or was 7% based on birth rate. There were 46 pregnancies with fetal heart motion in these 234 patients, giving a pregnancy rate of 20%. There was one triplet pregnancy, and the woman underwent selective reduction to twins. These were 10 miscarriages (22%). Thirty-six women gave birth; this was 15% of patients receiving treatment. No patient had premature birth.

We concluded that a regimen for COH–IUI using a starting dose of 112 IU, maintaining that dose for 5 days at least with small stepwise increments in a step up mode and administration of hCG at a 14-mm-diameter lead follicle was effective. We found that a woman's chance of giving birth to one normal term baby was 6% per cycle commenced with this regimen. There was a 20% chance of twins should pregnancy occur. With these guidelines, we have experienced only one triplet pregnancy in 510 cycles of treatment.

## 4. In vitro fertilisation

One approach to minimize IVF twins is to randomise IVF patients into research studies. The Australian Study of Single Embryo Transfer (ASSET) headed by Prof. Rob Norman and colleagues is a randomised controlled trial in women under 35 years who have three or more excellent embryos from their fresh IVF or ICSI cycle (personal communication). Patients are randomised to one- or two-embryo transfer. Recruitment to the ASSET trial has been unexpectedly slow. Our IVF or ICSI patients, once told of the risks of twins, are reluctant to be randomised due to fear of being randomised into the two-embryo arm of the study.

For IVF or ICSI patients, another way to minimize twins is to have an elective single embryo transfer (eSET) policy. This should minimize twin gestations while maintaining pregnancy rates in selected patients group. Unfortunately, a policy of single embryo transfer in a few programmes will have only a small impact on pooled data unless it is globally adopted.

The main strategy to combat multiple gestation associated with IVF and ICSI is to limit the maximum number of embryos transferred for any particular cycle. In many centres, the transfer of no more than two embryos is considered standard [5]. Unfortunately, the most recent reports from the Society for Assisted Reproductive Technology Registry in the United States of America and the European IVF Monitoring Program Registry, and the Australian National Perinatal Statistics Unit have failed to demonstrate a reduction in multiple delivery rate from 1998 to 1999. In the United States of America, this rate was 36.5%, in Europe, it was 26.3% [19] and in Australia, it was 20.9%.

We retrospectively examined all ART cycles initiated by the Monash IVF program, Monash University, Melbourne, Victoria, Australia in 2001. We defined assisted reproductive technology as any treatment involving oocyte retrieval, for subsequent manipulation in vitro, and their replacement into the female reproductive tract either as oocytes or embryos. This definition would include: IVF, with or without ICSI, gamete intrafallopian transfer (GIFT), zygote intrafallopian transfer (ZIFT) and microinjection intrafallopian transfer (MIFT). 'Cycle' described any ART treatment regimen started with the intended goal of oocyte retrieval, regardless of whether the retrieval was actually performed.

Included in our analysis were all gonadotrophin-stimulated cycles involving oocyte retrieval and insemination with either partner or donor sperm. Excluded from the analysis were: unstimulated or natural cycles, clomiphene citrate stimulated cycles, cycles utilizing donor oocytes or embryos, and frozen oocytes. Frozen–thawed embryo transfer cycles were excluded since those cycles were not stimulated. Controlled ovarian hyperstimulation cycles, which do not employ oocyte retrieval, were excluded by definition. Exclusions were not made based on female partner age, duration of infertility, aetiology of subfertility, or results of previous treatment cycles.

All women undergoing replacement of gametes or embryos had a maximum of three embryos transferred. All patients had quantitative determination of the βhCG 16 days following oocyte retrieval. Pregnancy was defined as two rising serum βhCG concentrations >5 IU/l. Those with positive pregnancy tests had transvaginal ultrasonography 6 weeks following oocyte retrieval to document the number of gestational sacs and the presence of fetal heart motion. A viable pregnancy was defined by the presence of at least one intrauterine gestational sac with fetal heart motion. Obstetric outcomes were monitored to determine pregnancy loss, preterm and term vaginal and caesarean birth rates.

Deliveries were classified as preterm if occurring between 20 and 36 6/7 completed weeks of gestation (between 18 and 34 6/7 completed weeks from the day of gamete or oocyte collection), and term if occurring after 37 completed weeks of gestation (after 35 completed weeks from the day of collection). Records of live birth or stillbirth were kept for each gestation.

Of all ART cycles initiated through Monash IVF programs in 2001, a total of 2600 cycles were identified in 1860 women for analysis by inclusion and exclusion criteria. Of the 2600 cycles initiated, 2214 oocyte retrievals (84%) and 2041 transfers (78%) of gametes or embryos were performed. IVF with or without ICSI accounted for 96.5% of all ART cycles conducted.

Of 644 preclinical pregnancies, 509 were viable on first-trimester ultrasound. Four hundred and forty-eight pregnancies continued past 20 weeks of gestation. Of these, 328 were singleton, 116 were twin and 4 were triplet pregnancies. Quadruplet or higher-order gestations did not occur.

Six pregnancies, one twin and five singleton, ended in stillbirth. All stillborn deliveries were preterm. The remaining 442 pregnancies resulted in live born neonates. One hundred and nineteen (28.2%) were multiple gestations. Of all live deliveries, 24.2% were preterm. Thirty-three singleton, 65 twin and all 4 triplet gestations delivered preterm. Multiples accounted for 67.6% of all preterm deliveries and 82.0% (150 of 183) of premature babies born. At term gestation, there were 50 twin and 290 singleton deliveries. Of pregnancies carrying to term, 85.3% were singleton.

Success rate varied widely depending upon the chosen endpoint. The rates for positive pregnancy test, fetal heart motion present on first trimester ultrasound and live delivery were 23.1%, 19.6% and 16.2%, respectively.

The singleton, term gestation, live birth rate of a baby was 11.1% per cycle initiated. One hundred and sixty-four (58.2%) of these babies delivered vaginally and 118 (41.8%) delivered by Caesarean section. The distribution into elective and emergency caesarean deliveries was not available.

## 5. Future directions

At Monash IVF, our typical woman was 35 years old (median; range 20–48 years) in 2001. Her prospect of a singleton, term gestation, live birth of a baby per cycle begun was 11.1%. We must note that this rate excludes frozen embryos. Outcomes derived from frozen embryo transfers would have contributed to the numerator but not the denominator, since the embryos used would have been obtained from oocytes collected in the original stimulation cycle. Subsequently, the success rate we report represents a minimum value.

ART techniques are now older than our patients. Clinical ART is now established worldwide in both developed and developing nations. The objective of treatment and reporting of endpoints must parallel this mature science. We propose the singleton, term gestation, live birth rate of a baby per cycle begun as the BESST measure of ART success.

## Acknowledgements

We are indebted to the staff at Monash IVF and our patients.

## References

[1] J.L.H. Evers, Female subfertility, Lancet 360 (2002) 151–159.
[2] M. Fathalla, Current challenges in assisted reproduction, in: E. Vayena, P.J. Rowe, P.D. Griffin (Eds.), Medical, Ethical and Social Aspects of Assisted Reproduction (2001: Geneva, Switzerland) Current Practices and Controversies in Assisted Reproduction: Report of a WHO Meeting. WHO Publications, Geneva, Switzerland, 2002, pp. 3–12.
[3] L.A. Schieve, L.S. Wilcox, J. Zeitz, G. Jeng, D. Hoffman, R. Brzyski, J. Toner, D. Grainger, L. Tatham, B. Younger, Assessment of outcomes for assisted reproductive technology: overview of issues and the US experience in establishing a surveillance system, in: E. Vayena, P.J. Rowe, P.D. Griffin (Eds.), Medical, Ethical and Social Aspects of Assisted Reproduction (2001: Geneva, Switzerland) Current Practices and Controversies in Assisted Reproduction: Report of a WHO Meeting. WHO Publications, Geneva, Switzerland, 2002, pp. 363–376.
[4] U.-B. Wennerholm, Obstetric and neonatal complications in multiple gestation, in: D.L. Healy, G.T. Kovacs, R. McLachlan, O. Rodriguez-Armas (Eds.), Reproductive Medicine in the Twenty-First Century. Proceedings of the 17th World Congress on Fertility and Sterility, Parthenon Publishing Group, London, England, 2002, pp. 182–193.

[5] O. Ozturk, A. Templeton, Multiple pregnancy in assisted reproduction techniques, in: E. Vayena, P.J. Rowe, P.D. Griffin (Eds.), Medical, Ethical and Social Aspects of Assisted Reproduction (2001: Geneva, Switzerland) Current Practices and Controversies in Assisted Reproduction: Report of a WHO Meeting. WHO Publications, Geneva, Switzerland, 2002, pp. 220–234.

[6] WHO Recommendations, in: E. Vayena, P.J. Rowe, P.D. Griffin (Eds.), Medical, Ethical and Social Aspects of Assisted Reproduction (2001: Geneva, Switzerland) Current Practices and Controversies in Assisted Reproduction: Report Of A WHO Meeting. WHO Publications, Geneva, Switzerland, 2002, pp. 381–396.

[7] G.T. Kovacs, V. MacLachlan, S.A. Breheny, What is the probability of conception for couples entering an IVF program? Aust. N. Z. J. Obstet. Gynaecol. 41 (2001) 207–209.

[8] H.W. Jones, J.A. Schnorr, Multiple pregnancies: a call for action, Correspondence 75 (2001) 11–13.

[9] M.R. Soules, J. Chang, L.I. Lipshultz, W.R. Keye, S. Carson, Multiple pregnancies: a call for action, Correspondence 75 (2001) 15–16.

[10] H.S. Jacobs, M.G.R. Hole, M.A.F. Murray, S. Franks, Therapy orientated diagnosis of secondary amenorrhea, Hum. Res. 6 (1975) 268–287.

[11] D.L. Healy, G.T. Kovacs, R.G. Pepperall, H.G. Burger, A normal cumulative conception rate after human pituitary gonadotrophin, Fertil. Steril. 34 (1980) 341–345.

[12] J.B. Brown, Pituitary control of ovarian function—concepts derived from gonadotrophin therapy, Aust. N. Z. J. Obstet. Gynaecol. 18 (1978) 4–54.

[13] D.M. White, D.W. Polson, D. Kiddy, P. Sagle, H. Watson, C. Gilling-Smith, D. Hamilton-Farley, S. Franks, Induction of ovulation with low dose gonadotrophins in polycystic ovary syndrome: an analysis of 109 pregnancies in 225 women, J. Clin. Endocrinol. Metab. 81 (1996) 3821–3824.

[14] A.O. Trounson, J.F. Leeton, C. Wood, J. Webb, J. Wood, Pregnancies in humans by fertilization in vitro and embryo transfer in the controlled ovulatory cycle, Science 212 (1981) 681–683.

[15] C.F. Wang, C. Gemzell, Pregnancy following treatment with human gonadotrophins in primary unexplained infertility, Acta Obstet. Gynecol. Scand. 58 (1979) 141–146.

[16] W.C. Dodson, A.F. Haney, Controlled ovarian hyperstimulation and intrauterine insemination for treatment of infertility (COH–IUI), Fertil. Steril. 55 (1991) 457–467.

[17] D.S. Guzick, S.A. Carspm, C. Coutifaris, J.W. Overstreet, Efficacy of superovulation in intrauterine insemination in the treatment of infertility, N. Engl. J. Med. 340 (1999) 177–183.

[18] N. Gleicher, D.M. Oleske, I. Tur-kaspa, A. Vidali, V. Karande, Reducing the risk of high order multiple pregnancy after ovarian stimulation with gonadotrophins, N. Engl. J. Med. 343 (2000) 2–7.

[19] K.C. Nygren, A.N. Andersen, Assisted reproductive technology in Europe, 1999. Results generated from European registers by ESHRE, Hum. Reprod. 17 (2002) 3260–3274.

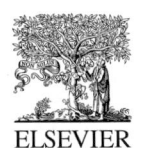

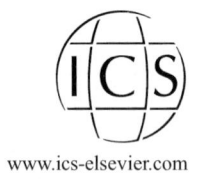

# Endocrine disrupters and ovarian function

Warren G. Foster*, Michael S. Neal, Edward V. YoungLai

*Department of Obstetrics and Gynecology, Division of Reproductive Biology, McMaster University Medical Center, 1200 Main Street West, Hamilton, Ontario, Canada L8N 3Z5*

**Abstract.** Endocrine disrupting chemicals are synthetic and naturally occurring chemicals that cannot be classified by any unique physical or chemical properties, but are characterized by their effects on the endocrine system. Recognition that environmental toxicants can mimic endogenous hormones and act as endocrine toxicants or "endocrine disrupters" has lead to concern that exposure to these compounds is linked to adverse health effects in humans. Although contemporary epidemiological studies fail to support an association between exposure to endocrine disrupters and infertility or decreased fecundity, quantification of endocrine toxicants in human ovarian follicular fluid, together with observed adverse effects in animals and in vitro studies, supports concerns that exposure to endocrine toxicants has the potential to adversely affect human ovarian function. Indeed, evidence that endocrine disrupting chemicals can bind with the estrogen receptor, change steroidogenic enzyme expression and activity, increase steroid hormone turnover, and induce ovarian follicle destruction supports the conclusion that these compounds are ovarian toxicants.
© 2004 Published by Elsevier B.V.

*Keywords:* Endocrine disrupter; Ovarian toxicity; Fecundity; Infertility; Toxicology

## 1. Introduction

Within the last decade, the terms *endocrine disrupter, endocrine modulator, hormonally active agents*, and *hormone mimics* have entered the lay and scientific press as terms, often used interchangeably, to describe exogenous chemicals that change the function(s) of the endocrine system and, consequently, cause adverse health effects in an organism, its progeny, or subpopulations [1]. Endocrine-disrupting chemicals include both synthetic and naturally occurring chemicals, such as the phytoestrogens, and cannot be classified on the basis of any unique common physical or chemical property. Rather, endocrine-disrupting chemicals are classified functionally on the basis of their biological activity. Specifically, endocrine disrupters can mimic [2] and antagonize the actions of endogenous hormones [3,4], induce changes in steroidogenic enzyme expression and/or activity [5,6], and alter circulating steroid hormone levels [5,7–9].

* Corresponding author. Tel.: +1-905-525-9140; fax: +1-905-524-2911.
  *E-mail address:* fosterw@mcmaster.ca (W.G. Foster).

0531-5131/ © 2004 Published by Elsevier B.V.
doi:10.1016/j.ics.2004.01.066

While endocrine disrupters have deleterious effects in wildlife and fish populations [1], adverse health effects in the human population have not been clearly demonstrated. However, an association between exposure to endocrine-disrupting chemicals and ovarian function is suggested by several distinct lines of evidence. Regional differences in infertility rates suggest that environmental toxicants may be contributing factors [10–13]. Furthermore, time-to-pregnancy (TTP) has been reported to be longer in couples in which the female partner has had exposure to endocrine-disrupting chemicals [14]. Ovarian toxicity of endocrine-disrupting chemicals has been documented in animal and in vitro studies, thus providing biological plausibility for the association between endocrine disrupter exposure and adverse effects on ovarian function. Herein, we review the evidence linking endocrine disrupting chemicals with adverse effects in the ovary.

## 2. Endocrine disrupters and fertility

Analyses of health trend data, such as infertility rates, are frequently used as an indicator of potential adverse health effects of environmental toxicants, including endocrine-disrupting chemicals, but these studies have not provided consistent results. For example, in the United States, the pregnancy rate in 1996 was 9% lower than in 1990 [15], whereas in Sweden, an analysis of birth registries has shown that the number of infertile couples (failure to conceive after 1 year of unprotected intercourse) decreased from 12.7% in 1983 to 8.3% in 1993 [16]. Analysis of fertility rates on a population basis, however, has the weakness of missing potential regional differences. For example, several studies conducted in a number of European cities have documented regional differences in TTP [10–12]. The greatest incidence of subfecundity was found in northern Italy, Germany, and Denmark [10,11], whereas the highest fecundity was observed in southern Italy and northern Sweden [10]. In another study [13], the incidence of infertility was greater in couples residing in heavily polluted areas (Superfund sites), compared with several reference populations that resided in relatively unpolluted areas in the rest of New York State. These studies, therefore, support the notion that subfecundity may be linked to exposure to environmental toxicants.

Actual toxicant exposure data in relation to fertility are limited; however, persistent organochlorine chemicals with documented endocrine-disrupting activity have been measured in ovarian follicular fluid of women undergoing in vitro fertilization [14,17,18]. In one study [17], levels of persistent organochlorine contaminants in ovarian follicular fluid were determined in women attending fertility clinics in three Canadian cities. Although some geographical differences in body burdens were observed, there was no association between exposure and adverse outcomes. In a larger study in Germany [14], elevated concentrations of chlorinated organic compounds with endocrine-disrupting characteristics, including pentachlorophenol, polychlorinated biphenyls (PCBs), dichlorodiphenyltrichloroethane (DDT), and hexachlorobenzene (HCB), were found in infertile women. Taken together, these reports demonstrate that there are regional differences in fertility rates and that endocrine-disrupting chemicals reach the ovary and can be measured in ovarian follicular fluid, raising concern that these chemicals are ovarian toxicants.

## 3. Ovarian toxicity of endocrine toxicants

Endocrine disrupters can affect fertility through multiple mechanisms, including effects on the hypothalamus, pituitary, gonad, and reproductive tract of members from both sexes, as well as direct toxic effects on the conceptus. The ovary is of particular interest, because it is a dynamic organ undergoing profound hormone-regulated changes with each menstrual cycle. The processes of recruitment of a cohort of growing follicles from the pool of primordial follicles, folliculogenesis, steroidogenesis, and ultimately ovulation of the dominant follicle represent targets for dysregulation by endocrine toxicants.

### 3.1. Follicle loss

With each menstrual cycle, a cohort of primordial follicles enters the growing pool of follicles, from which one follicle is selected to ovulate while the remainder become atretic. Thus, the primordial and growing follicles represent two distinct populations of follicles that are targeted by different endocrine-toxic chemicals. For example, chronic exposure to 4-vinylcyclohexane diepoxide (VCD) has been shown to induce apoptosis in primordial and primary follicles [19,20]. Elevated expression of Bax, a pro-apoptotic Bcl-2 family member, and increased caspase-3-like activity has been reported in VCD-treated ovaries [21,22]. In a subsequent study [23], loss of Bax, caspase-2, and caspase-3 activity conveyed only partial protection from the ovotoxic effects of VCD, suggesting that other pathways are also involved in VCD-mediated primordial and primary follicle apoptosis. Selective destruction of primordial follicles is a serious consequence of exposure to endocrine disrupters, as the number of follicles is set in utero and cannot be replaced. Hence, accelerated loss of primordial follicles can lead to premature ovarian failure in exposed women. In contrast, destruction of growing follicles and oocytes has been observed in several animal models following treatment with endocrine-disrupting chemicals. Dicofol, an estrogenic organochlorine pesticide, induced a significant decrease in healthy follicles and the number of estrous cycles [24]. Follicle destruction has also been reported for PCB-exposed rhesus monkeys [25]. In addition, there is a strong association between cigarette smoking and reduced fertility and earlier age at menopause, suggesting that smoking depletes ovarian follicle reserves and impairs oocyte competence [26]. Longer TTP in women exposed to cigarette smoke and reduced success rates of assisted reproductive technologies [27,28] illustrate the deleterious effects of environmental toxicants on ovarian function. The adverse effects of cigarette smoke on ovarian function are due, in part, to effects on follicle loss. Cigarette smoking in women significantly reduces their follicle reserves [29] and histological evaluation of ovaries from cigarette smoke-exposed mice reveals a reduction in the number of growing follicles, compared with controls (unpublished).

### 3.2. Steroidogenesis

Effects of endocrine disrupters on ovarian steroidogenesis can have serious consequences for ovulation, oocyte competence, and luteal phase competency. Endocrine disrupters alter ovarian steroidogenesis indirectly by attenuating pituitary gonadotropin levels in serum [5] and directly through changes in steroidogenic enzyme expression and/or activity [6,30] and steroid hormone turnover [7].

Circulating levels of estradiol were lower in bergaptin and xanthotoxin-treated rats [7]. Bergaptin and xanthotoxin are synthetic chemicals used in skin photochemotherapy and members of the psoralens family of chemicals that are found in many crop plants. In contrast, increased levels of circulating estradiol have been reported in DDE-treated rats, indicating that endocrine disrupters can modulate aromatase activity [8]. In perinatal and juvenile rats treated with the estrogenic pesticide methoxychlor (MXC), circulating levels of follicle stimulating hormone and progesterone were decreased in estrus [5]. Similarly, DDT treatment significantly reduced circulating progesterone levels in early pregnant rabbits [9]. Several cell-culture studies have demonstrated that environmental toxicants may exert adverse effects on gonadal function and gamete quality by altering the steroidogenic activity of reproductive cells [6,31–34]. In bis(2-diethylhexyl)phthalate (DEHP)-treated rats, there was a shift to production of more testosterone and estradiol during diestrus, compared with untreated controls in diestrus [35]. Similarly, treatment of human luteinized granulosa cells with TCDD, the pesticide Lindane, and mono(2-ethylhexyl) phthalate has been shown to decrease progesterone production by luteinized granulosa cells in culture [31,32,36,37]. While these studies demonstrate that endocrine toxicants can alter serum steroid levels, they fail to establish mechanisms of action. DDE, at concentrations detected in human reproductive fluids, has been shown to alter steroidogenesis in pig granulosa cells through altered expression of P450 side chain cleavage [6]. Taken together, these studies demonstrate that endocrine toxicants can affect ovarian steroidogenesis and suggest that ovarian steroidogenic enzyme expression and activity are important targets for their effects.

*3.3. Receptor signalling*

Hormone mimicry by endocrine-disrupting chemicals is well known. A growing number of chemicals have been shown to bind with estrogen and androgen receptors in receptor-binding studies [2–4,38], as well as gene-reporter assays [39,40]. From these studies, it is known that these chemicals can function as estrogens, anti-estrogens, and anti-androgens [3,4,40,41]. To date, there are no known androgen mimics. Recently, evidence has emerged that reveals divergent effects of toxicants depending upon dose. Dioxins are environmental toxicants for which anti-estrogenic effects are well documented [41]. However, it has recently been shown that the ligand activated arylhydrocarbon receptor nuclear translocator protein heterodimer directly associates with estrogen receptors ER$\alpha$ and ER$\beta$, leading to activation of transcription and estrogenic effects [42]. These data demonstrate that endocrine disrupting chemicals can exert opposite effects depending upon dose.

*3.4. Oocyte competence*

Specific PCB congeners, 153 (estrogenic) and 126 (dioxin-like), were shown to alter oocyte maturation and blastocyst development in bovine oocytes in culture [34]. While PCB 153 did not affect oocyte maturation, the highest concentration reduced the number of oocytes that cleaved. In contrast, PCB 126 had an adverse effect on oocyte maturation at the highest concentration, as well as on blastocyst development at all concentrations tested. These data provide insight into the potential mechanisms of contaminant action, but are of limited value, since the oocyte develops in a complex mixture of hormones, growth factors, and environmental agents. Campagna et al. [43] evaluated the effect of a mixture of environmental contaminants and demonstrated a dose-related decrease in the quality of cumulus expansion, a decrease in the viability of cumulus cells, and an increase in the number of incompletely matured oocytes. A dose-related decrease in the number of cells per blastocyst was also found in this study. Taken together, these data suggest that environmental toxicants may impair human fertility via altered gamete quality and/or embryo development.

## 4. Summary and conclusions

The role of endocrine disrupters in adverse human health outcomes and fertility remains highly controversial. Despite evidence in the human epidemiological and experimental animal literature, suggesting that endocrine disrupters are ovarian toxicants, the level of risk to the general population posed by unwitting exposure to these agents remains unknown. Several important questions remain and include the following:

1. Endocrine toxicants are almost exclusively tested alone or as dimeric mixtures, yet the human population is exposed to multiple toxicants throughout the day. Hence, there is a need to determine the consequences of exposure to environmentally relevant mixtures of endocrine toxicants. Will exposure to endocrine toxicants in complex mixtures result in additive, synergistic, or inhibitory effects on ovarian function?
2. Are there critical periods of folliculogenesis during which the follicle is at increased risk for adverse effects?
3. What are the cellular and molecular mechanisms underlying the observed effects of endocrine toxicants on ovarian function?
4. What is the biological relevance of endocrine disrupter effects on ovarian function documented in animal studies?

## References

[1] T. Damstra, S. Barlow, A. Bergman, R. Kavlock, G. Van Der Kraak, Global assessment on the state-of-the-science of endocrine disruptors. WHO publication no. WHO/PCS/EDC/02.2 World Health Organization, Geneva, Switzerland, 2002.
[2] A.M. Soto, C. Sonnenschein, K.L. Chung, M.F. Fernandez, N. Olea, F.O. Serrano, The E-Screen assay as a tool to identify estrogens: an update on estrogenic environmental pollutants, Environ. Health Perspect. 103 (Suppl. 7) (1995) 113–122.
[3] W. Kelce, C. Stone, S. Laws, L. Gray, J. Kemppainen, E. Wilson, Persistent DDT metabolite p,p'-DDE is a potent androgen receptor antagonist, Nature 375 (1995) 581–585.
[4] W.R. Kelce, C.R. Lambright, L.E. Gray Jr., K.P. Roberts, Vinclozolin and p,p'-DDE alter androgen-dependent gene expression: in vivo confirmation of an androgen receptor-mediated mechanism, Toxicol. Appl. Pharmacol. 142 (1997) 192–200.
[5] R.E. Chapin, M.W. Harris, B.J. Harris, S.M. Ward, R.E. Wilson, M.A. Mauney, A.C. Lockhart, R.J. Smialowicz, V.C. Moser, L.T. Burka, B.J. Collins, The effects of perinatal/juvenile methoxychlor exposure on adult rat nervous, immune, and reproductive system function, Fundam. Appl. Toxicol. 40 (1997) 138–157.
[6] N.K. Crellin, H.G. Kang, C.L. Swan, P.J. Chedrese, Inhibition of basal and stimulated progesterone synthesis by dichlorodiphenyldichloroethylene and methoxychlor in a stable pig granulosa cell line, Reproduction 121 (2001) 485–492.

[7] M.M. Diawara, K.J. Chavez, P.B. Hoyer, D.E. Williams, J. Dorsch, P. Kulkosky, M.R. Franklin, A novel group of ovarian toxicants: the psoralens, J. Biochem. Mol. Toxicol. 13 (1999) 195–203.
[8] L. You, S. Madhabananda, E. Bartolucci, S. Ploch, M. Whitt, Induction of hepatic aromatase by p,p'-DDE in adult male rats, Mol. Cell. Endocrinol. 178 (2001) 207–214.
[9] A. Lindeneau, B. Fischer, P. Seiler, H.M. Beier, Effects of persistent chlorinated hydrocarbons on reproductive tissues in female rabbits, Hum. Reprod. 9 (1994) 772–780.
[10] S. Juul, W. Karmaus, J. Olsen, Regional differences in waiting time to pregnancy: pregnancy-based surveys from Denmark, France, Germany, Italy and Sweden. The European Infertility and Subfecundity Study Group, Hum. Reprod. 14 (1999) 1250–1254.
[11] W. Karmaus, S. Juul, and The European Infertility and Subfecundity Study Group, Infertility and subfecundity in population-based samples from Denmark, Germany, Italy, Poland and Spain, Eur. J. Public Health 9 (1999) 229–235.
[12] T.K. Jensen, R. Slama, B. Ducot, J. Suominen, E.H. Cawood, A.G. Andersen, et al, Regional differences in waiting time to pregnancy among fertile couples from four European cities, Hum. Reprod. 16 (2001) 2697–2704.
[13] D.O. Carpenter, Y. Shen, T. Nguyen, L. Le, L.L. Lininger, Incidence of endocrine disease among residents of New York areas of concern, Environ. Health Perspect. 109 (Suppl. 6) (2001) 845–851.
[14] I. Gerhard, B. Monga, J. Krähe, B. Runnebaum, Chlorinated hydrocarbons in infertile women, Environ. Res. 80 (1999) 299–310.
[15] S.J. Ventura, W.D. Mosher, S.C. Curtin, J.C. Abma, S. Henshaw, Trends in pregnancies and pregnancy rates by outcome: estimates for the United States, 1976–96, Vital Health Stat. 56 (2000) 1–47.
[16] O. Akre, S. Cnattingius, R. Bergstrom, U. Kvist, D. Trichopoulos, A. Ekbom, Human fertility does not decline: evidence from Sweden, Fertil. Steril. 71 (1999) 1066–1069.
[17] J. Jarrell, D. Villeneuve, C. Franklin, S. Bartlett, W. Wrixon, J. Kohut, et al, Contamination of human ovarian follicular fluid and serum by chlorinated organic compounds in three Canadian cities, Can. Med. Assoc. J. 148 (1993) 1321–1327.
[18] E.V. Younglai, W.G. Foster, E.G. Hughes, K. Trim, J.F. Jarrell, Levels of environmental contaminants in human follicular fluid, serum, and seminal plasma of couples undergoing in vitro fertilization, Arch. Environ. Contam. Toxicol. 43 (2002) 121–126.
[19] P.B. Hoyer, I.G. Sipes, Assessment of follicle destruction in chemical induced ovarian toxicity, Annu. Rev. Pharmacol. Toxicol. 36 (1996) 307–331.
[20] B.J. Smith, D.R. Mattison, G.I. Sipes, The role of epoxidation in 4-vinylcyclohexene-induced ovarian toxicity, Toxicol. Appl. Pharmacol. 105 (1990) 372–381.
[21] X.M. Hu, P.J. Christian, I.G. Sipes, P.B. Hoyer, Expression and redistribution of cellular bad, bax, and bcl-xl protein is associated with VCD-induced ovotoxicity in rats, Biol. Reprod. 65 (2001) 1489–1495.
[22] X.M. Hu, P.J. Christian, K.E. Thompson, I.G. Sipes, P.B. Hoyer, Apoptosis induced in rats by 4-vinylcyclohexene diepoxide is associated with activation of the caspase cascades, Biol. Reprod. 65 (2001) 87–93.
[23] Y. Takai, J. Canning, G.I. Perez, J.K. Pru, J.J. Schlezinger, D.H. Sherr, R.N. Kolesnick, J. Yuan, R.A. Flavell, S.J. Korsmeyer, J.L. Tilly, Bax, caspase-2, and caspase-3 are required for ovarian follicle loss caused by 4-vinylcyclohexene diepoxide exposure of female mice in vivo, Endocrinology 144 (2003) 69–74.
[24] U.C. Jadaramkunti, B.B. Kaliwal, Effect of dicofol formulation on estrous cycle and follicular dynamics in albino rats, J. Basic Clin. Physiol. Pharmacol. 10 (1999) 305–314.
[25] W.F. Muller, W. Hobson, G.B. Fuller, W. Knauf, F. Coulston, F. Korte, Endocrine effects of chlorinated hydrocarbons in rhesus monkeys, Ecotoxicol. Environ. Saf. 2 (1978) 161–172.
[26] M.T. Zenzes, Smoking and reproduction: gene damage to human gametes and embryos, Hum. Reprod. Updat. 6 (2000) 122–131.
[27] M.S. Neal, A.C. Holloway, E.G. Hughes, W.G. Foster, Effect of sidestream and mainstream smoking on IVF outcomes, Canadian Fertility and Andrology Society Annual Meeting Abstract Book, 2003, Abs # TP-08.
[28] K.M. Curtis, D.A. Savitz, T.E. Arbuckle, Effects of cigarette smoking, caffeine consumption and alcohol intake on fecundability, Am. J. Epidemiol. 146 (1997) 32–41.
[29] A. El-Nemr, T. Al-Shawaf, L. Sabatini, C. Wilson, A.M. Lower, J.G. Grudzinskas, Effect of smoking on ovarian reserve and ovarian stimulation in in vitro fertilization and embryo transfer, Hum. Reprod. 13 (1998) 2192–2198.

[30] T. Sugawara, E. Nomura, N. Sakuragi, S. Fujimoto, The effect of the arylhydrocarbon receptor on the human steroidogenic acute regulatory gene promoter activity, J. Steroid Biochem. Mol. Biol. 78 (2001) 253–260.

[31] F.M. Morán, A.J. Conley, C.J. Corbin, C. VandeVoort, J.W. Overstreet, B.L. Lasley, 2,3,7,8-tetrachlorodibenzo-$p$-dioxin decreases estradiol production without altering the enzyme activity of cytochrome $P450$ aromatase of human luteinized granulosa cells in vitro, Biol. Reprod. 62 (2000) 1102–1108.

[32] L.P. Walsh, D.M. Stocco, Effects of lindane on steroidogenesis and steroidogenic acute regulatory protein expression, Biol. Reprod. 63 (2000) 1024–1033.

[33] S.D. Khokute, J. Rodriguez, W.R. Dukelow, Reproductive toxicity of aroclor-1254: effects on oocyte, spermatozoa, in vitro fertilization, and embryo development in the mouse, Reprod. Toxicol. 9 (1994) 487–493.

[34] A.K. Krogenaes, I. Nafstad, J.U. Skare, W. Farstad, A.L. Hafne, In vitro reproductive toxicity of polychlorinated biphenyl cogeners 153 and 126, Reprod. Toxicol. 12 (1998) 575–580.

[35] J.W. Laskey, E. Berman, Steroidogenic assessment using ovary culture in cycling rats: effects of bis(2-ethylhexyl)phthalate on ovarian steroid production, Reprod. Toxicol. 7 (1993) 25–33.

[36] J.A. Oduma, E.O. Wango, D. Oduor-Okelo, D.W. Makawiti, H. Odongo, In vivo and in vitro effects of graded doses of the pesticide heptachlor on female sex steroid hormone production in rats, Comp. Biochem. Physiol., Part C., Pharmacol., Toxicol. Endocrinol. 111 (1995) 191–196.

[37] K.A. Treimen, W.C. Dodson, J.J. Heindel, Inhibition of FSH-stimulated cAMP accumulation and progesterone production by mono(2-ethylhexyl)phthalate in rat granulosa cell cultures, Toxicol. Appl. Pharmacol. 106 (1990) 334–340.

[38] M.G. Wade, D. Desaulniers, K. Leingartnere, W.G. Foster, Interactions between endosulfan and dieldrin on estrogen-mediated processes in vitro and in vivo, Reprod. Toxicol. 11 (1997) 791–798.

[39] L.E. Gray Jr., W.R. Kelce, T. Wise, R. Tyl, K. Gaido, J. Cook, G. Kleinefelter, D. Desaulniers, E. Wilson, T. Zacharewski, C. Waller, P. Foster, J. Laskey, J. Reel, J. Giesy, S. Laws, J. McLachlan, W. Breslin, R. Cooper, R. Di Giulo, R. Johnson, R. Purdy, E. Mihaich, S. Safe, C. Sonnenschein, W. Welshons, R. McMaster, S. McMaster, T. Colborn, Endocrine screening methods workshop report: detection of estrogenic and androgenic hormonal and antihormonal activity for chemicals that act via receptor or steroidogenic enzyme mechanisms, Reprod. Toxicol. 11 (1997) 719–750.

[40] H. Kojima, M. Iida, E. Katsura, A. Kanetoshi, Y. Hori, K. Kobayashi, Effects of a diphenyl ether-type herbicide, chlornitrofen, and its amino derivative on androgen and estrogen receptor activities, Environ. Health Perspect. 111 (2003) 497–502.

[41] T. Zacharewski, K. Bondy, P. Mcdonell, Z. FenWu, Antiestrogenic effect of 2,3,7,8,-Tetrachlorodibenzo-p-dioxin on 17B-estradiol-induced pS2 expression, Cancer Res. 54 (1994) 2707–2713.

[42] F. Ohtake, K.-I. Takeyama, T. Matsumoto, H. Kitagawa, Y. Yamamot, K. Nohara, C. Tohyama, A. Krust, J. Mimura, P. Chambon, J. Yanagisawa, Y. Fujii-Kuriyama, S. Kato, Modulation of oestrogen receptor signalling by association with the activated dioxin receptor, Nature 423 (2003) 545–550.

[43] C. Campagna, M.A. Sirard, P. Ayotte, J.L. Bailey, Impaired maturation, fertilization, and embryonic development of porcine oocytes following exposure to an environmentally relevant organochlorine mixture, Biol. Reprod. 65 (2001) 554–560.

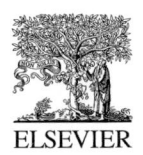

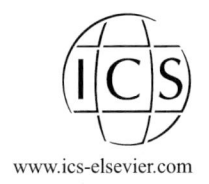

# Menopause-related definitions

## Wulf H. Utian*

*The North American Menopause Society, Reproductive Biology/Gynecology, 5900 Landerbrook Drive, Suite 195, Cleveland OH 44124, USA*

**Abstract.** *Introduction*: There is confusion in the use of terminology relating to the human female menopause. In turn, this can lead to misinterpretation of research publications and an adverse effect on health care provided to women. *Methods*: The history of attempts to define terminology related to the human menopause is reviewed and placed in scientific and clinical perspective. Appropriate terminology has been used in developing a staging system for reproductive aging. *Commentary*: The combination of appropriate definitions of the terminology around menopause with categorization in phases of the reproductive aging process allows for accurate selection of study populations in clinical research studies related to the menopause transition and beyond. In turn, this will allow for direct comparison of results of studies conducted in different geographic centers and cross-cultural populations. This is mandatory for future progress and to obviate errors that have occurred in translation of study results into guidelines for clinical practice. © 2004 Published by Elsevier B.V.

*Keywords:* Menopause; Definitions; Reproductive staging

The terminology relating to "menopause" that is utilized in the medical literature and subsequently by health providers, consumers and the media, represents a Tower of Babel! The research community involved in the area of the human female menopause has long recognized the need for both universality in utilization of menopause-related terminology and some form of a logical division of the 10–15 years of peripostmenopausal hypothalamic–pituitary–ovarian function into stages that could be primarily relevant to the research community, and that would also have clinical relevance.

Clearly, the primary objective for the specific use of menopause-related terminology and utilization of a substantiated staging system for reproductive aging is to allow researchers worldwide to enroll comparative populations into research studies that are well defined and similar to populations enrolled in other studies. The additional benefit is that clinicians would speak the same language when managing the health care of women through and beyond the menopause transition.

Despite several attempts by the scientific community to apply specific definitions to the menopause transition, the majority of published clinical studies do not clearly define their

---

* Tel.: +1-440-4427680; fax: +1-440-4422660.
*E-mail address:* utian@menopause.org (W.H. Utian).

0531-5131/ © 2004 Published by Elsevier B.V.
doi:10.1016/j.ics.2004.01.102

studied populations and conclusions drawn are therefore often of limited utility. For example, "menopause" is variously utilized to correctly refer to the final menstrual period (FMP) or incorrectly to the entire, menopause-related transition. Another example is "perimenopause" where late perimenopause is utilized by some investigators to refer to the final years of reproductive age, and others to the first 12 months after the FMP. A particularly egregious misuse of clear definitions of menopause-related terminology and reproductive staging occurs in the multiple publications from the terminated estrogen–progestin arm of the Women's Health Initiative. This has been reflected in the confusion sown among the medical profession, women in general and the media.

The concept of defining the terminology and stages of the menopause transition has been addressed specifically on only a few occasions.

## 1. First international menopause society definitions 1976

A workshop was convened during the first International Menopause Congress at LaGrande Motte in France in 1976 [1]. The definitions attempted to provide an explanation for the protean clinical presentation in the following terms:

1. The *climacteric*—the phase in the aging of women marking the transition from the reproductive phase to the nonreproductive state.
2. The *menopause*—the final menstrual period, which occurs during the climacteric, currently around the age of 51. The climacteric is sometimes, but not invariably, associated with symptomatology. When this occurs, it may be termed the *climacteric syndrome*.

Climacteric symptoms and complaints result from:

1. Decreased ovarian activity with subsequent hormonal deficiency causing early symptoms (hot flushes, perspiration, and atrophic vaginitis) and late symptoms related to changes in various end organs.
2. Sociocultural factors determined by the woman's environment.
3. Psychological factors, resulting from the individual woman's character.

The variety of symptomatology results from the interaction among these three components.

Review of the above definition illustrates that a staging system needs to be multidimensional. The 1976 IMS definition, in attempting to explain the protean associations with menopause, demonstrates an early attempt at multidimensional staging. The first level is chronological—the entire process labeled "climacteric" and the FMP (menopause) being time specific.

The second dimension addresses physical changes or symptoms. The third dimension involves integration of functional changes.

## 2. World Health Organization (WHO) scientific group definitions 1980, 1996

A World Health Organization (WHO) Scientific Group on Research in the Menopause met in 1980 and published recommendations in 1981 [2]. These definitions were revisited in 1994 and published in 1996 [3]. The scientific definitions were largely unidimensional with specific definitions for the phases of the life cycle being presented.

The 1994 WHO Scientific Group on Research in the Menopause [3] expanded on the relationship between different time periods surrounding the menopause, retained most of the 1980 definitions, and published the following statement in 1996:

1. The term *natural menopause* is defined as the permanent cessation of menstruation resulting from the loss of ovarian follicular activity. Natural menopause is recognized to have occurred after 12 consecutive months of amenorrhea for which there is no other obvious pathological or physiological cause. Menopause occurs with the final menstrual period (FMP), which is known with certainty only in retrospect a year or more after the event. An adequate independent biological marker for the event does not exist.
2. The term *perimenopause* should include the period immediately prior to the menopause (when the endocrinological, biological and clinical features of approaching menopause commence) and the first year after menopause. The term "climacteric" should be abandoned to avoid confusion.
3. The term *menopausal transition* should be reserved for that period of time before the FMP when variability in the menstrual cycle usually increases [13,14].
4. The term *premenopause* is often used ambiguously either to refer to the 1 or 2 years immediately before the menopause or to refer to the whole of the reproductive period prior to the menopause. The Group recommended that the term be used consistently in the latter sense to encompass the entire reproductive period up to the FMP.
5. The term *induced menopause* is defined as the cessation of menstruation, which follows either surgical removal of both ovaries (with or without hysterectomy) or iatrogenic ablation of ovarian function (e.g., by chemotherapy or radiation).
6. *Simple hysterectomy*, where at least one ovary is conserved, is used to define a distinct group of women in whom ovarian function may persist for a variable period after surgery.
7. The term *postmenopause* is defined as dating from the FMP, regardless of whether the menopause was induced or spontaneous.
8. Ideally, *premature menopause* should be defined as menopause that occurs at an age less than two standard deviations below the mean estimated for the reference population. In practice, in the absence of reliable estimates of the distribution of age at natural menopause in populations in developing countries, the age of 40 years is frequently used as an arbitrary cut-off point, below which menopause is said to be premature.

Of note, this group recommended dropping the term climacteric. In addition, the ambiguity of the terms premenopause and perimenopause were recognized.

## 3. Korpilampi definitions 1986

An important step forward was taken in Korpilampi in 1986 [4] when a time-related definition was suggested; and of particular significance, the necessity for separating a "normal" population from an "abnormal" population was explained.

1. Natural menopause was defined as at least 12 months of amenorrhea, not obviously attributable to other causes.

2. Recognition was given to the fact that surgical menopause could not be equated to spontaneous menopause, and these groups could not be combined in studies, particularly when health-related outcomes were under investigation.

## 4. Ovarian function/therapy-oriented definition 1991, 1994

A potential fourth dimension was recognized in 1991, namely, the possibility of addressing therapy through staging and definitions. Based on the premise that the above definitions did not take any potential residual ovarian activity into account and were thus of reduced value in describing populations either being considered for clinical study or for clarifying indications for postmenopausal hormone therapies, Utian [5,6] proposed an ovarian function, therapy-oriented definition of the postmenopause in 1991/1994.

The definition proposed was based on whether the postmenopausal ovary demonstrated functional ability (type B) or lack of activity (type A), or whether there was congenital absence of both ovaries (type C) or iatrogenic loss of ovarian function (type D), and in part was presented as follows:

This functional background allows integration into the definition a possible indication for hormone therapy ("estrogen dependent"), or a compensated type of climacteric (residual ovarian function) without clear indication for hormone replacement ("estrogen independent"). The suggested classification is thus as follows:

(Type A) Spontaneous estrogen-dependent climacteric (ovaries intact) (i.e., no ovarian compensation).
(Type B) Spontaneous estrogen-independent climacteric (ovaries intact) (i.e., ovarian compensation).
(Type C) Ovarian agenesis estrogen-dependent climacteric (ovaries absent).
(Type D) Iatrogenic estrogen-dependent climacteric (ovaries removed) (i.e., surgical menopause, chemotherapy).

## 5. The international menopause society definitions 1999

Through its internationally representative organ, the Council of Affiliated Menopause Societies, the IMS convened a working group to define the terminology. This group reported in 1999 [7].

Of note, the term climacteric was restored because of its international popularity and widespread usage outside of the United States. Much of the WHO 1996 terminology was retained and incorporated into the new recommendations:

Term    Source
*Menopause (natural menopause)* WHO; The term natural menopause is defined as the permanent cessation of menstruation resulting from the loss of ovarian follicular activity. Natural menopause is recognized to have occurred after 12 consecutive months of amenorrhea, for which there is no other obvious pathological or physiological cause. Menopause occurs with the final menstrual period which is

known with certainty only in retrospect a year or more after the event. An adequate independent biological marker for the event does not exist.

*Perimenopause* WHO; The term perimenopause should include the time immediately prior to the menopause (when the endocrinological, biological and clinical features of approaching menopause commence) and the first year after menopause.

*Menopausal transition* WHO; The term menopausal transition should be reserved for the time before the final menstrual period when variability in the menstrual cycle is usually increased. This term can be used synonymously with 'perimenopause,' although this latter term can be confusing and preferably should be abandoned.

*Climacteric* IMS; The phase in the aging of women marking the transition from the reproductive phase to the nonreproductive state. This phase incorporates the perimenopause, by extending for a longer variable period before and after the perimenopause.

*Climacteric syndrome* IMS; The climacteric is sometimes, but not necessarily always, associated with symptomatology. When this occurs, it may be termed the 'climacteric syndrome.'

*Premenopause* WHO; The term premenopause is often used ambiguously, either to refer to the 1 or 2 years immediately before the menopause or to refer to the whole of the reproductive period prior to the menopause. The group recommended that the term be used consistently in the latter sense to encompass the entire reproductive period up to the final menstrual period.

*Postmenopause* WHO; The term postmenopause is defined as dating from the final menstrual period, regardless of whether the menopause was induced or spontaneous.

*Premature menopause* WHO; Ideally, premature menopause should be defined as menopause that occurs at an age less than two standard deviations below the mean estimated for the reference population. In practice, in the absence of reliable estimates of the distribution of age at natural menopause in populations in developing countries, the age of 40 years is frequently used as an arbitrary cut-off point, below which menopause is said to be premature.

*Induced menopause* WHO; The term induced menopause is defined as the cessation of menstruation which follows either surgical removal of both ovaries (with or without hysterectomy) or iatrogenic ablation of ovarian function (e.g., by chemotherapy or radiation).

## 6. Stages of Reproductive Aging (STRAW) Workshop, Park City, UT, 2001

The most recent attempt to move this process forward was the Stages of reproductive Aging (STRAW) Workshop [9], at which an extremely representative group of experts attempted to tie all of the above together during the development of a staging system for reproductive aging. The anchor for the staging system is the Final Menstrual Period (FMP), represented as point zero (0). Prior to the FMP are five stages, and after the FMP there are two. Stages $-2$ and $-1$ are the menopausal transition, and $+1$ and $+2$ are the postmenopause. The participants agreed that menstrual cycle changes could be incorporated, but agreed that evidence was insufficient to allow for the categorization of any of the stages by presence or absence of specific symptoms. The value of STRAW is that it does classify the stages of reproductive aging and place the onus on researchers in describing study populations to clearly state the population they are investigating.

## 7. Commentary

The IMS nomenclature, unfortunately, remains unidimensional, and cannot be considered a real staging system, unless one-dimensional for the menopause transition. Moreover, confusion with terms like premenopause, perimenopause and the climacteric were not adequately addressed. Furthermore, the early attempt by Utian to relate ovarian endocrine status to terminology, function, and therapy, needs further elucidation. One attempt at this was presented by Prior [8], but her review only used a systematic literature research from 1990 and highlights the difficulty in relating what is known in the background endocrinology to change in reproductive function, menstruation, and symptom genesis.

The July 2001 joint working group (STRAW) convened by the NIH, NAMS, and ASRM, attempted to develop a workable staging system for reproductive aging, carefully considered the above menopause-related terminology, and utilized it in the staging system that resulted from the meeting. The STRAW reproductive staging system is a workable system that relies on investigators worldwide to utilize correct definitions. In particular, perimenopause (unless dropped from our lexicon) should be redefined so that it is synonymous with climacteric [9]. There should be no doubt that this new staging system is but one phase in an ongoing process. For the moment, it should provide a basis for researchers to be more uniform in population selection. Clinicians may find it of value in explaining the reproductive aging process to women.

With utilization of the scale should inevitably come greater detail of each of the stages, and ultimately refinement and perhaps even development of an enhanced system. Hopefully, as this process unfolds, we will eventually have a system that addresses all four dimensions: chronology, symptoms/physical changes, variance of functional groups, and finally, therapy orientation. Above all, there is now no excuse for investigators not to use correct terminology in selecting and describing their patient populations.

## References

[1] W.H. Utian, D. Serr, The climacteric syndrome, in: P.A. van Keep, R.B. Greenblatt, M. Albeavx-Fernet (Eds.), Consensus on Menopause Research, MTP Press, Lancaster, 1976, pp. 1–4.
[2] Research on the Menopause. Report of a WHO Scientific Group, Geneva, World Health Organization, WHO Technical Report Series 670, Geneva, Switzerland (1981).
[3] WHO Scientific Group on Research on the Menopause in the 1990's. WHO Technical Report Series 866. Geneva, Switzerland (1994).
[4] P. Kaufert, et al., A menopause research. The Korpilampi Workshop, Soc. Sci. Med. 22 (1986) 1285.
[5] W.H. Utian, Menopause—a proposed new functional definition, Maturitas 14 (1991) 1–2.
[6] W.H. Utian, Ovarian function–therapy oriented definition of menopause of menopause and climacteric, Exp. Gerontol. 29 (1994) 245–251.
[7] W.H. Utian, The International Menopause Society menopause-related terminology definitions, Climacteric 2 (1999) 284–286.
[8] J.C. Prior, Perimenopause: the complex endocrinology of the menopausal transition, Endocr. Rev. 19 (4) (1998) 397–428.
[9] Executive Summary: Stages of Reproductive Aging Workshop (STRAW) Park City Utah, July 2001, Menopause 8 (2001) 402–407.

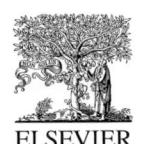

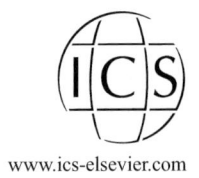

# Critique of the evidence from large trials of hormone replacement therapy

Henri Rozenbaum*

*Association Française pour l' Etude de la Menopause (AFEM), Menopause, 15 rue Daru, 75008 Paris, France*

**Abstract.** During several decades, hormone replacement therapy (HRT) was the only long-term treatment used by millions of women without any trial. A huge amount of observational studies performed on surrogate markers, animals or women has suggested that HRT reduces cardiovascular morbidity and mortality in postmenopausal women. Numerous observational studies have also suggested a slight increase of breast cancer risk. Other results from observational studies include prevention of osteoporosis, diminished colorectal cancer risk and increased venous thromboembolism risk. During the past decade, several trials have been set up, mostly to compare cancer and cardiovascular disease endpoints in HRT users and nonusers. With the early termination of part of the Women's Health Initiative (WHI) trial, the most important trial ever done on HRT, it is timely to review the evidence from such studies. Results from the main randomised trials broadly agree with findings from the majority of observational studies on the following points: reduction in incidence of osteoporotic fractures and colorectal cancer, increased incidence of venous thromboembolism and breast cancer risk and no significant change in endometrial cancer. However, the trials reported opposite results on the effect of HRT on cardiovascular risk, with a significantly increased incidence of coronary events and stroke. Furthermore, these trials tested only one drug regimen, and they do not necessarily apply to lower dosages of these drugs, to other formulations or methods of administering estrogen and progestins, or to estrogens alone. © 2004 Published by Elsevier B.V.

*Keywords:* HRT; Trials; WHI; HERS

## 1. Main potential bias of observational studies

Observational studies suffer from several types of bias, and each of these bias may lead to a spurious benefit of hormone replacement therapy (HRT) [1].

*1.1. Selection bias or the so-called "healthy users effect"*

Women who choose to take HRT differ from other women; they are healthier, more affluent and better educated than those who do not take these hormones. They are also

---

* Tel.: +33-14-2677747; fax: +33-14-6222027.
 *E-mail address:* henri.rozenbaum@wanadoo.fr (H. Rozenbaum).

younger, leaner, more likely to use alcohol, smoke cigarettes, have diabetes, be more physically active and less likely to have a worrisome family history [2–5]. How, and to what extent, do these differences account for the putative cardiac benefits of HRT seen in most observational studies?

### 1.2. Compliance bias

Compliance with the use of estrogen has also been considered as a marker for low risk of heart disease [6,7], suggesting to some that the behavioral characteristics of hormone users are more important to their decreased risk of coronary heart disease (CHD) than the estrogen that they are taking. This argument is based on findings from clinical trials, where subjects who were compliant placebo takers had a better outcome than noncompliant subjects on placebo [8].

Adherence with pill taking is a marker for personal characteristics that confer powerful protective effects, independent of the medication prescribed.

### 1.3. Surveillance bias

Surveillance bias may play a role in relation to HRT. For cardiovascular and breast cancer risk, women receiving HRT, available by prescription only, are likely to have more frequent contacts with clinicians and more frequent mammograms than women who do not take these hormones [3].

### 1.4. Survivor bias

Women who develop intercurrent illness are likely to stop their HRT, either on their own or at the direction of a clinician. Such women have a markedly increased risk of death [9]. Because of this selection, women who continue on HRT have a substantially lower risk of disease and death than do women not taking HRT.

### 1.5. Publication bias

To determine the extent to which publication is influenced by study outcome, a cohort of studies submitted to a hospital ethics committee over 10 years were examined retrospectively by Stern and Simes [10]. Of the 218 studies analysed with tests of significance, those with positive results were more likely to be published than those with negative results (HR: 2.32, 95% C.I.: 1.47–3.66, $p=0.0003$) and with a significantly shorter time to publication (median 4.8 vs. 8 years).

### 1.6. Incomplete capture of early clinical events

A major limitation of many prospective cohort studies is their limited ability to identify clinical events that occur early after the initiation of therapy. Most such studies collect information on hormone use only at baseline; thus, any immediate increase in the risk of coronary heart disease would not be detected since new users are usually not specifically enrolled and would constitute a minority of the study subjects.

Such a problem probably explains some of the discrepancies in the findings regarding heart disease in analyses of both primary and secondary prevention.

## 2. The large trials

During the past decade, several trials have been set up, mostly to compare cancer and cardiovascular disease endpoints in HRT users and nonusers.

### 2.1. The Postmenopausal Estrogen–Progestin Interventions trial [11]

The objective of the Postmenopausal Estrogen–Progestin Interventions (PEPI) trial was to assess pairwise differences between placebo, unopposed estrogen, and each of three estrogen–progestin regimens for selected heart disease risk factors in healthy postmenopausal women.

This 3-year, multicenter, randomized, double-blind, placebo-controlled trial involved 875 postmenopausal women aged 45–64 years.

Participants were randomly assigned in equal numbers to the following groups: placebo; conjugated equine estrogen (CEE), 0.625 mg/day; CEE, 0.625 mg/day plus cyclic medroxyprogesterone acetate (MPA), 10 mg/day for 12 days/month; CEE, 0.625 mg/day plus consecutive MPA, 2.5 mg/day; or CEE, 0.625 mg/day plus cyclic micronized progesterone (MP), 200 mg/day for 12 days/month.

The results were considered favourable for the surrogate markers studied; estrogen alone or in combination with a progestin improved lipoproteins and lowered fibrinogen levels without detectable effects on postchallenge insulin or blood pressure.

Excepting a high rate of endometrial hyperplasia in the group of women treated with unopposed estrogen, this study did not examine clinical outcomes.

### 2.2. The Heart and Estrogen–Progestagen Replacement Study

The Heart and Estrogen–Progestagen Replacement Study (HERS) trial was a randomized, double-blind, placebo-controlled clinical trial of secondary prevention [12]. The objective of the trial was to determine whether continuous treatment with 0.625 mg CEE and 2.5 mg MPA (PremPro) would reduce CHD events in women with preexisting coronary disease (CVD). The trial involved 2763 women (mean age 66.7 years) who were enrolled in 20 US clinical centers and randomized to treatment or placebo.

Follow-up averaged 4.1 years. Overall, there were 172 myocardial infarctions and coronary deaths in the hormone group and 176 in the placebo group, with no obvious, overall difference. Over time, differences were recorded: there was an increase in events in the first year (mostly in the first 4 months), and after 2 years of treatment, the appearance of a beneficial impact of HRT (although the annual relative risks did not achieve statistical significance, the test for the trend was significant).

The later decrease in CHD events led to the recommendation that women with CVD should not start treatment with hormones for the purpose of preventing CHD events, but that those who were already taking hormones could continue. Disease surveillance continued in HERS II for an additional 2.7 years, during which many of the women randomized to hormones took open-label estrogen prescribed by their personal physicians, but only a few of those assigned to placebo did. Lower rates of CHD events among women in the hormone group in the final years of HERS did not persist during additional years of follow-up ; RH=1(95% C.I., 0.77–01.29) [13].

## 2.3. The Women's Health Initiative

The Women's Health Initiative (WHI) [14], the largest preventive study of its kind, was launched by the National Institutes of Health (NIH) in 1993 to focus on defining the risks and benefits of strategies that could potentially reduce the incidence of heart disease, breast and colorectal cancer and fractures in postmenopausal women. Between 1993 and 1998, the WHI enrolled 161,809 postmenopausal women aged 50–79 into a set of clinical trials (trials of low-fat dietary pattern, calcium and vitamin D supplementation and postmenopausal hormone use) and an observational study at 40 clinical centers in the United States.

One treatment arm of the trial included postmenopausal women who were taking continuous, combined estrogen–progestogen hormone replacement therapy, using CEE 0.625 mg plus MPA 2.5 mg daily ($n$=8506) tested against placebo ($n$=8102). This primary prevention study was due to run for 8.5 years.

On May 31, 2002, after a mean of 5.2 years of follow-up, the data and safety monitoring board recommended stopping this arm because the test statistic for invasive breast cancer exceeded the stopping boundary for this adverse effect and the global index statistic supported risks exceeding benefits.

Estimated hazard ratios (HRs) (nominal 95% confidence intervals (CIs) for the major clinical outcomes were as follows: CHD, 1.29 (1.02–1.63) with 286 cases; breast cancer, 1.26 (1.00–1.59) with 290 cases; stroke, 1.41 (1.07–1.85) with 212 cases; pulmonary embolism (PE), 2.13 (1.39–3.25) with 101 cases; colorectal cancer, 0.63 (0.43–0.92) with 112 cases; endometrial cancer, 0.83 (0.47–1.47) with 47 cases; hip fracture, 0.66 (0.45–0.98) with 106 cases; and death due to other causes, 0.92 (0.74–1.14) with 331 cases.

Absolute excess risks per 10,000 person years, attributable to estrogen plus progestin, were 7 more CHD events, 8 more strokes, 8 more Pes and 8 more invasive breast cancers, while absolute risk reductions per 10,000 person years were 6 fewer colorectal cancers and 5 fewer hip fractures. The absolute excess risk of events included in the global index was 19 per 10,000 person years.

All-cause mortality was not affected during the trial.

It was concluded that overall health risks exceeded benefits from the use of combined estrogen plus progestin for an average 5.2-year follow-up among healthy, postmenopausal US women, and that this regimen should not be initiated or continued for primary prevention of CHD.

The estrogen trial alone, involving 10,739 women with prior hysterectomy, is still scheduled to continue until March 2005. During the year 2003, several detailed and updated analyses were published, focusing on breast cancer risk [15], coronary heart disease [16], gynecologic cancer [17] and risk of fracture and bone mineral density [18].

In May 2003, the results of the Women's Health Initiative Memory Study (WHIMS), an ancillary study to the two larger WHI hormone trials were published [19]. Among the women receiving estrogens plus progestogen, the hazard ratio (HR) for probable dementia was 2.05 (1.21–3.48); 45 vs. 22 per 10,000 person years; $p=0.01$). Treatment effects on mild cognitive impairment did not differ between groups: HR, 1.07 (0.74–1.55); 63 vs. 59 cases per 10,000 person years; $p=0.72$).

It was concluded that estrogen plus progestin therapy increased the risk for probable dementia in postmenopausal women aged 65 years or older. In addition, estrogen plus progestin therapy did not prevent mild cognitive impairment in these women.

### 2.4. The Women's International Study for Long-Duration Oestrogen after Menopause

The Women's International Study for Long-Duration Oestrogen after Menopause (WISDOM) [20,21] was the world's only remaining trial, and perhaps the last chance, to examine the long-term effects of combined HRT. It was planned to involve 22,000 postmenopausal women being treated with placebo, estrogen alone or combined HRT for 10 years with 5 years of further follow-up.

After the early termination of the WHI study, the steering committee of WISDOM recommended to continue. However, the Medical Research Council (UK) (MRC) called for an urgent separate report from an international committee of its choice. The WISDOM (UK) team had little time to justify the continuation of WISDOM, and WISDOM (Australia) and WISDOM (New Zealand) were not invited to contribute to the advisory committee's deliberations or the MRC decision. In October 2002, the MRC (UK) decided to withdraw funding for scientific and practical reasons. It stressed that there were no safety concerns for the women in WISDOM, but it cited the findings of WHI as the main influence for its decision.

### 2.5. Other trials

The other main trials performed on HRT with their outcomes and results are summarized in Table 1.

The EPAT study is the only trial on the primary prevention of CVD [22]. The result was a slower progression of subclinical atherosclerosis as measured by the intima-media thickness of the right distal common carotid artery.

Thickening of the intima-media of the arterial wall is the earliest detectable anatomic change in the development and progression of atherosclerosis.

All the other trials were secondary prevention studies [23–30]. They show no significant effect of ERT or HRT.

The only trial performed on venous thromboembolism (EVTET) [31] showed an increased risk of recurrence in women with previous thromboembolism on HRT.

## 3. Is it possible to compare observational studies and randomized, controlled trials?

Benson and Hartz [32] compared the results of observational studies published after 1984 with those of randomized controlled trials. There were 136 reports about 19 diverse treatments, such as calcium-channel blocker therapy for coronary artery disease, appendectomy, etc.

Table 1
Randomized trials of HRT or ERT vs. placebo set up to study vascular events and/or cancers as endpoints

| Study | Women recruited | Mean age (years) | Number | Treatment | Follow-up (years) | Outcomes | Results |
|---|---|---|---|---|---|---|---|
| *Primary prevention* | | | | | | | |
| Estrogen in the Prevention of Atherosclerosis Trial (EPAT) (22) | healthy postmenopausal women without preexisting cardiovascular disease | 60.9<br>62.1 | 97<br>102 | 1 mg E2<br>placebo | 2 | rate of change in intima-media thickness of the right distal common carotid artery far wall | average rate of progression of subclinical atherosclerosis slower with 1 mg E2 in women who did not take lipid-lowering drug |
| Women's International Study of Long-Duration Oestrogen after the Menopause (WISDOM) (20) | healthy women | | ~22,000 | as for WHI, except 0.625 mg CEE and 2.5 mg MPA also used in hysterectomised women | 10 (planned) | CHD, osteoporotic fractures, dementia, breast cancer | interrupted after the early termination of the WHI study |
| *Secondary prevention CVD* | | | | | | | |
| Estrogen Replacement and Atherosclerosis (ERA) (23) | with previous heart disease | 65.8 | 100<br>104<br>105 | 0.625 mg CEE<br>0.625 mg CEE+2.5 mg MPA<br>placebo | 3.2 | progression of coronary atherosclerosis | no significant effect |
| Women's Estrogen–Progestin Lipid-Lowering Hormone Atherosclerosis Regression Trial (WELL-HART) (24) | with previous heart disease | 63.5 | 54<br>53<br>59 | 1 mg oral E2<br>1 mg oral E2+5 mg MPA/12 days<br>placebo | 3.3 | average per-participant change between baseline and follow-up coronary angiograms in the percent stenosis measured by quantitative coronary angiography | no significant effect on the progression of atherosclerosis |

| Study | Population | Age | N | Treatment | Duration (years) | Endpoints | Results |
|---|---|---|---|---|---|---|---|
| Postmenopausal Hormone Replacement Against Atherosclerosis (PHOREA) (25–26) | with previous increased intima-media thickness in carotid arteries | 40.70 | 171 / 93 | 1 mgE2+0.025 mg gestodene 12 days/month or every 3 days/month no treatment | 1 | rate of change in intima-media thickness of carotid arteries or of femoral arteries | no significant effect on the progression of atherosclerosis |
| Papworth HRT Atherosclerosis (PHASE) study (27) | postmenopausal women with angiographically proven ischaemic heart disease | 66.3 / 67 | 42 / 39 / 113 | 80 µg E2 transd. "+120 µg NET/14 days no treatment | 30.8 months | CHD events | the HRT group had a higher, but not statistically significant, event rate than the control group |
| Estrogen in the Prevention of Reinfarction Trial (ESPRIT) (28) | postmenopausal women with first myocardial infarction | 62.3 / 62.9 | 513 | 2 mg E2 valerate placebo | 2 | CHD events or deaths | no significant effect of ERT |
| Women's Angiographic Vitamin and Estrogen (WAVE) trial (29) | women with previous coronary stenosis | 65 | 423 | 0.625 CEE alone or +2.5 mg MPA vitamin E+vitamin C placebo | 2.8 | change in minimum lumen diameter of coronary arteries; CHD events | no cardiovascular benefit with HRT or vitamin supplements; potential for harm suggested with each treatment |
| *Stroke* | | | | | | | |
| Womens's Estrogen for Stroke Trial (WEST) study (30) | postmenopausal women with preexisting stroke or transient ischemic attack | 71 | 337 / 327 | 1 mg E2 placebo | 2.8 | stroke, mortality, CHD | no reduction in mortality or the recurrence of stroke no difference in CHD, breast cancer, thromboembolic events |
| *Thromboembolism* | | | | | | | |
| Estrogen in Venous Thromboembolism Trial (EVTET) (31) | women with previous thromboembolism | 55.8 / 55.7 | 71 / 69 | 2 mg E2+1 mg NETA placebo | 1.3 | recurrent deep venous thrombosis or pulmonary embolism | increased risk of recurrence on HRT |

In most cases, the estimates of treatment effect from observational studies and randomized, controlled trials were similar. In only 2 of the 19 analyses of treatment effect did the combined magnitude of the effect in observational studies lie outside the 95% confidence interval for the combined magnitude in the trials.

Oncato et al. [33] performed a search of the midline database for articles published in five major medical journals from 1991 to 1995 and identified meta-analyses of trials and meta-analyses of either cohort or case-control studies that assessed the same intervention. For the 5 clinical topics and 99 reports evaluated, the average results of well-designed observational studies were remarkably similar to those of trials.

## 4. Limitations of trials

"My proposal is that the clinical trial is a very good study design, but not *necessarily* the ultimate study design" said Trudy Bush in an editorial following the publication of the HERS study [34].

Randomized, controlled trials have two types of validity: internal and external.

### 4.1. Internal validity

Internal validity implies that the trial answered the question it set out to answer. Major elements include a sample size large enough to find important differences, truly random assignment to treatments, concealment of the upcoming assignment from those involved with the trial, use of a placebo treatment, minimizing losses to follow-up and use of an intention-to-treat analysis.

In these important respects, the WHI trial used excellent methods.

### 4.2. External validity

External validity is the ability to extrapolate the trial's results to other women. By design, trials include a group of people that do not resemble any population on whom the drug is going to be used. Trials are designed that exclude people from participating in them for a wide variety of reasons.

There is also volunteer bias. People who participate in trials are different from those who do not, and they differ in ways that may affect their outcome.

### 4.3. Problems linked with the placebo

According to T. Bush, the placebo is not nothing, it is a powerful drug. Therefore, in a trial, one powerful drug is compared with another powerful drug, and it is more difficult to determine differences between two drugs than it is between a drug and nothing. In cohort studies, the exposure is compared with no exposure.

The other thing that can happen in clinical trials is that the placebo group may in fact not remain a true placebo group. This happened in HERS: Because estrogens have a very marked effect on lipids, women on HRT had beneficial HDL and LDL changes, while women on placebo did not. The women on placebo were referred back to their cardiologists, who put them on statins. Thus, during the course of HERS, significantly more women on placebo adopted statins than women on HRT, and according to T. Bush, HERS ended up not with a hormone vs. placebo test, but a hormone vs. statin test.

### 4.3.1. Problems specifically linked with WHI

The early cessation of the combined HRT arm of WHI caused fear and ill-advised responses in many HRT users.

However, some results from this trial may be questioned as there are large inconsistencies in the year-to-year estimates (Table 4 of the WHI paper). For example, for CHD, the HR was 0.99 for year 4, while that for year 5 was 2.38 and that for year 6 and later was 0.78. Similarly, they showed a more than twofold difference for breast cancer; 2.54 for year 5 and 1.12 for year 6 or later.

Furthermore, at 5 years, there was an unexpected temporary decrease in adverse events in the placebo group.

Indeed, the Writing Group for the WHI investigators indicated "possible narrowing of the difference by year 6;" however, they minimise the significance of this observation by further stating "HR estimates tend to be unstable beyond 6 years after randomization." So what? If this is true, the same can be said for all of their estimates.

The statistical relevance of the data from this trial is also puzzling. When adjusted confidence intervals reach unity, as is the case in WHI, is it statistically significant?

Other puzzling aspects of this study are

- the high dropout rate of 42% in the HRT group and
- the high unblinding rate of 40.5% in the HRT group vs. 6.8% in the placebo group.

Another difficulty with this study is the presentation of results for a population of a wide age range without stratification according to the various decades.

In fact, women between the ages of 50 and 59 accounted for only 33% of the women admitted into the study, while women between 60 and 69 represented 45% of the subjects and those between 70 and 79 years contributed the remaining 21%.

The women selected for the WHI study were considered to be healthy. Nearly 70% of the women were overweight, and of these, half were obese (body mass index≥30), 36% were treated for hypertension and only 50% had never smoked.

WHI was a mixed primary and secondary cardiovascular prevention study, which was not able to test the hypothesis that HRT may be cardioprotective when started around menopause.

It is possible that to have an effect in delaying the onset of CVD, there may exist a narrow window of only a few years after the menopause and before the development of significant atherosclerosis in which hormones may prevent the pathological processes. Supporting that suggestion are the striking findings from Clarkson's group of experiments in monkeys. Newly postmenopausal monkeys given hormone therapy have marked protection from coronary disease. However, when such therapy is initiated 2 years after ovariectomy (equivalent of about 6 human years), no protection is observed. In WHI, the vast majority of the women were initiated with the hormone therapy many years after menopause. Interestingly, in the recent WHI paper of Manson [16], one finds that in a group that initiated hormone therapy closest to the time of menopause (within 10 years), the relative risk was 0.89.

The same remarks apply to the effects of long-term HRT on cognitive function and dementia. A recent report of women using HRT for more than 10 years has shown an associated reduction in Alzheimer's disease (odds ratio 0.31, 95% C.I. 0.17–0.86) [35].

Some comments in the WHI papers issued in 2003 are strange. For example, Manson et al. [16] wrote, "A substantial elevation in the risk of CHD with estrogen plus progestin occurred in year 1, and a smaller and nonsignificant excess risk occurred in years 2 through 5. In year 6 and beyond, the increased rates in the placebo group resulted in an apparent risk reduction." Why not suppose a decreased risk induced by HRT, instead of an "increased rate," in the placebo group?

Last but not least, women included in HERS and WHI were asymptomatic and older than women usually using HRT. The dose of estrogen (0.625 mg CEE), appropriate for relieving hot flushes in 50-year-old women, may be inappropriate for those in their late 60s or 70s. This is a much higher dose than would normally be used clinically when starting older women on HRT.

## 5. Conclusion

In light of the findings of the WHI and HERS trials, the use of an HRT regimen containing CEE 0.625 mg together with MPA (at any dose?) should be avoided in the long term.

HRT, using different estrogens and progestogens and different doses and routes of administration, may be similar in its effects on the breast, bowel and skeleton. However, the metabolic effects of different molecules and/or different regimens being clearly different, this is most likely to have a different impact on their cardiovascular or neurologic effects.

As far as breast cancer risk is concerned, it seems mandatory to test the effects of other progestogens on the breast. Progesterone and norpregnane derivatives do not have the same effects on the enzymatic systems of the breast cells as MPA or nortestosterone derivatives.

## References

[1] D.A. Grimes, R.A. Lobo, Perspectives on the women's health initiative trial of hormone replacement therapy, Obstet. Gynecol. 100 (2002) 1344–1353.
[2] L.L. Humphrey, B.K.S. Chan, H.C. Sox, Postmenauposal hormone replacement therapy and the primary prevention of cardiovascular disease, Ann. Intern. Med. 137 (2002) 273–284.
[3] J.E. Rossouw, Debate: the potential role of estrogen in the prevention of heart disease in women after menopause, Curr. Control Trials Cardiovasc. Med. 1 (2000) 135–138.
[4] D.B. Petitti, Hormone replacement therapy and heart disease prevention: experimentation trumps observation, JAMA 280 (1998) 650–652.
[5] K.A. Matthews, et al., Prior to use of estrogen replacement therapy, are users healthier than nonusers? Am. J. Epidemiol. 143 (1996) 971–978.
[6] E. Barrett-Connor, Postmenopausal estrogen and prevention bias, Ann. Intern. Med. 115 (1991) 455–456.
[7] R.I. Horwitz, S.M. Horwitz, Adherence to treatment and health outcomes, Arch. Intern. Med. 153 (1993) 1863–1868.
[8] Coronary Drug Project Research Group, Influence of adherence to treatment and response of cholesterol on mortality in the coronary drug project, N. Engl. J. Med. 303 (1980) 1038–1041.

[9] S.R. Sturgeon, et al., Evidence of a healthy estrogen user survivor effect, Epidemiology 6 (1995) 227–231.
[10] J.M. Stern, R.J. Simes, Publication bias: evidence of delayed publication in a cohort study of clinical research projects, BMJ 315 (1997) 640–645.
[11] The Writing Group for the PEPI Trial, Effects of estrogen or estrogen/progestin regimens on heart disease risk factors in postmenopausal women. The Postmenopausal Estrogen/Progestin Interventions (PEPI) trial, JAMA 273 (1995) 199–208.
[12] S. Hulley, et al., for the Heart and Estrogen/Progestin Replacement Study (HERS) Research Group. Randomized trial of estrogen plus progestin for secondary prevention of coronary heart diseases in postmenopausal women, JAMA 280 (1998) 605–613.
[13] D. Grady, et al., Cardiovascular disease outcomes during 6.8 years of hormone therapy. Heart and Estrogen/Progestin Replacement study follow-up (HERS II), JAMA 288 (2002) 49–57.
[14] Writing Group for the Women's Health Initiative Investigators, Risks and benefits of estrogen plus progestin in healthy postmenopausal women: principal results from the Women's Health Initiative randomized controlled trial, JAMA 288 (2002) 321–333.
[15] R.T. Chlebowski, et al., Influence of estrogen plus progestin on breast cancer and mammography in healthy postmenopausal women. The Women's Health Initiative randomized trial, JAMA 289 (2003) 3243–3253.
[16] J.E. Manson, et al., Estrogen plus progestin and the risk of coronary heart disease, N. Engl. J. Med. 349 (2003) 523–524.
[17] G.L. Anderson, et al., Effects of estrogen plus progestin on gynecologic cancers and associated diagnostic procedures. The Women's Health Initiative randomized trial, JAMA 290 (2003) 1739–1748.
[18] J.A. Cauley, et al., Effects of estrogen plus progestin on risk of fracture and bone mineral density. The Women's Health Initiative randomized trial, JAMA 290 (2003) 1729–1738.
[19] S.A. Shumaker, et al., Estrogen plus progestin and the incidence of dementia and mild cognitive impairment in postmenopausal women. The Women's Health Initiative Memory Study: a randomized controlled trial, JAMA 289 (2003) 2651–2662.
[20] M.R. Vickers, N. Collins, Progress on the WISDOM trial—Women's International Study of long Duration Oestrogen after the Menopause, Climacteric 5 (Suppl. 1) (2002) 133–134.
[21] A. MaClennan, D. Sturdee, Editorial: the end of WISDOM, Climacteric 5 (2002) 313–316.
[22] H.N. Hodis, et al., for the estrogen in the prevention of atherosclerosis trial research group. Estrogen in the prevention of atherosclerosis. A randomized, double-blind, placebo-controlled trial, Ann. Intern. Med. 135 (2001) 939–953.
[23] D.M. Herrington, et al., Effects of estrogen replacement on the progression of coronary artery atherosclerosis, N. Engl. J. Med. 343 (2000) 522–529.
[24] H.N. Hodis, et al., Hormone therapy and the progression of coronary-artery atherosclerosis in postmenopausal women, N. Engl. J. Med. 349 (2003) 535–545.
[25] P. Angerer, et al., Effect of oral postmenopausal hormone replacement on progression of atherosclerosis: a randomized, controlled trial, Arterioscler. Thromb. Vasc. Biol. 21 (2001) 262–268.
[26] P. Angerer, et al., Effect of postmenopausal hormone replacement on atherosclerosis in femoral arteries, Maturitas 41 (2002) 51–60.
[27] S.C. Clarke, et al., A study of hormone replacement therapy in postmenopausal women with ischaemic heart disease: the Papworth HRT atherosclerosis study, BJOG 109 (2002) 1056–1062.
[28] N. Cherry, et al., Oestrogen therapy for the prevention of reinfarction in postmenopausal women: a randomised placebo controlled trial, Lancet 360 (2002) 2001–2008.
[29] D.D. Waters, et al., Effects of hormone replacement therapy and antioxidant vitamin supplements on coronary atherosclerosis in postmenopausal women: a randomized controlled trial, JAMA 288 (2002) 2432–2440.
[30] C.M. Viscoli, et al., A clinical trial of estrogen-replacement therapy after ischemic stroke, N. Engl. J. Med. 345 (2001) 1243–1249.
[31] E. Hoibraaten, et al., Increased risk of recurrent venous thromboembolism during hormone replacement therapy: results of the randomized, double-blind, placebo-controlled Estrogen in Venous Thromboembolism Trial (EVTET), Thromb. Haemost. 84 (2000) 961–967.
[32] K. Benson, A.J. Hartz, A comparison of observational studies and randomized controlled trials, N. Engl. J. Med. 342 (2000) 1878–1886.

[33] J. Concato, N. Shah, R.I. Horwitz, Randomized controlled trials, observational studies, and the hierarchy of research designs, N. Engl. J. Med. 342 (2000) 1887–1892.
[34] T. Bush, Beyond HERS: some (not so) random thoughts on randomized clinical trials, Int. J. Fertil. 46 (2001) 55–59.
[35] P.P. Zandi, et al., for the cache county memory study investigators. Hormone replacement therapy and incidence of Alzheimer disease in older women: the Cache County Study, JAMA 288 (2002) 2123–2129.

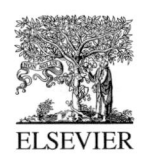

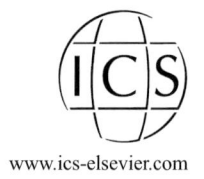

# Health in the menopause: advances in management

Sven O. Skouby*

*OB/GYN Department, Frederiksberg Hospital, NDR Fasanjev, DK 2000 F, Copenhagen, Denmark*

**Abstract.** Reliable estimates show that 10% of the global female population is currently either going through menopause or have already gone through it, and at least another 2% will reach this stage of life in the next decade. The average woman who reaches menopause has a life expectancy of nearly 30 years, and many of the causes of morbidity in older women appear to be influenced by the subsequent decline in oestrogen levels. Cardiovascular disease is the leading cause of death among women in industrialised countries and accounts for more than 40% of all deaths among women on a global scale. The probability that a menopausal woman will develop coronary heart disease (CHD) is 46% and 20% for stroke. Postmenopausal hormone therapy (HT) is one of the most frequently prescribed drug regimens for women after the age of 50. Traditionally, the primary indication for HRT is to treat symptoms of menopause. Over the past decades, however, publicity about the possible ability of HT to prevent CHD, apart from also preventing bone loss, has contributed to increased HT use. Most recently, however, the HT paradigm on the balance of costs and benefits has been impacted by puzzling information from several major randomized clinical trials. On a growing list, these studies have not shown any cardiovascular benefits from HT intervention. Epidemiological studies are essential for generating new hypotheses, and in many situations, they will provide the best information. Considering primary prevention of CHD, the strengths of the largest study conducted to date, the WHI study, are obvious but several shortcomings exist. Moreover, the clinical interpretation is influenced by the fact that we are on a steep learning curve in pharmacoepidemiology and pharmacogenetics. This points to the clinical relevance of also applying new findings from clinical studies on bio-markers and in vitro and animal research models. The research priority has been to identify the mechanisms and markers of risk and this represents one of the greatest potential scientific advances today. It can lead to the identification of women who will benefit from HT by preventing CHD, and also improve testing of hormones that do not trigger any pro-thrombotic activity. © 2004 Published by Elsevier B.V.

*Keywords:* Menopause; Cardiovascular disease; Risk markers; New developments; Risk groups

## 1. The epidemiological information

For more than two decades, it was the conventional belief that HRT would provide relative protection from ischemic heart disease in pre-menopausal women, compared with men of a similar age. This notion has been backed up by numerous observational studies

* Tel.: +45-38163390; fax: +45-38163399.
*E-mail address:* sven.skouby@fh.hosp.dk (S.O. Skouby).

that together include several hundred thousand women, years of follow-up and is supported by risk findings in women with an early compared with a late menopausal age. In 1992, Grady et al. [1] concluded from a well-conducted meta-analysis a 35% risk reduction of coronary heart disease (CHD) from oestrogen use. The more recent, extensive Nurses' Health Study (>400,000 women and years of follow-up) confirmed the substantial reduction in cardiovascular disease from intake of HRT [2]. Observational studies have the advantages of being able to include large numbers and long term follow-up, but the disadvantages of incomplete adjustment for confounders such as time trends, heterogeneity between users and non-users (*healthy user effect*) and imprecise information on HRT dosage and type. In general, observational studies tend to give a more positive finding of intervention compared with randomized placebo-controlled studies.

The first prospective randomized trial of HRT, the Heart and Oestrogen/Progestin Replacement Study (HERS) on clinical endpoints assessed the efficacy of HRT for *secondary prevention*, that is, the ability to prevent new CHD events in women with established coronary disease. The study included 2763 women from 20 centres, with a mean age of 67 years, followed up for an average of 4.1 years. In contrast to the large bulk of observational data, the HERS proved negative demonstrating that the fixed combination of 0.625 mg/day of conjugated equine oestrogen (CEE) and 2.5 mg/day of medroxyprogesterone acetate (MPA) had no effect on fatal or non-fatal cardiac events compared with placebo [3]. In 2002, less than 1 week after the updated publication of the HERS results [4], the U.S. National Heart Lung and Blood Institute (NHLBL) announced that it had stopped a trial of oestrogen–progestin versus placebo in healthy postmenopausal women. The trial was one component of the Women's Health Initiative (WHI), the first randomized primary prevention trial of postmenopausal hormones for CHD. The WHI was planned as a 15-year endeavour and one of the largest U.S. prevention studies of its kind. For this study, 16,608 women, aged between 50 and 79 years with an intact uterus, were enrolled in the trial component of oestrogen and progestin. The participants were randomized to a continuous combined combination of 0.625 mg/day of CEE and 2.5 mg/day of MPA or placebo. The primary outcome for the hormone therapy (HT) trials component was designated as CHD. The effect of hormones on overall health was also an important consideration. In an attempt to summarize important aspects of health benefits vs. risks, a global index was defined as the earliest occurrence of CHD, invasive breast cancer, stroke, pulmonary embolism, endometrial cancer, colorectal cancer, hip fracture, or death due to other causes The trial was stopped early based on health risks that exceeded health benefits over an average follow-up of 5.2 years [5]. A parallel trial of oestrogen alone in women who have had a hysterectomy is being continued, and the planned end of this trial is March 2005, by which time the average follow-up will be about 8.5 years.

The most striking result of the WHI was the lack of cardiovascular prevention in women receiving the combined hormone therapy as compared with those receiving placebo. The strengths of the WHI study are obviously related to its size, its design (a properly randomized controlled study), and its long-term duration, although the study was prematurely stopped. Several shortcomings of the trial, however, have been addressed that are inconsistent with criteria for a primary prevention study. First, the mean age of the trial population was 63 years, with 70% of the women aged 60 and over and a rather low percentage of young post-menopausal women. These "elderly" women, although considered healthy at enrolment, do not reflect the actual clinical setting when hormones are administered to menopausal women seeking therapy for recent development of the menopausal syndrome. Also, chronic diseases, such as atherosclerosis, are more likely to become complicated in women over 60 years of age than in women aged 50 to 59. Second, the enrolled population, which was considered healthy at the start of the study, had the baseline characteristics: 36% of women had prior therapy for hypertension; 34% had a body mass index (BMI) of 30 or above; 4% received prior treatment for diabetes; and no external validation on prevalence of index variables in similar age groups in the background population was performed.

Epidemiological studies are essential for generating new hypotheses, and in many situations, they will provide the best information, but to some extent the new epidemiological information has added complexity and uncertainty to the prescription of HT. Reasonable suggestions about possible explanations for understanding the paradox differences in results between cohort studies and randomized trials executed so far can be evaluated, and include among others: early start of treatment as more dominant in the cohort study is of importance; start of the use of HRT because of perimenopausal complaints identifies a subgroup with increased basal risk and a subsequent benefit of treatment; and cardiovascular changes that have been developed postmenopausally when no hormones are used responds deleteriously to hormones and prevention is different from treatment. Moreover, the clinical interpretation of the epidemiological studies is also influenced by the fact that we are on a steep learning curve in pharmacoepidemiology and pharmacogenetics. This points to the clinical relevance of also applying new findings from clinical studies on bio-markers and in vitro and animal research models.

## 2. Use of bio-markers

Atherosclerosis, characterised by the accumulation of lipids and fibrous elements in the large arteries, constitutes the single most important contributor to the growing burden of CHD, the leading cause of death in women. Overviews on the pathophysiology of atherosclerosis/thrombosis have evolved substantially over the past decades. The link between lipids and atherosclerosis dominated in the 1970s, supported by experimental and clinical observations and had deterioration in glucose metabolism/insulin sensitivity as an independent co-player. The emerging knowledge of vascular biology led to a focus on growth factors and the proliferation of smooth muscle cells in the 1980s. Over the past decades, we have come to appreciate a prominent role for inflammation in atherosclerosis, also involving a change in the haemostatic balance. This changing paradigm may also explain why earlier studies on metabolic risk markers in relation to HT were so coincidental with the preventive findings in the original observational studies on cardiovascular risk. Studies on surrogate markers may still be valid but as laboratory advances in vascular biology show, it has become evident that "real world" markers are subject to continuous evaluation and review. Perfect biomarkers that can serve as surrogate end-points are currently not known. Following the results of the WHI study, the research priority has been to identify the mechanisms and markers of risk, which will represent one of the most potential scientific advances today.

Traditionally, the metabolic effects of HT are divided into the impact on lipids, glucose and the haemostatic system, although an interdisciplinary approach should be warranted.

*Lipids*: HRT have independent effects on many aspects of lipid and lipoprotein metabolism, leading to changes in the concentration and/or composition of all lipoprotein species. Changes include a fall in low-density lipoprotein (LDL) and a rise in high-density lipoprotein (HDL). In addition, oral administration of oestrogens results in an increase in triglycerides and very low-density lipoprotein and an increase in the proportion of small, dense LDL, effects which are not seen with transdermal administration. In general, progestagens oppose the effects of oestrogens on HDL and triglycerides to an extent that depends on their type and dose and on the type and dose of oestrogen they are combined with. Some progestagens cause a net lowering of HDL in the presence of oestrogen. Both oestrogens and progestagens lower lipoprotein (a). Areas of investigation where clarification is needed include: interactions between triglycerides and VLDL and the haemostatic system; the impact of small dense LDL on endothelial damage; and the effects of sex steroids on HDL function rather than concentration.

*Glucose*: Postmenopausal women display some features of the metabolic syndrome, mainly insulin resistance. Oestrogen in replacement dosages improves the insulin secretion, sensitivity and elimination rate in normal and hyperinsulinaemic, postmenopausal women while added androgenic progestins may reverse part of this improvement, which does not seem to be the case for progesterone-derived progestins. Fasting glucose, insulin and HbA1C levels are not impaired in current HRT users versus nonusers, and HRT improves glycaemic control in postmenopausal women with type-2 diabetes. Accordingly, HRT may improve some aspects of the "menopausal metabolic syndrome."

*Haemostasis*: Sex steroids may increase fibrinogen consumption, as can be deduced from increased levels in the blood of degradation products (D-dimers) and/or activation markers of coagulation (fragment 1+2). Most of the documented changes within the haemostatic system, however, are minor or moderate and in normal subjects within the normal physiological ranges, and the deviations related to diseased states conjectural. The apparent increased fibrinogen consumption might be relevant in women with increased susceptibility, such as those with clinical thrombophilia. Notably, estradiol administered transdermally does not induce significant changes in coagulation or fibrinolysis. The presence of congenital thrombophilia increases the risk of venous thrombosis more than additive during HRT treatment, and the presence of an increased risk of VTE in the first time users indicates a group of susceptible individuals who are presently insufficiently detected.

Future development is mainly to be sought in unravelling cardiovascular mechanisms related to sex steroids, where we should avoid simplification in pharmacology, treat all preparations separately and also separate and allow for subgroups in the population to be different in responding to the medications.

*New potential markers*: *APC*: The protein C activation complex appears to be downregulated by inflammation in diabetes and atherosclerosis. *Leptin*: Platelets have leptin receptors. Leptin is increased in obese people and leptin limiting to platelets increases the sensitivity to platelet agonists and could contribute to arterial thrombosis. *Protein Z*: Protein Z binds to ZPI, a plasma protease. The complex inactivates factor $X_a$ on phospholipids. Protein Z levels seem to be a risk factor for DVT, MCP-1 A propagator of atherosclerosis and a key modulator of monocyte activity [6].

## 3. Conclusion

Use of the metabolic or biomarkers of cardiovascular disease during HT may lead to an increased understanding of the association of CHD and the use of hormones in normal, as well as high risk, groups. Despite the pessimistic findings in recent epidemiological studies, there are reasons to believe that in the years to come hormonal treatment with lower doses, new updated biomarkers, a wider range of progestins and tissue-specific products will enable reinforced possibilities for avoiding individual risk, and even reestablish the perception of generally beneficial effects on the occurrence of ischemic heart diseases.

## References

[1] D. Grady, et al., Hormone therapy to prevent disease and prolong life in postmenopausal women, Ann. Intern. Med. 117 (1992) 1016–1037.
[2] F. Grodstein, et al., Postmenopausal hormone therapy and mortality, N. Engl. J. Med. 336 (1997) 1769–1775.
[3] S. Hulley, et al., for the HERS Research Group, Randomized trial of estrogen plus progestin for secondary prevention of coronary heart disease in postmenopausal women: Heart and Estrogen/progestin Replacement Study (HERS) Research Group, JAMA 280 (1998) 605–613.
[4] D. Grady, et al., Cardiovascular Disease Outcomes During 6.8 Years of Hormone Therapy. Heart and Estrogen/Progestin Replacement Study Follow-up (HERS II), JAMA 288 (1) (2002) 49–57.
[5] Writing Group for the Women's Health Initiative Investigators, Risks and benefits of estrogen plus progestin in healthy postmenopausal women, JAMA 288 (3) (2002) 321–333.
[6] The European Consensus Development Conference 2002: Sex Steroids and Cardiovascular diseases. On the route to combined evidence from OC and HRT/ERT, Maturitas 44 (2003) 69–82.

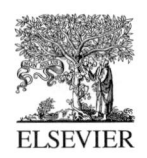

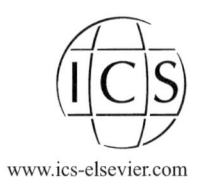

# Embryo selection and health

Anna Veiga*, Gemma Arroyo, Pere N. Barri

*Servei de Medicina de la Reproducció, Intitut Universitari Dexeus, P/Bonanova 89-91, Barcelona 08017, Spain*

**Abstract.** In order to achieve adequate pregnancy and implantation rates in In Vitro Fertilisation (IVF) programmes and to decrease multiple pregnancies, it is essential to be able to choose viable embryos for transfer. Different morphological criteria for oocyte, zygote, early cleavage embryo and blastocyst evaluation have been described and are currently used to select embryos for transfer or cryopreservation. © 2004 Published by Elsevier B.V.

*Keywords:* Embryo quality; Embryo selection criteria

## 1. Introduction

Human reproduction is very inefficient when compared with other animal species. Embryo loss is a very common event in human pregnancies. In some cases, this is evidenced by the occurrence of a miscarriage, either in the first or second trimester of the pregnancy, and may even be unnoticed if it occurs before or around implantation time.

The selection of viable embryos is a crucial point in order to achieve adequate pregnancy and implantation rates in In Vitro Fertilisation (IVF) programmes.

Embryo quality can only be defined in absolute terms as the potentiality to contribute to the birth of a healthy baby. It has to be taken into account that 60% to 75% of the embryos obtained in IVF laboratories will not be able to implant. This fact is not only due to embryonic factors as the endometrial receptivity has also to be considered.

IVF has made it possible to study early embryo stages and it has been reported that 40–60% of the embryos generated in vitro are aneuploid and up to 50% are mosaics [1]. The situation in vivo has not been studied as no in vivo early embryos are available.

The potential for normal embryo development originates in the oocyte and correct ovarian stimulation and the production of "good quality" oocytes is determinant in order to achieve success in an IVF cycle. Many implantation failures are a consequence of deficient oocyte production, and the relationship between those distant events has to be reminded to improve results.

The first developmental stages of the embryo are dependent on maternal mRNA and on oocyte reserves. The activation of the embryonic genome takes place at the four-to-eight-

---

\* Corresponding author. Tel.: +34-93-2274716; fax: +34-93-2057966.
*E-mail address:* anavei@dexeus.com (A. Veiga).

0531-5131/ © 2004 Published by Elsevier B.V.
doi:10.1016/j.ics.2004.01.118

cell stage in the human embryo [2], and it has been demonstrated that factors affecting oocyte development and maturation are related to embryo development as well. Some of the oocytes produced in vitro present biochemical, cellular or genetic defects at the time of ovulation.

## 2. Embryo selection

There are objective and subjective strategies to select the correct embryo for transfer or cryopreservation; in all cases, the selection has to be safe, non-invasive, as well as easy to carry out in a busy laboratory.

Some objective methods for embryo quality assessment are:

- High resolution videocinematography
- Polar body or embryo biopsy
- Metabolic evaluation in the culture medium
- Transfer after prolonged culture
- Cumulus cell culture and evaluation of steroid production
- O2 level in follicular fluid/perifollicular vascularisation
- Mitochondrial distribution, ATP levels
- Gene expression studies

Most of these techniques are high tech, expensive and some are invasive. They require specific instruments and experience. The results obtained have contributed to improve knowledge in the mechanisms that control embryo development.

*2.1. Oocyte evaluation*

In the morphologic evaluation of the oocyte, cytoplasmic defects, such as granularity and vacuolisation have been described. The morphology of the polar body has also been related to oocyte quality [3].

*2.2. Zygote evaluation*

Different classifications of zygotes, depending on pronuclear evaluation, have been described [4,5] and related to embryo development and to chromosomal abnormalities. Pronuclear patterns that give rise to good quality embryos with high implantation potential have been identified. In a study performed in our laboratory, it has been confirmed that certain pronuclear patterns lead to more favourable embryo development in terms of pregnancy and implantation rates.

*2.3. Embryo evaluation*

Many different scores have been described to quantify embryo quality, and every laboratory classifies embryos according to the one that correlates the best with embryo implantation.

All scores rate based on subjective morphological features of the embryo, such as the number of blastomeres (cleavage rate), the symmetry of the cells, the degree of cytoplasmic fragmentation and the aspect of the cytoplasm. Recently the early cleavage rate (at 25 to 29 h after insemination or ICSI) has been incorporated for embryo quality evaluation. It seems that embryos showing early cleavage get to the blastocyst stage at a higher rate. It has also been shown that embryos that cleave earlier give better pregnancy rates [6,7] even though an accelerated cleavage may be associated with embryo mosaicism [1]. According to morphological features, embryos have to be selected when they have two cells at the end of day 1, four to six cells at day 2, seven to nine cells or signs of compaction at day 3.

Different fragmentation patterns have been described [8,9] and correlated to embryo development. The cause or origin of such phenomenon is still unknown and it could be limited to in vitro culture conditions.

Multinucleation, in one or more blastomeres of an embryo, is observed mainly on day-2 embryos at a rate of 10–15%, and such embryos have a decreased implantation potential [10,11]. Multinucleated embryos have an increased rate of chromosomal abnormalities [12].

## 2.4. Blastocyst evaluation

Culture to the blastocyst stage has been used as a method to select the most viable embryos and only good quality embryos at day 3 become blastocysts, probably as a result of still inadequate culture conditions [13].

Embryos that reach the blastocyst rate at day 5 have a better prognosis than those at day 6. Few day-7 blastocysts can implant.

A good quality blastocyst has a well-defined and compact inner cell mass and a well-structured trophectoderm. The number of cells is also an important parameter; an expanded blastocyst should have between 150 and 200 cells.

The criteria actually used to evaluate embryo quality are subjective, have a number of limitations and do not always correlate with embryo development and implantation potential. It is essential to establish adequate patterns that define a "good quality" embryo. The evaluation must start with the oocyte (and even with the follicle), and proceed through pronuclear, early cleavage, embryo and blastocyst evaluation. Up to now, the sequential assessment of individually cultured embryos is a valuable tool to select the most suitable for transfer [14–16].

## References

[1] S. Munné, M. Sandalinas, J. Cohen, Chromosome abnormalities in human embryos, in: D. Gardner, A. Weissman, C. Howles, Z. Shoham (Eds.), Textbook of Assisted Reproductive Techniques. Laboratory and clinical perspectives, Martin Dunitz, London, 2001, pp. 297–318.
[2] P.R. Braude, V.N. Bolton, S. Moore, Human gene expression first occurs before the four-and-eight-cell stages o preimplantation development, Nature 332 (1988) 459–461.
[3] T. Ebner, et al., First polar body morphology and blastocyst formation rate in ICSI patients, Hum. Reprod. 17 (2002) 2415–2418.
[4] L. Scott, Pronuclear scoring as a predictor of embryo development, RBM Online 6 (2003) 201–214.
[5] J. Tesarik, E. Greco, The probability of abnormal preimplantation development can be predicted by a single static observation on pronuclear stage morphology, Hum. Reprod. 14 (1999) 1318–1323.
[6] D. Sakkas, et al., Early cleavage of human embryos to the two-cell stage after ICSI as an indicator of embryo viability, Hum. Reprod., (1998) 182–187.

[7] K. Lundin, C. Bergh, T. Hardarson, Early embryo cleavage is a strong indicator of embryo quality in human IVF, Hum. Reprod. 16 (2001) 2652–2657.
[8] M. Antczak, J. VanBlerkhom, Temporal and spatial aspects of fragmentation in early human embryos: possible effects on developmental competence and association with the differential elimination of regulatory proteins from polarized domains, Hum. Reprod. 14 (1999) 429–447.
[9] M. Alikani, et al., Human embryo fragmentation in vitro and its implications for pregnancy and implantation, Fertil. Steril. 71 (1999) 836–842.
[10] S. Pickering, et al., An analysis of multnucleated blastomere formation in human embryos, Mol. Hum. Reprod. 10 (1995) 1912–1922.
[11] E. Van Royen, et al., Multinucleation in cleavage stage embryos, Hum. Reprod. 18 (2003) 1062–1069.
[12] C. Staessen, A. van Steirteghem, The genetic constitution of multinuclear blastomeres and their derivative daughter blastomeres, Hum. Reprod. 13 (1998) 1625–1631.
[13] C. Rackowsky, Day 3 and day 5 morphological predictors of embryo viability, RBM Online 6 (2003) 323–331.
[14] E. Neuber, et al., Sequential assessment of individually cultured human embryos as an indicator of subsequent good quality blastocyst development, Hum. Reprod. 18 (2003) 1307–1312.
[15] L. Scott, The biological basis of non invasive strategies for selection of human oocytes and embryos, Hum. Reprod. Updat. 9 (2003) 237–249.
[16] T. Ebner, et al., Selection based on morphological assessment of oocytes and embryos at different stages of preimplantation development: a review, Hum. Reprod. Updat. 9 (2003) 251–262.

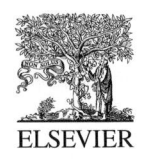

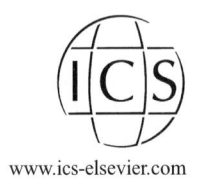

# In vitro maturation of human ova

Anne Lis Mikkelsen*

*The Fertility Clinic, Herlev University Hospital, DK-2730, Herlev, Denmark*

**Abstract.** The basis of IVM is the maturing in vitro of oocytes from Germinal Vesicle (GV) stage of development to the metaphase II stage. Oocytes are retrieved for IVM from antral follicles 2–10 mm diameter and matured in vitro for 24 to 52 h. A high proportion of the in vitro matured oocytes is able to resume meiosis and reach the MII stage in vitro. Their ability to be fertilized after 48–56 h of IVM is also high and a similar proportion is able to undergo early cleavage stage development comparable with conventional IVF and ICSI embryos. It has been questioned whether in vitro matured human oocytes are intrinsically compromised or whether culture conditions are inadequate to support the developmental capacity of the oocytes. However, recent data taken together suggest that in future immature oocyte retrieval combined with IVM could possibly replace standard stimulated IVF in selected patients. Women suffering from polycystic ovarian syndrome (PCOS) are extremely sensitive to stimulation with exogenous gonadotrophins in assisted reproduction, and they have a significant risk of developing OHSS. An attractive alternative to ovarian stimulation in women with PCOS would therefore be to retrieve immature oocytes. Immature oocyte retrieval combined with IVM could also replace standard stimulation in healthy regularly cycling women referred for IVF (ICSI) due to severe male infertility. In both groups, clinical pregnancy rates of 24% per aspiration has been obtained. The reported children born after IVM are healthy. © 2004 Published by Elsevier B.V.

*Keywords:* Maturation in vitro; Human oocytes

## 1. Introduction

In fully grown oocytes, resumption of meiosis in vivo is triggered by luteinizing hormone (LH) surge. Removal of the oocyte from the follicle is the corresponding in vitro signal.

Oocyte maturation includes nuclear and cytoplasmic events. The end point whether in vivo or in vitro is a metaphase II (MII) oocyte which can be fertilized and which can support normal embryonic development [1,2].

IVM studies in human have generally used fully grown oocytes removed from antral follicles of 2–10 mm and these experiments have dealt with the final maturation of the oocyte. Even in fully grown oocytes which are able to mature to MII the developmental potential after fertilization has been low compared with in vivo matured oocytes [3].

---

* Tel.: +45-44-88-32-16; fax: +45-44-88-39-01.
  E-mail address: anlimi@herlevhosp.kbhamt.dk (A.L. Mikkelsen).

In this chapter, the maturation in vitro of human oocytes is described and the experiences obtained in handling immature human oocytes for in vitro fertilization and embryo transfer are summarized.

## 2. Maturation and developmental competence of the oocyte

Nuclear maturation is characterized by breakdown of the nuclear membrane, separation of homologous chromosomes and extrusion of the first polar body into the perivitelline space.

Beyond these nuclear aspects of oocyte maturation, cytoplasmic events occur and they seem to be important for fertilization and developmental ability of the oocyte [4]. These aspects have been termed cytoplasmic maturation.

Nuclear and cytoplasmatic maturation are normally highly co-ordinated during normal reproductive cycles, but this co-ordination can be uncoupled by in vitro maturation technologies. Most deficiencies in oocytes during in vitro maturation are associated with cytoplasmic reprogramming rather than meiotic progression, for reasons, which remain unknown.

Evaluation of the development of oocytes following fertilization is generally considered being a valid criterion for developmental competence of the oocyte [5]. The effects of cytoplasmic aberrations are seldom expressed at an early stage of development but instead more frequently associated with cleavage and peri-implantation stages [4]. Therefore, fertilization and pronuclear development may occur in a wide spectrum of eggs, which lack the capacity to develop normally to term and the guide to the full developmental capacity is delivery of healthy infants.

## 3. IVM followed by IVF-ET

The ability of immature oocytes to spontaneously resume meiosis when removed from the follicle was first demonstrated by Pincus and Enzman in 1935. This was later confirmed by Edwards [6]. In 1969, Edwards et al. [7] were able to demonstrate for the first time the fertilization of in vitro matured human oocytes.

A high proportion of the in vitro matured oocytes are able to resume meiosis and reach the MII stage in vitro. Their ability to be fertilized after 48–56 h of IVM is also high and a similar proportion is able to undergo early cleavage stage development comparable with conventional IVF and ICSI embryos. Despite this, reported implantation results have been lower than expected from the apparent quality of the transferred embryos. It is uncertain whether in vitro matured human oocytes are intrinsically compromised or whether culture conditions are inadequate to support the developmental capacity of the oocytes.

## 4. Sources of oocytes for IVM

Sources of oocytes used for IVM include four main groups of patients: (1) Natural cycles (±FSH in vivo primed); (2) PCOS patients (±FSH primed or ±HCG primed); (3) stimulated ovaries from patients undergoing routine controlled ovarian hyperstimulation for IVF or ICSI (rescue IVM) and (4) cryopreserved and thawed oocytes.

### 4.1. Immature oocytes from natural cycles

In regularly cycling women with normal ovaries, a low basal level on day 3 of oestradiol (<200 pmol/l) [8] has been found to be a predictor of success. A clinical pregnancy rate of 14% per aspiration was obtained in 106 cycles. The concentration of FSH and the number of follicles on day 3 predicted the number of oocytes retrieved, whereas these parameters did not predict the subsequent development of oocytes [8].

Few prospective studies have examined the effect of priming with FSH before aspiration of immature oocytes in regularly menstruating women [9–11]. The series are small, a variety of stimulation regimens have been used. Similar rates of maturation, fertilization, cleavage and pregnancy were observed, if oocytes were obtained after a follicle of 10 mm was observed by ultrasound. FSH priming had to be followed by deprivation for 2–3 days [12].

In unprimed natural cycles, the oocytes have been retrieved at different moments in the menstrual cycle and probably from follicles of different sizes [13,14]. The recruitment and growth of numerous follicles characterize each menstrual cycle. One or two selected follicles continue to grow until the day of ovulation, while the remaining follicles undergo atresia. Mikkelsen et al. [15] aimed at oocyte collection to coincide with selection of the dominant follicle. Oocytes were aspirated after a leading follicle of 10 mm and an endometrial thickness of at least 5 mm were observed at ultrasound and in 87 cycles a pregnancy rate of 12.6% per aspiration was obtained. Serum levels of oestradiol and inhibin A were evaluated retrospectively. Significantly more oocytes were obtained in cycles with a detected increase in the level of oestradiol from day 3 to the day of aspiration (19% per aspiration) compared with cycles without such an increase. A higher pregnancy rate was observed after an increase in the level of inhibin A concentration (24% vs. 0%) per aspiration.

### 4.2. Immature oocytes from PCOS patients

Although pregnancy rates of 27% have been reported, the implantation rate has been low (6.9%) for embryos obtained after IVM on immature oocytes from unstimulated PCO patients [16]. To compensate for this, endogenous hCG [17] has been shown to improve the maturation rate of immature oocytes in PCOS patients. Furthermore, priming with rec-FSH followed by coasting for 2–3 days before aspiration of immature oocytes may improve the maturational potential of the oocytes [18].

### 4.3. Immature oocytes obtained from women undergoing routine superovulated IVF ("rescue IVM")

During controlled ovarian hyperstimulation, the oocyte population at the time of hCG administration may be heterogeneous and this leads to retrieval of oocytes at different stages of maturation. About 15% of the oocytes will remain in prophase I of meiosis. These oocytes can mature in vitro and develop into viable embryos. However, these oocytes may represent an inferior population as they failed to mature although the follicles were exposed to supra-physiological concentrations of gonadotrophins.

Immature oocytes have been retrieved and matured in vitro from patients at risk of hyperstimulation after gonadotrophin injections [19,20]. This could be adopted as an option to prevent occurrence of OHSS.

## 4.4. Cryopreserved and thawed immature oocytes

Freezing of immature oocytes may be an alternative approach to the cryopreservation of female gamete. Cryopreservation of immature prophase I oocytes and subsequent fertilization but without transfer have been described [21] and birth after cryopreservation of immature oocytes with subsequent IVM has been obtained [22]. Successful oocyte cryopreservation has the potential to provide more options for patient treatment, e.g. storage of oocytes from patients who have the risk of loss of ovarian function. Human oocyte cryopreservation is still under development.

## 5. Culture medium

Very few reports based on human data are available on the composition of culture media for human oocyte maturation. Furthermore, often too few GV oocytes have been available for stating significant comparisons [23–26].

Studies in human provide support for the responsiveness of human oocytes to gonadotrophins during IVM. Improvements in human oocyte maturation and embryo cleaving in the presence of FSH and LH have been reported [27]. Culture medium for human IVM is usually supplemented with serum. The most commonly used protein sources in human IVM are fetal cord serum [28] and fetal bovine serum [17,26,28]. Due to potential sources of infectious agents, it has been advised not to supplement with serum sources from other patients or from animals, and therefore the patient's serum has been used [29]. Significantly increased rates of maturation [47/74 (63%) vs. 26/63 (41%), $p<0.05$], pregnancy [6/28 (21.4%) vs. 0/23 (0%), $p<0.05$] and implantation [5/20 (30%) vs. 0/15 (0%), $p<0.05$] have been obtained from oocytes matured in culture medium with serum supplementation compared with oocytes matured in medium supplemented with HSA [30]. The reasons for the higher performance of serum supplemented media in the IVM system remain to be elucidated. Serum may contain growth factors such as epidermal growth factor or insulin-like growth factor-I, which are thought to be important for cytoplasmic maturation [31]. Other factors such as inhibins and activins may also improve nuclear maturation and subsequent fertilization of immature oocytes [32].

## 6. Time interval of maturation

Previous studies have shown, that 80% of immature human oocytes show nuclear maturation (extrusion of a polar body) and will be at MII by 48–54 h of culture [26,33]. A considerable asynchrony of the maturation has been observed and a number of MII oocytes can be obtained already after 24 h of maturation. If these oocytes are inseminated after 48 h they have been at MII arrest for 20–30 h, which places them well past the optimal fertilization time and may compromise their developmental competence.

To ensure that early matured oocytes do not remain in metaphase arrest for a prolonged period, Smith et al. [29] evaluated the effects of shortening the duration of oocyte maturation from 36 to 28 h. No significant difference in rates of maturation [78/107 (73%) vs. 65/84 (77%)], fertilization [56/78 (72%) vs. 51/65 (78%)] or pregnancy [4/29 (14%) vs. 4/26 (15%)], was observed, when oocytes were matured for 28 h compared with 36 h. The optimal time of insemination has not yet been established. The 28-h IVM period had a significant benefit in that it allowed the insemination to be performed during working hours; it had to be performed at night when the 36-h IVM schedule was used.

## 7. Safety of the IVM procedure and effects on offspring

Pregnancies resulting from in vitro derived cattle embryos have been characterized by sex ratio skewed in favour of males, increased spontaneous abortion rate throughout gestation, reduced intensity of labour and "Large Offspring Syndrome", including the following features: alteration in organ and tissue development, placental anomalies, increases in birth weight together with a high incidence of polyhydramnios and hydrops fetalis. The biological mechanisms that underlie these conditions remain to be uncovered [34–36].

In previous human IVM investigations, the delivery of about 300 babies have been reported after IVM followed by IVF and ET. There has been no report of malformations or "Large Offspring Syndrome".

Forty-one children have been born in our center. The median weight was 3650 g (range 1745–4690 g). One child was delivered at gestational age 32+4 weeks by cesarean section due to severe pre-eclampsia. The birth weight was 1745 g. The remaining children were born between 38 and 42 gestational weeks.

One girl had a soft cleft palate, the remaining had no malformations and they are all healthy, the oldest child being 3 years old. They are all followed up by examination when they are 6 months, 1 year and 2 years old.

## 8. Future perspectives

The extensive use of drugs for ovarian hyperstimulation has been questioned. The IVM protocol is relative simple with a shorter period of treatment. In addition, the side effects of stimulation, in particular OHSS, are eliminated and costs are reduced compared with conventional IVF.

Human oocytes are difficult to obtain and of variable quality and normality. This paucity of material forces us to draw conclusions from fewer oocytes (patients) than is ideal. Nevertheless, the results have some relevance in order to improve clinical procedures to obtain immature oocytes. The data taken together suggest that in future immature oocyte retrieval combined with IVM could possibly replace standard stimulated IVF in selected patients.

Before considering IVM as an alternative treatment in ART, the efficiency of the IVM protocol should be compared with those obtainable from the present "gold standard", the long down-regulated protocol also in terms of economy and patient attitudes.

Through further research, it may be possible to refine and optimize the conditions for IVM. In the future, in vitro follicle culture in combination with IVM may have advantages in assisted reproductive technologies and may help to restore fertility in the treatment of cancer in children and young women. Research is continuing in optimizing the methods for the freezing of isolated immature oocytes and of a complete human ovary, and progress is being made towards complete development of follicular oocytes in vitro [37]. Complete in vitro follicle growth from primordial follicle up to Grafian stage has been achieved only in mice [38]. Methods for long-term in vitro follicle growth of human primordial follicles are at present under development [23–25], but a successful culture system has not yet been reported. Human primordial follicles have been found to proliferate up to secondary follicles even after freeze-storage [39] and grow to antral stages when grafted under the renal capsule of immunodeficient mice [40].

While cryopreservation of reproductive cells and tissue is already becoming established, in vivo preservation will be a key goal in the future when the implications of inhibiting apoptosis or oocyte quality are better understood. Research is continuing in optimizing the methods for the freezing of isolated immature oocytes and of a complete human ovary. This may have advantages in assisted reproductive technologies and may help to restore fertility in the treatment of cancer in children and young women.

## References

[1] A. Gougeon, Regulation of ovarian follicular development in primates: facts and hypothesis, Endocr. Rev. 17 (1996) 121–155.
[2] M.-A. Driancourt, B. Thuel, Control of oocyte growth and maturation by follicular cells and molecules present in follicular fluid. A review, Reprod. Nutr. Dev. 38 (1998) 345–362.
[3] R.M. Moor, et al., Oocyte maturation and embryonic failure, Hum. Reprod. Updat. 4 (1998) 223–236.
[4] J.J. Eppig, et al., Relationship between the developmental programs controlling nuclear and cytoplasmic maturation of mouse oocytes, Dev. Biol. 164 (1994) 1–9.
[5] J.J. Eppig, et al., Factors affecting the developmental competence of mouse oocytes grown in vitro: follicle stimulation hormone and insulin, Biol. Reprod. 59 (1998) 1445–1453.
[6] R.G. Edwards, Maturation in vitro of human ovarian oocytes, Lancet II (1965) 926–929.
[7] R.G. Edwards, B.D. Bavister, P.C. Steptoe, Early stages of fertilization in vitro of human oocytes matured in vitro, Nature 221 (1969) 632–635.
[8] A.L. Mikkelsen, et al., Basal concentrations of oestradiol may predict the outcome of IVM in regular menstruating women, Hum. Reprod. 16 (2001) 862–867.
[9] A. Trounson, et al., Oocyte maturation, Hum. Reprod. 13 (Suppl. 3) (1998) 52–62.
[10] A.-M. Suikkari, et al., Lutheal phase start of low-dose FSH priming of follicles results in an efficient recovery, maturation and fertilization of immature human oocytes, Hum. Reprod. 15 (2000) 747–751.
[11] P. Wynn, et al., Pretreatment with follicle stimulating hormone promotes the number of human oocytes reaching metaphase II by in-vitro maturation, Hum. Reprod. 13 (1998) 3132–3138.
[12] A.I. Mikkelsen, S.D. Smith, S. Lindenberg, In vitro maturation of human oocytes from regular menstruating women may be successful without FSH priming, Hum. Reprod. 14 (1999) 1847–1851.
[13] M.H. Thornton, M.M. Francis, R.J. Paulson, Immature oocyte retrieval: lessons from unstimulated IVF cycles, Fertil. Steril. 70 (1998) 647–650.
[14] A.C. Cobo, et al., Maturation in vitro of human oocytes from unstimulated cycles: selection of the optimal day for ovum retrieval based on follicular size, Hum. Reprod. 14 (1999) 1864–1868.
[15] A.L. Mikkelsen, S. Smith, S. Lindenberg, Impact of oestradiol and inhibin A concentrations on pregnancy rate in in-vitro oocyte maturation, Hum. Reprod. 15 (2000) 1685–1690.
[16] K.Y. Cha, et al., Pregnancies and deliveries after in vitro maturation culture followed by in vitro fertilization and embryo transfer without stimulation in women with polycystic ovary syndrome, Fertil. Steril. 73 (2000) 978–983.
[17] R.C. Chian, et al., Prospective randomized study of human chorionic gonadotrophin priming before immature oocyte retrieval from unstimulated women with polycystic ovarian syndrome, Hum. Reprod. 15 (2000) 165–170.
[18] A.L. Mikkelsen, S. Lindenberg, Benefit of FSH priming of women with PCOS to the in-vitro maturation procedure and the outcome. A randomized prospective study, Reproduction 122 (2001) 587–592.
[19] S. Coskun, et al., Recovery and maturation of immature oocytes in patients at risk for ovarian hyperstimulation syndrome, J. Assist. Reprod. Genet. 15 (1998) 372–377.
[20] K.A. Jaroudi, et al., Embryo development and pregnancies from in-vitro matured and fertilized human oocytes, Hum. Reprod. 14 (1999) 1749–1751.

[21] T.L. Toth, et al., Fertilization and in vitro development of cryopreserved human prophase I oocytes, Fertil. Steril. 61 (1994) 891–894.
[22] M.J. Tucker, et al., Birth after cryopreservation of immature oocytes with subsequent in vitro maturation, Fertil. Steril. 70 (1998) 578–579.
[23] J. Smitz, R. Cortvridt, Oocyte in-vitro maturation and follicle culture: current clinical achievements and future directions, Human Reprod. 14 (Suppl. 1) (1999) 145–161.
[24] O. Salha, N. Abusheika, V. Sharma, Dynamics of human follicular growth and in-vitro oocyte maturation, Hum. Reprod. Updat. 4 (1998) 816–832.
[25] R. Van den Hurk, et al., Primate and bovine immature oocytes and follicles as sources of fertilizable oocytes, Hum. Reprod. Updat. 6 (2000) 457–474.
[26] A. Trounson, C. Anderiesz, G. Jones, Maturation of human oocytes in vitro and their developmental competence, Reproduction 121 (2001) 51–75.
[27] C. Anderiesz, et al., Effect of recombinant human gonadotrophins on human, bovine and murine oocyte meiosis, fertilization and embryonic development in-vitro, Hum. Reprod. 15 (2000) 1140–1148.
[28] K.Y. Cha, R.C. Chian, Maturation in vitro of immature human oocytes for clinical use, Hum. Reprod. Updat. 4 (1998) 103–120.
[29] S.D. Smith, A.L. Mikkelsen, S. Lindenberg, Development of human oocytes matured in vitro for 28 or 36 hours, Fertil. Steril. 73 (2000) 541–544.
[30] A.L. Mikkelsen, et al., Maternal serum supplementation in culture medium benefits maturation of immature human oocytes, Reprod. Biomed. Online 2 (2001) 112–116.
[31] E. Gomez, J.J. Tarin, A. Pellicer, Oocyte maturation in humans: the role of gonadotropins and growth factors, Fertil. Steril. 60 (1993) 40–46.
[32] B.M. Alak, et al., Enhancement of primate oocyte maturation and fertilization in vitro by inhibin A and activin A, Fertil. Steril. 66 (1996) 646–653.
[33] J.B. Russell, et al., Unstimulated immature oocyte retrival: early versus midfollicular endometrial priming, Fertil. Steril. 67 (1997) 616–620.
[34] A.M. Van Wagtendonk-de Leeuw, B.J.G. Aerts, J.H.G. den Daas, Abnormal offspring following in vitro production of bovine preimplantation embryos: a field study, Theriogenelogy 49 (1998) 883–894.
[35] J.F. Hasler, In-vitro production of cattle embryos: problems with pregnancies and parturition, Hum. Reprod. 15 (S5) (2000) 47–58.
[36] P.W. Farin, A.E. Croisier, C.E. Farin, Influence of in vitro systems on embryo survival and fetal development in cattle, Theriogenology 55 (2001) 151–170.
[37] R. Cortvrindt, J. Smitz, In vitro follicle growth: achievements in mammalian species, Reprod. Domest. Anim. 36 (2001) 3–9.
[38] J.J. Eppig, M.J. O'Brien, Development in-vitro of mouse oocytes from primordial follicles, Biol. Reprod. 54 (1996) 197–207.
[39] O. Hovatta, et al., Extracellular matrix improves survival of both stored and fresh human primordial and primary ovarian follicles in long-term culture, Hum. Reprod. 12 (1997) 1032–1036.
[40] K. Oktay, et al., Development of human primordial follicles to antral stages in SCID/hpg mice stimulated with follicle stimulating hormone, Hum. Reprod. 13 (1998) 1133–1138.

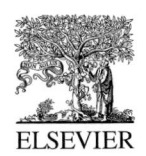

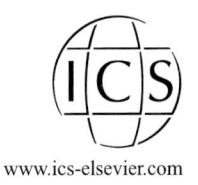

# Basic science issues in assisted reproduction: gamete interaction

Santiago Brugo Olmedo*

*Andrology and Embryology, CEGYR, Center for Gynecology and Reproduction Studies, Viamonte 1438, Buenos Aires, Capital Federal C1055ABB, Argentina*

*Keywords:* Assisted reproduction; Gamete interaction; Fertilization

Fertilization is the process that culminates in the union of one sperm nucleus with the egg nucleus within the activated egg cytoplasm.

This is a complex process of molecular events involving matured haploid male and female gametes, their mutual recognition and fusion.

Fertilization starts with: sperm activation; incorporation of the sperm into the egg cytoplasm, which includes binding and fusion of the plasma membranes; egg activation; formation of the sperm and egg nuclei; migrations of the pronuclei that should lead to genomic union; and, finally, initiation of the first division and development.

The union of the sperm and egg nuclei during fertilization is poorly understood in primates, including humans, mostly because the deliberate creation of human zygotes and embryos for scientific research is complicated by ethical and moral issues.

The process of fertilization is initiated upon certain modification of the spermatozoa in order to acquire fertilization ability. This requires three steps:

- Capacitation
- Hyperactivation
- Acromosome reaction

Capacitation is a calcium-dependent process that involves activation of adenosine triphosphatase (ATPase) and changes in the properties of the membranes, mainly due to redistribution of mannose receptors, glycolipids and glycoproteins.

The acquisition of hyperactivated motility results in enhanced lateral head displacement, reduced linearity, flagelar curvature and beat frequency.

---

* Tel.: +54-1-4372-8289; fax: +54-11-4371-7275.
  *E-mail address:* sbo@cegyr.com (S. Brugo Olmedo).

The acrosome reaction involves fusion of outer and inner membranes of acrosomal membranes, which results in the externalization of the contents of the acrosomal vesicle.

These contents include hydrolytic enzymes that permit the sperm to penetrate the outer investments of the egg.

The acrosome reaction is accompanied by modifications in the sperm plasma membrane, which exposes receptors for zona binding and possibly factors exposed on the equatorial segment in preparation for sperm–oocyte fusion.

Before hyperactivation, sperm swims in long curvilinear tracks, probably to span the distances within the female reproductive tract.

The spermatozoan binds to the zona pellucida, which contains three sulphated proteins:

- ZP1
- ZP2
- ZP3

with differing molecular weights and regulated by their corresponding genes.

The most important receptor for spermatozoa on the zona pellucida seems to be ZP3, which induces the acrosome reaction.

ZP2 may bind spermatozoa after their acrosome reaction has occurred.

Capacitation and the acrosome reaction last for 2 h and sperm passage through the zona may require another hour. Spermatozoa pass through the zona pellucida into the perivitelline space.

The sperm tail can be seen still beating outside the zona, after it head and midpiece have entered the perivitelline space and the equatorial segment has made an initial contact with the oolema.

From the egg's perspective, the sperm is essential for contributing with three components:

1. The paternal genome
2. The signal to initiate the metabolic activation of the egg
3. The centrosome, which directs microtubule assembly

Oocytes are metabolically quiescent, sperm–egg binding and fusion initiates a cascade of events that transforms the dormant egg, through an elevation in intracellular calcium ion concentration, as the central messenger.

In order to prevent polyspermy, there is a secretion of cortical granules, which prevents this condition by proteolytically digesting the sites for sperm binding and also enzymatically modifying the egg's coat to toughen and harden it.

Fertilization leads to the decondensation and remodeling of the paternal genome.

Following the incorporation of the sperm into the egg and after egg activation, a new motility system assembles within the egg and its organization is directed by the newly introduced sperm centrosome.

Male pronucleus formation occurs simultaneously with the disappearance of the nuclear membrane, decondensation of the chromosomes and reformation of the pronuclear membrane from oocyte endoplasmic reticulum. This coincides with decondensation of the maternal chromatin and the formation of the female pronucleus.

An inability of the centrosome to function normally leads to developmental arrest just before syngamy begins.

The role of microtubules and other structures and the motility of the sperm and egg nuclei within the oocyte is not well know.

A full understanding of the cellular and molecular events during fertilization is critical.

In order to dilucidate different aspects during fertilization and early development, we analyzed "non-fertilized" and "abnormally fertilized" human oocytes after in vitro fertilization (IVF) and intracytoplasmic sperm injection (ICSI).

We focused on the cytoskeletal architecture, chromatin configuration, aster organization and the presence of abortive activations.

We analyzed 815 "non-fertilized" and 153 "abnormally fertilized" oocytes after IVF and ICSI. The material was processed for immunofluorescence to detect $\beta$ tubulins and $\alpha$ acetylated tubulins. DNA was studied using Hoescht. Chromosomal spreads were performed by Tarkowski's air-drying method in 189 IVF and ICSI oocytes.

During fertilization failure, the main reason after IVF procedure was no sperm penetration (59.2%). The remaining oocytes showed different abnormal patterns: oocyte activation failure (10.5%) and defects in pronuclei (PNs) apposition (15.2%).

On the other hand, fertilization failure after ICSI technique was mainly associated to incomplete oocyte activation (36.5%). An 18.5% of the studied oocytes stopped their development at the metaphase of the first mitosis of the pre-embryo. The chromosomal spreads allowed identifying abortive activations, including metaphase III and others.

Immunofluorescence analysis of abnormal fertilization showed that the most frequent abnormal fertilization pattern found after IVF was the presence of three or four PNs (77.4%). On the other hand, the presence of one PN (65.2%) was the main pattern found after ICSI. No differences between both groups were seen in terms of subnuclei development.

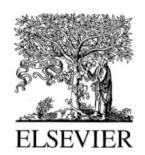

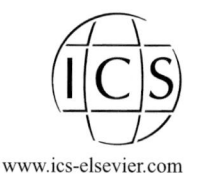

# Apoptosis in testicular germ cells

Dominique Royere*, Fabrice Guérif, Véronique Laurent-Cadoret, Marie-Thérèse Hochereau de Reviers

*Biologie de la Reproduction, UMR 6073 "Physiologie de la Reproduction et des Comportements" Inra/Cnrs/ Université de Tours, Chu Bretonneau 37 044 Tours cedex, France*

**Abstract.** Onset of spermatogenesis is associated with an apoptosis wave that limits its efficiency during the first cycles in most mammals. Beyond the first cycles the actual efficiency of spermatogenesis remains always under the theoretical one. Such physiological apoptosis depends partly upon the relationships between germinal cells and Sertoli cells. Since the steps of spermatogenesis require a continuous progression of the cell cycle rather than any arrest, germ cells might therefore be more sensitive to apoptosis. Moreover, this may lead to severe disturbances between proliferation and cell death. The first experiments designed to understand the mechanisms of germ cell apoptosis were based on hormonal deprivation or cryptorchidism. However, the link between hormonal or cellular action and cell survival remained to be established. The involvement of bcl-2 family genes has been confirmed, whereas the place of Fas/Fas ligand system during the first cycles of spermatogenesis remains a matter of debate. Factors involved in Tumor Necrosis Factor (TNF)/TNF R1 are under study. Among the oncogenes, which may modulate the apoptotic process, Kit/Stem Cell Factor has a peculiar interest, since Kit is expressed in germ cells to some extent and Leydig cells, whereas SCF is expressed in Sertoli cells. Using a transgenic mice model where Kit gene was inactivated by the insertion of a nls-lacZ sequence in its first exon, we showed that one single copy of the gene was unable to sustain at a physiological level both spermatogenesis and fertility in the male mice. Finally, the analysis of the signal transduction pathways involved in testicular apoptosis and their mechanisms of control are key steps in understanding both the impairment of spermatogenesis and the genesis of some germ cell tumours. © 2004 Published by Elsevier B.V.

*Keywords:* Apoptosis; Spermatogenesis; Bcl2; Fas; TNF; Kit; SCF

## 1. Introduction

Spermatogenesis is a highly synchronized dynamic process which involves division and differentiation steps with recovery rates that control its final efficiency. Cell loss was clearly stated for many years; however the concept of apoptosis or programmed cell death more recently substituted to cell degeneration [1,21]. Among germ cells, spermatogonia and spermatocytes are the main targets of apoptosis both in physiological

---

* Corresponding author. Tel.: +33-2-47-47-47-46; fax: +33-2-47-47-84-99.
 *E-mail address:* royere@med.univ-tours.fr (D. Royere).

or extra-physiological conditions (radiations, chemotherapy, and hyperthermia). The aim of this review is to focus on the physiological impact of germ cell apoptosis on the initiation and maintenance of spermatogenesis, using animal models and human data when available.

### 1.1. Hormonal deprivation, experimental cryptorchidism

The first experiments combined hypophysectomy or GnRH antagonists with hormonal supplementation to demonstrate the promoting effect of FSH and testosterone on germ cell survival [6,9,20,38,39]. The dual action of testosterone on germ cell apoptosis, depending both on experimental conditions and spermatogenetic stages, was reported [20,40], while caspase 3 was recently reported to be involved in apoptosis following testosterone deprivation [22]. Experimental cryptorchidism was reported to enhance germ cell apoptosis in some specific stages (XII–XIV, rat [19]) and to involve local factors [37]. However, such an integrative approach needed to be sustained by the analysis of signal transduction pathways of apoptosis that might be active in the testis.

### 1.2. Bcl-2 and spermatogenesis

Among cell death modulators, *Bcl-2* gene family shares some homology with the *CED-9* gene which encodes for the first natural repressor of cell death in *C elegans*. Three distinct subfamilies merged with different impact on cell survival, the *Bcl-2* subfamily that promote cell survival (*Bcl-2, Bcl-x long, Bcl-w, Mcl-1, A1/Bfl1, Nr13*), the *Bax* subfamily (*Bax, Bcl-x short, Bak, Bok*) and the BH3 subfamily which includes proteins with only the conserved BH3 (*Bcl-2* homology) domain (*Bik, Hrk, Bim, Bad, Bid*), both promoting cell apoptosis.

#### 1.2.1. Transgenic mice models misexpressing Bcl-2 genes

The physiological relevance of the apoptotic wave at the onset of spermatogenesis was clearly stated by misexpression of *Bcl-2* [14] or overexpression of *Bcl-Xl* [33] in spermatogonia. An increase in spermatogonia density was first observed in seminiferous tubules while apoptotic cells were rarely observed at day 21. Contrastingly, seminiferous tubules in adult males were partly deleted in germ cells with giant multinucleated cells. Interestingly, such phenotype was also reported in *bax* deficient mice [25,35].

#### 1.2.2. Expression pattern of Bcl-2 proteins in rat testis

During the onset of spermatogenesis, the expression of both anti (bcl-xl and bcl-w) and pro-apoptotic bcl-2 proteins was reported to increase around day 20 [41].

#### 1.2.3. Expression pattern of Bcl-2 proteins in man

Scant data are available in humans. Bcl-x protein was reported to be expressed in spermatogonia, whereas bcl-2 and bak were mainly observed in spermatocytes and spermatids in normal testicular tissue from necro-donors, suggesting some specific function for these proteins during the differentiation and maturation process in human spermatogenesis [29]. More recently an increase in apoptosis in primary spermatocytes was reported in aging men, with a decrease in bcl-xl expression in these cells [23].

## 1.3. TNF family and spermatogenesis

### 1.3.1. Fas, Fas ligand and spermatogenesis

Fas L is a member of a protein family which includes Tumour Necrosis factor (TNF), αlymphotoxine, APO3L, APO2L and TRAIL (TNF-related apoptosis inducing ligand). These proteins bind specific receptors (Fas, TNF-R1, TNF-R2, DR3, DR4, DR5) sharing a common segment with around 80 amino-acids inside their intracytoplasmic region, named Death Domain (DD). Their trimerization allows them to recruit effectors that combine a similar domain (DD) with a Death Effector Domain (DED) that will recruit procaspases. The whole is considered as Death Inducing Signalling Complex (DISC).

*1.3.1.1. Experimental data in murine.* Initially, Fas protein was detected in germ cells, while Fas L was detected in Sertoli cells, with an increase in their expression following Sertoli cell toxicant administration [26]. The physiological impact of Fas–Fas L on spermatogenesis was deduced from their increased expression in rat testis from day 16 to day 32 when an apoptosis wave may be observed [8]. However, conflicting data were reported in rat, where no Fas L mRNA was observed in Sertoli cells from day 10 onwards, whereas it was detected in testis from day 30. In addition, male rats issued from in utero irradiated females were reported to recover their spermatogenesis at day 63, whereas Fas L was only detected at this date [10]. Spermatocytes and round spermatids expressed Fas L at the mRNA level, while only elongated spermatids and spermatozoa expressed Fas L at the protein level. Such results did not support a physiological role for Fas–Fas L at onset of spermatogenesis, whereas they did not exclude some immunoprotective role in female genital tract [32].

*1.3.1.2. In vitro and in vivo human data.* Segments of seminiferous tubules from testicular biopsies were reported to have a drastic increase in germ cell apoptosis during in vitro culture without serum or hormones [30]. Such event might be prevented by the addition of an anti-Fas L antibody or a caspase inhibitor. Fas and Fas L were reported to be expressed at the mRNA level in human adult testis, not in foetal testis. Another report focused on the increased number of germ cells expressing the Fas protein when spermatogenesis was arrested at the post-meiotic level [13].

### 1.3.2. TNF, TRAIL and spermatogenesis

Similarities between Fas and TNF were previously underlined about trimerization and death domains. Although the recruited proteins may differ between both systems (TNFR associated death domain protein=TRADD; Fas associated death domain protein=FADD) the signal transduction lead to procaspase 8 activation. Contrastingly, TNF may mobilize an alternate anti-apoptotic signal transduction pathway that involves another protein (TNFR associated factor 2) able to recruit RIP (Receptor Interacting Protein) then activate NF-κB signalling to initiate the transcription of inhibitors of apoptosis (cIAP 1 et 2=cellular inhibitor of apoptosis). Thus, depending on the situation and the cell compartment, TNF may behave as a pro-or anti-apoptotic factor.

*1.3.2.1. Experimental data in rats.* Ontogenesis of TRAIL and its receptors was studied in rats. TRAIL was detected both at the mRNA and protein level in foetal and adult testis, within Leydig and germ cells. Additionally, type 1 receptors were observed in Leydig cells (DR5) and post-meiotic germ cells (DR4), whereas other expressed receptors were incomplete or decoy receptors [16]. Such results do not support a physiological role for TRAIL in spermatogonia apoptosis while it might influence later stages.

*1.3.2.2. In vitro human data.* Type 1 TNF receptors were detected in Sertoli and Leydig cells on adult human testis biopsies. Conversely, TNF was detected in germ cells (pachytene spermatocytes and round spermatids). During in vitro culture of segments of seminiferous tubules, addition of TNFα dose dependently inhibited germ cell apoptosis induced by hormonal or serum deprivation [31]. A partial decrease in Fas L expression was concomitantly observed, suggesting a possible involvement of TNFα in germ cell apoptosis via the control of Fas L expression.

## 1.4. P53 and spermatogenesis

Most data were reported in murine. P53 was first reported to be expressed and to promote apoptosis in primordial germ cells [27], type A1 spermatogonia [5] and primary spermatocytes [42]. Several lines of evidence support a physiological role for p53 in spermatogenesis. On one side, its expression was reported to increase in the first 4 weeks of life in mice [34] while p53 k.o. mice exhibited a doubling of undifferentiated spermatogonia compared with wild type mice [5]. On the other side, over-expression of p53 in post-meiotic cells was reported to generate a phenotype varying from a normal fertility to a severely altered spermatogenesis, depending on the level of over-expression [2], suggesting some dose-effect of this oncogene on spermatogenesis.

All the data presented here support the concept of density dependent regulation of germ cell population that was proposed in the early eighties to further underline the importance of an equilibrated ratio between somatic (Sertoli) and germinal component in the testis to ensure an efficient spermatogenesis [11]. This "germ cell homeostasis" will involve factors promoting germ cell apoptosis (Fas, TRAIL, TNFα, Bcl-2, p53) and factors promoting cell survival (Bcl-2, TNFα and Kit/SCF).

## 1.5. Kit/SCF and spermatogenesis

The impact of Kit/Stem Cell Factor (SCF=Kit ligand) on spermatogenesis was deduced from several data. Kit was reported to be expressed in germ cells and Leydig cells, while its ligand SCF was expressed in Sertoli cells. Natural mutations of the genes encoding these two proteins (White Spotting for Kit, Steel for SCF) are most often characterized by a common phenotype with a defect in migration and survival of primordial germ cells. Additionally Kit/SCF was reported to promote the survival of differentiated spermatogonia, while a truncated form might play some role in post-meiotic germ cells.

*1.5.1. Data on structure, expression and function of Kit/SCF*
*Kit* gene, corresponding to W locus, is situated on chromosome 4 in human (4q12), 5 in mouse and includes 21 exons. Three different mRNA result from transcription

depending on which promoter (main or alternative located in the 16th intron) is controlled. Among the resulting proteins, the longer one (140–160 kDa) is a member of tyrosine kinase receptors family, while the truncated one (tr-Kit, 24–30 kDa) is restricted to the second catalytic domain with phosphotransferase activity and the cytoplasmic end of the receptor [36].

SCF gene, corresponding to Steel locus, is located on chromosome 12 in human, 10 in mouse and includes nine exons. mRNA result form alternative splicing including exon 6 or not. Two transmembranal proteins are translated, the longer one (45 kDa) with a site for proteolytic cleavage allowing delivery in a soluble form, while the shorter one (32 kDa) does not [3], depending on age, development and FSH environment.

Kit was reported to promote both migration and survival of primordial germ cells [15]. Kit was also reported to be expressed in differentiated spermatogonia where it promotes their proliferation [28]. Additionally, the truncated form (tr-Kit) might be involved in oocyte activation following the fertilization [36]. Contrastingly, few data are available in human, since piebaldism which is characterized by a partial forehead depigmentation is the sole reported phenotype of loss of function kit mutations without any alteration in haematopoiesis or germ line [12].

### 1.5.2. Experimental data on gonadal functions of Kit/SCF in kit haplodeficient mice

In this study, we addressed the consequences of kit haplodeficiency on gonadal development and spermatogenesis in mice. By using transgenic mice resulting from nls-lacZ insertion in the first exon of kit gene [4], phenotypic analysis was combined with the follow-up of reporter gene expression under the control of Kit main promoter with inbred wild mice as controls.

$Kit^{+/+}$ and $Kit^{WlacZ/+}$ mice shared some similar characteristics such as weight, behaviour, undifferentiated spermatogonia density, meiosis recovery and spermiogenesis recovery [17]. However, an increase in apoptosis was observed in differentiated spermatogonia while transition from type A to type B spermatogonia was severely impaired in $Kit^{WlacZ/+}$ mice. This led to a decrease in sperm production with subfertility. This unusual "dose-effect" of Kit deficiency was enriched by two original observations. First, reporter gene expression was observed at two distinct stages of spermatogenesis, differentiated spermatogonia and late pachytene/diplotene spermatocytes, without any expression in between. Then male subfertility was confirmed both in vivo and in vitro, the latter with the same number of motile sperm inseminated. Altered motility and acrosomal reaction might suggest a possible role of Kit at the post-meiotic level, since the expression of the truncated form was not altered in our model [18].

Thus Kit/SCF seemed to have some pleiotropic effect on the gonad, since their expression will vary all along the gonadal development. Particularly, Kit expression is discontinuing, whereas signal transduction pathways may differ. For instance, PI3K pathway was reported to mediate Kit effect on differentiated spermatogonia proliferation [7,24] but not the promoting effect of kit on their survival. Additionally, during meiosis Kit expression was not relied on to any effect for proliferation or survival. Taken together these data suggest various control of gene expression as well as various signalling pathways depending on the development stage for kit/SCF system as part of the dialog between Sertoli cells and germ cells.

## 2. Conclusion

Thus apoptosis was shown to play a major role in onset and maintenance of spermatogenesis. This will lead to maintenance of a germ cell to Sertoli cell ratio between limits allowing spermatogenesis to go on. Any alteration (decrease or increase) will be followed by a severe impairment in gamete production. Although this brief review was limited to onset and maintenance of spermatogenesis, many data support a role for apoptosis as an answer to "germ cell homeostasis" disruption, whatever the factors, either endogenous factors like cell cycle defects, DNA damage, lack of growth factors, hormones or exogenous factors like ionizing radiations, chemotherapy, or endocrine disruptors. Although its impact in pathological processes, from infertility to tumour genesis, is highly probable, apoptosis in human testis need further studies.

## References

[1] D.J. Allan, B.V. Harmont, S.A. Roberts, Spermatogonial apoptosis has three morphologically recognizable phases and shows no circadian rhythm during normal spermatogenesis in the rat, Cell Prolif. 25 (1992) 241–250.
[2] I. Allemand, et al., Testicular wild-type p53 expression in transgenic mice induces spermiogenesis alterations ranging from differentiation defects to apoptosis, Oncogene 18 (1999) 6521–6530.
[3] L.K. Ashman, The biology of stem cell factor and its receptor C-kit, Int. J. Biochem. Cell Biol. 31 (1999) 1037–1051.
[4] F. Bernex, et al., Spatial and temporal patterns of c-kit-expressing cells in $W^{lacZ/+}$ and $W^{lacZ}/W^{lacZ}$ mouse embryos, Development 122 (1996) 3023–3033.
[5] T.L. Beumer, et al., The role of the tumour suppressor p53 in spermatogenesis, Cell Death Differ. 5 (1998) 669–678.
[6] H. Billig, et al., Apoptosis in testis germ cells: developmental changes in gonadotropin dependence and localization to selective tubule stages, Endocrinology 136 (1995) 5–12.
[7] P. Blume-Jensen, et al., Kit/stem cell factor receptor-induced activation of phosphatidylinositol 3′-kinase is essential for male fertility, Nat. Genet. 24 (2000) 157–162.
[8] K. Boekelheide, et al., Expression of Fas system-related genes in the testis during development after toxicant exposure, Toxicol. Lett. 102–103 (1998) 503–508.
[9] M.H. Brinkworth, et al., Identification of male germ cells undergoing apoptosis in adult rats, J. Reprod. Fertil. 105 (1995) 25–33.
[10] A. D'Alessio, et al., Testicular Fas L is expressed by sperm cells, PNAS 98 (2001) 3316–3321.
[11] D.G. De Rooij, A. Grootegoed, Spermatogonial stem cells, Curr. Opin. Cell Biol. 10 (1998) 694–701.
[12] R.A. Fleischman, Human piebald trait resulting form a dominant negative mutant allele of the c-kit membrane receptor gene, J. Clin. Invest. 89 (1992) 1713–1717.
[13] S. Francavilla, et al., Fas and Fas ligand expression in foetal and adult human testis with normal or deranged spermatogenesis, J. Clin. Endocrinol. Metab. 85 (2000) 2692–2700.
[14] T. Furuchi, et al., Inhibition of testicular germ cell apoptosis and differentiation in mice misexpressing Bcl-2 in spermatogonia, Development 122 (1996) 1703–1709.
[15] I. Godin, et al., Effects of the steel gene product on mouse primordial germ cells in culture, Nature 352 (1991) 807–809.
[16] R. Grataroli, et al., Expression of tumor necrosis factor-α-related apoptosis inducing ligand and its receptors in rat testis during development, Biol. Reprod. 66 (2002) 1707–1715.
[17] F. Guerif, et al., Apoptosis, onset and maintenance of spermatogenesis: evidence for the involvement of Kit in Kit-haplodeficient mice, Biol. Reprod. 67 (2002) 70–79.
[18] F. Guerif, et al., Characterization of the fertility of Kit-haplodeficient male mice, Int. J. Androl. 25 (2002) 358–368.
[19] K. Henriksen, H. Hakovirta, M. Parvinen, In-situ quantification of stage-specific apoptosis in the rat

seminiferous epithelium: effects of short-term experimental cryptorchidism, Int. J. Androl. 18 (1995) 256–262.
[20] K. Henriksen, et al., In vitro, follicle-stimulating hormone prevents apoptosis and stimulates deoxyribonucleic acid synthesis in the rat seminiferous epithelium in a stage-specific fashion, Endocrinology 137 (1996) 2141–2149.
[21] J.F. Kerr, A.H. Wyllie, A.R. Currie, Apoptosis: a basic biological phenomenon with wide-ranging implications in tissue kinetics, Br. J. Cancer 26 (1972) 239–257.
[22] J.M. Kim, et al., Caspase-3 and caspase-activated deoxyribonuclease are associated with testicular germ cell apoptosis resulting from reduced intratesticular testosterone, Endocrinology 142 (2001) 3809–3916.
[23] M. Kimura, et al., Balance of apoptosis and proliferation of germ cells related to spermatogenesis an aged men, J. Androl. 24 (2003) 185–191.
[24] H. Kissel, et al., Point mutation in kit receptor tyrosine kinase reveals essential roles for kit signalling in spermatogenesis and oogenesis without affecting other kit responses, EMBO J. 19 (2000) 1312–1326.
[25] C.M. Knudson, et al., Bax-deficient mice with lymphoid hyperplasia and male germ cell death, Science 270 (1995) 96–99.
[26] J. Lee, et al., Fas system, a regulator of testicular germ cell apoptosis, is differentially up-regulated in sertoli cell versus germ cell injury of the testis, Endocrinology 140 (1999) 852–858.
[27] Y. Matsui, R. Nagano, M. Obinata, Apoptosis of fetal testicular cells is regulated by both p53-dependent and independent mechanisms, Mol. Reprod. Dev. 55 (2000) 399–405.
[28] H. Ohta, et al., Regulation of proliferation and differentiation in spermatogonial stem cells: the role of c-kit and its ligand SCF, Development 127 (2000) 2125–2131.
[29] N.B. Oldereid, et al., Expression of Bcl-2 family proteins and spontaneous apoptosis in normal human testis, Mol. Hum. Reprod. 7 (2000) 403–408.
[30] V. Pentikäinen, K. Erkkilä, L. Dunkel, Fas regulates germ cell apoptosis in the human testis in vitro, Am. J. Physiol. 276 (1999) E310–E316. Endocrinol. Metab. 39.
[31] V. Pentikäinen, et al., TNFα down regulates the Fas ligand and inhibits germ cell apoptosis in the human testis, J. Clin. Endocrinol. Metab. 86 (2001) 4480–4488.
[32] A. Riccioli, et al., The Fas system in the seminiferous epithelium and its possible extra-testicular role, Andrologia 35 (2003) 64–70.
[33] I. Rodriguez, et al., An early and massive wave of germinal cell apoptosis is required for the development of functional spermatogenesis, EMBO J. 16 (1997) 2262–2270.
[34] P. Rossi, et al., Role of c-kit in mammalian spermatogenesis, J. Endocrinol. Invest. 23 (2000) 609–615.
[35] L.D. Russell, et al., Bax dependent spermatogonia apoptosis is required for testicular development and spermatogenesis, Biol. Reprod. 66 (2002) 950–958.
[36] C. Sette, et al., Tr-kit induced resumption of the cell cycle in mouse eggs requires activation of a Src-like kinase, EMBO J. 21 (2002) 5386–5395.
[37] T. Shikone, H. Billig, A.J.W. Hsueh, Experimentally induced cryptorchidism increases apoptosis in rat testis, Biol. Reprod. 51 (1994) 865–872.
[38] A.P. Sinha Hikim, et al., Involvement of apoptosis in the induction of germ cell degeneration in adult rats after gonadotropin releasing hormone antagonist treatment, Endocrinology 136 (1995) 2770–2775.
[39] J.S. Tapanainen, et al., Hormonal control of apoptotic cell death in the testis: gonadotropins and androgens as testicular cell survival factors, Mol. Cell. Endocrinol. 7 (1993) 643–650.
[40] L. Troiano, et al., Apoptosis and spermatogenesis: evidence from an in vivo model of testosterone withdrawal in the adult rat, Biochem. Biophys. Res. Commun. 202 (1994) 1315–1321.
[41] W. Yan, et al., Bcl-w forms complexes with Bax and Bak, and elevated ratios of Bax/Bcl-w and Bak/Bcl-w correspond to spermatogonial and spermatocyte apoptosis in the testis, Mol. Cell. Endocrinol. 14 (2000) 682–699.
[42] Y. Yin, et al., P53-mediated germ cell quality control in spermatogenesis, Dev. Biol. 204 (1998) 165–171.

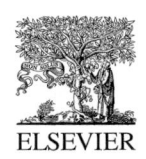

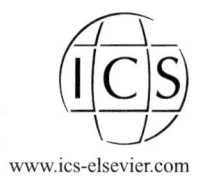

# Implantation and uterine receptivity

José A. Horcajadas[a], Francisco Domínguez[a],
Julio Martín[a], Antonio Pellicer[a,b,*], Carlos Simón[a,b,*]

[a] IVI Foundation, C/ Guadassuar, 1, 46015 Valencia, Spain
[b] Department of Pediatrics, Obstetrics and Gynecology, Faculty of Medicine, Valencia University,
Av. Blasco Ibáñez 17, 46010 Valencia, Spain

**Abstract.** The knowledge of the gene expression profile of the endometrium during the window of implantation is fundamental for the understanding of human reproduction. The genomics approach allows us now to investigate the hierarchical contribution of a high number of genes to a specific function in a metabolic or pathologic situation. In this work, we have compared gene expression profiles of prereceptive (day LH+2) with receptive (LH+7) endometrium in well-characterized human endometrial biopsies of five women, and we have compared our results with similar works published in the literature. Although all the studies have used the Affymetrix HG-95A array, the differences in the approaches have generated different results. Collectively, these studies identify new candidate markers that may be used to diagnose unequivocally the receptive endometrium.
© 2004 Published by Elsevier B.V.

*Keywords:* Endometrial receptivity; Gene expression profile; Microarray

## 1. Introduction

The human endometrium is a complex tissue and its cyclic regulation requires the successful interaction of hundreds of factors. The endometrial receptivity is a self-limited period, in which the endometrial epithelium acquires a functional and transient ovarian steroid-dependent status that allows blastocyst adhesion [1]. The scientific knowledge of the endometrial receptivity process is fundamental for the understanding of the mechanisms that govern embryonic implantation and human reproduction [2]. This important knowledge can potentially be used to improve fertility in infertile women, whereas the opposite can be applied as an interceptive approach to prevent embryo implantation [3].

Normal human endometrium is controlled by the ovarian sex steroid hormones, estrogen and progesterone. The steroid hormones elicit their actions by binding to specific high-affinity receptors. These act as ligand-dependent transcription factors [4], modulating the transcription of a large amount of proteins. The action of these hormones produces a

---

\* Corresponding authors. Department of Pediatrics, Obstetrics and Gynecology Research Division, Valencia University, C/ Guadassuar, 1, 46015 Valencia, Spain. Tel.: +34-96-345-55-60; fax: +34-96-345-55-12.
*E-mail address:* csimon@interbook.net (A. Pellicer).

0531-5131/ © 2004 Published by Elsevier B.V.
doi:10.1016/j.ics.2004.01.063

period of receptivity between 7 and 9 days postovulation during the midsecretory or midluteal phase [5]. In response to ovarian steroids, characteristic morphological changes occur in the endometrium, and these are responses routinely used to stage the human endometrium [6]. These changes include modifications in plasma membrane [7] and cytoskeleton [8,9]. The apical plasma membrane develops transitional adhesive properties by undergoing structural changes; long, thin, regular microvilli are gradually converted in irregular, flattened projections and this process is named plasma membrane transformation [7].

But the best markers of a true receptive state would be those molecules directly involved in the initial stages of the implantation process; however, functional testing of these marker molecules would need to be done, an impractical approach in humans. Until now, in most cases, the identification of these markers has been the result of careful examination of the expression of particular proteins or mRNAs, based on preconceived ideas or results obtained in animal models. The recent advent of high throughput microarray screening for the expression of human genes has allowed an unevaluated approach toward identifying changes in global gene expression in a concrete physiological or pathological situation [10]. This technology has made it possible to study the endometrial receptivity process from a global genomic perspective [11–14]. In this study, we show the results obtained comparing the mRNA expression profile of five women at LH+2 with LH+7, i.e., 2 and 7 days, respectively, after the LH surge [14]. We also show the comparison between our results and the results of other similar works published previously [11–13].

## 2. Results and discussion

### 2.1. Data analysis

Samples were taken from the same women on LH+2 and LH+7 of consecutive cycles, frozen at $-70$ °C and stored until further processing. After RNA extraction, the probe was performed as described [15]. The microarray chosen for this study was the Affimetrix HG-U95A that contains more than 12,000 human genes. Only those genes that had a ratio of at least threefold between LH+7 and LH+2 were considered regulated. And only those genes that appear in at least four out five women were selected. Using these criteria, we identified 211 regulated genes; 153 of these genes were specifically upregulated on LH+7 and 58 downregulated.

In the complete lists of regulated genes, we identified genes that were already known to be differentially expressed during the receptive phase, compared with the prereceptive phase such as glycodelin (107 foldup), osteopontin (11 foldup), IGF-BP-3 (5.4 foldup), crystallin alphaB (4.4 foldup) and integrin, alpha 3 (4.3 foldup). However, we also identified a number of genes for which the differential expression between the prereceptive (LH+2) and the receptive (LH+7) endometria or even the presence in human endometrium has not been described before. These genes can be classified into different groups such as immune modulatory genes, adhesion molecules, genes related to oxidative stress, cytoskeletal proteins, and others (see complete tables of regulated genes in Riesewijk et al. [14]).

## 2.2. Validation studies

Some of these genes, three upregulated (glutation peroxidase-3, claudin-4 and solute carrier 1 A1) and one downregulated (alpha catenin), were selected for the validation studies. These studies were carried out by Quantitative PCR (Q-PCR). The system used was the ABI PRISM™ 7700 Sequence Detection System from Applied Biosystems, Foster City, CA. The average values obtained for LH+2 and LH+7 by this technique were in accordance with the regulation observed in the five studied women by microarray for the four selected genes. However, patient-to-patient variation was observed, probably due to the differences in the cell populations present in the different biopsies.

## 2.3. Menstrual cycle studies

The three selected upregulated genes were studied throughout the menstrual cycle. All of them were shown to be regulated, increasing their expression at the beginning of the midsecretory phase. It is remarkable that claudin-4 declines in the last phase of the cycle, while the other two genes have a sharp increase in the late luteal phase [14].

## 2.4. In situ hybridization

Localization of the mRNA of glutathione peroxidase 3 and SLC1A1 was carried out by in situ hybridization in natural menstrual cycles, labeling the sense and antisense probes with digoxigenin (DIG). With this type of experiment, it is possible to detect in which compartment of the tissue the increase or decrease of mRNA takes place. We observed that, in the case of glutathione peroxidase 3, the increase in the mRNA expression occurred in glandular and luminal epithelium during the secretory phase, consistent with the pattern observed in the Q-PCR analysis [14]. The results for SLC1A1 were also consistent with the Q-PCR data.

## 2.5. Comparative studies

Microarray technology is one of the most recent and recognized tools in research nowadays. There are many different types of arrays available, depending on the needs of the researchers and the topic being studied.

This technique has erupted so suddenly in the scientific world that some requirements remain unclear, such as the minimum number of arrays necessary for solid data, the best way for validating the array's data, or the correct cut-off for considering that a gene is regulated.

In a short period of time, four works focusing on endometrial gene expression profile during receptivity have been published: Carson et al. [11], Kao et al. [12], Borthwick et al. [13] and our own work, Riesewijk et al. [14]. All of them used the same technology and, even more, the same array of the same company. However, some variations in the experimental design and data analysis make the studies different. Table 1 summarizes the main differences among these four works.

The menstrual day for sample collection, pooling or not of the RNA isolated, and the number of samples used in the study are the main differences among the four approaches. Furthermore, the cut-off used for considering a gene to be regulated is different. Three of

Table 1

| Study | Samples | RNA pooled | First sample | Second sample | Fold change | Up | Down | Microarray |
|---|---|---|---|---|---|---|---|---|
| Kao | 11 | NO | Proliferative phase (8–10) | LH+(8–10) | >2.0 | 156 | 377 | AFFIMETRIX HG-U95A |
| Carson | 6 | YES | LH+(2–4) | LH+(7–9) | >2.0 | 323 | 370 | AFFIMETRIX HG-U95A |
| Borthwick | 10 | YES | Proliferative phase (9–11) | LH+(6–8) | >2.0 | 90 | 46 | AFFIMETRIX HG-U95A-E |
| Riesewijk | 10 | NO | LH+2 | LH+7 | >3.0 | 153 | 58 | AFFIMETRIX HG-U95A |

them [11–13] established a minimal fold increase of 2.0 as evidence of gene regulation. Only Riesewijk et al. [14] used a threefold increase. It is important to remark that, in that latter work, the samples used came from the same woman at two different stages of the menstrual cycle. The differences in study design are reflected in the lists of differentially expressed genes identified.

We have compared the results all together, just considering those genes upregulated or downregulated in the receptive phase with a fold change of >3.0. Only one downregulated gene is present in all four studies, the *olfactomedin*, a tissue-specific secreted glycoprotein involved in the maintenance, growth, or differentiation of chemosensory cilia on the apical dendrites of olfactory neurons [16]. In the lists of upregulated genes, three of them appeared in all four works: *osteopontin* [17], *apoliprotein D* [18], and *Dickkopf*. It is interesting to note the presence of the latter protein in all the works. Dickkopf-1 belongs to the human Dickkopf gene family [19] and is an inhibitor of Wnt signaling; it is known that Wnt7A (−/−) null mice are infertile [20]. The role of the Wnt family in human endometrium and implantation has to be considered in future investigations and, recently, the identification, characterization, and regulation of the canonical Wnt signaling pathway in human endometrium have been published [21]. In addition, it is remarkable that glycodelin (also

Table 2

| Accesion number (function) | Gene name | Riesewijk | Kao | Carson | Borthwick |
|---|---|---|---|---|---|
| *Upregulated genes present in the four works* | | | | | |
| AF052124 (Structural protein) | Osteopontin | ✓ | ✓ | ✓ | ✓ |
| J02611 (Trasporter) | Apolipoprotein D | ✓ | ✓ | ✓ | ✓ |
| AB020315 (Signalling) | Dickkopf/DKK1 (hdkk-1) | ✓ | ✓ | ✓ | ✓ |
| *Upregulated genes present in Riesewijk's works and in two out of the other three works* | | | | | |
| J04129 (Secretary protein) | Placental protein-14/Glycodelin | ✓ | ✓ | | ✓ |
| M31516 (Immunomodulator) | Decay accelerating factor for complement (CD55, Cromer blood group system) | ✓ | ✓ | | ✓ |
| M84526 (Complement protein) | Adipsin/complement factor D | ✓ | ✓ | | ✓ |
| M55543 (GTP-Binding protein) | Guarrylate binding protein 2, interferon-inducible | ✓ | | ✓ | ✓ |
| AB000712 (Receptor) | Claudin 4/CEP-R | ✓ | ✓ | ✓ | |
| AA420624 (Signalling) | Monoamine oxidase A (MAOA) | ✓ | ✓ | | ✓ |
| M60974 (Regulatory protein) | Growth arrest and DNA-damage-inducible protein (gadd45) | ✓ | ✓ | | ✓ |
| AB002365 (Cell death factor) | Nip2 | ✓ | | ✓ | ✓ |
| Total genes analyzed (>3.0) | | 153 | 60 | 120 | 85 |
| *Downregulated genes present in the four works* | | | | | |
| U79299 (Secretory protein) | Olfactomedin-related ER localized protein | ✓ | ✓ | ✓ | ✓ |
| Total genes analyzed (>3.0) | | 58 | 87 | 153 | 40 |

called placental protein 14) [22], a secreted protein, was the most upregulated gene in two of the four works, appearing in three of the four works. The complete comparison of these studies is represented in Table 2. We have also included those genes that appeared in our work and in two of the other three works (eight genes in total).

Recently, another work has been published on endometrial receptivity. Domínguez et al. [23] compared the gene expression pattern in receptive with prereceptive human endometria, and contrasted the results with gene expression in the highly adhesive cell line RL95-2 vs. HEC-1A, a cell line with markedly less adhesiveness. They used a macroarray containing 375 human cytokines, chemokines, and related factors and they found a new gene implicated in human endometrial receptivity, the Insulin-Like Growth Factor-Binding Protein Related 1 (IGFBP-rP1) [17]. This last publication reveals that a predesigned strategy for getting useful results does not exist in genomics. All the data of the five works that have published wide genomic analysis [11–14,17] offer the opportunity to develop an endometrial database of genes expressed during the window of implantation.

We consider that all the published data are complementary, due not only to differences in study design, but also to differences in the software and statistics used for analysis of the hybridization data. All together, these results contribute to provide an insight into the complexity of endometrial receptivity and the large number of known and unknown factors involved in achieving a successful embryo implantation.

## References

[1] A. Psychoyos, Endocrine control of egg implantation, in: R.O. Greep, E.B Astwood (Eds.), Handbook of Physiology, Section 7, Endocrinology, vol. II (pt. II), American Physiological Society, Washington, DC, 1973, pp. 187–215.
[2] K. Yoshinaga, Maternal and fetal endocrinology, in: D. Tulchinsky, A.B. Little (Eds.), Maternal–fetal Endocrinology, Saunders, Philadelphia, 1994, pp. 336–349.
[3] C. Simón, Potential molecular mechanisms for the contraceptive control of implantation, Mol. Hum. Reprod. 2 (1996) 475–480.
[4] B.M. O'Malley, M.J. Tsai, Molecular pathways of steroid receptor action, Biol. Reprod. 2 (1992) 163–167.
[5] A.J. Wilcox, D.D. Baird, C.R. Weinberg, Time of implantation of the conceptus and loss of pregnancy, N. Engl. J. Med. 340 (1999) 1796–1799.
[6] R.N. Noyes, A.T. Hertig, J. Rock, Dating the endometrial biopsy, Fertil. Steril. 1 (1950) 3–25.
[7] C.R. Murphy, The plasma membrane transformation of uterine epithelial cells during pregnancy, J. Reprod. Fertil. Suppl. 55 (2000) 23–28.
[8] M. Thie, et al., Cell adhesion to the apical pole of epithelium: a function of cell polarity, Eur. J. Cell Biol. 66 (1995) 180–191.
[9] J.C. Martín, et al., Increased adhesiveness in cultured endometrial-derived cells is related to the absence of moesin expression, Biol. Reprod. 63 (2000) 1370–1376.
[10] M. Schena, et al., Quantitative monitoring of gene expression patterns with a complementary DNA microarray, Science 270 (1995) 467–470.
[11] D.D. Carson, et al., Changes in gene expression during the early to mid-luteal (receptive phase) transition in human endometrium detected by high-density microarray screening, Mol. Hum. Reprod. 8 (2002) 879–971.
[12] L.C. Kao, et al., Global gene profiling in human endometrium during the window of implantation, Endocrinology 143 (2002) 2119–2138.
[13] J.M. Borthwick, et al., Determination of the transcript profile of human endometrium, Mol. Hum. Reprod. 9 (2003) 19–33.
[14] A. Riesewijk, et al., Gene expression profiling of human endometrial receptivity on days LH+2 versus LH+7 by microarray technology, Mol. Hum. Reprod. 9 (2003) 253–264.

[15] D. Tackels-Horne, et al., Identification of differentially expressed genes in hepatocellular carcinoma and metastatic liver tumors by oligonucleotide expression profiling, Cancer 92 (2001) 395–405.
[16] H. Yokoe, R.R.H. Anholt, Molecular cloning of olfactomedin, an extracellular matrix protein specific to olfactory neuroepithelium, Proc. Natl. Acad. Sci. U. S. A. 90 (1993) 4655–4659.
[17] K.B. Apparao, et al., Osteopontin and its receptor alphavbeta3 integrin are coexpressed in the human endometrium during the menstrual cycle but regulated differentially, J. Clin. Endocrinol. Metab. 86 (2001) 4991–5000.
[18] D. Drayna, et al., Cloning and expression of human apolipoprotein D cDNA, J. Biol. Chem. 261 (1986) 16535–16539.
[19] E. Krupnik, et al., Functional and structural diversity of the human Dickkopf gene family, Gene, (1999) 301–313.
[20] A. Miller, A. Pabloba, D.A. Sassoon, Differential expression patterns of Wnt genes in the murine female reproductive tract during development and the estrous cycle, Mech. Dev. 76 (1998) 91–99.
[21] S. Tulac, et al., Identification, characterization, and regulation of the canonical Wnt signalling pathway in human endometrium, J. Clin. Endocrinol. Metab. 88 (2003) 3860–3866.
[22] M. Julkunen, et al., Secretory endometrium synthetizes placental protein 14, Endocrinology 118 (1986) 1782–1786.
[23] F. Domínguez, et al., A combined approach for gene discovery identifies insulin-like growth factor-binding protein-related protein 1 as a new gene implicated in human endometrial receptivity, J. Clin. Endocrinol. Metab. 88 (2003) 1849–1857.

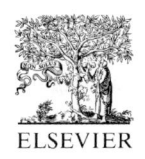

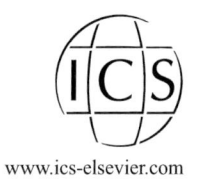

# Fibroids: basic science and etiology

Shingo Fujii*, Ayako Suzuki, Noriomi Matsumura,
Takanobu Kanamori, Hiroaki Shime, Ken Fukuhara,
Kenji Takakura, Masatoshi Kariya

*Department of Gynecology and Obstetrics, Faculty of Medicine, Kyoto University, Sakyoku,
Kyoto 606-8507, Japan*

**Abstract.** Uterine leiomyomas, commonly called fibroids, are the most common smooth muscle tumor in women. However, the etiology of leiomyomas remains largely unknown. Leiomyomas have been considered to grow under the influence of ovarian steroids, such as estrogen and progesterone. However, leiomyomas show more increased cell proliferation than the myometrium with abnormalities of factors such as cytokines, growth factors, and cell cycle regulatory factors. As the intermediate elements, cytokines and growth factors regulated by the ovarian steroids are now considered to exert their growth-stimulatory effects on leiomyomas. Leiomyomas are also characterized by increased cell proliferation and tissue fibrosis. Recently, it has been proposed that smooth muscle cells respond to injury or ischemia with increased cell proliferation and production of extracellular matrix that are critical for the pathogenesis of uterine leiomyomas. We speculate that myometrial contraction for cessation of menstrual bleeding could induce ischemic injury or ischemic–reperfusion injury to the myometrial smooth muscle cells that are proliferating during the luteal phase of the menstrual cycle. These cells could be candidates for progenitor cells of leiomyomas. If this is the case, repetition of the menstrual cycle itself is important for the pathogenesis of uterine leiomyomas. © 2004 Published by Elsevier B.V.

*Keywords:* Leiomyoma; Fibroid; Cytokine; Growth factor; Histogenesis

## 1. Introduction

Uterine leiomyomas, commonly called fibroids, are the most common tumor in women, with a reported incidence of 20–25% [1,2]. The tumors are defined as benign, solid tumors composed of smooth muscle cells with variable amounts of fibrous tissue and collagen matrix [3]. Leiomyomas are clinically important because they are associated with a number of reproductive problems, such as infertility, pregnancy loss, and menorrhagia, and are the primary cause of hysterectomy [1]. However, the etiology of leiomyomas remains largely unknown.

---

\* Corresponding author. Tel.: +81-75-751-3267; fax: +81-75-751-3247.
  *E-mail address:* sfu@kuhp.kyoto-u.ac.jp (S. Fujii).

In recent years, a large number of studies have appeared in the literature examining the basic biology of leiomyomas. This brief review begins with an overview of recent basic studies that describe the growth activity and pathogenesis of uterine leiomyomas. The review then discusses the histogenesis of uterine leiomyoma through the analyses of the unusual clinical entity, leiomyomatosis peritonealis disseminata (LPD) [4–6], the development of smooth muscle in the human fetal uterus [7–9], and the proliferative mechanism of myometrial smooth muscle during the reproductive period [10–12], because the progenitors of leiomyomas have not been clearly identified.

## 2. Basic biology of uterine leiomyoma

### 2.1. Neoplastic characteristics

Leiomyomas are true neoplasms, as detected by X-linked glucose-6-phosphate dehydrogenase (G6PD) isoenzyme analysis [13] and by androgen receptor gene analysis [14], which have shown they are clonal population of cells. Approximately 40% of leiomyomas have been reported to have nonrandom chromosomal abnormalities [15]. However, it is important to note that the majority (60%) of leiomyomas are chromosomally normal. This finding suggests that cytogenetic abnormalities are secondary changes in tumorigenesis, and that a primary genetic change may be responsible for tumor growth in genetically susceptible cells [15].

### 2.2. Growth-promoting factors

Clinical observations of the development of uterine leiomyomas usually after menarche, their enlargement and growth during pregnancy, and their remarkable shrinkage in menopause and in the pseudo-menopause state created by the use of gonadotrophin-releasing hormone analogue (GnRH-a) treatment [16] have suggested that the growth of leiomyomas depends on ovarian steroids, such as estrogen and progesterone [10,11]. Indeed, leiomyomas have significantly increased levels of both estrogen and progesterone receptors, compared with normal myometrium [11,17,18]. Moreover, in situ synthesis of estrogen by the enzyme aromatase P450 is suggested to promote cell growth of uterine leiomyoma [19]. However, the intermediate elements, such as cytokines and growth factors, which may be regulated by the ovarian steroids may be exerting their growth-stimulatory effects on leiomyomas [20,21].

A number of cytokines and growth factors have been investigated in leiomyomas to determine which cytokine(s)/growth factor(s) may be responsible for mediating the growth-promoting effects of ovarian hormones. Recently, Sozen and Arici [21] reviewed the literature and found that transforming growth factor β (TGF-β), insulin-like growth factor-1 (IGF-1), prolactin, basic fibroblast growth factor (bFGF), platelet-derived growth factor (PDGF), human chorionic gonadotrophin (hCG) [22], and interleukin-8 (IL-8) are either over-expressed in leiomyomas, compared with myometrium, or their receptors have been identified in leiomyoma, or both. In addition, they are reported to have mitogenic action [21].

Recently, we found that redox factor 1 (Ref-1), a DNA repair enzyme and redox-modifying factor, is associated with the growth regulation of leiomyomas. We detected two forms of Ref-1 protein and found that leiomyomas have an abundance of the large form of Ref-1, which has a correlation with increased proliferation. The results suggested that altered posttranslational modification of Ref-1 is involved in uterine smooth muscle tumorigenesis [23].

Collectively, leiomyomas show more increased cell proliferation than the myometrium, with abnormalities of growth promoting factors, such as cytokines, growth factors, and cell cycle regulatory factors (cdc2, cdk2 [24], cyclin G1 [25]). However, the growth rate is moderate and not unrestricted, like that of uterine leiomyosarcomas that show an accumulation of genetic alterations, such as tumor suppressor gene p53 and/or calponin h1 [24,26–28]. Moreover, leiomyomas grow mainly during the luteal phase of the menstrual cycle [10]. The growth activity of leiomyomas controlled under the hormonal milieu of the menstrual cycle is an important expression of a benign neoplasm.

Recently, we have produced immortalized uterine leiomyoma and myometrial cell lines after induction of telomerase activity, as reported by Carney et al. [29]. These cells are expressing both estrogen and progesterone receptors and the phenotypic characteristics are close to those of leiomyoma and myometrium in vivo [29]. Further analysis using these cell lines is necessary to confirm the relationship between the ovarian steroids and growth factor(s)/cytokines in the growth of leiomyomas.

## 2.3. Growth-inhibitory factors

### 2.3.1. Heparin

Mast cells are widely distributed in human tissues, including the human uterus and leiomyomas [30–32]. However, the function of mast cells in uterine smooth muscle has not been clearly established. Mast cells possess secretory granules containing such substances as heparin, serotonin, histamine, and many cytokines. To understand the role of mast cells in the human myometrium and leiomyomas, the action of heparin was investigated using smooth muscle cells (SMC) from normal myometrium and from leiomyoma. Then, heparin inhibited the proliferation of myometrial and leiomyoma SMC through the induction of $\alpha$-smooth muscle actin, calponin h1, and p27 [33]. Mason et al. [34] also reported that heparin inhibits the motility and proliferation of human myometrial and leiomyoma SMC. These results suggest that heparin might be useful in the treatment of uterine leiomyomas.

### 2.3.2. Antifibrotic agents

Pirfenidone is an antifibrotic agent that is being tested for use in patients with pulmonary fibrosis. Because leiomyomas are characterized also by increased cell proliferation and tissue fibrosis, Lee et al. [35] examined the effects of pirfenidone on cell proliferation and collagen expression in cultured myometrial and leiomyoma smooth muscle cells, finding that it is an effective inhibitor of myometrial and leiomyoma cell proliferation in vitro.

Tranilast is known to suppress fibrosis or to work as a mast cell stabilizer and is reported to inhibit proliferation of vascular smooth muscle cells [36]. Therefore, we examined the effects of tranilast on cultured human leiomyoma cells in vitro and concluded that it is a potent agent for the inhibition of proliferative activity of uterine leiomyoma cells [37]. These results suggest that antifibrotic agents might be useful in the treatment of uterine leiomyomas.

## 2.4. Differential gene expression in leiomyoma

Recently, our microarray analysis revealed that genes, such as PEP-19 (Purkinje cell protein 4), secreted frizzled related protein 1 (sFRP1), stromelycin 3, IGF 2, TGF-$\beta$-3, and IGFBP 5 are upregulated in leiomyoma, relative to matched normal myometrium [38]. These results were similar to the report of Tsibris et al. [39] that showed that the expression of PEP-19, stromelycin 3, IGF 2, IGFBP 5, versican, and TGF-$\beta$-3 was upregulated in leiomyoma, relative to matched myometrium.

Among these genes, PEP-19, a calmodulin regulatory protein found within neurons, exhibited the most striking difference in expression between leiomyoma and normal myometrium. The function of PEP-19 in the pathogenesis of uterine leiomyoma is unknown; however, it might be involved in the control of apoptosis of leiomyoma cells [38].

We also found that secreted frizzled related protein 1 (sFRP1), a modulator of Wnt signaling, was over-expressed in uterine leiomyoma, with the strongest expression in the late follicular phase (high estrogenic milieu) of the menstrual cycle [40]. However, sFRP1 expression was not associated with cell proliferation, but rather occurred during cell protection against apoptosis in vitro. Strong sFRP1 expression under high estrogenic conditions is suggested to contribute to the development of uterine leiomyomas through the anti-apoptotic effect of sFRP1, which appears to be independent of cell proliferation [40].

## 3. Histogenesis of uterine leiomyoma

Regarding the histogenesis of uterine leiomyoma, Mayer [41] suggested that the cells of leiomyoma originate from myoblasts of uterine musculature, and his theory has been generally accepted. However, the progenitors of leiomyomas still have not been clearly identified.

Although smooth muscle tissues are widely distributed within the body, approximately 95% of leiomyomas occur within the female genital tract [42]. It remains unclear why neoplastic transformation of smooth muscle cells predominantly occurs in the uterus and how the progenitors of leiomyomas appear in the myometrium.

### 3.1. Leiomyomatosis peritonealis disseminata (LPD) and development of smooth muscle cells in the human fetal uterus

An unusual clinical entity, leiomyomatosis peritonealis disseminata (LPD), occurs in women associated with pregnancy or use of oral contraceptive steroids and is characterized by multiple leiomyoma-like nodules scattered throughout the abdominal cavity, which regress after withdrawal of reproductive steroids [4,6]. The analysis of this clinical entity [4,6] and experimental LPD [5] suggested to us the possibility of smooth muscle cell differentiation and leiomyoma-like nodule formation from undifferentiated mesenchymal cells in the subperitoneal mesenchyme. The embryonic kinship between the mullerian ducts (fetal uterus) and the peritoneum encouraged us to study the development of smooth muscle cells in the fetal uterus.

A study of the prenatal development of uterine smooth muscle revealed that smooth muscle differentiation begins at 18 weeks of gestation and is completed by 31 weeks [7,8]. If we may compare the development of smooth muscle cells of the uterus (mesoderm-derived duct) with that of the endoderm-derived duct, such as fetal urinary bladder and digestive tracts, there is a significant difference between these ducts in the period of smooth muscle differentiation. The latter completes smooth muscle differentiation by 14 weeks, but in the former this process is gradual until 31 weeks of gestation [7,8]. The slower differentiation of fetal uterine smooth muscle suggests that undifferentiated cells that proliferate and differentiate into smooth muscle in the uterus have a longer duration of instability during the fetal life. Some unknown maternal factors may affect the undifferentiated mesenchymal cells during the fetal period. Initial neoplastic transformation, involving as yet undetermined predisposing genetic factors, might occur during the development of smooth muscle cells in the fetal uterus. As the progenitors of leiomyomas, they could reside in the myometrium and begin to grow after menarche, and thrive during the years of greatest ovarian activity under the hormonal influence of both estrogen and progesterone [12].

### 3.2. Smooth muscle proliferation in the myometrium during the menstrual cycle and pregnancy

During the menstrual cycle, the myometrial smooth muscle cells express both estrogen receptors (ER) and progesterone receptors (PR), with scarce positive cells for the cell proliferation-associated antigen Ki-67 in the follicular phase [11]. However, in the luteal phase, the expression of PR is maintained with slight increase of positive cells for Ki-67. During pregnancy, they continue to express PR with significant increase of positive cells for Ki-67. ER expression is suppressed in the luteal phase and during pregnancy [11]. Consequently, myometrial smooth muscle cells show proliferative activity in the luteal phase and mainly during pregnancy, but little in the follicular phase.

Therefore, in each luteal phase of the menstrual cycle, myometrial smooth muscle cells are exhibiting proliferative activity, expecting an establishment of pregnancy. However, if no pregnancy occurs, the proliferative activity of the myometrial smooth muscle cells is interrupted at the time of menstruation. Myometrial contraction for cessation of menstrual bleeding could induce an ischemic and hypoxic state in the myometrial smooth muscle cells. Ischemic injury or ischemic–reperfusion injury could occur to the myometrial smooth muscle cells that are proliferating. We speculate that these cells are candidates for the progenitor cells of leiomyomas [12]. If this is the case, repetition of the menstrual cycle itself is very important for the pathogenesis of uterine leiomyomas.

To confirm this hypothesis, we investigated the expression of apoptotic-positive cells, p53-positive cells, p21-positive cells, and Ki-67-positive cells in the myometrium during the menstrual cycle. The apoptotic-positive cells, p53-positive cells, and p21-positive cells were only observed in the follicular phase of the menstrual cycle. Ki-67 positive cells are mainly observed in the luteal phase of the menstrual cycle. Therefore, the smooth muscle cells that are injured during menstruation seem to be eliminated in the follicular phase of the menstrual cycle, as apoptotic cells or cell cycle arrested cells expressing either p53 or p21. The majority of injured cells would be eliminated as apoptotic cells or cell cycle-arrested cells, but some injured cells may survive, acquiring a protective mechanism against oxidative stress and apoptosis. These cells might be a candidate for the progenitor cell of uterine leiomyoma. Indeed, uterine leiomyoma cells have a protective mechanism against oxidative stress expressing manganese superoxide dismutase (MnSOD) and against apoptosis expressing Bcl-2 [43], PEP-19 [38], and sFRP-1 [40].

Stewart and Nowak [44] also suggested that the pathogenesis of uterine leiomyomas might be similar to the response to injury. Analogous situations include the formation of keroids after surgery and atherosclerotic plaques after vascular injury. Smooth muscle cells respond to injury or ischemia with increased cell proliferation and production of extracellular matrix that are critical for the pathogenesis of uterine leiomyomas.

## 4. Summary

Recent investigations with advanced molecular techniques suggest that a leiomyoma might arise from a single parent cell derived from the smooth muscle elements of the myometrium, involving somatic mutations and the complex interactions of reproductive steroids and local growth factors and cytokines [20,21] during the repetition of the menstrual cycle [12].

## References

[1] V.C. Buttram Jr., R.C. Reiter, Uterine leiomyomata: etiology, symptomatology, and management, Fertil. Steril. 36 (1981) 433–445.
[2] B.J. Vollenhoven, A.S. Lawrence, D.L. Healy, Uterine fibroids: clinical review, Br. J. Obstet. Gynaecol. 97 (1990) 258–298.
[3] I. Konishi, et al., Ultrastructural study of minute uterine leiomyomas, Int. J. Gynecol. Pathol. 2 (1983) 113–120.
[4] S. Fujii, et al., Leiomyomatosis peritonealis disseminata, Obstet. Gynecol. 55 (1980) 79S–83S.
[5] S. Fujii, et al., Progesterone-induced smooth muscle-like cells in the subperitoneal nodules produced by estrogen. Experimental approach to leiomyomatosis peritonealis disseminata, Am. J. Obstet. Gynecol. 139 (1981) 164–172.
[6] S. Fujii, Leiomyomatosis peritonealis disseminata, in: C.J. Williams, J.G. Krikorian, M.R. Green, D. Raghavan (Eds.), Textbook of Uncommon Cancer, Wiley, Chichester, 1988, pp. 133–149.
[7] I. Konishi, et al., Development of smooth muscle in the human fetal uterus: an ultrastructural study, J. Anat. 139 (1984) 239–252.
[8] S. Fujii, et al., Ultrastructure of smooth muscle tissue in female genital tract: uterus and oviduct, in: P.M. Motta (Ed.), Ultrastructure of Smooth Muscle: Electron Microscopy in Biology and Medicine, Series in Current Topics of Ultrastructural Research, Martinus Nijhoff, The Hague, 1990, pp. 197–220.
[9] S. Fujii, I. Konishi, T. Mori, Smooth muscle differentiation at endometrio-myometrial junction: an ultra-structural study, Virchows Arch., A, Pathol. Anat. Histopathol. 414 (1989) 105–112.
[10] K. Kawaguchi, et al., Mitotic activity in uterine leiomyomas during the menstrual cycle, Am. J. Obstet. Gynecol. 160 (1989) 637–641.
[11] K. Kawaguchi, et al., Immunohistochemical analysis of oestrogen receptors, progesterone receptors and Ki-67 in leiomyoma and myometrium during the menstrual cycle and pregnancy, Virchows Arch., A, Pathol. Anat. Histopathol. 419 (1991) 309–315.
[12] S. Fujii, et al., Mesenchymal differentiation—speculation about the histogenesis of uterine leiomyomas, in: L.A. Brosen, B. Lunenfeld, J. Donnez (Eds.), Pathogenesis and Medical Management of Uterine Fibroids, Parthenon Publishing Group, London, 1999, pp. 3–15.

[13] D.E. Townsend, et al., Unicellular histogenesis of uterine leiomyomas as determined by electrophoresis of glucose-6-phosphate dehydrogenase, Am. J. Obstet. Gynecol. 107 (1970) 1168–1173.
[14] R.D. Mashal, et al., Analysis of androgen receptor DNA reveals the independent clonal origins of uterine leiomyomata and the secondary nature of cytogenetic aberrations in the development of leiomyomata, Genes Chromosomes Cancer 11 (1994) 1–6.
[15] K.L. Gross, C.C. Morton, Genetic and the development of fibroids, Clin. Obstet. Gynecol. 44 (2001) 335–349.
[16] O. Oguchi, et al., Prediction of histopathologic features and proliferative activity of uterine leiomyoma by magnetic resonance imaging prior to GnRH analogue therapy: correlation between T2-weighted images and effect of GnRH analogue, J. Obstet. Gynaecol. 21 (1995) 107–117.
[17] D.D. Brandon, et al., Estrogen receptor gene expression in human uterine leiomyomas, J. Clin. Endocrinol. Metab. 80 (1995) 1876–1881.
[18] B. Viville, et al., Distribution of the A and B forms of the progesterone receptor messenger ribonucleic acid and protein in uterine leiomyoma and adjacent myometrium, Hum. Reprod. 12 (1997) 817–822.
[19] H. Sumitani, et al., In situ estrogen synthesized by aromatase P450 in uterine leiomyoma cells promotes cell growth probably via an autocrine/paracrine mechanism, Endocrinology 141 (2000) 3852–3861.
[20] J. Andersen, Growth factors and cytokines in uterine leiomyoma, Semin. Reprod. Endocrinol. 14 (1996) 269–282.
[21] I. Sozen, A. Arici, Interactions of cytokines, growth factors, and the extracellular matrix in the cellular biology of uterine leiomyomata, Fertil. Steril. 78 (2002) 1–8.
[22] A. Horiuchi, et al., S. Fujii, HCG promotes proliferation of uterine leiomyomal cells more strongly than that of myometrial smooth muscle cells in vitro, Mol. Hum. Reprod. 6 (2000) 523–528.
[23] A. Orii, et al., Altered post-translational modification of redox factor 1 protein in human uterine smooth muscle tumors, J. Clin. Endocrinol. Metab. 87 (2002) 3754–3759.
[24] Y.L. Zhai, et al., Expression of cyclins and cyclin-dependent kinases in smooth muscle tumors of the uterus, Int. J. Cancer 84 (1999) 244–250.
[25] W.K. Baek, et al., Increased expression of cyclin G1 in leiomyoma compared with normal myometrium, Am. J. Obstet. Gynecol. 188 (2003) 634–639.
[26] Y.L. Zhai, et al., Frequent occurrence of loss of heterozygosity among tumor suppressor genes in uterine leiomyosarcoma, Gynecol. Oncol. 75 (1999) 453–459.
[27] A. Horiuchi, et al., Reduced expression of calponin h1 in leiomyosarcoma of the uterus, Lab. Invest. 78 (1998) 839–846.
[28] A. Horiuchi, et al., Possible role of calponin h1 as a tumor suppressor in human uterine leiomyosarcoma, J. Natl. Cancer Inst. 91 (1999) 790–796.
[29] S.A. Carney, et al., Immortalization of human uterine leiomyoma and myometrial cell lines after induction of telomerase activity: molecular and phenotypic characteristics, Lab. Invest. 82 (2002) 719–728.
[30] A. Mori, et al., Distribution and heterogeneity of mast cells in the human uterus, Hum. Reprod. 12 (1997) 368–372.
[31] A. Orii, et al., Mast cells in smooth muscle tumors of the uterus, Int. J. Gynecol. Pathol. 17 (1998) 336–342.
[32] A. Mori, et al., Analysis of stem cell factor for mast cell proliferation in the human myometrium, Mol. Hum. Reprod. 3 (1997) 411–418.
[33] A. Horiuchi, et al., Heparin inhibits proliferation of myometrial and leiomyomal smooth muscle cells through the induction of alpha-smooth muscle actin, calponin h1 and p27, Mol. Hum. Reprod. 5 (1999) 139–145.
[34] H.R. Mason, et al., Heparin inhibits the motility and proliferation of human myometrial and leiomyoma smooth muscle cells, Am. J. Pathol. 162 (2003) 1895–1904.
[35] B.S. Lee, S.B. Margolin, R.A. Nowak, Pirfenidone: a novel pharmacological agent that inhibits leiomyoma cell proliferation and collagen production, J. Clin. Endocrinol. Metab. 83 (1998) 219–223.
[36] H. Kusama, et al., Tranilast inhibits the proliferation of human coronary smooth muscle cell through the activation of p21waf1, Atherosclerosis 143 (1999) 307–313.
[37] H. Shime, et al., Tranilast inhibits the proliferation of uterine leiomyoma cells in vitro through G1 arrest associated with the induction of p21(waf1) and p53, J. Clin. Endocrinol. Metab. 87 (2002) 5610–5617.

[38] T. Kanamori, et al., PEP-19 overexpression in human uterine leiomyoma, Mol. Hum. Reprod. 9 (2003) 709–717.
[39] J.C. Tsibris, et al., Insights from gene arrays on the development and growth regulation of uterine leiomyomata, Fertil. Steril. 78 (2002) 114–121.
[40] K. Fukuhara, et al., Secreted frizzled related protein 1 is overexpressed in uterine leiomyomas, associated with a high estrogenic environment and unrelated to proliferative activity, J. Clin. Endocrinol. Metab. 87 (2002) 1729–1736.
[41] R. Mayer, Die pathologische Anatomie der Gebarmutter, Handbuch der speziellen pathologischen Anatomie und Histologie, Bd VII/I, Springer-Verlag, Berlin, 1930, pp. 213–249.
[42] A.G. Farman, Benign smooth muscle tumors, S. Afr. Med. J. 48 (1974) 1214.
[43] Z. Gao, et al., Up-regulation by IGF-I of proliferating cell nuclear antigen and Bcl-2 protein expression in human uterine leiomyoma cells, J. Clin. Endocrinol. Metab. 86 (2001) 5593–5599.
[44] E.A. Stewart, R.A. Nowak, New concepts in the treatment of uterine leiomyomas, Obstet. Gynecol. 92 (1998) 624–627.

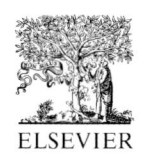

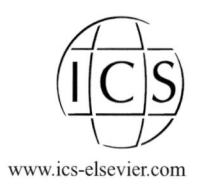

# Fibroids: effect on infertility and assisted reproduction

Cynthia M. Farquhar*

*Obstetrics and Gynaecology, National Women's Hospital, University of Auckland, Claude Road, Auckland 1105, New Zealand*

**Abstract.** Uterine fibroids (leiomyomata) are the most common pelvic tumours found in women. Twenty to fifty percent of women are estimated to have fibroids, and their incidence increases with age until the time of the menopause. There has been considerable speculation that fibroids cause infertility. In order to establish causality between pathology and symptoms, it has been suggested that certain criteria must exist. These include evidence of benefit in removing fibroids in experimental studies, a strong association between fibroids and infertility, a temporal relationship in detection of the fibroids preceding onset of infertility, the epidemiological and biological plausibility of fibroids causing infertility and whether or not the association of fibroids is specific to infertility. Although more than 40 case series of myomectomy have been reported, only seven of them are prospective and only one reports a comparison group. Another approach to establishing causality in the absence of experimental human studies is to consider the impact of fibroids on assisted reproductive technology (ART) cycles. Fibroids have been associated with poor outcomes in assisted reproductive technology cycles. However, it is not clear if the position of the fibroid influences the outcome. Given the frequency with which fibroids are found, well-designed experimental studies are needed to establish fibroids as a factor in infertility. © 2004 Published by Elsevier B.V.

*Keywords:* Leiomyomata; Fibroids; Infertility; Causality

## 1. Introduction

Uterine fibroids (leiomyomata) are the most common pelvic tumours found in women. Twenty to fifty percent of women are estimated to have fibroids, and their incidence increases with age until the time of the menopause [1]. There has been considerable speculation that fibroids cause infertility. The impression that fibroids are related to infertility has arisen from a number of reported case series where removal of fibroids resulted in subsequent conception rates between 30% and 80% [2–4]. However, such studies do not establish causality and it is generally agreed that it is yet to be established whether or not fibroids cause infertility [3–5].

\* Tel.: +64-9-630-9943x3243; fax: +64-9-630-9858.
*E-mail address:* c.farquhar@auckland.ac.nz (C.M. Farquhar).

## 2. Establishing causality: do fibroids cause infertility?

In order to establish causality between pathology and symptoms, it has been suggested that certain criteria must exist [6,7] (Table 1). The following questions have been suggested as a guide to establishing causality:

Is there experimental evidence from human studies?
Is the association between the proposed cause and effect strong?
Is the association consistent from study to study?
Is the temporal relationship correct?
Is there a dose–response relationship?
Is the association consistent with existing biological and environmental knowledge?
Does the association make biological sense?
Is the association specific?
Is there a similar accepted link between an exposure and a disease?

The first of the nine questions posed above, *Is there experimental evidence from human studies?* refers to the need for studies with an experimental design in which the cause is removed and the disease rates are studied. Although such a study is often done in the context of a randomised controlled trial (RCT), the use of this design is not always possible. For example, in trying to establish the link between lung cancer and cigarette smoking, it was not feasible to do an RCT. However, in the example of fibroids and infertility, it would help to establish if fibroids had a role in infertility by evaluating pregnancy rates following surgical removal of the fibroids with a randomised controlled trial comparing myomectomy with no surgical intervention for infertility. Unfortunately, no randomised controlled trial of

Table 1
The relationship between fibroids and infertility

| Question | Explanation of question | Role of fibroids in infertility |
| --- | --- | --- |
| Is there experimental evidence from human studies? | What happens to the pregnancy rate if fibroids are removed? | Only one comparative study available. |
| Is the association strong? | Large relative risk from well designed studies; in this case, ideally RCTs are required. | No well designed studies available. |
| Is the association consistent from study to study? | Repeated observations by different studies. | Yes, although mostly case series of fertility following myomectomy and fertility outcomes with ART cycles. |
| Is the temporal relationship correct? | Does the occurrence of the fibroids precede the occurrence of infertility? | No, as fibroids are frequently diagnosed at the same time as infertility. |
| Is there a dose–response relationship? | Is infertility more likely with increasing number or size of fibroids? | Few studies have addressed this question and do not show an effect. |
| Is there coherence of the evidence? | Is the association between fibroids and infertility consistent with biological and environmental knowledge? | Possibly, although fibroids are more common than infertility. |
| Does the association make biological sense? | Is it likely that fibroids could interfere with fertility? | Yes, especially if they cause distortion of the uterine cavity. |
| Is the association specific? | Do fibroids often lead to infertility? | No, women with fibroids conceive and deliver mostly without any problems. |
| Is there a similar accepted link between an exposure and a disease? | Is there another example of cause for infertility that is analogous to fibroids? | Example of anovulation and infertility given. |

this intervention exists. If one did exist, then an increase in pregnancy rate in the surgical arm of the study would suggest a role for fibroids in causing infertility.

In the absence of randomised controlled trials, it is necessary to rely on the evidence from case series or case-control studies. There are more than 40 reports of myomectomy and subsequent pregnancy rates in the published literature, and the pregnancy rates vary from 10% to 77% [5]. However, few of these studies are prospective and only one includes a comparison or control group [8]. The large variation in pregnancy rates following myomectomy is likely to reflect differences in patient characteristics—the size and position of the fibroids, the duration of infertility and the age of the women. It is also likely to reflect differences in the skill of the surgeon. In the one study that compared the pregnancy rates between women who had undergone myomectomy with those who had not, there was an increased pregnancy rate in the surgery group [8].

Another approach to establishing causality in the absence of experimental human studies is to consider the impact of fibroids on assisted reproductive technology (ART) cycles. A number of studies have consistently shown a decrease in pregnancy rates in women with fibroids, particularly in women who have a distorted uterine cavity, when compared with women without distortion of the cavity and women with no fibroids [5,9]. Most of these studies concluded that pregnancy and implantation rates were significantly lower in the groups of women with intramural and submucous fibroids. In two studies, a subgroup of women with submucosal fibroids was considered and the results suggested that hysteroscopic myomectomy was beneficial, although the total number of women included was small (33 in one study and 5 in the other) [10,11]. However, even when there was no deformation of the uterine cavity, the pregnancy rates were lower [9,10]. These results are in contrast to a retrospective case series of women with fibroids undergoing intracytoplasmic sperm injection (ICSI) cycles, compared with women without fibroids, which did not demonstrate an effect of intramural or subserous fibroids (women with submucous fibroids were excluded from the study) [12].

The second and third questions of causality ask, *Is the association strong and consistent?* In relation to fibroids and infertility, the association cannot be described as either strong or consistent, as there are few studies that report a comparison or control group [10,11] and the total numbers of women included are small [13]. Although most of the results from the many case series are consistent, not much weight can be given to studies that do not include a comparison group. Even in those studies that do include a comparison group, there are some conflicting reports about the role of intramural fibroids in ART cycles [10,12].

The fourth causality question asks, *Is the temporal relationship correct?* This question relates to the relationship between time and the onset of disease and symptoms. Unfortunately, this chronology is difficult to establish in women with infertility, as fibroids may be undiagnosed until infertility is diagnosed. Furthermore, as the incidence of fibroids increases with age and many women present for infertility care at an age when fibroid incidence is particularly high, it is not surprising that fibroids are a relatively common finding in women with infertility.

The next question of causality reads, *Is there a dose–response relationship?* Do women with several fibroids have more problems conceiving than women with only one or two fibroids? Does the size of the fibroid influence the outcome? No study was found that specifically addressed these questions, although many studies excluded women with large fibroids. In one retrospective study, neither the size nor the number of fibroids influenced the pregnancy rate in women undergoing ICSI [12]. In studies of myomectomy, a lower pregnancy rate was reported in some studies when more fibroids were removed, although other authors noted no difference [5]. Altogether, it would seem that the evidence on the influence of size and number of fibroids on pregnancy rates is contradictory and no conclusions can be drawn.

The next two questions of causality are, *Is the association consistent with existing biological and environmental knowledge?* and *Does the association make biological sense?* The idea that a condition as common as fibroids could cause infertility appears, at first, to be unlikely. For example, if as many as half of all women have fibroids and infertility occurs only in 10–20% of couples, then it would seem unlikely that fibroids play a major role in infertility. However, with many women delaying childbearing until the fourth decade, it is possible that a higher proportion of the female population has fibroids. Unfortunately, as mentioned previously, increasing age confounds this association. With regard to the question of biological plausibility, there are several possibilities. For example, it is possible that fibroids that distort the cavity do adversely affect fertility rates and it is generally agreed that anatomical location of the fibroid is an important factor. Six studies have reported lower pregnancy rates among women with fibroids that distort the cavity [5,11,12,14–16]. Other mechanisms that could affect fertility include the possibility that fibroids may cause dysfunctional uterine contractility, thus interfering with sperm migration, ovum transport or nidation [2,17,18]. Fibroids have also been implicated in implantation failure or pregnancy loss due to focal endometrial vascular disturbance, endometrial inflammation, secretion of vasoactive substances and enhanced endometrial androgen environment [2,19].

The next question of causality asks, *Is the association specific?* Many women with fibroids, even large ones, conceive and deliver without difficulty. The reported prevalence of fibroids in pregnancy (detected by ultrasonography) is 4–5%, although this figure will be strongly influenced by maternal age [20,21]. Most fibroids remain uncomplicated in pregnancy and most do not increase in size. Up to 10% of fibroids undergo red degeneration, typically in the second trimester [21].

The final question of causality asks, *Is the association analogous to a previously proven causal association?* One such example in the field of infertility is anovulation, for which many of the above questions can be adequately answered from the literature. For example, there are experimental studies for the role of clomiphene citrate in women with anovulation [22] and, although there is no study comparing follicle-stimulating hormone with placebo for anovulation, the effect size is sufficiently large not to require RCTs. Similarly, the association between anovulation and infertility is strong and consistent, has obvious temporal and dose–response relationships, is specific and makes both epidemiological and biological sense.

## 3. Conclusions

This chapter has attempted to establish a link between fibroids and infertility, using the causality criteria adapted from Bradford-Hill [6]. While it is not necessary to prove all nine criteria in order to establish the causal link, it can be seen that the majority of the criteria have not been met (Table 1). Thus, the case for fibroids causing infertility remains to be established. It is generally agreed that applying these criteria results in concluding that fibroids probably do not cause infertility in most cases. For example, a recent review concluded, "the relationship between leiomyomas and infertility remains a subject of debate" [5]. Although the prevalence of fibroids in infertile women can be high, no causal relationship between fibroids and infertility has been demonstrated. Given the frequency with which fibroids are found, the establishment of fibroids as a factor in infertility and the role of myomectomy as a management strategy should be possible with well-designed experimental studies. Future studies, ideally, should be randomised controlled trials of myomectomy in women with fibroids and should report live birth outcomes. In the absence of undertaking randomised controlled trials, at the very least, prospective observational studies should include a control group of women who do not have fibroids. Such studies are long overdue.

## References

[1] B.S. Verkauf, Myomectomy for fertility enhancement and preservation, Fertil. Steril. 58 (1992) 1–15.
[2] V.C. Buttram, R.C. Reiter, Uterine leiomyomata: etiology, symptomatology, and management, Fertil. Steril. 36 (1981) 433–445.
[3] N. Bajekal, T.C. Li, Fibroids, infertility and pregnancy wastage, Hum. Reprod. Updat. 6 (2000) 614–620.
[4] M.A. Lumsden, E.M. Wallace, Clinical presentation of uterine fibroids, Bailliere's Clin. Obstet. Gynaecol. 12 (1998) 177–195.
[5] J. Donnez, P. Jadoul, What are the implications of myomas on fertility? A need for a debate? Hum. Reprod. 17 (2002) 1424–1430.
[6] A. Bradford Hill, The environment and disease: association or causation? Proc. R. Soc. Med. 58 (1965) 295–300.
[7] K.J. Rothman, Modern Epidemiology, Little and Brown and Co., Boston, 1996, Chap. 2.
[8] C. Bulletti, D. De Ziegler, V. Polli, L. Diotallevi, E. Del Ferro, C. Flamigni, The role of leiomyomas in infertility, J. Am. Assoc. Gynecol. Laparosc. 6 (1999) 441–445.
[9] R. Hart, Y. Khalaf, C.T. Yeong, P. Seed, A. Taylor, P. Braude, A prospective controlled study of the effect of intramural uterine fibroids on the outcome of assisted conception, Hum. Reprod. 16 (2001) 2411–2417.
[10] T. Eldgar-Geva, S. Meagher, D.L. Healy, V. MacLachlan, S. Breheny, C. Wood, Effect of intramural, subserosal and submucosal uterine fibroids on the outcome of assisted reproductive technology treatment, Fertil. Steril. 70 (1998) 687–691.
[11] J. Farhi, J. Ashkenazi, D. Feldberg, D. Dicker, R. Orvieto, Z. Ben Rafael, Effect of uterine leiomyomata on the results of in vitro fertilization treatment, Hum. Reprod. 10 (1995) 2576–2578.
[12] H. Yarali, Bukulmez, The effect of intramural and subserous uterine fibroids on implantation and clinical pregnancy rates in patients having intracytoplasmic sperm injection, Arch. Gynecol. Obstet. 266 (2002) 30–33.
[13] E.A. Pritts, Fibroids and infertility: a systematic review of the evidence, Obstet. Gynecol. Surv. 56 (2001) 483–491.
[14] S.H. Jun, E.S. Ginsburg, C. Racowsky, L.A. Wise, M.D. Hornstein, Uterine leiomyomas and their effect on in vitro fertilization outcome: a retrospective study, J. Assist. Reprod. Genet. 18 (2001) 139–143.
[15] A.M. Ramzy, M. Satta, Y. Amin, R.T. Mansour, G.I. Serour, M.A. Aboulghar, Uterine myomata and outcome of assisted reproduction, Hum. Reprod. 13 (1998) 198–202.
[16] D.W. Stovall, S.B. Parrish, B.J. Van Voorhis, S.J. Hahn, A.E. Sparks, C.H. Syrop, Uterine leiomyomas reduce the efficacy of assisted reproduction cycles: results of a matched follow-up study, Hum. Reprod. 13 (1998) 192–197.
[17] E.S. Surrey, A.K. Liez, W.B. Schoolcraft, Impact of intramural leiomyomata in patients with a normal

endometrial cavity on in vitro fertilization-embryo transfer cycle outcome, Fertil. Steril. 75 (2001) 405–410 (Hunt and Wllach).
[18] B.J. Vollenhoven, A.S. Lawrence, D.L. Healy, Uterine fibroids: a clinical review, Br. J. Obstet. Gynaecol. 97 (1990) 285–288.
[19] L. Deligdish, M. Lowenthal, Endometrial changes associated with myomata of the uterus, J. Clin. Pathol. 23 (1970) 676–680.
[20] S.F. Cramer, A. Patel, The frequency of uterine leiomyomas, Am. J. Clin. Pathol. 94 (1990) 435–438.
[21] C. Exacoustos, P. Rosati, Ultrasound diagnosis of uterine myomas and complications in pregnancy, Obstet. Gynecol. 82 (1993) 97–101.
[22] E. Hughes, J. Collins, P. Vandekerckhove, Clomiphene citrate for ovulation induction in women with oligo-amenorrhoea (Cochrane Review), The Cochrane Library, Issue 4, Wiley, Chichester, UK, 2003.

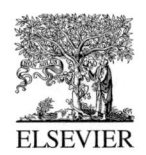

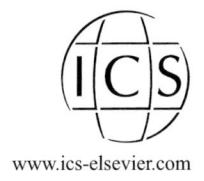

# Treatment options for uterine myoma

Raedah Al-Fadhli, Togas Tulandi*

*Department of Obstetrics and Gynecology, McGill University, Montreal, Quebec, Canada*

**Abstract.** Leiomyoma or fibroid is the most common benign tumor occurring in the uterus and female pelvis. Fibroids are the primary indication for hysterectomies and they represent over 30% of the total number of hysterectomies. There are other treatments for uterine fibroids, including expectant management, medical treatment, conservative surgical treatment and recently, uterine fibroid embolization. For women of reproductive age, myomectomy is an option and in selected cases it can be done by laparoscopy. Submucus myoma should be treated by the hysteroscopic approach. Uterine fibroid embolization carries the risk of premature ovarian failure in 1% of women. Myolysis is associated with adhesion formation that might further decrease fertility. For women who have completed their family, supracervical hysterectomy is a viable option. © 2004 Published by Elsevier B.V.

*Keywords:* Leiomyoma; Myoma; Fibroid; Myomectomy; Uterine fibroid embolization; Uterine artery embolization; Myolysis; Hysterectomy

Uterine leiomyoma or fibroids are the most common pelvic tumors in women. Its incidence in women of reproductive age is estimated to be 20–25%. Because most uterine fibroids are asymptomatic, the actual incidence is much higher. In one study, histopathological examination of the hysterectomy specimen revealed that 77% of the uteri contained fibroids [1–3]. The main symptoms of uterine fibroid are excessive menstrual bleeding and pressure symptoms.

## 1. Uterine fibroids and reproduction

Submucous fibroid is associated with a higher risk of miscarriage, whereas subserous myoma has no deleterious effect. The effect of fibroids on fertility is unclear. Hassan et al. [4] showed that 43% of pregnant women with fibroids have a history of infertility before pregnancy. Impaired gamete transport, distorted uterine cavity, and abnormal blood supply to the endometrium may be a reason for poor implantation in patients with fibroids [5–9].

---

* Corresponding author. Tel.: +514-842-1231; fax: +514-843-1448.
*E-mail address:* togas.tulandi@muhc.mcgill.ca (T. Tulandi).

0531-5131/ © 2004 Published by Elsevier B.V.
doi:10.1016/j.ics.2004.01.112

The role of uterine fibroids on infertility has been indirectly evaluated. In a review, 54% of patients conceived after abdominal myomectomy [8]. Verkauf [10] reported a pregnancy rate of 59.5% after myomectomy. Eldar-Geva et al. [11] found that pregnancy and implantation rates were significantly lower in patients with intramural and submucous fibroid even when there was no deformity of the uterine cavity. In their opinion, surgical or medical treatment should be considered in infertile women who have intramural or submucous fibroid. However, removal of intramural myoma is associated with adhesion formation that might further lead to infertility.

The relationship between submucous myoma and infertility or miscarriages is more definitive. In infertile women with submucous myoma, we recommend hysteroscopic myomectomy. Asymptomatic infertile women with intramural or subserous myoma are managed expectantly, and those with symptoms are treated conservatively by myomectomy.

## 2. Abdominal myomectomy

In women with multiple fibroids or deep intramural fibroid, abdominal myomectomy is the treatment of choice. Compared with hysterectomy, myomectomy is associated with more blood transfusion, and a higher rate of febrile morbidity. Another common complication is postoperative adhesions [12].

## 3. Laparoscopic myomectomy

Compared with laparotomy, laparoscopic procedures are associated with less postoperative pain, shorter hospital stay, rapid recovery and reduced adhesion formation [13]. In a randomized study, Seracchioli et al. [14] found no significant difference in the rates of abortion, preterm delivery, and cesarean section between laparoscopic myomectomy and abdominal myomectomy.

Despite their benefits, laparoscopic myomectomy is technically demanding, and the surgeon should be familiar with laparoscopic suturing. Furthermore, Dubuisson et al. [15] reported a 1.0% risk of uterine rupture among 100 deliveries. This could be related to inadequate closure of the uterine defect or poor healing. Patients with more than three fibroids of ≥5 cm or a fibroid of >15 cm are better treated by laparotomy. We recommend multilayered suturing of the uterine defect.

## 4. Hysteroscopic myomectomy

Hysteroscopic myomectomy is the standard treatment for submucous fibroids of <5 cm in diameter. It is associated with a pregnancy rate of up to 73% in women with infertility [16]. Long-term complications include intrauterine adhesions in 10% of cases [17]. In women with submucous myoma of >3 cm, we prefer to reduce the size of the myoma using three doses of gonadotropin-releasing hormone analog [18] before the surgery.

## 5. Uterine fibroid embolization (UFE)

Uterine fibroid embolization is one of the newest treatments of uterine fibroids without surgery. The main purpose is to reduce the size of the fibroids and to treat excessive uterine bleeding. In a review of 119 cases of UFE [19], the authors reported that about 70% of the patients had an immediate cessation of menorrhagia and improvement of pain and pressure symptoms after the procedure. At 6 months follow-up, the total uterine volume decreased by 56% and the average diameter of the largest myoma decreased by 36%.

Due to reports of ovarian failure resulting from UFE, there has been uncertainty in prescribing this treatment for younger women [20–24]. However, a few investigators recently reported that ovarian function, especially in young women, is not affected by UFE [25]. There are also several reports of pregnancy following UFE [26].

It is clear that UFE is an alternative treatment for women who do not wish to undergo a hysterectomy. However, following this procedure several women have become menopausal [25]. It seems that premature menopause following embolization occurs predominantly in the older age group. This is due to embolization of the utero-ovarian collateral circulation compromising the blood supply to the ovaries. Although, perimenopausal women with declining ovarian function tend to be more affected than younger women, it has also been reported in women less than 40 years. The estimated risk is about 1%. Similar to others, we have encountered permanent ovarian failure with severe menopausal symptoms in a 40-year-old woman immediately after UFE.

It appears that myomectomy is a better alternative than UFE in women of reproductive age who have not completed their family.

### 6. Laparoscopic bipolar uterine artery coagulation as an alternative to UFE

A group from Taiwan recently introduced laparoscopic bipolar coagulation of uterine vessels as an alternative to UFE [27]. Of the total 87 patients undergoing the procedure, the average fibroid volume and uterine volume reductions were 76% and 46%, respectively. The FSH levels in three patients were >30 mIU/ml, postoperatively. However, their ages were 46, 48 and 53 years, respectively. Two patients conceived after the procedure.

Because this procedure does not interrupt the utero-ovarian collaterals, it is unlikely that the treatment would be associated with premature ovarian failure or decreased ovarian function. Further study is needed to clarify this matter.

### 7. Laparoscopic myolysis

Myolysis is done by coagulating the central part of the myoma either with a long bipolar needle or with laser. Coagulating necrosis of the fibroid results in vascular damage and changes of the collagen leading to shrinkage of the fibroid. A 41% mean decrease of the fibroid volume has been reported [28]. The main disadvantage of this procedure is adhesion formation that could lead to infertility and pelvic pain. A case of uterine rupture has also been described. In our institution, myolysis is not done anymore.

### 8. Hysterectomy

Following the childbearing period, symptomatic women with uterine fibroids could be offered a hysterectomy or UFE. For diseases above the cervix such as uterine fibroids, a subtotal or supracervical hysterectomy is particularly suitable. However, cervical cytology should be normal for at least 3 years. Otherwise, a total hysterectomy can be considered.

Vaginal hysterectomy appears to be associated with less morbidity than abdominal hysterectomy, but a uterine weight of >500 g is associated with complications. With improvement in laparoscopy techniques, the use of GnRHa to decrease the uterine and fibroid size, and the ease of uterine removal with morcellation, more hysterectomies can be performed by laparoscopy giving patients the advantages of minimally invasive surgery [29]. The ultimate results depend on the proper patient selection, and surgeon's experience, expertise, and preference.

## References

[1] S.F. Cramer, A. Patel, The frequency of uterine leiomyomas, Am. J. Clin. Pathol. 94 (1990) 435–438.
[2] M.P. Vessey, et al., The epidemiology of hysterectomy: findings in a large cohort study, Br. J. Obstet. Gynaecol. 99 (1992) 402–407.
[3] F. Parazzini, et al., Reproductive factors and risk of uterine fibroids, Epidemiology 7 (1996) 440–442.
[4] F. Hasan, K. Arumugan, V. Sivanesaratnam, Uterine leiomyomata in pregnancy, Int. J. Gynecol. Obstet. 34 (1990) 45–48.
[5] L. Deligdish, M. Lowenthal, Endometrial changes associated with myomata of the uterus, J. Clin. Pathol. 23 (1970) 676–680.
[6] D.S.F. Settladge, M. Motoshima, D.R. Tredway, Sperm transport from the external os to the fallopian tubes in women: a time and quantitation study, Fertil. Steril. 24 (1972) 655–658.
[7] C.S. Losif, M. Akerland, Fibromyomas and uterine activity, Acta Obstet. Gynecol. Scand. 62 (1983) 165–167.
[8] J.E. Hunt, E.F. Wallach, Uterine factor in infertility: an overview, Clin. Obstet. Gynecol. 17 (1974) 44–64.
[9] V.C. Buttram, R.C. Reiter, Uterine leiomyomata: etiology, symptomatology and management, Fertil. Steril. 36 (1981) 433–435.
[10] B.S. Verkauf, Myomectomy for fertility enhancement and preservation, Fertil. Steril. 58 (1992) 1–15.
[11] T. Eldar-Geva, et al., Effect of intramural, subserosal, and submucosal uterine fibroids on the outcome of assisted reproductive technology treatment, Fertil. Steril. 70 (1998) 687–691.
[12] J. Sanfilippo, M. Haggerty, Abdominal myomectomy, in: T. Tulandi (Ed.), Uterine Fibroids. Embolization and other treatment, Cambridge Univ. Press, London, 2003, pp. 31–40.
[13] D. Seidman, et al., Abdominal myomectomy, in: T. Tulandi (Ed.), Uterine Fibroids. Embolization and other treatment, Cambridge Univ. Press, London, 2003, pp. 41–49.
[14] R. Seracchioli, et al., Fertility and obstetric outcome after laparoscopic myomectomy of large myomata: a randomized comparison with abdominal myomectomy, Hum. Reprod. 15 (2000) 3663–3668.
[15] J.B. Dubuisson, et al., Fertility after laparoscopic myomectomy of large intramural myomas: preliminary results, Human. Reprod. 11 (1996) 518–522.
[16] D.R. Phillips, et al., Transcervical electrosurgical resection of submucous leiomyomas for chronic menorrhagia, J. Am. Assoc. Gynecol. Laparosc. 2 (1995) 147–153.
[17] J.P. Hallez, Single-stage total hysteroscopic myomectomies: indications, techniques, and results, Fertil. Steril. 63 (1995) 703–708.
[18] A. Gervaise, H. Fernandez, Abdominal myomectomy, in: T. Tulandi (Ed.), Uterine Fibroids. Embolization and other treatment, Cambridge Univ. Press, London, 2003, pp. 50–56.
[19] B. McLucas, L. Adler, Uterine artery embolization as therapy for myomata, Infertil. Reprod. Med. Clin. North Am. 11 (2000) 77–94.
[20] S.C. Goodwin, et al., Uterine artery embolization for the treatment of uterine leiomyomata midterm results, J. Vasc. Interv. Radiol. 10 (1999) 1159–1165.
[21] J.B. Spies, et al., Initial results from uterine fibroid embolization as primary treatment for symptomatic uterine leiomyomata, J. Vasc. Interv. Radiol. 10 (1999) 1149–1157.
[22] E.A. Bradley, et al., Transcatheter uterine artery embolization to treat large uterine fibroids, Br. J. Obstet. Gynaecol. 105 (1998) 235–240.
[23] H. Chrisman, et al., The impact of uterine fibroid embolization on resumption of menses and ovarian function, J. Vasc. Interv. Radiol. 11 (2000) 699–703.

[24] N.H. Stringer, et al., Ovarian failure after uterine artery embolization for treatment of myomas, J. Am. Assoc. Gynecol. Laparosc. 7 (2000) 395–400.
[25] T. Tulandi, Reproductive function after uterine fibroid embolization, in: T. Tulandi (Ed.), Uterine Fibroids. Embolization and Other Treatment, Cambridge Univ. Press, London, 2003, pp. 119–124.
[26] J.H. Ravina, et al., Pregnancy after embolization of uterine myoma: report of 12 cases, Fertil. Steril. 73 (2000) 1241–1243.
[27] W.M. Liu, et al., Laparoscopic bipolar coagulation of uterine vessels: a new method for treating symptomatic fibroids, Fertil. Steril. 75 (2001) 417–422.
[28] M. Nisolle, et al., Laparoscopic myolysis with the Nd:YAG laser, J. Gynecol. Surg. 37 (1992) 636–638.
[29] H. Al-fozan, T. Tulandi, Hysterectomy for uterine fibroid, in: T. Tulandi (Ed.), Uterine Fibroids. Embolization and other treatment, Cambridge Univ. Press, London, 2003, pp. 74–79.

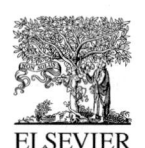

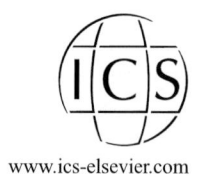

# Guidelines in the treatment of male infertility

## Stewart Irvine*

*MRC Human Reproductive Sciences Unit, Centre for Reproductive Biology,
The University of Edinburgh Chancellor's Building, 49 Little France Crescent, Edinburgh EH16 4SB, UK*

**Abstract.** Information overload is a major problem facing those caring for patients, and there is evidence that much patient care is not based on the best available evidence. Many strategies have been deployed to improve translation of the evidence base into clinical practice, key amongst which is the development of clinical practice guidelines. In the field of male subfertility, several such guidelines exist, many based on expert review of the evidence, but lacking the rigour of a systematic review of evidence and synthesis of recommendations. Some examples of formally evidence-based guidelines do exist. However, they serve to demonstrate that the strength of the evidence base in the field is not good, with fewer than one in five recommendations in a recent evidence-based guideline being based on grade A (RCT) evidence. Given this state of the evidence, there will continue to be a place for a range of guideline development strategies for the foreseeable future. © 2004 Published by Elsevier B.V.

*Keywords:* Infertility; Male infertility; Guidelines; Evidence-based medicine

## 1. Introduction

Information overload is a serious problem facing clinicians, the nature of which was highlighted by the editor of the British Medical Journal, reflecting recently on the issues which confront new medical undergraduates [1]:

> In particular, avoid the trap of thinking you need to know everything. Even if you knew everything at 6 o'clock this morning (which of course you never could), you won't by midday—because a thousand new studies will have been published. ... We need the help of machines. Ask travel agents the time of planes from Shanghai to Hong Kong, and they will not quote from their heads. They will use information tools. Doctors must learn to do the same.

The scale of the problem is illustrated by the fact that about 10,000 new randomised, controlled trials are included in MEDLINE each year [2], and almost 380,000 trials have been identified by the Cochrane collaboration [3]. However, major difficulties arise in introducing these innovations into daily clinical practice. The gap between evidence and

---

\* Tel.: +44-131-242-2483; fax: +44-131-242-2487.
*E-mail address:* d.s.irvine@ed.ac.uk (S. Irvine).

0531-5131/ © 2004 Published by Elsevier B.V.
doi:10.1016/j.ics.2004.01.071

practice is all too apparent [4], with studies suggesting that 30–40% of patients do not receive care according to current scientific evidence, and 20–25% of care provided is either not needed or is potentially harmful [5].

## 2. Guidelines

Approaches to improve the uptake of research findings, and their implementation into routine clinical practice, have focused on improving the availability and presentation of evidence by identifying, synthesizing, and disseminating evidence to clinicians through reviews, clinical guidelines, electronic sources, continuing medical education (CME) courses, and conferences. This paper will focus on guidelines in the management of male subfertility.

Guidelines have been defined as "systematically developed statements to assist practitioner and patient decisions about appropriate health care for specific clinical circumstances" [6]. They provide recommendations for effective practice in the management of clinical conditions where variations in practice are known to occur and where effective care may not be delivered uniformly. There are many guidelines available, most being based on a consensus of 'expert opinion' or a non-systematic review of the scientific literature. Increasingly, however, we see the development of formally evidence-based guidelines, derived from a systematic review of the scientific evidence, and therefore (arguably) less susceptible to bias in their conclusions and recommendations [7]. Evidence-based medicine, defined as the process of systematically finding, appraising, and using contemporaneous research findings as the basis for clinical decisions, asks questions, finds and appraises the relevant data, and harnesses that information for everyday clinical practice [8]. A large number of organisations worldwide are now engaged in the development and promulgation of evidence based-guidelines, and these organisations are increasingly collaborating across national boundaries [9,10].

## 3. Guidelines in male infertility

To date, comparatively few guideline development organisations have produced guidelines relevant to the field of subfertility, and few of these in turn are 'evidence-based' in the formal sense. For example, the World Health Organization (WHO) has produced expert guidance in the field of semen analysis [11], the investigation of the infertile couple [12] and the investigation and management of the infertile male [13]. In the USA, the American Urological Association (AUA) and the American Society for Reproductive Medicine (ASRM) have produced a series of four reports, based on expert opinion, covering the optimal evaluation of the infertile male [14], the evaluation of the azoospermic male [15], the management of obstructive azoospermia [16], and varicocele [17]. In Europe, the European Association of Urology (EAU) has produced detailed and extensively referenced guidelines on male infertility [18], and the European Academy of Andrology (EAA) [19] and the European Molecular Genetics Quality Network (EMQN) [20] have produced expert guidance on the laboratory diagnosis of Y-Chromosome microdeletions [21]. Lastly, within the UK, the Royal College of Obstetricians and Gynaecologists (RCOG) has produced more formally evidence based guidelines on the initial investigation and management of infertility [22], the management of infertility in

Table 1
Cochrane reviews of male infertility [27]

*Current reviews*
- Timed intercourse versus intra-uterine insemination with or without ovarian hyperstimulation for subfertility in men [35]
- Surgery or embolization for varicocele in subfertile men [36]
- Intra-uterine versus cervical insemination of donor sperm for subfertility [37]
- Techniques for surgical retrieval of sperm prior to ICSI for azoospermia [38]

*Reviews withdrawn (not updated since 1996)*
- Androgens versus placebo or no treatment for idiopathic oligo/asthenospermia [39]
- Bromocriptine for idiopathic oligo/asthenospermia [40]
- Clomiphene or tamoxifen for idiopathic oligo/asthenospermia [41]
- Kinin-enhancing drugs for unexplained subfertility in men [42]

secondary care [23], and in tertiary care [24]. These guidelines will shortly be superseded by a single guideline currently under development by the UK NHS National Institute for Clinical Excellence (NICE), and due for publication in February 2004. The final draft of this guideline was made available for consultation in August 2003 [25].

### 3.1. Expert guidance and review

The majority of published and electronically available guidance in the field falls into this category. As mentioned above, WHO, the EAU and the AUA/ASRM have provided detailed and comprehensive guidance on the investigation and management of the infertile male [11–18]. Although these documents are clearly based on a review of the available evidence by recognized and authoritative international experts, they tend not to contain explicit evidence of several of the domains outlined in the AGREE guideline appraisal document [26], such as evidence of a systematic literature review.

### 3.2. Evidence-based reviews

Against a background of evidence of varying quality, the Cochrane reviews [27] are widely regarded as the gold standard in the hierarchy of evidence-based medicine [28]. Regrettably, but perhaps unsurprisingly in view of the comments above, the current Cochrane database contains only four active reviews directly relevant to subfertility in the male. A similar number of reviews have been withdrawn, not having been updated since 1996 (Table 1). Other electronic sources of evidence-based clinical guidance, for example Clinical Evidence [29], provide similarly limited coverage (Table 2).

Table 2
Clinical evidence [29]

In couples with male factor infertility
- *Donor insemination*: We found no good evidence on the effects of donor insemination [43]
- *Intracytoplasmic sperm injection plus in vitro fertilisation*: One systematic review found insufficient evidence on the effects of intracytoplasmic sperm injection plus in vitro fertilisation versus in vitro fertilisation alone [44]
- *Intrauterine insemination*: Two systematic reviews have found that intrauterine insemination significantly increases pregnancy rate compared with intracervical insemination or natural intercourse [45]
- *In vitro fertilisation versus gamete intrafallopian transfer*: One RCT found insufficient evidence on the effects of in vitro fertilisation versus gamete intrafallopian transfer [46]

## 3.3. Evidence-based guidelines

The RCOG Guidelines [22–24] probably represented the first attempt to construct a systematic, evidence-based guideline for the field. These have all now passed their 'review by dates,' and will shortly be replaced by guidance from NICE (available in draft form at the time of writing this manuscript) [25].

## 4. Quality of evidence

Whilst there are some areas of practice where evidence is probably not required (as suggested in the recently published systematic review of randomised controlled trials of the parachute [30]), in general it is inevitable that evidence-based guidelines are only as good as the evidence on which they are based, and this is frequently limited either in quantity or in quality. This is certainly true in the field of male subfertility. For example, as Barlow has pointed out [31], when the UK Evidence-Based Clinical Guidelines on the Management of Subfertility were published by the RCOG [22–24] it was noticeable that many of the recommendations for practice could not be based on evidence classifiable as level A (RCT-based). Johnson et al. [32] have identified the many significant gaps in the evidence for fertility treatment, based upon an analysis of the Cochrane Menstrual Disorders and Subfertility Group database, and have demonstrated that of 38 subfertility reviews in the Cochrane Library, there was insufficient evidence of effectiveness in 26 of them. The reviewers in 23 of these reviews called for further research to address their respective questions, despite the large volume of papers published on subfertility topics over many years. This is perhaps not surprising since, as Vail and Gardener [33] have shown, the standards of design, analysis and reporting of many subfertility trials are not sufficient to allow reliable interpretation of results, or inclusion in meta-analyses. Many of the issues to arise have been discussed by Daya [34].

The UK RCOG Guidelines [22–24], published between 1998 and 2000, made 153 recommendations. Of these, 22% were based on grade A evidence, 32% on Grade B, and 45% on Grade C evidence—which relies on expert opinion and has the endorsement of respected authorities. In the final draft of the UK NICE guideline [25] (which makes some 165 recommendations, and was issued in August 2003), 31% are based on Grade A evidence, 24% on grade B and 44% are grade C or less. Looking specifically at those recommendations that focus on the male partner, only 16% of 50 recommendations in the RCOG guidelines, and only 20% of 41 recommendations in the NICE guideline are based on Grade A evidence. Almost one in five recommendations were based on the expert opinion of the guideline development group alone.

## 5. Conclusion

Evidence-based clinical practice guidelines offer an important tool to facilitate the translation of research evidence into clinical care. It is important to recognize that such guidelines are inevitably limited by the extent and quality of the evidence base on which they draw. Even in a rigorously evidence-based guideline, a significant number of recommendations will continue to rely upon expert opinion.

## References

[1] R. Smith, Thoughts for new medical students at a new medical school, BMJ 327 (2003) 1430–1433.
[2] M.R. Chassin, Is health care ready for Six Sigma quality? Milbank Q. 76 (1998) 565-91, 510.
[3] Cochrane Collaboration, The Cochrane Central Register of Controlled Trials, http://www.cochrane.org.
[4] J.M. Grimshaw, et al., Changing physicians' behavior: what works and thoughts on getting more things to work, J. Contin. Educ. Health Prof. 22 (2002) 237–243.
[5] R. Grol, J. Grimshaw, From best evidence to best practice: effective implementation of change in patients' care, Lancet 362 (2003) 1225–1230.
[6] M. Field, K. Lohr, Clinical Practice Guidelines: Directions for a New Program, National Academy Press, Washington, DC, 1990.
[7] Scottish Intercollegiate Guidelines Network (SIGN), SIGN 50: A Guideline Developer's Handbook, SIGN, Edinburgh, 2002.
[8] W. Rosenberg, A. Donald, Evidence based medicine: an approach to clinical problem-solving, BMJ 310 (1995) 1122–1126.
[9] Guidelines International Network, http://www.g-i-n.net/.
[10] The AGREE Collaboration, http://www.agreecollaboration.org/.
[11] World Health Organization, WHO Laboratory Manual for the Examination of Human Semen and Sperm–Cervical Mucus Interaction, Cambridge Univ. Press, Cambridge, 1999.
[12] P.J. Rowe, et al., WHO Manual for the Standardized Investigation and Diagnosis of the Infertile Couple, Cambridge Univ. Press, Cambridge, 1993.
[13] P.J. Rowe, et al., WHO Manual for the Standardized Investigation, Diagnosis and Management of the Infertile Male, Cambridge Univ. Press, Cambridge, 2000.
[14] I.D. Sharlip, et al., Report on Optimal Evaluation of the Infertile Male, American Urological Association & American Society for Reproductive Medicine, Baltimore, MO, USA and Birmingham, AL, USA, 2001, pp. 1–10.
[15] I.D. Sharlip, et al., Report on Evaluation of the Azoospermic Male, American Urological Association & American Society for Reproductive Medicine, Baltimore, MO, USA and Birmingham, AL, USA, 2001, pp. 1–7.
[16] I.D. Sharlip, et al., Report on the Management of Obstructive Azoospermia, American Urological Association & American Society for Reproductive Medicine, Baltimore, MO, USA and Birmingham, AL, USA, 2001, pp. 1–5.
[17] I.D. Sharlip, et al., Report on Varicocele and Infertility, American Urological Association & American Society for Reproductive Medicine, Baltimore, MO, USA and Birmingham, AL, USA, 2001, pp. 1–5.
[18] G.M. Colpi, et al., Guidelines on Infertility, European Association of Urology, Arnhem, Netherlands, 2004, pp. 1–58.
[19] European Academy of Andrology (EAA), http://www.uni-leipzig.de/~eaa/index.html.
[20] European Molecular Genetics Quality Network (EMQN), http://www.emqn.org/emqn.php.
[21] M. Simoni, et al., Laboratory guidelines for molecular diagnosis of Y-chromosomal microdeletions, Int. J. Androl. 22 (1999) 292–299.
[22] The Royal College of Obstetricians and Gynaecologists, The Initial Investigation and Management of the Infertile Couple, RCOG Press, London, 1998.
[23] The Royal College of Obstetricians and Gynaecologists, The Management of Infertility in Secondary Care, RCOG Press, London, 1998.
[24] The Royal College of Obstetricians and Gynaecologists, The Management of Infertility in Tertiary Care, RCOG Press, London, 2000.
[25] National Institute for Clinical Excellence (NICE) (UK), Fertility: assessment and treatment for people with fertility problems: final draft for consultation, The National Collaborating Centre for Women and Children's Health 2003.
[26] The AGREE Collaboration, AGREE instrument training manual, Appraisal of Guidelines for Research and Evaluation, AGREE, London, 2003, pp. 1–73.
[27] The Cochrane Collaboration, http://www.cochrane.org.
[28] P. Glasziou, J. Vandenbroucke, I. Chalmers, Assessing the quality of research, BMJ 328 (2004) 39–41.

[29] Clinical Evidence, http://www.clinicalevidence.com/.
[30] G.C. Smith, J.P. Pell, Parachute use to prevent death and major trauma related to gravitational challenge: systematic review of randomised controlled trials, BMJ 327 (2003) 1459–1461.
[31] D.H. Barlow, The design, publication and interpretation of research in subfertility medicine: uncomfortable issues and challenges to be faced, Hum. Reprod. 18 (2003) 899–901.
[32] N.P. Johnson, M. Proctor, C.M. Farquhar, Gaps in the evidence for fertility treatment—an analysis of the Cochrane Menstrual Disorders and Subfertility Group database, Hum. Reprod. 18 (2003) 947–954.
[33] A. Vail, E. Gardener, Common statistical errors in the design and analysis of subfertility trials, Hum. Reprod. 18 (2003) 1000–1004.
[34] S. Daya, Pitfalls in the design and analysis of efficacy trials in subfertility, Hum. Reprod. 18 (2003) 1005–1009.
[35] B. Cohlen, et al., Timed intercourse versus intra-uterine insemination with or without ovarian hyperstimulation for subfertility in men (Cochrane Review), The Cochrane Library.
[36] J. Evers, J. Collins, P. Vandekerckhove, Surgery or embolization for varicocele in subfertile men (Cochrane Review), The Cochrane Library.
[37] P. O'Brien, P. Vandekerckhove, Intra-uterine versus cervical insemination of donor sperm for subfertility (Cochrane Review), The Cochrane Library.
[38] A. Van Peperstraten, et al., Techniques for surgical retrieval of sperm prior to ICSI for azoospermia (Cochrane Review), The Cochrane Library.
[39] P. Vandekerckhove, et al., Androgens versus placebo or no treatment for idiopathic oligo/asthenospermia (Cochrane Review, Withdrawn), The Cochrane Library.
[40] P. Vandekerckhove, et al., Bromocriptine for idiopathic oligo/asthenospermia (Cochrane Review, Withdrawn), The Cochrane Library.
[41] P. Vandekerckhove, et al., Clomiphene or tamoxifen for idiopathic oligo/asthenospermia (Cochrane Review, Withdrawn), The Cochrane Library.
[42] P. Vandekerckhove, et al., Kinin-enhancing drugs for unexplained subfertility in men (Cochrane Review, Withdrawn), The Cochrane Library.
[43] K. Duckitt, What are the effects of treatments for male infertility : donor insemination, Clinical Evidence, http://www.clinicalevidence.com.
[44] K. Duckitt, What are the effects of treatments for male infertility: Intracytoplasmic sperm injection plus in vitro fertilisation, Clinical Evidence, http://www.clinicalevidence.com.
[45] K. Duckitt, What are the effects of treatments for male infertility: intrauterine insemination, Clinical Evidence, http://www.clinicalevidence.com.
[46] K. Duckitt, What are the effects of treatments for male infertility: in vitro fertilisation versus gamete intrafallopian transfer, Clinical Evidence, http://www.clinicalevidence.com.

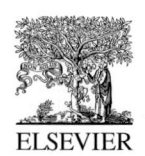

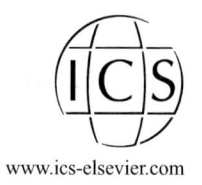

# Intrauterine insemination for idiopathic male subfertility

## B.J. Cohlen*

*Department of Obstetrics and Gynaecology, Isala Clinics Zwolle, Sophia, P.O. Box 10400, Dr. van Heesweg 2, 8000 GK Zwolle, The Netherlands*

**Abstract.** Using evidence from randomized trials, systematic reviews and meta-analyses only, the following conclusions can be drawn regarding intrauterine insemination (IUI) for male subfertility:

1. Compared with timed intercourse, IUI significantly increases the probability of conception [Peto OR with 95% CIs: 3.1 (1.5–6.3)].
2. Mild ovarian hyperstimulation does not increase pregnancy rates, except for couples with a mild semen factor [Peto OR with 95% CIs: 1.4 (0.86–2.4)].
3. In cases where mild ovarian hyperstimulation (MOH) is applied, gonadotropins seem to be more effective compared with clomiphene citrate [Peto OR with 95% CIs: 2.2 (1.2–3.9)].
4. Prevention of multiplets is a major issue when applying MOH. A strategy to prevent multiple pregnancies is proposed.
5. Only a few randomized trials exist that compare the cost-effectiveness of MOH/IUI with IVF-ET and/or ICSI. From the available evidence, it can be concluded that IUI is the most cost-effective treatment option when multiple pregnancies are prevented.
6. There is no difference in treatment outcome after IUI between gradient techniques and swim-up for semen preparation [Peto OR with 95% CIs: 0.55 (0.17–1.76)].
7. Up till now it has been impossible to predict treatment outcome on an individual basis.
8. The post-wash total motile count is a good predictor of non-pregnancy. The optimal cut-off level is between 0.8 and 5 million. Below these levels, ICSI should be considered the treatment option of first choice. © 2004 Published by Elsevier B.V.

*Keywords:* Male subfertility; Intrauterine insemination; Mild ovarian hyperstimulation; Multiple pregnancy; Cost-effectiveness; Predicting factors

## 1. Introduction

In this era of new therapeutic options for couples with male subfertility, "old-fashioned techniques" like intrauterine insemination (IUI), with or without mild ovarian hyperstimulation (MOH), become a matter of debate [1]. Why not offer all couples ICSI or similar

---

* Tel.: +31-38-4245000; fax: +31-38-4247676.
*E-mail address:* b.cohlen@isala.nl (B.J. Cohlen).

techniques, thus offering high perspectives of pregnancy [2]? Or, is new not always better? Is IUI in couples with a male factor cost-effective at all and can we identify those couples that will become pregnant with this non-invasive technique? What is the most optimal semen preparation technique? When should we apply MOH, with which drugs and can we prevent multiple pregnancies?

Using evidence from randomized trials and systematic reviews only, we will try to find answers for these important clinical questions.

## 2. Strength of existing evidence

Ideally, all evidence is gained from large, multi-center studies that provide clear results from well-designed trials in clearly defined populations of subfertile couples. These trials should have adequate power to detect clinical relevant differences in live birth rates per couple. They should have used well-defined 'materials and methods,' applicable in various centers. Intention-to-treat analysis should have been performed and blinding should have been applied when possible.

Regretfully, these trials hardly exist. Most randomized trials (especially those from before the start of the era of evidence-based medicine) are single center, small, without sufficient power, combining various subfertile populations. Results are mostly expressed as pregnancy rates per completed cycle without intention-to-treat analysis. Reasons for drop-out or cancellation of cycles remains unclear, if stated at all. Complications of treatment like multiple or ectopic pregnancies are often not mentioned.

We can only rely on these trials to draw our conclusions from the best available evidence. To increase power, it is sometimes possible to combine the results of several randomized studies into a meta-analysis. However, we should always keep in mind that the quality of any systematic review and meta-analysis depends upon the quality of the trial with the lowest methodological quality.

## 3. Is IUI effective in couples with idiopathic male subfertility?

The rationale for performing IUI is that it increases the number of motile spermatozoa with a high proportion of normal forms at the site of fertilization.

To (dis)prove a beneficial effect of IUI, it should be compared with (timed) intercourse, and the results of these randomized trials should show a statistical significant difference favoring IUI. Furthermore, the material and methods should be applicable in daily practice and the differences in live birth rates (or pregnancy rates) found should have clinical value. To (dis)prove a beneficial effect of ovarian hyperstimulation, MOH should be compared with natural cycles, in combination either with timed intercourse or IUI [3] (Fig. 1).

Comparison 1 of Fig. 1 in couples with a male factor has been the subject of several RCTs. Table 1 shows the results of a meta-analysis [3]. The combined OR with 95% CIs shows a statistically significant improvement of conception rates favoring IUI [Peto OR with 95% CIs: 3.1 (1.5–6.3)]. The pregnancy rates per completed IUI cycle varied between 0% and 8.7%.

Comparison 2 of Fig. 1 in couples with a male factor has been performed in six RCTs. The combined OR with 95% CIs shows a statistically significant improvement of

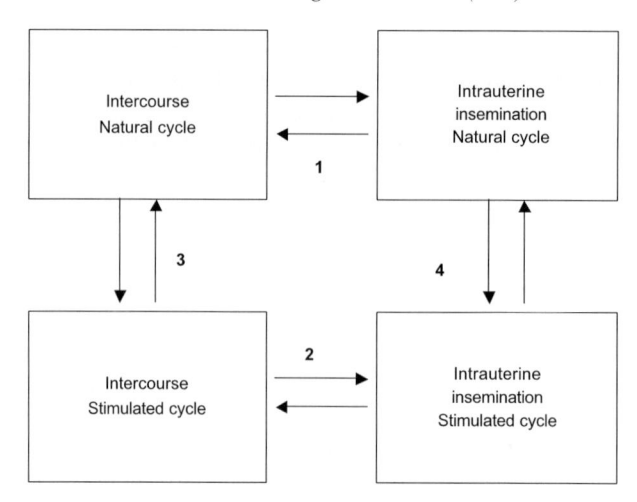

Fig. 1. Comparisons to be performed in randomized trials to (dis)prove a beneficial effect of IUI and/or MOH.

conception rates favoring IUI (Table 2) [Peto OR with 95% CIs: 2.1 (1.3–3.5)]. The pregnancy rates per completed IUI cycle varied considerably: between 0% and 25%.

From these meta-analyses it can be concluded that IUI is effective in the case of a male factor, although pregnancy rates might vary considerably between centers, depending on the definition of male subfertility and, perhaps, different 'materials and methods'.

## 4. Should we apply MOH in the case of male subfertility treated with IUI?

Mild ovarian hyperstimulation might improve timing, corrects subtle cycle disorders and might increase the number of available oocytes. On the other hand, it significantly increases the risks of multiple pregnancies and/or ovarian hyperstimulation syndrome. It should, therefore, be applied only after being proven effective, in experienced hands, with adequate monitoring, strict cancellation criteria and using low-dose step-up protocols [4].

Table 1
Intrauterine insemination (IUI) versus timed intercourse in natural cycles in couples with male subfertility (comparison I, Fig. 1)

| Reference | IUI | | Intercourse | | Peto OR | 95% CIs |
|---|---|---|---|---|---|---|
| | n pregnancies | n cycles | n pregnancies | n cycles | | |
| Kerin and Quinn [27] | 9 | 103 | 0 | 80 | 6.4 | 1.7–24 |
| Glazener et al. [28] | 1 | 87[a] | 1 | 100 | 1.2 | 0.1–19 |
| Ho et al. [29] | 0 | 114 | 1 | 124 | 0.2 | 0.0–7.4 |
| te Velde et al. [30] | 3 | 112 | 2 | 90 | 1.2 | 0.2–7.2 |
| Martinez et al. [31] | 2 | 13[b] | 0 | 13[b] | 8.0 | 0.5–135 |
| Kirby et al. [32] | 10 | 179 | 2 | 154 | 3.4 | 1.1–0.86 |
| Total | 25 | 608 | 6 | 561 | 3.1 | 1.5–6.3 |

Statistical homogeneous ($\chi^2$ 5.47).
[a] High intracervical insemination with unprepared semen.
[b] Assuming an equal number of treatment cycles in each group.

Table 2
Intrauterine insemination (IUI) versus timed intercourse in cycles with mild ovarian hyperstimulation (MOH) in couples with male subfertility (comparison 2, Fig. 1)

| Reference | MOH with IUI | | MOH with intercourse | | Peto OR | 95% CIs |
|---|---|---|---|---|---|---|
| | n pregnancies | n cycles | n pregnancies | n cycles | | |
| Evans et al. [33] | 0 | 22 | 1 | 22 | 0.14 | 0.00–6.8 |
| Martinez et al. [34] | 2 | 28 | 0 | 28 | 7.6 | 0.5–125 |
| Crosignani and Walters [35] | 7 | 48 | 0 | 49 | 8.6 | 1.9–39 |
| Nan et al. [36] | 11 | 107 | 4 | 95 | 2.4 | 0.8–6.9 |
| Melis et al. [37] | 11 | 103 | 12 | 110 | 0.98 | 0.4–2.3 |
| Gregoriou et al. [38] | 15 | 130 | 5 | 128 | 2.9 | 1.2–7.2 |
| Total | 46 | 438 | 22 | 432 | 2.1 | 1.3–3.5 |

Statistical homogeneous ($\chi^2$ 9.54).

Table 3 shows the pregnancy rates per completed cycle of five trials that compared IUI in stimulated cycles with IUI in natural cycles in couples with male subfertility (comparison 4, Fig. 1). The Peto odds ratio is 1.4 with a 95% confidence interval of 0.86–2.4. Thus, in the case of a male factor, MOH does not seem to improve the probability of conception.

The study by Cohlen et al. [5] differentiates between couples with a severe or moderate male factor (total motile sperm count on average below $10 \times 10^6$) and those with a mild male factor (total motile sperm count above $10 \times 10^6$). In couples with a mild male factor, MOH with low-dose gonadotropins significantly improves the probability of conception, whereas in couples with a severe or moderate male factor, it does not. It is suggested that in the case of a severe male factor the subfertility of the couple is solely due to the male factor. In these couples, IUI alone significantly increases the chance to conceive (see Table 1) and ovarian hyperstimulation does not further improve treatment outcome. In couples with a less severe semen defect, almost resembling couples with unexplained subfertility, the subfertility of the couple is probably due to a combination of male and subtle female factors. For such couples, ovarian hyperstimulation might improve the quality of the cycle as it has been proven effective in couples with unexplained subfertility [6].

Table 3
Intrauterine insemination (IUI) in natural cycles versus IUI in cycles with mild ovarian hyperstimulation (MOH) in couples with male subfertility (comparison 4, Fig. 1)

| Reference | IUI with MOH | | IUI in natural cycles | | Peto OR | 95% CIs |
|---|---|---|---|---|---|---|
| | n pregnancies | n cycles | n pregnancies | n cycles | | |
| Arici et al. [39] | 1 | 26 | 1 | 26 | 1.0 | 0.06–16 |
| Cohlen et al. [5] | 21 | 153 | 13 | 155 | 1.7 | 0.84–3.5 |
| Goverde et al. [15][a] | 9 | 102 | 11 | 105 | 0.83 | 0.33–2.1 |
| Martinez et al. [31] | 2 | 14 | 2 | 10 | 0.67 | 0.08–5.7 |
| Nulsen et al. [40] | 7 | 54 | 1 | 41 | 3.9 | 0.90–16 |
| Total | 40 | 349 | 28 | 337 | 1.4 | 0.86–2.4 |

Statistically homogeneous ($\chi^2$ 3.94).
[a] Results are given as pregnancies per started cycle.

## 5. When MOH is applied: clomiphene citrate or gonadotropins?

Clomiphene citrate (CC) is used extensively in subfertility treatment, being cheap, easy to apply and probably effective. Gonadotropins are effective, however, also more expensive and only applicable as subcutaneous injections. Since MOH turns out to be a major risk factor for multiple pregnancies in IUI, this side effect should be included in the overall decision of which drug to choose as the one of first choice. Both Hughes [6] and Cohlen [3] discussed the use of CC in IUI cycles in their systematic reviews and concluded that CC seemed less effective.

The comparison between CC and gonadotropins has been the subject of several small RCTs [7–10]. Regretfully, the conclusions are contradictory and the trials are too small to draw any firm conclusion, let alone for couples with male subfertility only. When the results, expressed as pregnancy rate per couple, of these four small RCTs are combined in a meta-analysis, a statistically significant difference is found in favor of gonadotropins [Peto OR with 95% CIs: 2.2 (1.2–3.9)] (unpublished data). Multiple pregnancies are not always mentioned and cost-effectiveness has not been an outcome of interest. Therefore, we have to wait until the final results are published of a large ongoing multi-center study in the Netherlands in which the cost-effectiveness of CC is compared with that of gonadotropins, also in couples with male subfertility.

## 6. Can we prevent multiple pregnancies after MOH/IUI?

Cycles with ovarian hyperstimulation are usually monitored by ultrasound assessment of follicular number and size and/or estradiol measurements. Several large retrospective trials have been published on this subject [11–14]. Although these trials were clinically heterogeneous, the probability of achieving a multiple pregnancy seemed to be related to the age of the woman, the total number of follicles and/or the number of follicles larger than 11 mm at hCG administration. The parameters found in these retrospective trials should be checked in large prospective trials using ROC curves to determine optimal cut-off values. From several randomized trials on COH/IUI, it can be concluded that the probability of achieving a multiple pregnancy is correlated with the aggressiveness of the stimulation protocol and the applied cancellation criteria [5,7,15,16]. Randomized trials comparing different low-dose stimulation protocols for IUI (for instance, 50 IU FSH per day versus 75 IU FSH per day) in a well-defined, subfertile population using strict cancellation criteria should be conducted to define the optimal stimulation protocol-acceptable pregnancy rates with only very few, or even zero, multiple pregnancies. Fig. 2 shows a proposed strategy to prevent multiple pregnancies after MOH/IUI [4].

## 7. MOH/IUI versus IVF-ET: comparison of cost-effectiveness

Only a few trials have been performed that compared the cost-effectiveness of MOH/IUI with IVF-ET. The elegant RCT of Goverde et al. [15] clearly showed MOH/IUI to be more cost-effective compared with IVF/ET. The cost per live birth after MOH/IUI was approximately US$5000, whereas after IVF-ET it was approximately US$13,000. A randomized trial comparing IUI with IVF by Karande et al. [17] came to the same

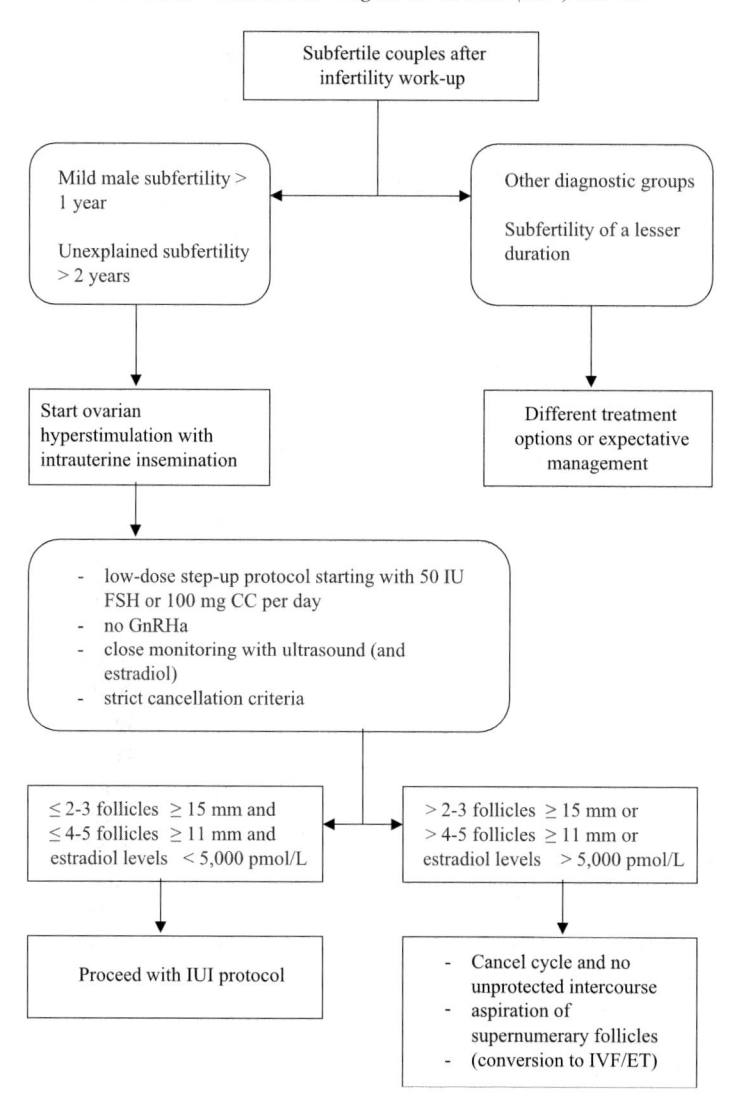

Fig. 2. Proposed strategy to prevent multiple pregnancies in ovarian stimulation in combination with intrauterine insemination.

conclusion, although both costs were considerably higher. Unfortunately, both trials did not include the neonatal costs of preterm birth of multiple pregnancies. A recent published abstract showed that the high costs of MOH/IUI are directly correlated with the number of multiple pregnancies, thus preventing multiplets should be a major goal when applying MOH/IUI [18]. Only then MOH/IUI seems to be more cost-effective. A review on the published literature up to 1998 also concluded that in the absence of a severe male factor IUI, or the combination of MOH and IUI, is more cost-effective than IVF [19]. The investigators calculated the cost per delivery for hMG/IUI to be approximately US$10,000 compared with US$43,000 for IVF-ET. In this review, the costs of multiple pregnancies and premature deliveries is discussed but not incorporated in the numbers mentioned above.

Using modeling techniques with data derived from a systematic review, national UK data and expert opinion, Philips et al. [20] concluded that in case of moderate male subfertility, IUI in cycles with MOH is more cost-effective compared with ICSI (average cost per pregnancy: MOH/IUI, US$9450; ICSI, US$17,000–15,300).

To further reduce costs, only one insemination per cycle should be offered. We have shown in a recently published systematic review that a second insemination per cycle does not improve treatment outcome, and is therefore not cost-effective [Peto OR with 95% CIs: 1.45 (0.78–2.7)] [21]. It has been suggested that MOH/IUI treatment should be limited to three treatment cycles only [22].

## 8. Semen preparation technique for IUI in case of a semen defect

Several semen preparation techniques have been described in the literature. The techniques used most often include gradient techniques, swim-up and simple wash and centrifugation. At the moment we are preparing a systematic Cochrane review on this subject (Boomsma et al., unpublished data). The first conclusion should be that the methodological quality of the published trials on this subject is very low. Only two trials can be included for meta-analysis. There seems to be no statistical, significant difference in IUI outcome (pregnancy rate per couple) after swim-up or gradient techniques [Peto OR with 95% CIs: 0.55 (0.17–1.76)]. Regarding recovery rates after semen preparation, gradient techniques seem to result in the highest recovery rates. However, whether this results in higher pregnancy rates after IUI needs to be further investigated in a large randomized trial.

## 9. Can we predict the outcome of IUI with or without MOH?

Up till now it has been impossible to counsel subfertile couples on an individual basis about their probability of success or failure after IUI, with or without MOH. Several prediction models have been proposed to predict the probability of spontaneous conception [23,24]. Based on prospectively collected data of very large subfertile populations undergoing IUI treatment such models might be constructed to predict IUI outcome. However, the outcome after IUI seems to be related to various factors, including age of the woman, duration of subfertility, history of pelvic inflammation, timing of insemination and parameters related to the inseminate [25]. The latter factor has been the subject of a recently performed meta-analysis (van Weert and co-workers, unpublished data). The investigators found that the post-wash total motile count at insemination has potential in predicting IUI outcome. At cut-off levels between 0.8 and 5 million motile spermatozoa, the specificity of the post-wash total motile count defined as the ability to predict non-pregnancy was as high as 100%, while the sensitivity of the test, defined as the ability to predict pregnancy, was limited.

Others performed a meta-analysis on the role of normal morphology using strict criteria on IUI outcome [26]. They concluded that a poor ($\leq 4\%$) sperm morphology significantly reduces the chance of achieving pregnancy after IUI.

## 10. Conclusion

There seems to be robust evidence to support the conclusion that compared with timed intercourse, IUI is cost-effective for couples with male subfertility. After semen preparation with a gradient technique, at least 0.8–5 million motile spermatozoa should be obtained to make the procedure useful. In cases of severe semen defects with less than 1 million motile spermatozoa after semen preparation, ICSI should probably be the treatment option of first choice. In cases of a moderate semen defect with a total motile sperm count of less than 10 million, IUI in natural cycles should be offered. In cases of only a mild semen defect, almost resembling unexplained subfertility, IUI should be combined with MOH.

Compared with IVF-ET all RCTs published up till now consider IUI to be more cost-effective, although various indications for treatment were combined and neonatal costs of multiple birth were not included. Costs after IUI/MOH rise tremendously when multiple pregnancy rates are high. We should therefore focus on preventing multiplets without compromising pregnancy rates. A strategy has been proposed (Fig. 2). Costs can be further reduced by performing only one insemination per cycle and restricting the number of treatment cycles to three. Whether clomiphene citrate or gonadotropins should be used when MOH is applied is the subject of an ongoing multi-center trial. The existing evidence is in favor of gonadotropins.

Because it is at the moment not possible to give individualized advice based on several clinical parameters, couples should be able to make judgments about what they consider reasonable perspectives for pregnancy themselves. When costs are not an issue for the couple, new techniques like IVF-ET or ICSI might be first line treatment options. Otherwise, an "old-fashioned technique" like IUI, with or without MOH, is still a very effective tool in treating subfertile couples with a male factor.

## References

[1] J.A. Stewart, Stimulated intra-uterine insemination is not a natural choice for the treatment of unexplained subfertility. Should the guidelines be changed? Hum. Reprod. 18 (2003) 903–907.
[2] S. Fishel, et al., Should ICSI be the treatment of choice for all cases of in vitro conception? Hum. Reprod. 15 (2000) 1278–1283.
[3] B.J. Cohlen, et al., Timed intercourse versus intra-uterine insemination with or without ovarian hyperstimulation for subfertility in men, Cochrane Database Syst. Rev. (2) (CD000360).
[4] B. Cohlen, P. van Dop, Prevention of multiple pregnancies after non-in vitro fertilization treatment, in: J. Gerris, F. Olivennes, P. de Sutter (Eds.), Assisted Reproductive Technologies. Quality and Safety, The Parthenon Publishing Group, London, 2004, pp. 39–48.
[5] B.J. Cohlen, et al., Controlled ovarian hyperstimulation and intrauterine insemination for treating male subfertility: a controlled study, Hum. Reprod. 13 (6) (1998) 1553–1558.
[6] E.G. Hughes, The effectiveness of ovulation induction and intrauterine insemination in the treatment of persistent infertility: a meta-analysis, Hum. Reprod. 12 (1997) 1865–1872.
[7] J. Balasch, et al., Late low-dose pure follicle stimulating hormone for ovarian stimulation in intra-uterine insemination cycles, Hum. Reprod. 9 (10) (1994) 1863–1866.
[8] R. Matorras, et al., Ovarian stimulation in intrauterine insemination with donor sperm: a randomized study comparing clomiphene citrate in fixed protocol versus highly purified urinary FSH, Hum. Reprod. 17 (8) (2002) 2107–2111.
[9] R. Ecochard, et al., A randomized prospective study comparing pregnancy rates after clomiphene citrate and human menopausal gonadotropin before intrauterine insemination, Fertil. Steril. 73 (2000) 90–93.

[10] P.O. Karlstrom, T. Bergh, O. Lundkvist, A prospective randomized trial of artificial insemination versus intercourse in cycles stimulated with human menopausal gonadotropin or clomiphene citrate, Fertil. Steril. 59 (1993) 554–559.
[11] R.P. Dickey, et al., Relationship of follicle numbers and estradiol levels to multiple implantation in 3608 intrauterine insemination cycles, Fertil. Steril. 75 (2001) 69–78.
[12] R. Tur, et al., Risk factors for high-order multiple implantation after ovarian stimulation with gonadotrophins: evidence from a large series of 1,878 consecutive pregnancies in a single centre, Hum. Reprod. 16 (2001) 2124–2129.
[13] P.F. Kaplan, et al., Assessing the risk of multiple gestation in gonadotropin intrauterine insemination cycles, Am. J. Obstet. Gynecol. 186 (2002) 1244–1249.
[14] N. Gleicher, et al., Reducing the risk of high-order multiple pregnancy after ovarian stimulation with gonadotropins, N. Engl. J. Med. 343 (2000) 2–7.
[15] A.J. Goverde, et al., Intrauterine insemination or in vitro fertilisation in idiopathic subfertility and male subfertility: a randomized trial and cost-effectiveness analysis, Lancet 355 (2000) 13–18.
[16] D.S. Guzick, et al., Efficacy of superovulation and intrauterine insemination in the treatment of infertility, National Cooperative Reproductive Medicine Network, N. Engl. J. Med. 340 (1999) 177–183.
[17] V.C. Karande, et al., Prospective randomized trial comparing the outcome and cost of in vitro fertilization with that of a traditional treatment algorithm as first-line therapy for couples with infertility, Fertil. Steril. 71 (1999) 468–475.
[18] S.K. Kalra, M.P. Milad, W.A. Grobman, In vitro fertilization versus COH/IUI as first line treatment for unexplained infertility in women under 35: a cost-based decision analysis, Fertil. Steril. 80 (Suppl. 3) (2003) P47.
[19] B.J. Van Voorhis, et al., Cost-effective treatment of the infertile couple, Fertil. Steril. 70 (1998) 995–1005.
[20] Z. Philips, M. Barraza-Llorens, J. Posnett, Evaluation of the relative cost-effectiveness of treatments for infertility in the UK, Hum. Reprod. 15 (2000) 95–106.
[21] A.E.P. Cantineau, M.J. Heineman, B.J. Cohlen, Single versus double intrauterine insemination in stimulated cycles for subfertile couples: a systematic review based on a Cochrane review, Hum. Reprod. 18 (2003) 941–946.
[22] M. Aboulghar, et al., Controlled ovarian hyperstimulation and intrauterine insemination for treatment of unexplained infertility should be limited to a maximum of three trials, Fertil. Steril. 75 (2001) 88–91.
[23] J.M. Eimers, et al., The prediction of the chance to conceive in subfertile couples, Fertil. Steril. 61 (1994) 44–52.
[24] J.A. Collins, E.A. Burrows, A.R. Wilan, The prognosis for live birth among untreated infertile couples, Fertil. Steril. 64 (1995) 22–28.
[25] H.E. Duran, et al., Intrauterine insemination: a systematic review on determinants of success, Hum. Reprod. Updat. 8 (2002) 373–384.
[26] J. Van Waart, et al., Predictive value of normal sperm morphology in intrauterine insemination (IUI): a structured literature review, Hum. Reprod. Updat. 7 (2001) 495–500.
[27] J.F.P. Kerin, P. Quinn, Washed intrauterine insemination in the treatment of oligospermic infertility, Semin. Reprod. Endocrinol. 5 (1987) 23–33.
[28] C.M.A. Glazener, et al., The value of artificial insemination with husband's semen in infertility due to failure of postcoital sperm-mucus penetration-controlled trial of treatment, Br. J. Obstet. Gynaecol. 94 (1987) 774–778.
[29] P.-C. Ho, et al., Intrauterine insemination is not useful in oligoasthenospermia, Fertil. Steril. 51 (1989) 682–684.
[30] E.R. te Velde, R.J. van Kooij, J.J.H. Waterreus, Intrauterine insemination of washed husband's spermatozoa: a controlled study, Fertil. Steril. 51 (1989) 182–185.
[31] A.R. Martinez, et al., Intrauterine insemination does and clomiphene citrate does not improve fecundity in a prospective, randomized, controlled study, Fertil. Steril. 53 (1990) 847–853.
[32] C.A. Kirby, et al., A prospective trial of intrauterine insemination of motile spermatozoa versus timed intercourse, Fertil. Steril. 56 (1991) 102–107.
[33] J. Evans, et al., A comparison of intrauterine insemination, intraperitoneal insemination, and natural intercourse in superovulated women, Fertil. Steril. 56 (1991) 1183–1187.

[34] A.R. Martinez, et al., Pregnancy rates after timed intercourse or intrauterine insemination after human menopausal gonadotropin stimulation of normal ovulatory cycles: a controlled study, Fertil. Steril. 55 (1991) 258–265.
[35] P.G. Crosignani, D.E. Walters, Clinical pregnancy and male subfertility: the ESHRE multicentre trial on the treatment of male subfertility, Hum. Reprod. 9 (1994) 1112–1118.
[36] P.M. Nan, et al., Intra-uterine insemination or timed intercourse after ovarian stimulation for male subfertility? A controlled study, Hum. Reprod. 9 (1994) 2022–2026.
[37] G.B. Melis, et al., Ovulation induction with gonadotropins as sole treatment in infertile couples with open tubes: a randomized prospective comparison between intrauterine insemination and timed vaginal intercourse, Fertil. Steril. 64 (1995) 1088–1093.
[38] O. Gregoriou, et al., Pregnancy rates in gonadotrophin stimulated cycles with timed intercourse or intrauterine insemination for the treatment of male subfertility, Eur. J. Obstet. Gynecol. Reprod. Biol. 64 (1996) 213–216.
[39] A. Arici, et al., Evaluation of clomiphene citrate and human chorionic gonadotropin treatment: a prospective, randomized, crossover study during intrauterine insemination cycles, Fertil. Steril. 61 (1994) 314–318.
[40] J.C. Nulsen, et al., A randomized and longitudinal study of human menopausal gonadotropin with intrauterine insemination in the treatment of infertility, Obstet. Gynecol. 82 (1993) 780–786.

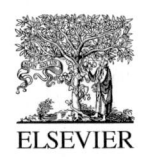

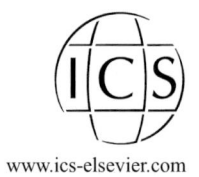

# Leukocytospermia

## Roelof Menkveld*

*Andrology Laboratory E3, Reproductive Biology Unit, Department of Obstetrics and Gynaecology, Tygerberg Hospital and University of Stellenbosch, Tygerberg, 7505, South Africa*

**Abstract.** The role of leukocytes in semen (leukocytospermia) is still controversial. Contradictory reports on leukocytospermia have been published indicating negative effects on semen parameters and even in vitro fertilization (IVF) results, while other investigators did not find any negative influences of leukocytospermia on semen parameters. A few papers indicated a positive role for seminal leukocytes by elimination of morphological abnormal spermatozoa by phagocytosis. However, from the most recent literature, it is now clear that the most important deleterious effect of leukocytospermia may be the production of reactive oxygen species (ROS) causing DNA fragmentation of spermatozoa, leading to significant reduced pregnancy rates with IVF and intracytoplasmic sperm injection (ICSI) when oocytes are inseminated with spermatozoa from leukocytospermic semen samples. Contradictive results on treatment of leukocytospermia by antibiotics have also been published. However, a survey of the literature indicated that more evidence is presented testifying that antibiotic treatment of leukocytospermia may be beneficial by lowering the number of seminal leukocytes and even improving semen parameters. Therefore, treating leukocytospermia seems indicated. © 2004 Published by Elsevier B.V.

*Keywords:* Leukocytospermia; Semen parameters; Antibiotic treatment; ROS production; DNA fragmentation

## 1. Introduction

The role, if any, played by the presence of white blood cells (WBC) in semen, called leukocytospermia, is a subject of great controversy, as illustrated in the following article titles:

- The removal of morphologically abnormal sperm forms by phagocytes: a positive role for seminal leukocytes? [1]
- Infection and pyospermia in male infertility. Is it really a problem? [2]
- Should male infertility patients be tested for leukocytospermia? [3]
- Semen leukocytes: friends or foes? [4]
- Seminal leukocytes: passengers, terrorist or good Samaritans? [5]

---

\* Tel.: +27-21-938-4851; fax: +27-21-9399345.
 *E-mail address:* rme@sun.ac.za (R. Menkveld).

0531-5131/ © 2004 Published by Elsevier B.V.
doi:10.1016/j.ics.2004.01.094

From these few titles, it is already clear that no consensus exists on the role and importance of leukocytospermia and that different studies have come to different conclusions. The matter is further complicated by the fact that leukocytospermia was found to be present in semen samples of men without diagnosed genital tract infections and vice versa. Matters are further complicated by the fact that different subpopulations of leukocytes and the manner in which leukocytospermia is diagnosed may also play roles in the outcome of a specific study [6,7].

The aim of this presentation is, therefore, to reevaluate the current status of leukocytospermia according to the more recent literature, with regard to the possible effect on semen parameters and sperm function and especially with emphasis on the role of treatment of leukocytospermia with antibiotics.

## 2. Controversy on leukocytospermia

Controversy exists on what can be regarded as leukocytospermia, sometimes also called pyospermia [8,9]. The WHO manual [10] defines leukocytospermia as the presence of excessive numbers of white blood cells (WBC) or leukocytes in the human ejaculate, which are predominantly granulocytes and, more specifically, of the neutrophil subtype [11], and states that, in a normal ejaculate, the number of WBC should be $<1\times10^6$/ml semen. However, this is an empirical value [5,6] and regarded in the more recent literature as being too high; lower cut-off values as low as $0.25\times10^6$ and $0.2\times10^6$ WBC/ml semen have been proposed [6,12]. To add further to the controversy, the published incidence of leukocytospermia, as found in infertile male populations, varies widely from 6.8% to 32.0% [12–16].

The notion that the presence of leukocytes in semen may have a negative impact on semen parameters and sperm function was published as early as 1980 by Comhaire et al. [14] and in 1982 by Berger et al. [8]. However, in 1992 and 1993, Tomlinson et al. [1,11,17] published three articles with an opposite view. The first article indicated that seminal leukocytes may play a positive role in male fertility through the removal of morphologically abnormal spermatozoa by phagocytosis [1]. The second suggested that the presence of immature germ cells, but not leukocytes, in semen is associated with reduced success rates of in vitro fertilization (IVF) [11]. The third, a prospective study, suggested that leukocytes and leukocyte subpopulations in semen do not act as a cause for male infertility [17].

In contrast to these publications by Tomlinson et al. [1,11,17], suggesting a positive role for leukocytes as a scavenger for abnormal spermatozoa, other papers have reported that normal sperm morphology is significantly reduced in the presence of leukocytospermia [6,7,18] and positively correlated with increased midpiece abnormalities [18] and elongated spermatozoa [6,7]. Matters are even more complicated by reports that inflammatory episodes in the male reproductive tract and leukocytospermia are temporary and self-limiting events that are probably common phenomena, even in fertile men [19,20].

## 3. Sources of seminal leukocytes

According to Barratt et al. [21], leukocytospermia has a heterogeneous etiology, including infections, inflammations, and autoimmunity, making the immediate cause for this condition quite complex and unclear. Most cases of leukocytes in semen are presumed to originate from some sort of infection, but most men with leukocytospermia have negative cultures of samples obtained from the seminal tract [3]. A very poor relationship exists between the presence of bacteriospermia and leukocytospermia [15]. It is thought that, in some males with leukocytospermia, the origin may be from sources outside the genital tract [19]. For instance, Close et al. [9] found that current cigarette smokers, marijuana users, and heavy alcohol users showed a statistically significant greater number of leukocytes in the seminal fluid than nonusers, while Trum et al. [15] concluded that leukocytospermia was associated with a history of gonorrhea, and Matthews et al. [22] found increased seminal leukocyte concentrations after clomiphene citrate treatment.

## 4. Detection of seminal leukocytes

The most basic method for detecting WBC in semen samples is by direct observation of semen-stained smears by bright field light microscopy [6,7,12]. However, the cytological identification of WBC has been regarded as an insufficient method by some investigators, the argument being the inability to distinguish between different WBC forms and immature germinal epithelium cells [23]. However, positive identification of both groups is possible with a good staining method such as the Papanicolaou method [6,7,24].

Two cytochemical techniques, based on the presence of intracellular peroxidase and on leukocytes-specific antigens, are given in the WHO manual [10]. The first is the leukocyte peroxidase technique and the other is the pan-leukocyte monoclonal antibody technique. According to the WHO manual [10], the leukocyte peroxidase technique gives estimates that are lower than those obtained using the monoclonal antibody technique. This difference may be due to the fact that the leukocyte peroxidase test cannot identify lymphocytes and monocytes that are identified with the monoclonal antibody tests, whereby granulocytes, lymphocytes, and macrophages are also detected [25,26]. Therefore, immunocytochemistry can be considered the gold standard [26], but these methods are time consuming and labour intensive, and are thus more suitable as a research tool than a routine method.

Flow cytometry using monoclonal antibodies is a simple and reproducible method for detecting and identifying WBC subpopulations without preliminary purification procedures [27]. Another method for the identification of the presence of leukocytospermia is the detection of PMN elastase [26]. The enzyme elastase is secreted by activated granulocytes, and can be measured in fresh or frozen seminal plasma; strong correlations were found between elastase levels and WBC numbers in semen [26,28].

However, for practical reasons, it has been proposed that the leukocyte peroxidase test can be considered as a reliable method and suitable for routine use [26], also seen in the light that polymorphonuclear granulocytes are the most prevalent WBC in semen and, furthermore, that the results of the leukocyte peroxidase test (Endtz test) are very strongly correlated with reactive oxygen species (ROS) formation in semen [29]. It appears, therefore, that the peroxidase test will be the method of choice for routine investigations. More experienced investigators can use the semen cytological method, as it has been shown that WBC identified in this manner are correlated with observed sperm morphological abnormalities [6,7].

## 5. Effect of leukocytospermia on semen parameters and sperm function

Apart from the negative effects as published by Comhaire et al. [14], Berger et al. [8], Wolff [23,26], Thomas et al. [18], and Menkveld and Kruger [6], many other negative reports have also been published. Chan et al. [30] found that leukocytospermia decreases sperm hyperactivation but not motility, and Arata de Bellabarba et al. [16] found it to have negative effects on sperm concentrations, motility, normal sperm morphology, and hypo-osmotic swelling tests scores, to mention a few.

No effect or positive effects of leukocytospermia, apart from Tomlinson et al. [1,11,17], have been published. Eggert-Kruse et al. [13] did not find any significant association between leukocytospermia and the production of IgA and IgG antisperm antibodies in semen. Kaleli et al. [31] found a significant positive correlation between increased leukocyte counts and increased hypo-osmotic swelling test scores, higher sperm concentrations, and enhanced acrosome reactions. Kiessling et al. [4] found higher frequencies of spermatozoa with normal morphology in the presence of leukocytospermia.

From the most recent literature, it is now clear that the main negative effect of leukocytospermia is the production of ROS, causing sperm DNA fragmentation [32–34]. It was found by Henkel et al. [33,34] that DNA fragmentation did not correlate with in vitro fertilization rates, but there was a significant reduced pregnancy rate after in vitro fertilization (IVF) and intracytoplasmic sperm injection (ICSI) when oocytes were inseminated by spermatozoa of samples showing DNA damage, compared with normal sperm samples. This finding implies that spermatozoa with damaged DNA are able to fertilize an oocyte, but that, at the time the parental genome is switched on, further development of the embryo stops, leading to a lower pregnancy rate [33,34].

## 6. Treatment of leukocytospermia

Leukocytospermia has routinely been treated by antibiotics [3,19] but this issue is also controversial. Skau and Folstad [35] performed a meta-analysis on the effectiveness of leukocytospermia treatment by broad-spectrum antibiotics. Following certain selection criteria and excluding men suffering from any other condition, including proven or suspected of genital tract infections, but including men showing bacteriospermia only, 12 studies were identified as suitable for analysis. The results of their study indicated that the most used antibiotics were doxycycline, erythromycin, and trimethoprim in combination with sulfamethoxazole, which are all considered as broad-spectrum antibiotics. After complex statistical manipulation of the data obtained from the 12 articles, Skau and Folstad [35] concluded that treatment of leukocytospermia by broad-spectrum antibiotics resulted in significant improvements in semen quality. When the results on the different semen parameters were expressed as weighted effect sizes, the smallest effect was found for sperm concentration with a mean weighted effect size of 0.16, followed by semen volume and sperm motility with a mean weighted effect of 0.20, and an improvement in normal sperm morphology with a weighted effect size of 0.22. The best response to antibiotic treatment was a significant reduction in the concentration of leukocytes in the semen samples with a mean weighted effect size of 0.23.

Table 1 represents the results of a literature survey [20,36–41], performed for this presentation, involving articles concentrating on treatment of leukocytospermia as the main parameter. Interesting was the observation by Branigan and Muller [36] that antibiotic treatment, together with higher ejaculation frequencies, enhanced the disappearance of leukocytes from semen samples. Similar results were also published by Yamamoto et al. [42].

According to Purvis and Christiansen [19], there may be several reasons for difficulties in showing an effect of antibiotic treatment on male infertility, one being that the type of antibiotic therapy may not have been appropriate for the organism responsible and another that the dose or duration of treatment may have been inadequate. Differences in, especially, the duration of treatment and the time lapse after treatment to the follow-up semen analyses also complicates the interpretation of treatment results, as well as differences on what can be regarded as a successful treatment end point. This issue has been illustrated in the study by Erel et al. [39] who found a significant reduction in the number of leukocytes but did not regard this as a positive response because leukocytospermia was still present in some of the males after treatment.

Some authors have indicated that men with symptoms of genital tract infection (leukocytospermia) should be treated as soon as possible, often as partner therapy, to avoid the severe sequelae of ascending infections [2,25]. However, these authors have also

Table 1
Results of a literature survey, performed for this presentation, of antibiotic treatment of males with leukocytospermia as primary target

| Authors | Number | Treatment | Outcome measurement |
|---|---|---|---|
| **Positive response** | | | |
| Branigan and Muller, 1994 [36] | 25 | Doxycycline | Decrease in leukocytes |
| | 25 | None | |
| | 22 | Frequent ejaculation | |
| | 23 | Doxycycline and frequent ejaculation[a] | |
| Branigan et al., 1995 [37] | 53 | Doxycycline | Increased pregnancy rate |
| | 42 | None | |
| Fedder, 1996 [38] | 11 | Not specified | Decrease in leukocytes/increased pregnancy rate |
| Erel et al., 1997 [39] | 24 | Placebo | Decrease in leukocytes |
| | 25 | Doxycycline | |
| | 21 | Doxycycline and ceftriaxone | |
| Montag et al., 1998[b] [40] | 1 | Doxycycline and diclofenac | Decrease in leukocytes/appearance of sperm |
| **No response** | | | |
| Yanushpolsky et al., 1995 [20] | 17 | None | Decrease in leukocytes |
| | 13 | Doxycycine | |
| | 11 | Trimethoprim and sulfamethoxazole | |
| Erel et al., 1997 [39] | 24 | Placebo | Disappearance of leukocytes |
| | 25 | Doxycycline | |
| | 21 | Doxycycline and ceftriaxone | |
| Krisp et al., 2003 [41] | 18 | Levofloxacine | Significant decrease in leukocytes |
| | 18 | None | |

[a] Results are better compared with antibiotic treatment alone.
[b] Case study of male with azoospermia.

strongly warned, like many others, that antibiotic treatment should be used with caution and only used when clearly indicated, especially in healthy individuals. The reason being that the noncritical use of antibiotics may result in resistant strains of bacteria and that certain antibiotics may also have a possible toxic effect on spermatogenesis.

## 7. Conclusion

From the literature, it appears that the arbitrary value of $>1 \times 10^6$ WBC /ml semen, indicated in the WHO manual [10], may be too high to be of clinical value. It seems that the most pronounced negative effect of leukocytospermia is the production of ROS causing sperm DNA fragmentation, which in turn can causes lower pregnancy rates after IVF or ICSI. Therefore, although there still seems to be controversy over the treatment of leukocytospermia with board spectrum antibiotics, it may well be indicated to treat men with leukocytospermia with antibiotics, as the main effect of treatment, seems to be a reduction in the amount of WBC present in semen samples. This reduction can decrease ROS production and, although not seen in increased fertilization rates, can lead to higher pregnancy rates.

## References

[1] M.J. Tomlinson, et al., The removal of morphologically abnormal sperm forms by phagocytes: a positive role for seminal leukocytes? Hum. Reprod. 10 (1992) 517–522.
[2] N. Bar-Chama, E. Goluboff, H. Fisch, Infection and pyospermia in male infertility. Is it really a problem? Urol. Clin. North Am. 21 (1994) 469–475.
[3] D.J. Anderson, Should male infertility patients be tested for leukocytospermia? Fertil. Steril. 63 (1995) 246–248.
[4] A.A. Kiessling, et al., Semin leukocytes: friends of foes? Fertil. Steril. 64 (1995) 196–198.
[5] R.J. Aitken, H.W.G. Baker, Seminal leukocytes: passengers, terrorists or good Samaritans? Hum. Reprod. 10 (1995) 1736–1739.
[6] R. Menkveld, T.F. Kruger, Sperm morphology and male urogenital infections, Andrologia 30 (Suppl. 1) (1998) 49–53.
[7] R. Menkveld, et al., Morphological sperm alternations in different types of prostatitis, Andrologia 35 (2003) 288–293.
[8] R.E. Berger, et al., The relationship of pyospermia and seminal fluid bacteriology to sperm function as reflected in the sperm penetration assay, Fertil. Steril. 37 (1982) 557–564.
[9] C.E. Close, P.A. Roberts, R.E. Berger, Cigarettes, alcohol and marijuana are related to pyospermia in infertile men, J. Urol. 144 (1990) 900–903.
[10] World Health Organization, WHO Laboratory Manual for the Examination of Human Semen and Sperm–Cervical Mucus Interaction, Third ed., Cambridge Univ. Press, Cambridge, 1999.
[11] M.J. Tomlinson, C.L.R. Barratt, I.D. Cooke, Prospective study of leukocytes and leukocytes subpopulations in semen suggest they are not a cause of male infertility, Fertil. Steril. 60 (1993) 1069–1075.
[12] M. Punab, et al., The limit of leukocytospermia from the microbiological viewpoint, Andrologia 35 (2003) 271–278.
[13] W. Eggert-Kruse, et al., Induction of immunoresponse by subclinical male genital tract infection? Fertil. Steril. 65 (1996) 1202–1209.
[14] F. Comhaire, G. Verschraegen, L. Vermeulen, Diagnosis of accessory gland infection and possible role in male infertility, Int. J. Androl. 3 (1980) 32–45.
[15] J.W. Trum, et al., Value of detecting leukocytospermia in the diagnosis of genital tract infection in subfertile men, Fertil. Steril. 70 (1998) 315–319.
[16] G. Arata de Bellabarba, et al., Nonsperm cells in human semen and their relationship with semen parameters, Arch. Androl. 45 (2000) 131–136.

[17] M.J. Tomlinson, et al., Round cells and sperm fertilizing capacity: the presence of immature germ cells but not seminal leukocytes are associated with reduced success of in vitro fertilization, Fertil. Steril. 58 (1992) 1257–1259.
[18] J. Thomas, et al., Increased polymorphonuclear granulocytes in seminal plasma in relation to sperm morphology, Hum. Reprod. 12 (1997) 2418–2421.
[19] K. Purvis, E. Christiansen, Infection in the male reproductive tract. Impact, diagnosis and treatment in relation to male fertility, Int. J. Androl. 16 (1993) 1–13.
[20] E.H. Yanushpolsky, et al., Antibiotic therapy and leukocytospermia: a prospective, randomized, controlled study, Fertil. Steril. 63 (1995) 142–147.
[21] C.L.R. Barratt, A.E. Bolton, I.D. Cooke, Functional significance of white blood cells in the male and female reproductive tract, Hum. Reprod. 5 (1990) 639–648.
[22] G.J. Matthews, M. Goldstein, H.J.M. Schlegel, Nonbacterial pyospermia: a consequence of clomiphene citrate therapy, Int. J. Menopausal Stud. 40 (1995) 187–191.
[23] H. Wolff, The biologic significance of white blood cells in semen, Fertil. Steril. 63 (1995) 1143–1157.
[24] E. Johanisson, et al., Evaluation of 'round cells' in semen analysis: a comparative study, Hum. Reprod. Updat. 6 (2000) 404–412.
[25] W. Eggert-Kruse, et al., Differentiation of round cells by means of monoclonal antibodies and relationship with male fertility, Fertil. Steril. 58 (1992) 1046–1055.
[26] H. Wolff, Methods for the detection of male genital tract inflammation, Andrologia 30 (Suppl. 1) (1998) 35–39.
[27] G. Ricci, et al., Leukocyte detection in human semen using flow cytometry, Hum. Reprod. 15 (2000) 1329–1337.
[28] M. Ludwig, et al., Evaluation of seminal plasma parameters in patients with chronic prostatitis or leukocytospermia, Andrologia 30 (Suppl. 1) (2003) 41–47.
[29] M. Shekarriz, et al., Positive myeloperoxidase staining (Endtz test) as an indicator of excessive reactive oxygen species formation in semen, J. Assist. Reprod. Genet. 12 (1995) 70–74.
[30] P.J. Chan, et al., White blood cells in semen affect hyperactivation but not sperm membrane integrity in the head and tail regions, Fertil. Steril. 61 (1994) 986–989.
[31] S. Kaleli, et al., Does leukocytospermia associate with poor semen parameters and sperm function in male fertility? The role of different seminal leukocytes concentrations, Eur. J. Obstet. Gynecol. Reprod. Biol. 89 (2000) 185–191.
[32] J.G. Alvarez, et al., Increased DNA damage in sperm from leukocytospermic semen samples as determined by the sperm chromatin structure assay, Fertil. Steril. 78 (2002) 319–329.
[33] R. Henkel, et al., DNA fragmentation of spermatozoa and assisted reproduction technology, RBM Online 7 (2003) 477–484.
[34] R. Henkel, et al., Urogenital inflammation: changes of leukocytes and ROS, Andrologia 35 (2003) 309–313.
[35] P.A. Skau, I. Folstad, Do bacterial infections cause reduced ejaculate quality? A meta-analysis of antibiotic treatment of male infertility, Behav. Ecol. 14 (2003) 40–47.
[36] E.F. Branigan, C.H. Muller, Efficacy of treatment and recurrence rate of leukocytospermia in infertile men with prostatitis, Fertil. Steril. 62 (1994) 580–584.
[37] E.F. Branigan, L.R. Spadoni, C.H. Muller, Identification and treatment of leukocytospermia in couples with unexplained infertility, J. Reprod. Med. 40 (1995) 625–629.
[38] J. Fedder, Nonsperm cells in human semen: with special reference to seminal leukocytes and their possible influence on fertility, Arch. Androl. 36 (1996) 41–65.
[39] C.T. Erel, et al., Antibiotic treatment in men with leukocytospermia, Int. J. Fertil. 42 (1997) 206–210.
[40] M. Montag, H. van der Ven, G. Haidl, Recovery of ejaculated spermatozoa for intracytoplasmic sperm injection after anti-inflammatory treatment of an azoospermic patient with genital tract infection: a case report, Andrologia 31 (1999) 179–181.
[41] A. Krisp, et al., Treatment with levofloxcin does not resolve asymptomatic leukocytospermia—a randomized controlled study, Andrologia 35 (2003) 244–247.
[42] M. Yamamoto, et al., Antibiotic and ejaculation treatments improve resolution rate of leukocytospermia in infertile men with prostatitis, Nagoya J. Med. Sci. 58 (1995) 41–45.

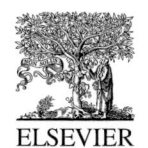

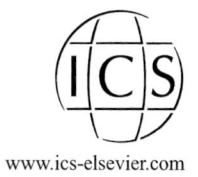

# Polycystic ovary syndrome—diagnosis and etiology

R.J. Norman*, T. Hickey, L. Moran, J. Boyle, J. Wang, M. Davies

*Reproductive Medicine Unit and Repromed, Adelaide Hormone and Menopause Centre, The Queen Elizabeth Hospital, Department of Obstetrics and Gynaecology, University of Adelaide, 28 Woodville Road, Woodville SA 5011, Australia*

**Abstract.** Polycystic ovary syndrome (PCOS) is a heterogenous condition with signs and symptoms including menstrual dysfunction, weight disorders, hirsutism, acne, endometrial hyperplasia, diabetes mellitus, metabolic syndrome and hyperlipidemia. As such, diagnosis is controversial and differs between countries and communities. By consensus, recent definitions highlight ovarian morphology, hyperandrogenism and menstrual dysfunction. Etiology is undetermined and may include genetic and environmental aspects, including lifestyle factors such as reduced activity and high caloric diet. Hyperinsulinaemia is common, even in the absence of obesity, and may be one of the causes for hyperandrogenism. Genetic causes are ill-determined at present but may include genes related to insulin secretion, insulin receptor function, ovarian steroidogenesis and paracrine regulators of ovarian function. © 2004 Published by Elsevier B.V.

*Keywords:* Polycystic ovary syndrome; Androgens; Etiology; Diagnosis

## 1. Introduction

Interest in polycystic ovary syndrome (PCOS) has increased considerably in recent years with the concept that it is a condition involving more than the reproductive system. Initially called the Stein-Levinthal syndrome after its discovery in the 1930s, the term PCOS does not do justice to the multisystem involvement including hyperinsulinism, hyperlipidaemia, increased androgens, cosmetic problems, endometrial hyperplasia, diabetes mellitus, infertility, obesity, anovulation and possible cardiac disease [1,2]. The diagnosis is controversial but is generally based on peri-pubertal onset of menstrual problems with clinical or biochemical hyperandrogenism. The presence of polycystic ovaries (PCO) on ultrasound as a diagnostic criterion remains controversial particularly as the ultrasound characteristics are subjective: up to 25% of the normal female population have PCO on ultrasound and most publications on PCOS do not include PCO as diagnostic criteria.

---

\* Corresponding author. Tel.: +1-61-8-8222-6788; fax: +1-61-8-8222-7521.
*E-mail address:* robert.norman@adelaide.edu.au (R.J. Norman).

## 2. The polycystic ovary

Polycystic ovaries are characteristically larger in volume, have a different surface appearance and have a ring of peripheral follicles less than 10 mm around the periphery. Webber et al. [3] took cortical biopsies during routine laparoscopy from 24 women with normal ovaries and regular cycles and from 32 women with polycystic ovaries, 16 of whom had regular, ovulatory cycles and 16 of whom had oligomenorrhoea. Using computerised image analysis to assess the density and developmental stage of small preantral follicles in serial sections of fixed tissue, it was shown that the median density of small preantral follicles, including those at primordial and primary stages, was six-fold greater in biopsies from polycystic ovaries in anovulatory women than in normal ovaries. In women with polycystic ovaries, a significant increase in the percentage of early growing (primary) follicles was noted and a reciprocal decrease in the proportion of primordial follicles was seen compared with normal ovaries. A number of candidate molecules such as anti-mullerian hormone (AMH) and GDF-9 could explain this difference. Histology reveals that PCO is associated with an increase in the size of the theca cells that envelop the follicle. These cells overproduce androgens such as testosterone and androstenedione, hormones normally used by the ovary to make oestrogen. In PCOS, there are generally higher circulating concentrations of insulin and luteinizing hormone and the theca cells are over responsive to this stimulation. A state of high oestrogen, androgens, insulin and LH, would explain the classic PCOS presentation of hirsutism, anovulation or dysfunctional bleeding and glucose dysfunction. Paradoxically, the insulin regulatory molecules on the theca are responsive to insulin while those in the muscle and liver are resistant.

## 3. Diagnosis of PCOS

Originally PCOS was diagnosed on the basis of clinical features of menstrual dysfunction, obesity, infertility and direct visualisation of the ovaries at laparotomy. Subsequently, biochemical markers such as high LH/FSH ratio and increased testosterone were introduced. In the early 1990s, an attempt was made to rationalise the

Table 1
Classification of PCOS (based on NIH recommendations)

PCO
  Presence of polycystic ovaries on ultrasound
  Absence of menstrual or cosmetic symptoms
  Absence of biochemical hyperandrogenaemia
PCOS
  Presence of menstrual abnormalities and anovulation
  Presence of clinical and/or biochemical hyperandrogenaemia
  Absence of hyperprolactinaemia or thyroid disease
  Absence of late-onset congenital adrenal hyperplasia
  Absence of Cushing's syndrome
  Idiopathic hirsutism
  Presence of excess hair growth (e.g. Ferriman–Gallwey score >8)
  Absence of biochemical hyperandrogenaemia

Table 2
ESHRE/ASRM guidelines for PCOS

Two of the following
 Presence of polycystic ovaries on ultrasound
 Presence of clinical or biochemical hyperandrogenism
 Presence of menstrual dysfunction with anovulation and
 Absence of hyperprolactinaemia or thyroid disease
 Absence of late-onset congenital adrenal hyperplasia
 Absence of Cushing's syndrome

diagnosis at an NIH conference where certain agreed criteria were given precedence over other more controversial features (Table 1) [4]. Ultrasound was not included at that time as it did not have wide use in North America. A further attempt to bridge the Atlantic divide was made by ASRM and ESHRE in 2003 at a conference in Rotterdam [5]. The proponents of ultrasound were able to introduce this diagnostic tool added to the list of features and now two of the three criteria have to be accepted for a diagnosis (Table 2). This change has had the effect of widening the inclusion criteria to incorporate many more women than would have been considered previously. Several studies have shown that the three criteria do not necessarily overlap and there needs to be care in publications and clinical endeavours to define patients more completely.

## 4. Prevalence of PCOS

Several studies have suggested a prevalence of PCOS of between 5% and 10% in women of reproductive age and PCO alone is found in 20–25% of women. While women with PCO and no evidence of menstrual problem or hyperandrogenism appear to be normal, they do have an over-exaggerated response to hormone stimulation by gonadotrophins (follicle stimulating hormone) seen in cycles of assisted reproduction (IVF and stimulated intra-uterine insemination). PCOS is generally under-diagnosed in women and teenagers where menstrual abnormalities such as cycles <21 and >35 days are often associated with the condition [6,7]. Many of these young women are given the oral contraceptive pill, which masks the condition until the drug is stopped to try and achieve pregnancy.

## 5. PCOS as a life-long condition

PCOS may have its origins in fetal life with either intra-uterine growth retardation or post-term birth. Ibanez et al. [8] have claimed that these children are more prone to hyperinsulinism, premature pubarche and signs of PCOS early in reproductive life. Teenagers with this condition will often have oligo-amenorrhoea, hirsutism, acne and weight disorders. There is some controversy over whether eating disorders are associated with PCOS [9]. Women seeking to become pregnant will have difficulties because of anovulation and later may be concerned about weight and hirsutism. Endometrial cancer is alleged to be at least four times more common because of unopposed oestrogen action on the uterus and may appear in women as young as their early 20s (although this is controversial) [10]. Diabetes mellitus and impaired glucose tolerance is a major complication in the overweight person and features of the metabolic syndrome are common with raised fasting and stimulated insulin, hypertriglyceridemia, low HDL cholesterol and increased plasminogen activator inhibition in the circulation. There is no firm evidence for an increase in cardiac disease based on a large retrospective study of death in women with histologically proven PCOS [11–13] although other studies have shown accelerated narrowing of major blood vessels [14,15]. Because of the potential complications across the lifespan, there should be an awareness of the possible diagnosis.

## 6. Clinical aspects of polycystic ovary syndrome

PCOS is a heterogeneous condition that presents in various combinations of a wide variety of physical and biochemical symptoms. Many of these symptoms arise shortly after menarche, which frequently occurs at a younger age in this population of women. Approaching menopause many of the symptoms of PCOS are ameliorated [16].

### 6.1. Polycystic ovaries

Transvaginal utrasonography is the gold standard for detection of polycystic ovarian morphology. Although opinions vary, $\geq 10$ peripherally arranged follicular cysts <10 mm in diameter, with a minimum ovarian volume >5.5cm$^3$ are commonly used criteria [17]. With the widespread use of transvaginal scanning, the ultrasound criteria need to be somewhat different [18].

### 6.2. Hirsutism, acne, seborrhoea, and alopecia

Women with PCO have a higher incidence of all of these cutaneous symptoms compared with women with normal ovaries.

### 6.3. Menstrual irregularity

Chronic amenorrhoea, oligomenorrhoea, and prolonged, erratic menstrual bleeding are characteristic of women with PCOS. Cycles with an interval greater than 35 days are likely to be anovulatory, and are reported in 50–90% of women with PCO. In addition, a number of normal cycling women with PCO may also be anovulatory if signs of hyperandrogenism are also present [19].

### 6.4. Biochemical features

Women with PCOS commonly have elevated serum androgen levels of either testosterone or androstenedione compared with normal cycling women. Largely due to obesity, sex-hormone binding protein (SHBG) values are often low, leading to an increased free androgen index (FAI).

### 6.5. Metabolic symptoms

A large proportion (40–60%) of women with PCOS will be obese, and a greater proportion (40–80%) will demonstrate insulin resistance. While most obese PCOS patients are insulin resistant, this feature is also a characteristic of lean PCOS patients [20]. Approximately 40% of obese North American women with PCOS will develop type II diabetes before the age of 40 [21].

## 7. Pathophysiology

The pathophysiology of PCOS remains unclear despite intense research. Recent studies provocatively suggest that initiation of a pathological mechanism may occur during fetal life, with high maternal serum levels of androgen and/or insulin that may influence genetic programming in a manner that predisposes the developing individual to PCOS and associated metabolic diseases [22,23]. Hyperandrogenism and hyperinsulinaemia may represent two independent modalities that are common enough to coexist in a syndrome that afflicts a relatively large portion of the female population [24].

### 7.1. Hyperandrogenism

The ovary is accepted as the main source of excess androgens in women with PCOS, although excess adrenal androgen production may also occur. Ovarian theca cells produce androgen under the influence of LH, and can be modulated by a number of local growth factors, hormones, and cytokines. Theca cells from polycystic ovaries maintain increased androgen production over long-term culture conditions with normal doses of gonadotrophin [25]. These cells display intrinsic alterations in steroidogenic activities, including increased expression and differential regulation of genes required for steroidogenesis, that are suggestive of underlying genetic causes. In addition to excess androgen production, a functional state of hyperandrogenaemia can occur in PCOS via increased androgen sensitivity, availability or clearance. Anomalies in the activity, but not the expression levels, of both 5-alpha-reductase and aromatase have been implicated in PCOS. Polymorphic variants of the androgen receptor represent another means of altering tissue sensitivity to androgens. We have found an association between high serum androgens and increased frequency of a less aggressive AR variant [26]. It is feasible that an androgen dependant activity influences the secretion of androgen at the follicular level, or influences LH secretion at the hypothalamic or pituitary level.

### 7.2. Hyperinsulinaemia

Insulin resistance and pancreatic beta cell dysfunction, both found in women with PCOS, can result in abnormal insulin secretion. Acting on the liver, insulin inhibits production of sex-hormone binding globulin (SHBG) and IGF-1 binding protein (IGFBP-1), resulting in increased bioavailability of these substances. Increased bioavailability of testosterone may result in increased androgen activity at the tissue level despite normal levels of serum androgen. In the ovary, IGF-1 is secreted by granulosa cells and acts in both an autocrine and paracrine manner to modulate the stimulatory effects of gonadotropins during many phases of follicle development [27]. In theca cells, IGF-1 may indirectly augment androgen production by increasing mRNAs for LH receptors and enzymes involved in steroidogenesis. Post-receptor signal abnormalities have been demonstrated for the insulin receptor in women with PCOS, but the abnormality is extrinsic to the receptor, and specific for different tissues. A defective serine kinase common to both insulin and androgen activity has been proposed as a potential cause of PCOS that would marry these two hormone activities but to date none have been found. Insulin action in the ovary remains undefined, although insulin resistance has clear adverse effects on ovulation.

### 7.3. Genetics of PCOS

#### 7.3.1. Inheritance

The familial clustering of PCOS described by many studies clearly indicates a genetic foundation for susceptibility to this disorder [28]. At least 50%, and as high as 87% of first-degree relatives of women with PCOS will have some symptom manifestation. Many modes of inheritance have been suggested by these studies with the result that no convincing inheritance pattern has emerged. Indeed twin studies do not support the concept of a single gene defect leading to PCOS. Discrepancies between studies for affected status criteria, lack of a male phenotype, ascertainment bias, and study sizes, have severely compromised the findings of most segregation analyses. In addition, the well-documented effects of environmental factors in determining phenotype expression increase the difficulty of achieving consistent results. There is no evidence that chromosomal abnormalities are found in PCOS.

#### 7.3.2. Candidate genes

The search for genes involved in PCOS has mainly involved association and linkage analyses for selected candidates. These candidates reflect what is known of the pathophysiology of PCOS to date and include genes involved in: (1) steroid hormone synthesis and action, (2) gonadotrophin action and regulation, (3) energy metabolism and homeostasis, and (4) immune function. The most thorough and highly acclaimed linkage analysis identified follistatin as the most likely gene to be involved in PCOS [29]. Subsequent larger linkage and mutation analyses failed to detect abnormalities in the follistatin gene that would incur physiological consequences [30], although our group has demonstrated increased follistatin in the blood of women with polycystic ovaries [31]. Other genes implicated in the aetiology of PCOS that have well-characterised polymorphic sites are the AR and the VNTR, both of which remain strong contenders as causal genes. Recently, an area near the insulin receptor gene has been shown to be linked to PCOS [32].

## 8. PCOS phenotype in the male

Because males do not have ovaries and have high androgens, the typical markers of PCOS are not applicable in men. Several years ago, we showed that brothers had hyperinsulinaemia and hypertriglyceridemia when their sister was affected [33].

## 9. Environmental aspects of PCOS

Obesity is common in patients with PCOS from North America and Northern Europe but less so in those from other areas and ethnic backgrounds. It is uncertain whether obesity is a cause or effect of PCOS. What is certain is that it complicates the clinical presentation by enhancing insulin resistance, glucose intolerance and hyperlipidaemia. The effects of obesity in this condition have been well documented and the benefits of weight loss established [34–36]. Lifestyle modification leads to reduction in insulin resistance, improved spontaneous and induced ovulation, less miscarriage and better pregnancy outcomes [2,36–38]. Fat produces hormones such as leptin and adiponectin, which may have direct effects on the ovary in addition to those on the hypothamus and pituitary. Leptin levels in PCOS women are not different from non-PCOS of comparable body mass index, so cannot explain the ovarian features easily.

Exposure of monkeys to androgens in pregnancy leads to offspring that exhibit many of the features of PCOS including hormone and metabolic disorders [23]. This has led to the thought that excess placental or maternal androgens may program the egg or embryo to develop an ovarian phenotype analogous to that found in PCOS. Alternatively, androgens could change the hypothalamic-pituitary functioning to alter control of the ovary. There is little evidence yet to support this in human PCOS although several authors have looked at androgen receptor polymorphisms in subjects with this condition.

## Acknowledgements

National Health and Medical Research Council (Australia) through project and program funding.

## References

[1] R.A. Lobo, Priorities in polycystic ovary syndrome, Med. J. Aust. 174 (2001) 554–555.
[2] R.J. Norman, Obesity, polycystic ovary syndrome and anovulation—how are they interrelated? Curr. Opin. Obstet. Gynecol. 13 (2001) 323–327.
[3] L.J. Webber, et al., Formation and early development of follicles in the polycystic ovary, Lancet 362 (2003) 1017–1021.
[4] J.K. Zawadzki, A. Dunaif, Diagnostic criteria for polycystic ovary syndrome; towards a rational approach, in: A. Dunaif, J.R. Givens, F.P. Haseltine, G.R. Merriam (Eds.), Current Issues in Endocrinology and Metabolism, Blackwell, 1992, pp. 377–384.
[5] The Rotterdam ESHRE/ASRM-sponsored PCOS consensus workshop group, Revised 2003 consensus on diagnostic criteria and long-term health risks related to polycystic ovary syndrome (PCOS), Hum. Reprod. 19 (1) (2004 January) 41–47.
[6] M.H. van Hooff, et al., Polycystic ovaries in adolescents and the relationship with menstrual cycle patterns, luteinizing hormone, androgens, and insulin, Fertil. Steril. 74 (2000) 49–58.
[7] M.H. van Hooff, et al., Relationship of the menstrual cycle pattern in 14–17 year old adolescents with gynaecological age, body mass index and historical parameters, Hum. Reprod. 13 (1998) 2252–2260.
[8] L. Ibanez, et al., Polycystic ovary syndrome after precocious pubarche: ontogeny of the low-birthweight effect, Clin. Endocrinol. (Oxf.) 55 (2001) 667–672.
[9] K.F. Michelmore, A.H. Balen, D.B. Dunger, Polycystic ovaries and eating disorders: are they related? Hum. Reprod. 16 (2001) 765–769.
[10] P. Hardiman, O.C. Pillay, W. Atiomo, Polycystic ovary syndrome and endometrial carcinoma, Lancet 361 (2003) 1810–1812.
[11] R.A. Wild, Polycystic ovary syndrome: a risk for coronary artery disease? Am. J. Obstet. Gynecol. 186 (2002) 35–43 (t&artType=abs&id=a119180&target=).
[12] R.A. Wild, Long-term health consequences of PCOS, Hum. Reprod. Updat. 8 (2002) 231–241.
[13] T. Pierpoint, et al., Mortality of women with polycystic ovary syndrome at long-term follow-up, J. Clin. Epidemiol. 51 (1998) 581–586.

[14] E.O. Talbott, et al., Cardiovascular risk in women with polycystic ovary syndrome, Obstet. Gynecol. Clin. North Am. 28 (2001) 111–133 (vii).
[15] C.G. Solomon, et al., Menstrual cycle irregularity and risk for future cardiovascular disease, J. Clin. Endocrinol. Metab. 87 (2002) 2013–2017.
[16] S.J. Winters, et al., Serum testosterone levels decrease in middle age in women with the polycystic ovary syndrome, Fertil. Steril. 73 (2000) 724–729.
[17] J. Adams, D.W. Polson, S. Franks, Prevalence of polycystic ovaries in women with anovulation and idiopathic hirsutism, Br. Med. J. (Clin. Res. Ed.) 293 (1986) 355–359.
[18] D. Dewailly, et al., Interrelationship between ultrasonography and biology in the diagnosis of polycystic ovarian syndrome, Ann. N.Y. Acad. Sci. 687 (1993) 206–216.
[19] M.G. Hull, Epidemiology of infertility and polycystic ovarian disease: endocrinological and demographic studies, Gynecol. Endocrinol. 1 (1987) 235–245.
[20] A. Dunaif, et al., Profound peripheral insulin resistance, independent of obesity, in polycystic ovary syndrome, Diabetes 38 (1989) 1165–1174.
[21] R.S. Legro, Diabetes prevalence and risk factors in polycystic ovary syndrome, Obstet. Gynecol. Clin. North Am. 28 (2001) 99–109.
[22] M.J. Davies, R.J. Norman, Programming and reproductive functioning, Trends Endocrinol. Metab. 13 (2002) 386–392.
[23] D.H. Abbott, D.A. Dumesic, S. Franks, Developmental origin of polycystic ovary syndrome—a hypothesis, J. Endocrinol. 174 (2002) 1–5.
[24] R.S. Legro, Polycystic ovary syndrome. Phenotype to genotype, Endocrinol. Metab. Clin. N. Am. 28 (1999) 379–396.
[25] C. Gilling-Smith, et al., Hypersecretion of androstenedione by isolated thecal cells from polycystic ovaries, J. Clin. Endocrinol. Metab. 79 (1994) 1158–1165.
[26] T. Hickey, A. Chandy, R.J. Norman, The androgen receptor CAG repeat polymorphism and X-chromosome inactivation in Australian Caucasian women with infertility related to polycystic ovary syndrome, J. Clin. Endocrinol. Metab. 87 (2002) 161–165.
[27] L.C. Giudice, Growth factor action on ovarian function in polycystic ovary syndrome, Endocrinol. Metab. Clin. N. Am. 28 (1999) 325–339 (vi).
[28] R.S. Legro, The genetics of polycystic ovary syndrome, Am. J. Med. 98 (1995) 9S–16S.
[29] M. Urbanek, et al., Thirty-seven candidate genes for polycystic ovary syndrome: strongest evidence for linkage is with follistatin, Proc. Natl. Acad. Sci. U. S. A. 96 (1999) 8573–8578.
[30] M. Urbanek, et al., Allelic variants of the follistatin gene in polycystic ovary syndrome, J. Clin. Endocrinol. Metab. 85 (2000) 4455–4461.
[31] R.J. Norman, et al., Circulating follistatin concentrations are higher and activin concentrations are lower in polycystic ovarian syndrome, Hum. Reprod. 16 (2001) 668–672.
[32] R.S. Legro, J.F. Strauss, Molecular progress in infertility: polycystic ovary syndrome, Fertil. Steril. 78 (2002) 569–576.
[33] R.J. Norman, S. Masters, W. Hague, Hyperinsulinemia is common in family members of women with polycystic ovary syndrome, Fertil. Steril. 66 (1996) 942–947.
[34] D.S. Kiddy, et al., Improvement in endocrine and ovarian function during dietary treatment of obese women with polycystic ovary syndrome, Clin. Endocrinol. (Oxf.) 36 (1992) 105–111.
[35] R. Pettigrew, D. Hamilton-Fairley, Obesity and female reproductive function, Br. Med. Bull. 53 (1997) 341–358.
[36] R.J. Norman, et al., The role of lifestyle modification in polycystic ovary syndrome, Trends Endocrinol. Metab. 13 (2002) 251–257.
[37] M.M. Huber-Buchholz, D.G. Carey, R.J. Norman, Restoration of reproductive potential by lifestyle modification in obese polycystic ovary syndrome: role of insulin sensitivity and luteinizing hormone, J. Clin. Endocrinol. Metab. 84 (1999) 1470–1474.
[38] L.J. Moran, et al., Dietary composition in restoring reproductive and metabolic physiology in overweight women with polycystic ovary syndrome, J. Clin. Endocrinol. Metab. 88 (2003) 812–819.

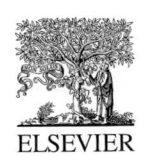

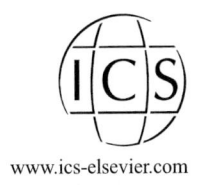

# Do women with polycystic ovary syndrome have an increased risk of cardiovascular disease: review of the evidence

Evelyn O. Talbott*, Jeanne V. Zborowski, Monique Y. Boudreaux

*Department of Epidemiology, University of Pittsburgh, GSPH, A526 Crabtree Hall, 130 DeSoto St., Pittsburgh, PA 15216, USA*

**Abstract.** Polycystic ovary syndrome (PCOS) is a reproductive endocrine disorder found in ~5% of the general population and is characterized by chronic anovulation, hyperandrogenism, and insulin resistance. Women with PCOS are at increased risk for the development of Type II diabetes and may represent a unique group of women at high risk for the development of coronary heart disease (CHD). More adverse CHD risk profiles of women with PCOS have been demonstrated in several studies, yet actual health outcome studies have been inconclusive as to whether this translates into increased rates of cardiovascular disease in PCOS cases when compared with controls. This review focuses on the controversy surrounding the potential relationship between cardiovascular disease outcomes and polycystic ovary syndrome. © 2004 Published by Elsevier B.V.

*Keywords:* Polycystic ovary syndrome; Coronary heart disease; Risk factors; Diabetes; Coronary calcium

## 1. Introduction

Polycystic ovary syndrome (PCOS) is a reproductive endocrine disorder characterized by chronic anovulation, hyperandrogenism, and insulin resistance. The estimated prevalence is 5–10% among women of reproductive age. Given this high population prevalence and the association of PCOS with an increased risk for the development of Type II diabetes, women with PCOS may represent a unique group of women at high risk for the development of coronary heart disease (CHD).

The literature describing CHD risk factors and PCOS has more recently expanded from case reports and clinical research involving women seen for infertility or androgen excess [1–5] to larger epidemiological studies [6–10]. PCOS has been linked to an increased risk of metabolic cardiovascular syndrome (MCS). MCS refers to a clustering within the same individual of hyperinsulinemia, mild glucose intolerance, dyslipidemia, and hypertension; all are CHD risk factors that are also associated with PCOS [11–13]. Therefore, the study of women with PCOS provides a natural experiment for evaluation of the effects of lipid

---

\* Corresponding author. Tel.: +1-412-624-3074; fax: +1-412-624-7397.
*E-mail address:* eot1@pitt.edu (E.O. Talbott).

0531-5131/ © 2004 Published by Elsevier B.V.
doi:10.1016/j.ics.2004.02.007

and hormonal abnormalities and altered glucose metabolism on cardiovascular risk factors and coronary artery disease.

## 2. CHD risk factors in PCOS

Wild et al. [2] were among the first investigators to report that women with PCOS had lower HDLc levels, higher LDLc/HDLc ratios, and higher triglyceride levels than regularly menstruating women. Subsequently, Slowinska-Srzednicka et al. [8] drew attention to the role of insulin in the lipid abnormalities observed in hyperandrogenic women with PCOS. These investigators compared 27 women with PCOS and 22 eumenorrheic controls, stratified by weight (obese, nonobese). After adjustment for age, BMI and sex steroids, fasting insulin (FI) was a significant explanatory variable for total triglycerides and apolipoprotein A-1, suggesting that hyperinsulinemia, independent of obesity, might play a role in the lipid disturbances of PCOS. Lipoprotein abnormalities appeared to be associated more with insulin levels than with alterations in androgens or estrogens.

In a large-scale epidemiological study of CHD risk factors in women with a diagnosis of PCOS, Talbott et al. [7] demonstrated that women with PCOS ($N=244$) have adverse lipid profiles, including elevated LDLc and triglycerides and decreased HDLc, compared with age-, race- and neighborhood-matched controls ($N=244$). After adjustment for BMI, fasting insulin independently contributed to the variation in HDLc, LDLc and triglycerides. In PCOS cases, decreased estradiol levels, but not androgen levels, were independently associated with increased LDLc.

In this same population, Talbott et al. [14] also evaluated the age-specific coronary heart disease risk profiles across four specific age groups (19–24, 25–34, 35–44 and 45+ years). Compared with controls, PCOS women had substantially higher LDLc and total cholesterol levels at each age group under 45+ years after adjustment for body mass index, hormone use, and insulin levels. After 45 years of age, little difference was noted between groups. These findings suggest that PCOS women exhibit significantly adverse lipid and coronary heart disease risk factors at a younger age compared with normally menstruating women. This 15–20-year excess in exposure to elevated LDLc and depressed HDLc levels could translate into premature coronary heart disease, morbidity and mortality in the PCOS population.

More recently, Dejager et al. [15] demonstrated that atherogenic modifications of LDLc, specifically a shift toward smaller, more dense particles, were evident among 31 women with PCOS compared with 27 controls (mean age $26.1\pm6.1$ years in total group; BMI=26.7 and 24.2 kg/m$^2$, respectively). LDLc particle size was significantly smaller among hyperandrogenic women with PCOS compared with regularly cycling women ($p=0.006$), suggesting a more atherogenic lipid profile and, potentially, a higher risk of CHD among PCOS women. After adjustment for potential confounders, only SHBG was an independent predictor of particle size.

### 2.1. Type 2 diabetes

An increased prevalence of Type II diabetes has been demonstrated retrospectively in both premenopausal and postmenopausal PCOS women ($N=47$) [10]. Women with PCOS also appear to develop Type II diabetes at a younger age than normal women [16–20]. Legro [21] observed that the prevalence of Type II diabetes and impaired glucose tolerance (IGT) was significantly higher in PCOS women than age-, weight- and ethnically similar normal cycling women. Thirty-one percent of the PCOS women had impaired glucose tolerance (IGT) and 7.5% overt diabetes vs. 15.7% IGT and 0% diabetes in controls. In our Pittsburgh cohort of PCOS subjects and controls (42.34 and 43.06 years, respectively), a total of 12.6% reported a physician diagnosis of Type 2 diabetes in contrast to 1.4% in the control group at the second follow-up visit, 1996–1999.

## 3. Subclinical atherosclerosis and PCOS

### 3.1. Coronary angiography

In a study of PCOS and coronary artery disease, Birdsall et al. [22] evaluated 143 women aged less than 60 years who had undergone coronary angiography for investigation of chest pain or valvular disease over a 2-year period. When the ovaries of these women were examined by transvaginal ultrasound, 42% were found to have polycystic-appearing ovaries—twice the background prevalence of polycystic-appearing ovaries reported in a general population of women [23]. Women with polycystic ovaries had more advanced coronary artery disease than women with normal ovaries ($p=0.01$).

### 3.2. Carotid ultrasonography

More recent studies have suggested that PCOS cases have increased subclinical atherosclerosis as evidenced by increased carotid intima media thickness (IMT). In a follow-up study of the total Pittsburgh PCOS cohort, Talbott et al. [24] evaluated carotid intima media thickness in 125 Caucasian women with PCOS and 142 age-matched controls. Among women 45 years of age and older, PCOS cases had a significantly greater mean IMT than control women (0.78 vs. 0.70 mm, $p=0.005$). This difference remained significant after adjustment for BMI ($p<0.05$). Regression modeling suggested that the PCOS–IMT association was mediated by central adiposity and increased fasting insulin concentrations. The findings also suggested that higher LDLc levels might independently mediate atherosclerotic potential in all younger women.

### 3.3. Electron beam tomography for coronary calcification

During the most recent follow-up visit (2000–2002) of our original Pittsburgh cohort, we evaluated the prevalence of coronary artery calcification (CAC), another surrogate for subclinical CHD, using electron beam tomography (EBT) among 102 middle-aged women with PCOS compared with 118 controls (mean aged 46.9 and 48.5 years, respectively). We also assessed the relationship of metabolic syndrome, insulin resistance and traditional CHD risk factors measured at baseline (1993–1994) with calcification in these middle-aged women [25]. The mean and median coronary calcium for cases and controls were 25.2 and 4.1 (range of 0–845.5) and 6.0 and 0 (range=0–204.6), respectively ($p<0.001$). Fasting insulin demonstrated the highest correlation with CAC. After adjustment for age and BMI, PCOS remained an independent predictor of coronary calcium ($p=0.015$). In subsequent regression models, only PCOS, age, BMI, smoking status, fasting insulin (FI), and $HDL_2$ contributed to the variability in coronary calcium and also mediated the PCOS–CAC association.

Christian et al. [26] also determined that the prevalence of coronary artery calcification in a cohort of 36 women with PCOS, aged 30–45 years, was higher than a control group of 71 women matched on BMI and age (39% vs. 21%, odds ratio=2.4, $p$=0.05). Mean CAC scores were also greater in PCOS women than in control women ($p$=0.04). After adjustment for BMI, however, PCOS was no longer a significant predictor of CAC (OR=1.99, $p$=0.21). In this study, although PCOS as an exposure was diagnosed years earlier, CHD risk factors were measured concurrently with EBT assessment of calcification.

## 4. C-reactive protein levels in PCOS and the relationship with SCA

Inflammatory markers and homocysteine have been postulated to have a more significant role in atherosclerosis than lipid levels [27]. Hemostatic abnormalities and inflammation have also been implicated as potential mediating factors in the PCOS–subclinical atherosclerosis association as measured by carotid IMT. Kelly et al. [28] studied CRP levels in women with PCOS to determine if CRP was increased in PCOS and related to risk for future cardiovascular events. After adjustment for BMI and age, women with PCOS ($N$=17) were found to have significantly elevated CRP levels compared with controls ($N$=15). The authors proposed low-grade chronic inflammation as a novel mechanism contributing to increased CHD and Type 2 diabetes risks in women with PCOS.

In a recent analysis, we examined the relationship between hemostatic and inflammatory markers and measures of subclinical atherosclerosis, including carotid IMT in 47 PCOS cases and 59 controls aged 45 years and older (mean=49.2 and 49.5 years, respectively). These factors included BMI, insulin, blood lipids and hemostatic factors [Factor VII, plasminogen activator inhibitor (PAI-1), TPA (tissue plasminogen activator), D-Dimer and fragment 1.2] and markers of inflammation (C-reactive protein). SCA was measured concurrently using B-mode ultrasonography. PAI-1, CRP and TPA were significantly greater among cases compared with controls upon univariate analysis. In univariate models, IMT was associated with PCOS, BMI, CRP, insulin and TPA ($p$<0.05). After adjustment for age, PCOS remained an independent predictor of carotid IMT ($p$=0.003). CRP made an additional contribution to the variation in IMT ($p$=0.04), independent of both PCOS status ($p$=0.019). The addition of BMI reduced the association of both PCOS ($p$=0.109) and CRP ($p$=0.739) with IMT. When insulin was included in the PCOS–age–CRP model, in lieu of BMI, the effect of CRP was again attenuated ($p$=0.197), but PCOS remained significant ($p$=0.025) [29]. These results suggest that (1) the influence of both PCOS and inflammation (CRP) on IMT is mediated by obesity (BMI); (2) insulin levels may also partially mediate the relationship between inflammation and increased IMT; however, (3) the hyperinsulinemia or IR in this cross-sectional analysis may be attributable to other dimensions of adiposity.

## 5. CHD endpoints in PCOS

Six studies conducted to date have focused on cardiovascular risk factors and endpoints in a middle-aged PCOS population. Dahlgren et al. [6,10] evaluated CHD risk in a cohort of 33 PCOS women (mean age of 50) with ovarian histopathology typical of PCOS at wedge resection, 22–31 years previously, and 132 age-matched controls (mean age 51.7±5.3). Compared with controls, PCOS patients had a higher prevalence of central obesity, a sevenfold higher prevalence of diagnosed diabetes, a threefold higher prevalence of treated hypertension and an average waist hip ratio higher by half a standard deviation. The results indicate that women with PCOS would potentially experience over time an increased risk of cardiovascular endpoints (angina, myocardial infarction, and sudden death).

Subsequently, Pierpoint et al. [30] conducted a long-term mortality study of women at least 45 years of age at the time of follow-up who were diagnosed with polycystic ovary disease by wedge resection in UK hospitals between 1930 and 1979. Of the initial sample of 1028, 786 women had a documented birth date and 668 (66%) could actually be traced and were included in the final age-specific comparison. There were 59 deaths from all causes [standardized mortality ratio (SMR)=0.90]; a total of 15 circulatory deaths were observed vs. 18.1 expected (SMR=0.83). The only noteworthy finding was an increase in the observed number of deaths in which diabetes mellitus was an underlying or contributing cause compared with expected (6 observed vs. 1.7 expected). Unfortunately, socioeconomic information and smoking histories were not available on this cohort. In addition, the possibility of selection bias is real because cases were identified only among women who had undergone an ovarian wedge resection.

In a more recent follow-up in the Pierpoint/McKeigue cohort, Wild et al. [31] compared both cardiovascular morbidity and mortality among subjects. Seven hundred eighty-six women (76% of the original cohort) were traced for mortality data. All cause and cardiovascular mortality in the PCOS cohort was similar to that observed in the general population. For the morbidity follow-up, data were collected on 319 women with PCOS and 1060 age-matched control women. The difference in CHD morbidity was not statistically different among PCOS women compared with the general population [crude odds ratio (95%)=1.5 (0.7–2.9)]. Women with PCOS were, however, more likely to experience nonfatal cerebrovascular disease [crude odds ratio (95%)=2.8 (1.1–7.1)]. Given that only 56% of the original PCOS cohort was evaluated, underestimation of CHD morbidity among the PCOS women is a legitimate concern.

Elting et al. [32] conducted a study of the prevalence of diabetes mellitus, hypertension, and coronary heart disease among 346 PCOS patients (mean age of 38.7 and body mass index of 24.4) compared with published data on the Dutch female population aged 25–54 years. Diabetes and hypertension were more prevalent in this relatively lean PCOS population compared with the Dutch female population ($p<0.05$), especially in women aged 45–54 years. The prevalence of cardiac events in the 45–54-year-old PCOS group was 3.1% compared with 0.9% in the Dutch population, suggesting a relative risk over 3.0. The effect was not significant, however, due to the small sample in this age subgroup ($N=32$).

Cibula et al. [33] also determined the prevalence of Type 2 diabetes, hypertension and coronary artery disease in 28 women with PCOS who had undergone wedge resection compared with 752 control women aged 45–54 years chosen as a probability sample from nine districts of the Czech Republic. PCOS women did not differ from the larger control group with regard to age, body mass index or waist hip ratio. No statistically significant difference between groups was noted in the prevalence of hypertension (50% of PCOS women and 39% of controls, respectively). However, a diagnosis of Type 2 diabetes was established in 32% of women with PCOS vs. only 8% of controls ($p<0.001$). Moreover, coronary artery disease (CAD) was diagnosed in 21% of PCOS women vs. 5% of controls ($p<0.001$). Despite the similar risk profile for the development of the disease studied, the prevalence of Type 2 diabetes and CAD was significantly higher in PCOS women. Although this was a cross-sectional study with a small sample size, this finding nonetheless suggests that women with markedly expressed clinical symptoms of PCOS may make up a subgroup in the general population at increased risk of heart disease.

During the second follow-up period in the Pittsburgh PCOS cohort (1997–1999), we obtained the most recent history of cardiovascular events, including myocardial infarction, doctor-diagnosed angina pectoris, coronary insufficiency, bypass and angioplasty as well as stroke ($N=127$ PCOS cases and 142 Caucasian controls). The population represented approximately 75% of the original cohort. Five cardiovascular events were identified among PCOS women (one myocardial infarction with bypass surgery, one angina with bypass surgery and three doctor-diagnosed and medically treated angina). Among Caucasian controls of similar age, no events were observed. The odds ratio of 5.86 ($p<0.05$) was similar to the projected risk estimate of earlier work Dahlgren's [20] involving 33 wedge-resected women with PCO followed for 20 or more years.

## 6. Conclusions

Although considerable previous research supports the finding of an increased risk of CHD in PCOS, controversy still remains concerning whether the adverse risk factor profile observed in PCOS translates into an increase in actual cardiovascular events. The previous large cohort analysis by Pierpoint et al. [30] was retrospective in nature and failed to demonstrate an increase in CHD mortality among women with PCOS. Some investigators suggest that the higher estrogen (estrone) levels observed among women with PCOS may play a protective role within the vascular endothelium. However, the rate of heart disease among premenopausal and perimenopausal women is very small; the Framingham Study reported an average annual CHD incidence rate among women aged 45–54 of seven per 1000 [34]. Given this low rate among women in the general population, it is not surprising that a study of the risk of MI and CHD in middle-aged women with PCOS is difficult at best. Continued follow-up of established cohorts of women with PCOS through menopause and aging, as well as the assembly of larger groups of women with and without PCOS for long-term surveillance, are necessary to answer this important question.

## Acknowledgements

Financial support for this study was provided by the National Heart, Lung, Blood Institute, a division of the National Institutes of Health (#R01 44664-09).

## References

[1] L.A. Mattsson, et al., Lipid metabolism in women with polycystic ovary syndrome: possible implications for an increased risk of coronary heart disease, Fertil. Steril. 42 (1984) 579–584.

[2] R.A. Wild, et al., Lipoprotein lipid concentrations and cardiovascular risk in women with polycystic ovary syndrome, J. Clin. Endocrinol. Metab. 61 (1985) 946–951.
[3] R.J. Chang, et al., Insulin resistance in nonobese patients with polycystic ovarian disease, J. Clin. Endocrinol. Metab. 57 (1983) 356–359.
[4] R. Pasquali, et al., C-peptide levels in obese patients with polycystic ovaries, Horm. Metab. Res. 14 (1982) 284–287.
[5] R. Pasquali, S. Venturoli, Hyperandrogenism, hyperinsulinism and polycystic ovarian disease, J. Endocrinol. Invest. 9 (1986) 531–533.
[6] E. Dahlgren, et al., Polycystic ovary syndrome and risk for myocardial infarction. Evaluated from a risk factor model based on a prospective population study of women, Acta Obstet. Gynecol. Scand. 71 (1992) 599–604.
[7] E. Talbott, et al., Coronary heart disease risk factors in women with polycystic ovary syndrome, Arterioscler. Thromb. Vasc. Biol. 15 (1995) 821–826.
[8] J. Slowinska-Srzednicka, et al., The role of hyperinsulinemia in the development of lipid disturbances in nonobese and obese women with the polycystic ovary syndrome, J. Endocrinol. Invest. 14 (1991) 569–575.
[9] G.S. Conway, et al., Risk factors for coronary artery disease in lean obese women with the polycystic ovary syndrome, Clin. Endocrinol. (Oxf.) 37 (1992) 119–125.
[10] E. Dahlgren, et al., Women with polycystic ovary syndrome wedge resected in 1956 to 1965: a long-term follow-up focusing on natural history and circulating hormones, Fertil. Steril. 57 (1992) 505–513.
[11] S. Franks, Polycystic ovary syndrome, N. Engl. J. Med. 333 (1995) 853–861.
[12] J.A. Eden, The polycystic ovary syndrome, Aust. N. Z. J. Obstet. Gynaecol. 29 (1989) 403–416.
[13] S.S. Yen, The polycystic ovary syndrome, Clin. Endocrinol. (Oxf.) 12 (1980) 177–207.
[14] E. Talbott, et al., Adverse lipid coronary heart disease risk profiles in young women with polycystic ovary syndrome: results of a case-control study, J. Clin. Epidemiol. 51 (1998) 415–422.
[15] S. Dejager, et al., Smaller LDL particle size in women with polycystic ovary syndrome compared to controls, Clin. Endocrinol. (Oxf.) 54 (2001) 455–462.
[16] A. Dunaif, et al., Profound peripheral insulin resistance, independent of obesity, in polycystic ovary syndrome, Diabetes 38 (1989) 1165–1174.
[17] A. Dunaif, Hyperandrogenic anovulation (PCOS): a unique disorder of insulin action associated with an increased risk of non-insulin-dependent diabetes mellitus, Am. J. Med. 98 (1995) 33S–39S.
[18] A. Dunaif, D.T. Finegood, Beta-cell dysfunction independent of obesity and glucose intolerance in the polycystic ovary syndrome, J. Clin. Endocrinol. Metab. 81 (1996) 942–947.
[19] D.A. Ehrmann, et al., Insulin secretory defects in polycystic ovary syndrome. Relationship to insulin sensitivity and family history of non-insulin-dependent diabetes mellitus, J. Clin. Invest. 96 (1995) 520–527.
[20] D.A. Ehrmann, et al., Prevalence of impaired glucose tolerance and diabetes in women with polycystic ovary syndrome, Diabetes Care 22 (1999) 141–146.
[21] R.S. Legro, Diabetes prevalence and risk factors in polycystic ovary syndrome, Obstet. Gynecol. Clin. North Am. 28 (2001) 99–109.
[22] M.A. Birdsall, C.M. Farquhar, H.D. White, Association between polycystic ovary extent of coronary artery disease in women having cardiac catheterization, Ann. Intern. Med. 126 (1997) 32–35.
[23] D.W. Polson, et al., Polycystic ovaries—a common finding in normal women, Lancet 1 (1988) 870–872.
[24] E.O. Talbott, et al., Evidence for association between polycystic ovary syndrome and premature carotid atherosclerosis in middle-aged women, Arterioscler. Thromb. Vasc. Biol. 20 (2000) 2414–2421.
[25] E. Talbott, et al., Metabolic cardiovascular syndrome and its relationship to coronary calcification in women with polycystic ovarian syndrome, 3rd International Workshop on Insulin Resistance, New Orleans, LA, 2003.
[26] R.C. Christian, et al., Prevalence and predictors of coronary artery calcification in women with polycystic ovary syndrome, J. Clin. Endocrinol. Metab. 88 (2003) 2562–2568.
[27] M.T. Magyar, et al., Early-onset carotid atherosclerosis is associated with increased intima-media thickness and elevated serum levels of inflammatory markers, Stroke 34 (2003) 58–63.
[28] C.C. Kelly, et al., Low grade chronic inflammation in women with polycystic ovarian syndrome, J. Clin. Endocrinol. Metab. 86 (2001) 2453–2455.

[29] E. Talbott, et al., The relationship between carotid intima media wall thickness and markers of inflammation and hemostasis in women with polycystic ovary syndrome, 4th Annual Conference on Arteriosclerosis, Thrombosis and Vascular Biology, Washington, DC, 2003.
[30] T. Pierpoint, et al., Mortality of women with polycystic ovary syndrome at long-term follow-up, J. Clin. Epidemiol. 51 (1998) 581–586.
[31] S. Wild, et al., Cardiovascular disease in women with polycystic ovary syndrome at long-term follow-up: a retrospective cohort study, Clin. Endocrinol. (Oxf.) 52 (2000) 595–600.
[32] M.W. Elting, et al., Prevalence of diabetes mellitus, hypertension and cardiac complaints in a follow-up study of a Dutch PCOS population, Hum. Reprod. 16 (2001) 556–560.
[33] D. Cibula, et al., Increased risk of non-insulin dependent diabetes mellitus, arterial hypertension and coronary artery disease in perimenopausal women with a history of the polycystic ovary syndrome, Hum. Reprod. 15 (2000) 785–789.
[34] W.B. Kannel, P.W.F. Wilson, Risk factors that attenuate the female coronary disease advantage, Arch. Intern. Med. 155 (1995) 57–61.

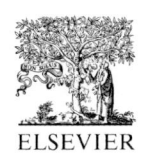

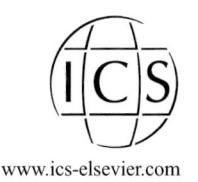

# Ovarian bone morphogenetic proteins in female reproduction

Shunichi Shimasaki*, R. Kelly Moore,
Gregory F. Erickson, Fumio Otsuka

*Department of Reproductive Medicine, University of California at San Diego, School of Medicine, 9500 Gilman Dr., La Jolla, CA 92093-0633, USA*

**Abstract.** Although bone morphogenetic proteins (BMPs) have been well-known regulators in ectopic formation of bone and cartilage, as well as in early embryonic development, nothing was known about the role of the BMP system in regulating ovarian function until recently. We demonstrated for the first time that the BMP system exists in the mammalian ovary and plays key roles in regulating important granulosa cell (GC) functions. Specifically, all BMPs we examined, including BMP-4, -6, -7, and -15, inhibit follicle-stimulating hormone (FSH)-dependent progesterone synthesis by primary cultures of rat granulosa cells. Thus, our observations provided experimental support for the hypothesis that BMPs may be a physiologically relevant luteinization inhibitor in growing ovarian follicles. BMP-7 and -15, but not BMP-6, are mitogens for granulosa cells. BMP-6 and BMP-15 are potent inhibitors of FSH action, by suppressing adenylate cyclase activity and FSH receptor expression, respectively. BMP-15 stimulates kit ligand (KL) expression, whereas kit ligand inhibits BMP-15 expression, thus forming a novel oocyte-somatic cell negative feedback loop. The physiological importance of the BMP system for normal mammalian reproduction has been established by the elucidation of the aberrant reproductive phenotypes of animals having mutated genes encoding BMP family members. Here we provide the recent advances in our understanding of the functions of BMPs in the ovary. © 2004 Published by Elsevier B.V.

*Keywords:* Bone morphogenetic protein; Fertility; ovary; Reproduction; Granulosa cell; Oocyte; Ovulation

## 1. Expression of BMP ligands, receptors, and a binding protein in the ovary

To study the expression of bone morphogenetic protein (BMP) system components in the ovary, we performed detailed in situ hybridization analyses of the spatiotemporal expression patterns of the BMP ligands (BMP-2, -3, -3b, -4, -6, -7, -15), receptors (BMPR-IA, -IB, -II), and a binding protein (follistatin) in rat ovaries throughout the normal estrous

---

*Abbreviations:* BMP, bone morphogenetic protein; FSH, follicle-stimulating hormone; GC, granulosa cell; KL, kit ligand.
* Corresponding author. Tel.: +1-858-822-1414; fax: +1-858-822-1482.
*E-mail address:* sshimasaki@ucsd.edu (S. Shimasaki).

0531-5131/ © 2004 Published by Elsevier B.V.
doi:10.1016/j.ics.2004.01.058

cycle [1]. Our collective conclusions from these studies are: (i) the mRNAs of each of these genes exhibit a cell-specific expression pattern in ovarian cells and each of the functional ovarian cell types expresses components of the BMP system, and (ii) the expression of BMP system components undergoes dynamic changes during follicular and corpora luteal morphogenesis and histogenesis [2]. The general principle to emerge from these studies is that the developmental programs of folliculogenesis (recruitment, selection, atresia), ovulation, and luteogenesis (luteinization, luteolysis) are accompanied by rather dramatic spatial and temporal changes in the expression patterns of these BMP genes. Therefore, these results have led us to hypothesize previously unanticipated roles for the BMP family in determining fundamental developmental events that ensure the proper timing and progression of cell division and differentiation during the estrous cycle.

## 2. BMP-4 and -7 differentially regulate follicle-stimulating hormone (FSH)-induced estradiol and progesterone synthesis

Using recombinant BMPs, we uncovered novel functions of BMP-4 and BMP-7, which are expressed in theca cells of the rat ovary. In these experiments, we found that BMP-4 and -7 are the first molecules known to differentially regulate follicle stimulating hormone (FSH)-induced estradiol and progesterone production by rat granulosa cells (GCs), in a way that reflects the normal steroidogenic physiology during the follicular phase of the cycle, i.e. these BMPs enhance and suppress FSH-induced estradiol and progesterone production, respectively [3]. These findings provide strong support for the new concept that BMPs play an important physiological role in regulating FSH action in the mammalian ovary. Because a precise temporal and quantitative pattern of FSH action is obligatory for normal folliculogenesis and cyclicity, this ovarian BMP system could have new implications for fertility and infertility [2].

## 3. BMP-7 regulates folliculogenesis and ovulation

We also demonstrated that BMP-7 exhibits pronounced activity when administered locally to rat ovaries in vivo, influencing multiple stages of folliculogenesis from initial recruitment through ovulation [2,4]. These studies revealed that BMP-7 decreases the number of primordial follicles, but increases the number of primary, secondary, and antral follicles. Thus, BMP-7 promotes the recruitment of primordial follicles into the growing follicle pool. The concurrent finding that BMP-7 stimulates GC mitosis in vitro suggests a possible mechanism by which BMP-7 stimulates this process. In contrast to the stimulatory role of BMP-7 in early folliculogenesis, BMP-7 reduced the number of ovulated oocytes. Because BMP-7 also caused a reduction in circulating progesterone, and given that progesterone is essential for ovulation, the inhibition of progesterone production by BMP-7 could be causally connected to the mechanisms of ovulation inhibition.

## 4. BMP-6 does not regulate GC proliferation

BMP-6 mRNA is strongly expressed in the oocytes and GCs of healthy Graafian follicles in the rat ovary [1]. Since BMP-7 has been shown to stimulate GC mitosis, we also examined whether BMP-6 is capable of regulating GC proliferation. Treatment of primary cultured rat

GCs with BMP-6 (0–300 ng/ml) produced no significant change in thymidine incorporation nor any change in GC numbers [5].

## 5. BMP-6 inhibits FSH action by suppressing adenylate cyclase activity

Similar to BMP-4 and -7, BMP-6 was found to inhibit FSH-induced progesterone synthesis in rat GCs [5]. Consistent with this effect, BMP-6 inhibits FSH-induced stimulation of StAR and P450scc mRNA expression. Interestingly, BMP-6 also inhibits forskolin-stimulated progesterone synthesis, as well as the corresponding expression of StAR and P450scc, but fails to inhibit progesterone synthesis and these steroidogenic parameters induced by 8-bromo cAMP (Br-cAMP). BMP-6 also inhibits the expression of mRNAs encoding other FSH-responsive genes, including the inhibin/activin subunits ($\alpha$, $\beta$A, and $\beta$B) and the luteinizing hormone (LH) receptor, when stimulated by forskolin or FSH, but not by Br-cAMP. These data, together with the fact that BMP-6 decreases FSH- and forskolin-induced cAMP production, are consistent with the proposal that BMP-6 inhibits FSH action by suppressing adenylate cyclase activity [5]. In terms of physiology, it should be noted that BMP-6 mRNA expression in GCs, but not oocytes, is rapidly decreased at the time the dominant follicle is selected during the normal estrous cycle in the rat [1]. The loss of the FSH action inhibitor, BMP-6, may be linked to the mechanism by which dominant follicles are selected in the rat. The finding that BMP-6 mRNA is strongly expressed in GCs during atresia is also consistent with this hypothesis.

A strain of sheep called Booroola, which are highly prolific due to an increased ovulation quota, has been found to carry a mutation in the kinase domain of activin-like receptor kinase-6 (ALK-6) [6–8], an established type I receptor for multiple BMPs. Our findings on the biological activities and cellular mechanism of BMP-6 suggest that the Booroola phenotype may be caused, at least in part, by the inability of Booroola GCs to properly elicit BMP-6 signaling [2]. This hypothesis is supported by the fact that Booroola GCs are more responsive to FSH than normal GCs, with respect to cAMP production, with no changes in FSH binding capacity [9]. Moreover, follicles dissected from the ovaries of Booroola ewes produce increased amounts of progesterone induced by FSH, compared with the comparable follicles from wild-type ewes, yet there is no change in estradiol production. Collectively, the enhanced gonadotropin responsiveness of the follicles from Booroola ewes, compared with those from wild-type ewes, could be explained by the incapable ALK-6 signaling triggered by endogenous BMP-6. Thus, BMP-6 may control fundamental physiological processes in follicular development that are vitally important for female fertility. However, since BMP receptors and ligands have broadly overlapping functions in redundant system, multiple ligands are likely to be involved in the aberrant phenotype of Booroola ewes.

## 6. BMP-15 stimulates GC proliferation

Since results from in situ hybridization and immunohistochemistry analyses indicated that BMP-15 is expressed exclusively in the oocyte in the rat ovary and its expression increases in association with follicle growth and development, we hypothesized that BMP-15 may be an important factor for regulating GC proliferation and/or differentiation. We first examined the mitotic activity of BMP-15 in cultured rat GCs. BMP-15 increased thymidine uptake of GCs in a dose-dependent manner [10]. This finding was not only the first reported biological activity of BMP-15, but it also indicates that GCs are target cells for BMP-15. BMP-15 increases GC number and, taken together, we concluded that BMP-15 is a mitogen for GCs. The fact that the mitotic activity of BMP-15 is FSH-independent suggests that it plays an important role in promoting early (FSH-independent) stages of follicle development.

## 7. BMP-15 inhibits FSH action by suppressing FSH receptor expression

Another important action of BMP-15 is its ability to inhibit FSH actions [2,11]. Namely, the FSH-induced expressions of StAR, P450scc, 3β-HSD, LH receptor, and inhibin/activin subunits (α, βA, and βB) are all inhibited by BMP-15. The finding that FSH-induced StAR, P450scc, and progesterone synthesis are inhibited by BMP-15 demonstrates that BMP-15, like BMP-4, -6, -7, and GDF-9, is a luteinization inhibitor. The BMP-15 suppression of FSH action on all these parameters is quite similar to that of BMP-6. However, the underlying mechanism by which BMP-6 and BMP-15 inhibit FSH action is different. BMP-6 inhibits FSH signaling by suppressing adenylate cyclase activity, whereas BMP-15 inhibits FSH signaling by suppressing FSH receptor expression. Indeed, BMP-15 does not inhibit the stimulatory action of forskolin. Regarding BMP-6 and BMP-15 action, it is noteworthy that neither ligand inhibits the stimulatory action of FSH on P450arom mRNA expression and estradiol production. In these in vitro cell culture experiments, androstenedione was added to the medium to serve as a substrate for P450arom. Interestingly, in the absence of androstenedione, both ligands inhibit FSH stimulation of P450arom mRNA expression [11]. Given the fact that, in vivo, FSH stimulates the expression of P450arom mRNA and estradiol production in dominant follicles replete with androstenedione in the follicular fluid, neither BMP-6 nor BMP-15 would be expected to affect FSH-dependent estradiol production in vivo. This action of BMP-6 and BMP-15 is clearly different from that of BMP-4 and BMP-7, both of which enhance FSH-induced estradiol production. Nonetheless, an important consensus is that all these BMPs are selective inhibitors of progesterone synthesis induced by FSH. Collectively, this provides strong support for our initial hypothesis that BMPs are the long sought luteinization inhibitors [3].

A strain of sheep, called Inverdale, has been shown to carry a single point mutation in the BMP-15 gene [12]. The investigation of the reproductive phenotype of the Inverdale ewe provides in vivo data that support our in vitro findings on the role of BMP-15 in regulating GC processes and establishes the importance of this oocyte-secreted factor in mammalian reproduction. Specifically, ewes that are homozygous carriers of the Inverdale mutation in the BMP-15 gene exhibit a block in folliculogenesis at the primary stage. Consequently, these animals fail to ovulate and are infertile. Surprisingly, the heterozygous mutants exhibit increased ovulation rates. In this connection, several interesting abnormal features of the ovaries of the heterozygotes have been identified: (i) there are more healthy estrogenic follicles, (ii) the number of GCs in these developing follicles is significantly smaller, (iii) these GCs have a higher mean LH responsiveness at smaller follicle stages, and (iv) the corpora lutea are smaller [13]. The fact that the plasma FSH and LH levels in the heterozygotes are normal would imply that the mechanisms responsible for these unusual features in the heterozygote reside in the ovary. Our observation that BMP-15 inhibits FSH receptor expression could explain the cause of the abnormal phenotype of the Inverdale ewe [2]. In the heterozygotes, we propose that reduced levels of intact BMP-15 result in higher levels of FSH receptors in the GCs, which, in turn, lead to more developing healthy estrogenic follicles with high expression levels of the LH receptor. The end result of this sequence of events would be precocious follicle maturation, leading to an increased ovulation rate. At the opposite extreme, follicle development in the homozygotes is arrested at the primary follicle (FSH-independent) stage. In these homozygous ewes, the impaired GC proliferation corresponds to our findings that BMP-15 is a potent GC mitogen [10] and stimulates the expression of kit ligand (KL) [14], which is also essential for normal folliculogenesis [15].

## 8. BMP-15 stimulates kit ligand expression, whereas kit ligand inhibits BMP-15 expression

A third important biological function of BMP-15 that we have uncovered is that BMP-15 stimulates the expression of kit ligand (KL) mRNA in rat GCs [14]. KL, in turn, caused a reduction in the expression of BMP-15 mRNA. Therefore, oocyte-derived BMP-15 and GC-derived KL form a novel negative feedback loop that is functionally linked to GC proliferation [2]. There is evidence that growing oocytes isolated from immature mouse ovaries enhance KL expression when co-cultured with GCs [16,17]. Therefore, it is possible that the KL-inducing factor secreted by growing oocytes is BMP-15.

## 9. Follistatin inhibits BMP-15 bioactivities

We also found that follistatin binds BMP-15 and inhibits its biological activities by forming an inactive complex. The binding of follistatin to BMP-15 was demonstrated directly using a surface plasmon resonance biosensor. The ability of follistatin to inhibit BMP-15 functions was demonstrated using our established BMP-15 bioassays in primary rat GC cultures. Specifically, follistatin attenuated BMP-15 stimulation of GC proliferation and reversed BMP-15 inhibition of FSH receptor mRNA expression and the subsequent suppression of FSH-induced progesterone synthesis. This was the first demonstration of the biochemical interaction between follistatin and BMP-15, as well as the biological antagonism of BMP-15 by follistatin. Follistatin is strongly expressed in dominant follicles of rat ovaries, whereas its expression in atretic follicles is very low or undetectable in rat ovaries [18,19]. Given that BMP-15 is an inhibitor of FSH receptor expression, it can be predicted that follistatin regulation of BMP-15 is important for normal folliculogenesis in vivo. The capacity of follistatin to inhibit the actions of both activin and BMP-15 in GCs, which have opposing influence on FSH-induced cytodifferentiation [3,10], begins to establish the complex, yet well-balanced, mechanisms by which folliculogenesis is precisely regulated in female mammals.

## 10. Conclusion

Collectively, recent research has demonstrated that the BMP system comprises a critical component of the local regulatory system by which ovarian processes are physiologically governed. Specifically, BMP ligands and receptors are powerful regulators of fundamental GC functions, including mitosis and FSH-mediated differentiation and steroidogenesis. Accordingly, further research in this field will, undoubtedly, greatly advance our understanding of ovarian physiology. It may also lead to novel targets for clinical regimens aimed at modulating female fertility for the purpose of developing new strategies to manage infertility, as well as for the development of novel nonsteroidal contraceptives.

## Acknowledgements

We thank Andrea Hartgrove for excellent editorial assistance. This work was supported in part by NIH Grant RO1 HD41494 and NICHD/NIH through cooperative agreement [U54HD12303] as part of Specialized Cooperative Centers Program in Reproduction Research. F. Otsuka was supported by a Fellowship Grant from The Lalor Foundation and R.K. Moore was supported by a Medical Research Fellowship from Giannini Family Foundation.

## References

[1] G.F. Erickson, S. Shimasaki, The spatiotemporal expression pattern of the bone morphogenetic protein family in rat ovary cell types during the estrous cycle, Reprod. Biol. Endocrinol. 1 (2003) 9.
[2] S. Shimasaki, R.K. Moore, F. Otsuka, G.F. Erickson, The bone morphogenetic protein system in mammalian reproduction, Endocr. Rev. 25 (2004) 72–101.
[3] S. Shimasaki, R.J. Zachow, D. Li, H. Kim, S.-I. Iemura, N. Ueno, K. Sampath, R.J. Chang, G.F. Erickson, A functional bone morphogenetic protein system in the ovary, Proc. Natl. Acad. Sci. U. S. A. 96 (1999) 7282–7287.
[4] W. Lee, F. Otsuka, R.K. Moore, S. Shimasaki, The effect of bone morphogenetic protein-7 on folliculogenesis and ovulation in the rat, Biol. Reprod. 65 (2001) 994–999.
[5] F. Otsuka, R.K. Moore, S. Shimasaki, Biological function and cellular mechanism of bone morphogenetic protein-6 in the ovary, J. Biol. Chem. 276 (2001) 32889–32895.
[6] T. Wilson, X.-Y. Wu, J.L. Juengel, I.K. Ross, J.M. Lumsden, E.A. Lord, K.G. Dodds, G.A. Walling, J.C. McEwan, A.R. O'Connell, K.P. McNatty, G.W. Montgomery, Highly prolific Booroola sheep have a mutation in the intracellular kinase domain of bone morphogenetic protein 1B receptor (ALK-6) that is expressed in both oocytes and granulosa cells, Biol. Reprod. 64 (2001) 1225–1235.
[7] P. Mulsant, F. Lecerf, S. Fabre, L. Schibler, P. Monget, I. Lanneluc, C. Pisselet, J. Riquet, D. Monniaux, I. Callebaut, E. Cribiu, J. Thimonier, J. Teyssier, L. Bodin, Y. Cognie, N. Chitour, J.-M. Elsen, Mutation in bone morphogenetic protein receptor-1B is associated with increased ovulation rate in Booroola Merino ewes, Proc. Natl. Acad. Sci. U. S. A. 98 (2001) 5104–5109.
[8] C.J.H. Souza, C. MacDougall, B.K. Campbell, A.S. McNeilly, D.T. Baird, The booroola (FecB) phenotype is associated with a mutation in the bone morphogenetic receptor type 1 B (BMPR1B) gene, J. Endocrinol. 169 (2001) R1–R6.
[9] K.P. McNatty, L.E. Kieboom, J. McDiarmid, D.A. Heath, S. Lun, Adenosine cyclic $3',5'$-monophosphate and steroid production by small ovarian follicles from booroola ewes with and without a fecundity gene, J. Reprod. Fertil. 76 (1986) 471–480.
[10] F. Otsuka, Z. Yao, T.H. Lee, S. Yamamoto, G.F. Erickson, S. Shimasaki, Bone morphogenetic protein-15: identification of target cells and biological functions, J. Biol. Chem. 275 (2000) 39523–39528.
[11] F. Otsuka, S. Yamamoto, G.F. Erickson, S. Shimasaki, Bone morphogenetic protein-15 inhibits folliclestimulating hormone (FSH) action by suppressing FSH receptor expression, J. Biol. Chem. 276 (2001) 11387–11392.
[12] S.M. Galloway, K.P. McNatty, L.M. Cambridge, M.P.E. Laitinen, J.L. Juengel, T.S. Jokiranta, R.J. McLaren, K. Luiro, K.G. Dodds, G.W. Montgomery, A.E. Beattie, G.H. Davis, O. Ritvos, Mutations in an

oocyte-derived growth factor gene (BMP15) cause increased ovulation rate and infertility in a dosage-sensitive manner, Nat. Genet. 25 (2000) 279–283.
[13] G.H. Shackell, N.L. Hudson, D.A. Heath, S. Lun, L. Shaw, L. Condell, L.R. Blay, K.P. McNatty, Plasma gonadotropin concentrations and ovarian characteristics in inverdale ewes that are heterozygous for a major gene (FecX1) on the X chromosome that influences ovulation rate, Biol. Reprod. 48 (1993) 1150–1156.
[14] F. Otsuka, S. Shimasaki, A negative feedback system between oocyte bone morphogenetic protein 15 and granulosa cell kit ligand: its role in regulating granulosa cell mitosis, Proc. Natl. Acad. Sci. U. S. A. 99 (2002) 8060–8065.
[15] M.A. Driancourt, K. Reynaud, R. Cortvrindt, J. Smitz, Roles of kit and kit ligand in ovarian function, Rev. Reprod. 5 (2000) 143–152.
[16] A.I. Packer, Y.C. Hsu, P. Besmer, R.F. Bachvarova, The ligand of the c-kit receptor promotes oocyte growth, Dev. Biol. 161 (1994) 194–205.
[17] I.M. Joyce, F.L. Pendola, K. Wigglesworth, J.J. Eppig, Oocyte regulation of kit ligand expression in mouse ovarian follicles, Dev. Biol. 214 (1999) 342–353.
[18] S. Shimasaki, M. Koga, M.L. Buscaglia, D.M. Simmons, T.A. Bicsak, N. Ling, Follistatin gene expression in the ovary and extragonadal tissues, Mol. Endocrinol. 3 (1989) 651–659.
[19] A. Nakatani, S. Shimasaki, L.V. DePaolo, G.F. Erickson, N. Ling, Cyclic changes in follistatin gene expression and translation in the rat ovary during the estrous cycle, Endocrinology 129 (1991) 603–611.

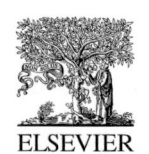

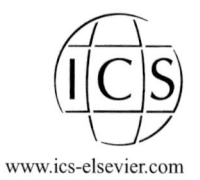

# Clinical use of cytokines in ovulation induction

Hitoshi Okamura[a,*], Takashi Ohba[a], Hidetaka Katabuchi[a], Nobuyuki Tanaka[a], Akihisa Takasaki[b,1]

[a]*Department of Reproductive Medicine and Surgery, Faculty of Medical and Pharmaceutical Sciences, Kumamoto University, Honjo 1-1-1, Kumamoto 860-8556, Japan*
[b]*Department of Obstetrics and Gynecology, Saiseikai Shimonoseki General Hospital, Kifune 3-4-1 Shimonoseki, Yamaguchi 751-8502, Japan*

**Abstract.** Ovarian dysfunction, which is resistant to normal ovulation induction therapies and known to the clinician as "poor response", is a heterogenic syndrome. Although most causes of ovarian dysfunction are unclear, recent molecular techniques have clarified the subtle defects in function of the cells surrounding the oocyte. Macrophages have been identified in growing follicles of humans and rats and they promote the proliferation of granulosa cells as local mediators. A hematopoietic growth factor, colony-stimulating factor-1 (CSF-1), is produced by granulosa cells and stimulates the follicular macrophages to enhance cytokine production. In CSF-1 null mice, characterized by severely depleted macrophage populations in many tissues, the numbers of both antral and mature follicles are significantly lower, but are recovered by administration of CSF-1. We have reported that gonadotropins lead to increased human ovarian CSF-1 production and that this augmentation of CSF-1 in response to human menopausal gonadotropins (hMG) administration is lost in poor responders. By concomitant administration of CSF-1 with hMG, follicle development is improved in poor responders who show low serum CSF-1 levels in the follicular phase. These women show normal responses to the examination of the growth hormone (GH) reserve. Thus, CSF-1 may be a useful therapeutic tool for selected poor responders. © 2004 Published by Elsevier B.V.

*Keywords:* CSF-1; Macrophage; Follicle development; Ovulation induction; Poor responder

## 1. Introduction

Macrophages, essential in the immune response, are also thought to have tropic roles, through their capabilities of cytokine production. They are abundant in the reproductive tract of both male and female and are in close proximity to steroidogenic cells. These observations have suggested that macrophages play important roles in reproductive processes.

---

\* Corresponding author. Tel.: +81-96-373-5269; fax: +81-96-363-5164.
*E-mail address:* hokamura@kaiju.medic.kumamoto-u.ac.jp (H. Okamura).
[1] Tel.: +81-832-5201; fax: +81-832-32-8209.

0531-5131/ © 2004 Published by Elsevier B.V.
doi:10.1016/j.ics.2004.01.067

Macrophages are found in the corpus luteum [1] and are also recognized in the developing follicle [2]. Fig. 1a shows the distribution of macrophages in the rat ovary. Macrophages were found in the granulosa layer of antral and mature follicles, as well as the stroma around the developing follicles and corpora lutea. The average ratios of macrophages to granulosa cells in preantral, antral and, mature follicles were 0.008, 0.007 and, 0.002, respectively. Macrophages promote the proliferation of granulosa cells as local mediators in developing follicles (Fig. 2) [3]. Labeling of granulosa cells with [$^3H$]thymidine was significantly greater and the labeling index peaked at 25.0% when the ratio of macrophages to granulosa cells was 0.01, compared with the value of 14.2% when the granulosa cells were cultured alone. This ratio of macrophages to granulosa cells was close to those found in preantral and antral follicles in vivo. These results suggest that macrophages participate in the proliferation of granulosa cells as local mediators in growing follicles.

Colony-stimulating factor-1 (CSF-1, also known as macrophage colony-stimulating factor, M-CSF) is a homodimeric glycoprotein that belongs to the family of hematopoietic growth factors [4]. CSF-1 mRNA can be detected in granulosa cells in mice and humans. Through alternative mRNA splicing and differential posttranslational proteolytic processing, CSF-1 can either be secreted into the circulation or be expressed as a membrane-spanning glycoprotein on the surface of CSF-1-producing cells. Its action is exerted via a transmembrane receptor tyrosine kinase, CSF-1R, encoded by the c-*fms* protooncogene product [5]. CSF-1 is a chemoattractant for macrophages [6], induces proliferation and differentiation of monocyte–macrophage progenitor cells [7] and acts on mature monocytes and macrophages to maintain their survival [8,9]. Additionally, CSF-1 has indirect effects on cellular proliferation through the stimulation of cytokine production and release by macrophages, such as epidermal growth factor (EGF) [10], tumor necrosis factor (TNF)

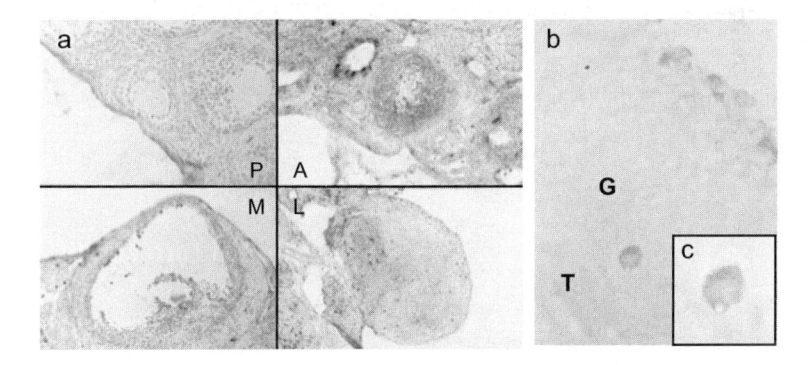

Fig. 1. (a) Distribution of macrophages in rat ovary. Immunohistochemistry was performed using mouse antirat macrophage monoclonal antibodies TRPM-3 (BMA Biomedicals, Augusto). Macrophages were found in the granulosa layer of antral (A) and mature (M) follicles and in corpora lutea (L) and stroma around the developing follicles. Methyl green. (P) Primordial follicle, ×40, (A) antral follicle, ×40, (M) mature follicle, ×20, (L) corpus luteum, ×20, (b and c) Double immunostaining of EGF and macrophages in rat ovary. The sections were incubated with mouse antirat EGF monoclonal antibody. After visualization of peroxydase activity with DAB–H$_2$O$_2$, the sections were stained with TRPM-3 by alkaline phosphatase antialkaline phosphatase (APAAP) method. (G) Granulosa cell layer, (T) theca cell layer, ×80 (b), ×200 (c).

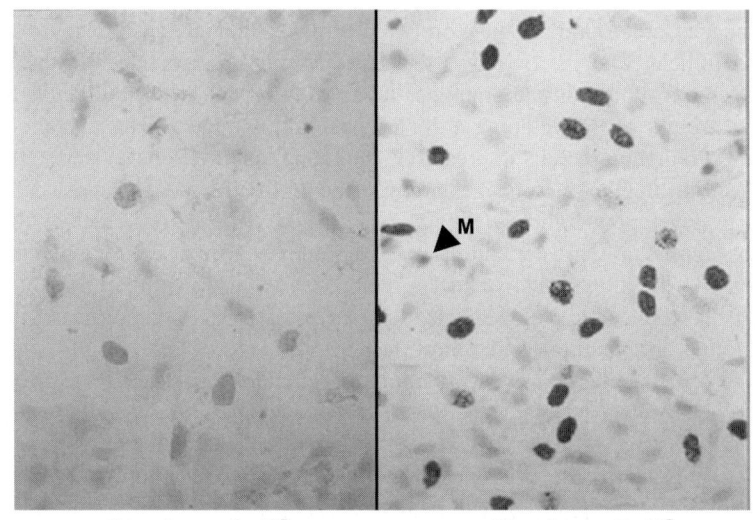

Granulosa cells 10⁵          Granulosa cells 10⁵
                               + Macrophages 10³

Fig. 2. [$^3H$]Thymidine autoradiography of $10^5$ rat granulosa cells cultured with $10^3$ macrophages. Rat granulosa cells were cocultured with rat peritoneal macrophages in various concentrations for 24 h. To examine the proliferative capacity of the granulosa cells, they were incubated in medium containing 1 μCi/ml of [methyl-$^3H$]thymidine for 2 h. Granulosa cells labeled with [$^3H$]thymidine have numerous grains on the nucleus. Macrophage (M, arrowhead) can be easily distinguished because they are smaller and rounder than granulosa cells, ×360.

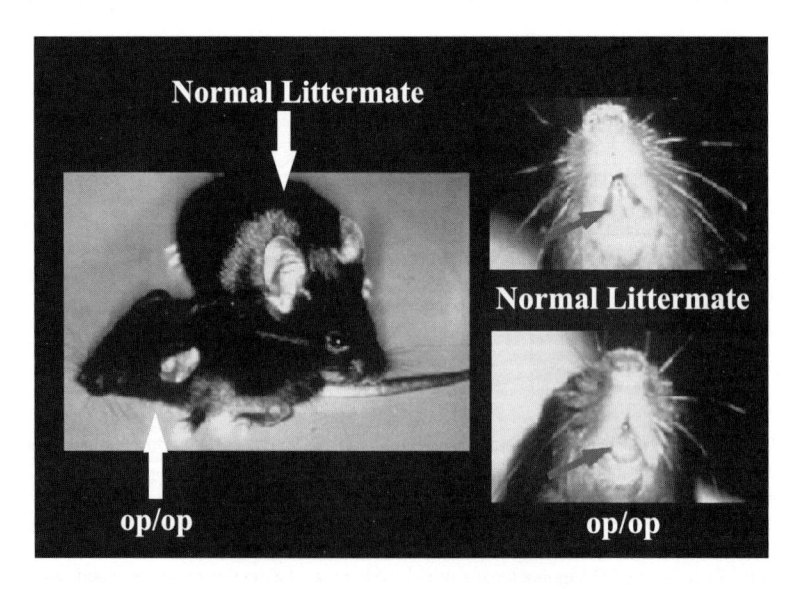

Fig. 3. Mice homozygous for the null mutation in the CSF-1 gene, osteopetrotic ($Csfm^{op}/Csfm^{op}$) mice. They have severely depleted macrophage populations and show osteopetrosis and low fertility.

alpha [11], transforming growth factor (TGF) beta [12], and fibroblast growth factor (FGF) [13]. Fig. 1b and c shows the double immunostaining in a rat antral follicle. The diffuse staining indicates immunoreactive EGF and the granules indicate that the cell is a macrophage.

## 2. The role of CSF-1 in osteopetrotic mice

Mice homozygous for the null mutation in the CSF-1 gene, osteopetrotic ($Csfm^{op}$/$Csfm^{op}$) mice (Fig. 3), have severely depleted macrophage populations in many tissues [14]. Female osteopetrotic mice have extended estrous cycles (approximately 14 days), compared with the normal 5-day cycle [15]. In $Csfm^{op}$/$Csfm^{op}$ mice, the numbers of both antral and mature follicles in the proestrous ovary were significantly lower (39.2±3.1 vs. 77.8±4.0 and 9.1±1.5 vs. 16.3±1.4, respectively), which lead to a decreased number of ovulations. The numbers of granulosa cells and macrophages in the antral follicles were significantly decreased and the proliferative capacity of granulosa cells in antral follicles was reduced in $Csfm^{op}$/$Csfm^{op}$ mice, compared with normal littermates. Administration of recombinant human CSF-1 (Mirimostim, Leukoprol®, Kyowa, Japan) to $Csfm^{op}$/$Csfm^{op}$ mice recovered the number of granulosa cells and macrophages, the proliferative capacity of granulosa cells, and the number of ovulations (Table 1) [16]. Although the effects of direct signaling of CSF-1 to the oocyte must be considered, these data suggest that macrophages are implicated in the process of folliculogenesis and ovulation.

Table 1
Manifestation of the follicles of $Csfm^{op}$/$Csfm^{op}$ mice undergoing CSF-1 treatment

|  | Normal littermates | $Csfm^{op}$/$Csfm^{op}$ | $Csfm^{op}$/$Csfm^{op}$ +CSF-1 |
| --- | --- | --- | --- |
| No. of antral follicles / ovaries examined | 20/5 | 20/6 | 20/6 |
| No. of follicles containing macrophages | 14 | 1 | 8 |
| No. of granulosa cells per section of one antral follicle | 525.1 ± 10.2 | 465.6 ± 19.7 | 516.3 ± 9.5 |
| No. of proliferating granulosa cells per section of one antral follicle | 45.3 ± 4.3 | 28.3 ± 3.4 | 39.4 ± 3.1 |
| No. of macrophages per section of one antral follicle | 1.8 ± 0.4 | 0.1 ± 0.1 | 0.6 ± 0.2 |
| No. of ovulated ova per animal | 11.1 ± 0.4 | 4.1 ± 0.9 | 8.1 ± 0.8 |

The number of antral follicles (200–400 μm in the greatest diameter) was counted microscopically in serial sections of each ovary stained with HE or immunohistochemically. Rat antimouse macrophage monoclonal antibody, F4/80 (kindly supplied by Dr. Simon Gordon, Oxford University, UK), was used in immunohistochemistry. [$^3H$]Thymidine autoradiography was performed to determine the proliferating granulosa cells. The metestrous oviducts were separated from the ovaries and uterus and the number of oocytes were enumerated under a dissecting microscope.
*p < 0.01, **p < 0.05.

## 3. Cotreatment with CSF-1 for ovulation induction; rat model

The effects of CSF-1 in folliculogenesis and ovulation were studied in gonadotropin-treated immature female rats. Folliculogenesis and ovulation were induced in immature female Wistar rats with a subcutaneous injection of equine chorionic gonadotropin (eCG), followed 48 h later by human chorionic gonadotropin (hCG). When CSF-1 was administered daily for three consecutive days (i.e., 48, 24, and 0 h before hCG injection), more than $30 \times 10^3$ IU of CSF-1 significantly increased, in a dose-dependent manner, the number of ovulations up to twofold compared with the controls that were stimulated with eCG/hCG alone [17]. This stimulatory effect was also observed when CSF-1 was administered between 96 and 49 h before hCG injection. To investigate the effect of CSF-1 on the number of macrophages in developing rat follicles, $100 \times 10^3$ IU of CSF-1 was administered intraperitoneally at 1 h before eCG injection and the ovaries were removed 24 h later. The number of follicular macrophages per section was counted using immunohistochemistry with mouse anti-rat macrophage monoclonal antibody, TRPM-3. CSF-1 significantly increased the number of ovarian macrophages in mature follicles ($3.4 \pm 0.7$ vs. $1.6 \pm 1.2$ in one section, $p<0.05$).

## 4. Changes of CSF-1 concentration in serum and follicular fluid in IVF cycles

CSF-1 concentration in follicular fluid is significantly higher than in the serum, at least in humans [18]. To examine the changes of CSF-1 concentrations in serum and follicles during the menstrual cycle, sera and matched follicular fluids were collected serially through in vitro fertilization (IVF) cycles ($n=126$). Serum CSF-1 concentration gradually increased throughout ovarian stimulation and reached a peak from the day of oocyte retrieval for 2 days. However, no significant change in CSF-1 was observed in women with poor ovarian response to hMG, in whom fewer than two developing follicles were observed by transvaginal ultrasonography on the day of hCG administration or the day of cancellation of IVF (Table 2) [19]. The concentrations of CSF-1 in follicles from which an oocyte could be retrieved were significantly higher than in those from which an oocyte could not be retrieved. These results suggest that follicle-synthesized CSF-1 may play a role in promoting follicular development.

Table 2
Serum CSF-1 concentrations (mean±S.E.M., U/ml) in IVF cycles

|  | Follicular phase ||  Days after hCG injection |||  Luteal phase |
| --- | --- | --- | --- | --- | --- | --- |
|  | Early | Mid | 0 | 1 | 2 | Mid |
| Total | 704.9±20.2 | 843.7±29.7 | 916.4±36.5 | 931.8±37.7 | 945.3±43.4* | 974.4±61.1 |
| Good responder | 770.9±60.3 | 1050±80.1 | 1213.2±80.9* | 1163.0±112.0* | 1278.6±111.7* | 1550.8±172.3* |
| Poor responder | 791.1±32.4 | 786.2±32.9 | 798.0±70.6 | 791.4±72.0 | 778.8±61.6 | 789.0±56.1 |

Total ($n=126$): All cycles examined undergoing IVF procedures. The mean age of patients was 33.8±4.6 years (range 25–42 years). Indication for IVF was tubal factor ($n=43$), male factor ($n=27$), endometriosis ($n=13$), functional infertility ($n=14$), and refractory infertility ($n=11$). Good responders ($n=8$): cycles in which more than 20 developing follicles were observed by transvaginal ultrasonography on the day of hCG administration. Poor responders ($n=9$): cycles in which less than two developing follicles were observed by transvaginal ultrasonography on the day of hCG administration or the day of cancellation of IVF. CSF-1 was assayed using ELISA for human CSF-1 established by Hanamura et al. [21].

* Significantly different from the value of each follicular phase ($p<0.05$).

## 5. Cotreatment with CSF-1 for ovulation induction for poor responders

To investigate the effect of cotreatment with CSF-1 for ovulation induction with hMG on conception in poor responders, follicular development, ovulation rate, and pregnancy rate were compared between groups of women who received either $8\times10^6$ IU/day of CSF-1 for 3 days concomitant with 150 IU/day of hMG, followed by hCG, or 150 IU/day of hMG alone, in a preliminary, prospective protocol of ovulation induction for either in vivo insemination or IVF. All of these women were normogonadotropic (mean serum FSH concentration $8.4\pm3.2$ mIU/ml) with long-standing infertility, despite many previous attempts at ovulation induction with hMG/hCG. All women were diagnosed as positive by clonidine test or growth hormone (GH)-releasing factor stimulation test, to eliminate systemic GH insufficiency, which is one of the possible causes of poor responses to gonadotropins [20].

In this study protocol, a total of 30 poor responders were pretreated with gonadotropin releasing hormone (GnRH) analog from the midluteal phase of the preceding cycle and received 150 IU of recombinant human follicle stimulating hormone (FSH, Fertinorm P®, Serono, Japan) daily from cycle day 3, followed by 150 IU of hMG (Humegon®, Teikoku Zouki, Japan) daily, with concomitant administration of $8\times10^6$ IU of recombinant human CSF-1 every other day up to four times (Fig. 4). HCG was administered when a leading follicle reached 18 mm in diameter. Oocyte retrieval was performed 35 h after the hCG injection in IVF cycles.

Controlled ovarian hyperstimulation was superior in GnRH/FSH/hMG plus CSF-1 stimulation cycles, compared with the prior cycles with GnRH/FSH/hMG. There were more mature follicles ($2.8\pm1.3$ vs. $0.36\pm0.5$), fewer cycle cancellations (8.3% vs. 83.3%), and lower doses of gonadotropin required ($1786.4\pm472.9$ vs. $2120.5\pm476.8$ IU). Five (16.7%) pregnancies were achieved in association with the CSF-1 cotreatment among 30 poor responders. We conclude that CSF-1 may increase the pregnancy rate when combined with hMG/hCG for ovulation induction.

Next, we performed a further study to identify the most suitable candidates among poor responders for cotreatment with CSF-1. Serum CSF-1 concentrations were assayed in 22 women on day 3 of the IVF cycle to determine endogenous CSF-1 secretion [21]. In this study, "CSF-1 effective" was defined as a case in which the number of mature oocytes was increased by 2 or more with CFS-1 cotreatment, compared with the number in the preceding

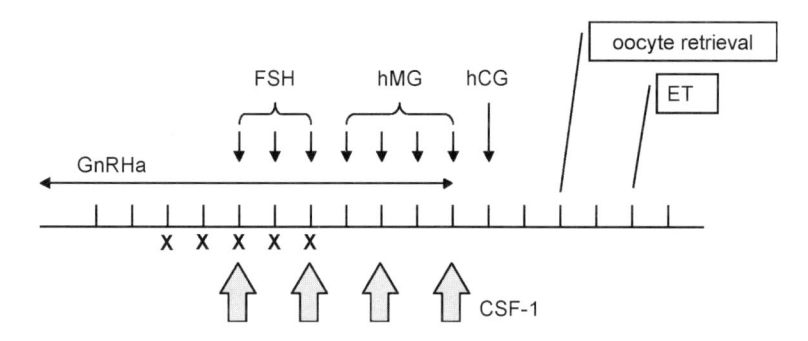

Fig. 4. Protocol of concomitant CSF-1 treatment with FSH/hMG in IVF cycles for poor responders.

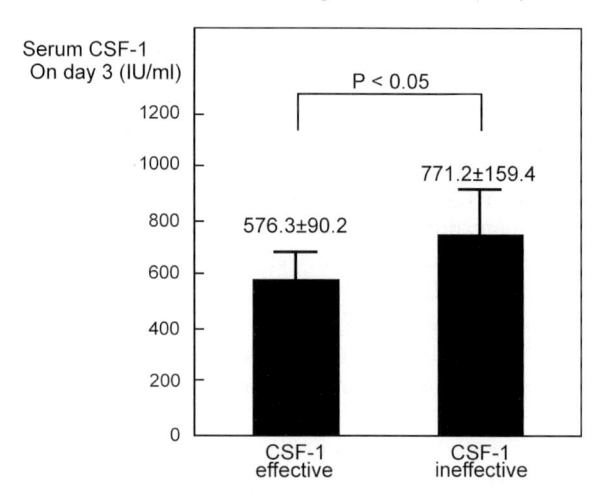

Fig. 5. Serum concentrations of CSF-1 on day 3 of the IVF cycle. "CSF-1 effective" was defined as cases in which the number of mature oocytes was increased by 2 or more, compared with the number in the preceding IVF cycle stimulated with hMG/hCG alone.

IVF cycle stimulated with hMG/hCG alone. The CSF-1 effective patients showed significantly lower serum CSF-1 concentrations on day 3 than the CSF-1 ineffective patients (576.3±90.2 vs. 771.2±159.4 IU/ml, $p<0.05$) (Fig. 5). We thereby determined the diagnostic potential and cut-off values for serum CSF-1 among poor responders using receiver operator characteristic (ROC) analysis, based on the serum concentrations of CSF-1 on day 3 of the cycle. The optimal cut-off value, 650 IU/ml, for serum CSF-1 concentration gave an efficiency of 77.8% (sensitivity of 63.6%, specificity of 81.8%). Four women (36.4%) conceived among the 11 poor responders who showed serum CSF-1 concentrations less than 650 IU/ml, in contrast to none of 11 women with higher serum CSF-1 concentrations.

## 6. Conclusion

Improving pregnancy rates in poor responders remains a challenge in treatment with controlled ovarian hyperstimulation and IVF. A variety of protocols has been used to improve responses in these women. Here we report an approach to poor responders, based upon our findings from basic research. Macrophages are considered as important accessory cells for reproductive function and CSF-1 may be a useful therapeutic tool for selected poor responders, particularly those who have insufficient serum levels of CSF-1 measured on day 3 of the cycle.

## References

[1] L.G. Paavola, C.O. Boyd, Surface morphology of macrophages in the regressing corpus luteum, as revealed by scanning electron microscopy, Anat. Rec. 195 (1979) 659–681.
[2] H. Katabuchi, et al., Distribution and fine structure of macrophages in the human ovary during the menstrual cycle, pregnancy and menopause, Endocr. J. 44 (1997) 785–795.

[3]  Y. Fukumatsu, et al., Effect of macrophages on proliferation of granulosa cells in the ovary in rats, J. Reprod. Fertil. 96 (1992) 241–249.
[4]  S.C. Clark, R. Kamen, The human hematopoietic colony-stimulating factors, Science 236 (1987) 1229–1237.
[5]  E.R. Stanley, et al., Biology and action of colony-stimulating factor-1, Mol. Reprod. Dev. 46 (1997) 4–10.
[6]  S.E. Webb, J.W. Pollard, G.E. Jones, Direct observation and quantification of macrophage chemoattraction to the growth factor CSF-1, J. Cell Sci. 109 (1996) 793–803.
[7]  E.R. Stanley, P.M. Heard, Factors regulating macrophage production and growth. Purification and some properties of the colony stimulating factor from medium conditioned by mouse L cells, J. Biol. Chem. 252 (1977) 4305–4312.
[8]  R.J. Tushinski, et al., Survival of mononuclear phagocytes depends on a lineage-specific growth factor that the differentiated cells selectively destroy, Cell 28 (1982) 71–81.
[9]  S. Becker, M.K. Warren, S. Haskill, Colony-stimulating factor-induced monocyte survival and differentiation into macrophages in serum-free cultures, J. Immunol. 139 (1987) 3703–3709.
[10] H. Katabuchi, et al., Role of macrophage in ovarian follicular development, Horm. Res. 46 (1996) 45–51.
[11] M.K. Warren, P. Ralph, Macrophage growth factor CSF-1 stimulates human monocyte production of interferon, tumor necrosis factor, and colony stimulating activity, J. Immunol. 137 (1986) 2281–2285.
[12] R.K. Assoian, et al., Expression and secretion of type beta transforming growth factor by activated human macrophages, Proc. Natl. Acad. Sci. U. S. A. 84 (1987) 6020–6024.
[13] A. Baird, P. Mormede, P. Bohlen, Immunoreactive fibroblast growth factor in cells of peritoneal exudate suggests its identity with macrophage-derived growth factor, Biochem. Biophys. Res. Commun. 126 (1985) 358–364.
[14] H. Yoshida, et al., The murine mutation osteopetrosis is in the coding region of the macrophage colony stimulating factor gene, Nature 345 (1990) 442–444.
[15] P.E. Cohen, L. Zhu, J.W. Pollard, Absence of colony stimulating factor-1 in osteopetrotic (csfmop/csfmop) mice disrupts estrous cycles and ovulation, Biol. Reprod. 56 (1997) 110–118.
[16] M. Araki, et al., Follicular development and ovulation in macrophage colony-stimulating factor-deficient mice homozygous for the osteopetrosis (*op*) mutation, Biol. Reprod. 54 (1996) 478–484.
[17] K. Nishimura, et al., Effects of macrophage colony-stimulating factor on folliculogenesis in gonadotrophin-primed immature rats, J. Reprod. Fertil. 104 (1995) 325–330.
[18] B.R. Witt, J.W. Pollard, Colony stimulating factor-1 (CSF-1) in human follicular fluid, Fertil. Steril. 68 (1997) 259–264.
[19] K. Nishimura, et al., Changes in macrophage colony-stimulating factor concentration in serum and follicular fluid in in-vitro fertilization and embryo transfer cycles, Fertil. Steril. 69 (1998) 53–57.
[20] Z. Blumenfeld, et al., Growth hormone co-treatment for ovulation induction may enhance conception in the co-treatment and succeeding cycles, in clonidine negative but not clonidine positive patients, Hum. Reprod. 9 (1994) 209–213.
[21] T. Hanamura, et al., Quantitation and identification of human monocytic colony-stimulating factor in human serum by enzyme-linked immunosorbent assay, Blood 72 (1988) 886–892.

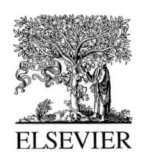

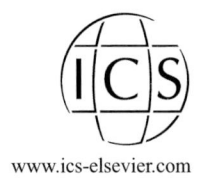

# Solo mothers: quality of parenting and child development

Susan Golombok*

*Family and Child Psychology Research Centre, City University, Northampton Square, EC1V OHB, London, UK*

**Abstract.** *Introduction:* Any consideration of the development of children in solo mother families is essentially addressing the more fundamental question "Do fathers really matter?" This presentation will explore the empirical evidence relating to the two areas of child development where fathers are generally considered to matter a great deal, (i) children's psychological adjustment and (ii) children's sex role development, and will examine whether fathers really do matter for these key aspects of children's lives. *Children's psychological adjustment:* The role of fathers in promoting children's psychological adjustment has been examined in the following ways: (i) Fatherless families have been studied to determine whether children without fathers differ from those who grow up with a father in the home; (ii) Lesbian families have been investigated to establish whether it is a father's maleness, or his role as an additional parent, that is important; (iii) Research has been carried out on families where the father is the primary caregiver to examine what effect this has on the child; and (iv) Traditional two-parent families have been studied to increase understanding of the processes through which fathers' relationships with their children influence children's psychological adjustment. *Children's sex–role development:* Whether or not fathers matter for children's sex–role development depends on the extent to which it is possible for parents to influence the gender development of their children. Different theoretical perspectives range from the view that fathers are essential to the position that fathers make no difference at all. Empirical evidence regarding the sex–role development of children in different family types will be presented to examine the role of fathers in children's gender development. *Solo mothers:* There has been much controversy in recent years about whether single heterosexual women should have access to assisted reproduction. The concerns that have been expressed center around the negative effects of growing up in a fatherless family following parental separation or divorce. However, children born to single mothers following assisted reproduction have not experienced the adverse factors associated with divorce, although they may be exposed to other pressures that may increase their vulnerability to emotional and behavioral problems. Findings will be presented from a controlled study of women who have had a child through donor insemination (DI) and who are raising that child without a father right from the start.
© 2004 Published by Elsevier B.V.

*Keywords:* Solo mothers; Parenting; Child development; Donor insemination

---

\* Tel.: +44-207-040-8510; fax: +44-207-040-8582.
*E-mail address:* s.e.golombok@city.ac.uk (S. Golombok).

0531-5131/ © 2004 Published by Elsevier B.V.
doi:10.1016/j.ics.2004.01.095

## 1. Introduction

Any consideration of the development of children in solo mother families is essentially addressing the more fundamental question "Do fathers really matter?" This presentation looks at the two areas where fathers are generally considered to matter a great deal: (i) children's psychological adjustment and (ii) children's gender development—and examines whether fathers really do matter for these key aspects of children's lives.

## 2. Children's psychological adjustment

The role of fathers in promoting children's psychological adjustment has been examined in four ways:

(1) Fatherless families have been studied to see whether children without fathers differ from those who grow up with a father in the home.
(2) Lesbian mother families have been investigated to establish whether it is a father's maleness, or his role as an additional parent, that is important.
(3) Research has been carried out on families where the father is the primary caregiver to examine what effect this has on the child. If children in these families differ from other children then this is informative about the nature of fathers' influences.
(4) Traditional nuclear families have been studied to increase understanding of the processes through which fathers' relationships with their children influence children's adjustment.

### 2.1. Father-absent families

Large-scale epidemiological studies of father-absent families consistently show that children raised by single mothers are more likely to show psychological problems, and are less likely to perform well at school, than their counterparts from two-parent homes. These include McLanahan and Sandefur's [1] examination of four nationally representative samples in the United States, Ferri's [2] investigation of father-absent children sampled from the National Child Development Study in the United Kingdom, and most recently, Dunn et al.'s [3] study of single mother families from the Avon Longitudinal Study of Pregnancy and Childhood. For example, McLanahan and Sandefur [1] have found that adolescents raised by single mothers during some period of their childhood were twice as likely to drop out of high school, twice as likely to have a baby before the age of 20, and one and a half times more likely to be out of work in their late teens or early twenties than those from a similar background who grew up with two parents at home. In Dunn et al.'s [3] study of 4 year olds and their siblings, children from single-parent families showed higher levels of psychological disorder than their counterparts from two-parent homes.

So why is it that children from single-mother families show poorer outcomes? Is it because of the absence of a father? Or are other factors involved? In examining why children in single-mother families are at risk, researchers have found that factors such as financial hardship and the mother's lack of social support are largely responsible for children's difficulties. Another important contributing factor is exposure to conflict and hostility between parents before, during, and sometimes after separation or divorce. The majority of single parent families result from marital breakdown. Hetherington and Stanley-Hagan [4] have carefully documented the negative effects of such conflict for children over several years. Interestingly, longitudinal studies have demonstrated that children can begin to show problems years before the divorce actually takes place, sometimes even before the parents have considered separation. This tells us that the psychological problems shown by children when their parents divorce do not simply result from the divorce itself but arise in response to the arguments and bitterness between parents that they experience at home.

Researchers have also looked at the impact of single parenthood on parenting, and have demonstrated that, on the average, children in single-parent homes experience a poorer quality of parenting than children who live with two parents. In Dunn et al.'s [3] study, scores on a scale of maternal negativity were higher for single mothers than for mothers in two-parent families. This scale included items such as "This child gets on my nerves" and "I have frequent battles of will with this child". Greater maternal negativity was associated with a higher rate of behavioral problems in children. Similarly, McLanahan and Sandefur [1] reported that single mothers exert less control over their children in terms of supervision and establishing rules than mothers in two-parent families. Not only do children with single parent experience less discipline and monitoring from their mother than children in two-parent families, but also they receive no discipline from their father, an aspect of parenting that is often associated with the paternal role.

The poorer quality of parenting shown by single mothers may be explained, in part at least, by the higher rates of psychological problems, particularly depression, found among single mothers. In Dunn et al.'s [3] study, depression was high among single mothers and was associated with psychological disorder in children. One explanation for the association between maternal depression and psychological disorder in children is that depression reduces the ability to be an effective parent. Depression is thought to interfere with parents' emotional availability and sensitivity to their children and also with their control and discipline of them. A number of studies have shown that depressed parents tend either to be very lenient with their children or very authoritarian, often switching between the two.

So what can we conclude about the importance of fathers from studies of father-absent families? There is no doubt that, overall, children raised by single mothers are more likely to develop psychological problems and are less likely to do well at school than children raised by both their mother and their father. However, it has been argued that it is not so much the absence of a father, but the difficulties that accompany father absence such as poverty and lack of social support, that lead to adverse outcomes for children. When these factors are controlled for in statistical analyses, the differences between children with and without fathers largely disappear. This has led some researchers to conclude that the problems faced by children living with single mothers do not result from the absence of a father in itself. Instead, it is the circumstances that are associated with single parenthood that are to blame. Others, such as McLanahan and Sandefur [1], take the view that it is completely inappropriate to treat low income or lack social support as factors to be controlled for in statistical analyses. Instead they concluded that "low income—and the sudden drop in income that is often associated with divorce—is the single most important factor in children's lower achievement in single-parent homes, accounting for about half of the disadvantage."

## 2.2. Lesbian mother families

In examining the consequences for children of growing up in single-mother families, it is not possible to disentangle the effects of father absence from the effects of the absence of a second parent. So we cannot say whether it is the lack of a parent in general, or the lack of a male parent in particular, that is associated with the difficulties faced by children in single-mother homes. Lesbian mother families provide an opportunity to investigate children who are raised without a father but with two parents, and can help shed light on the question of whether it is the fathers' maleness that is important, or his involvement as an additional parent in the home.

A number of studies have investigated children raised from birth by a lesbian couple in comparison with children raised by two heterosexual parents. There have been two studies in the United States [5,6], one in Belgium [7] and one in the United Kingdom [8]. These studies show that children in two-parent lesbian families do not differ from children in two-parent heterosexual families with respect to psychological adjustment, and suggest that it is the number of parents rather than the gender of parents that is important for children's development. Children who have two parents (whether of the same or opposite sex) appear to be better off in many ways than those with only one parent. Interestingly, the only clear difference to emerge from these studies was the greater involvement in the care of their children by comothers from lesbian families than by fathers from heterosexual homes. However, existing studies have only investigated children up to early school age. It remains to be seen what the outcomes will be for these children during their adolescent years.

## 2.3. Fathers as primary caregivers

In the third category of families, fathers are the primary caregivers. What can we learn from families where the father takes on what has traditionally been the mothers role? Although far less common than single-mother families, some children are brought up by single fathers. This is most likely to happen when the mother has died, or after the parents' separation or divorce. Because so few single fathers exist, there has been little research on what happens to the children. But the few studies that have been carried out show that most single fathers are able to care for their children well. However, it is important to remember that fathers who have custody of their children, particularly those who choose to have custody, are more likely to have had good relationships with their children before the divorce.

Studies of two-parent families where the father is the primary caregiver have involved comparisons between families where the father takes primary responsibility for childcare and traditional families where the mother takes the load. These studies show that having a highly involved father is not bad for children, and if anything, the effects are positive [9]. In addition to a better relationship with their father, children raised in this way have been found to be more independent, to see themselves as more in control of what happens to them, to show greater intellectual ability, and to be more accepting of nontraditional family roles. Thus, the findings of these studies suggest that children benefit from having a highly involved father, and that fathers may play a part in children's development of independence and intellectual skills. Once again, however, it may be the presence of a second highly involved parent rather than the sex of that parent that has the positive effect. Also, mothers in these families are likely to feel more satisfied with their lives and so family relationships in general may be more harmonious. Moreover, in all of these studies, the fathers were highly involved with their children because both parents wanted it that way. The picture is quite different when fathers are forced into this role, e.g., through unemployment. What seems to matter is not how much fathers are involved with their children, but how they feel about it. Nevertheless, the findings demonstrate that fathers who so wish can play an influential role in their children's lives.

*2.4. Traditional families*

Another way of examining the role of fathers is to study traditional two-parent families to determine whether different types of fathers have different influences on their children. For example, Cox et al. [10] have shown that fathers who are affectionate and encouraging with their 3-month-old infants are most likely to have securely attached 1 year olds. A 1995 review of 14 studies that assessed the security of children's attachment to both their mother and their father, involving almost 1000 families, demonstrated that the proportion of children securely attached to their father was almost identical to the proportion classified as securely attached to their mother [11]. Of the 38% of these children who obtained a different classification with each parent, half were securely attached to their father and not their mother. Thus, it seems that fathers are important attachment figures for young children.

It is not just the child's relationship with the father that is improved by the father's involvement; relationships with other children are better as well. In a study of preschool children, those who were securely attached to their father at age 1, were found to play more harmoniously with their peers [12]. Another study found that children who had a good relationship with their father at age 3 had better friendships when they were 5 [13]. Investigations of school age children have produced similar findings. The National Survey of Families and Households in the United States has shown that fathers who are actively involved with their 5–18-year-old children have sons and daughters with fewer emotional and behavioral problems [14]. Although these studies indicate that having a warm and involved father is beneficial to children's social and emotional development, it is possible that children who have a good relationship with their father are more sociable in general, and may well have had better relationships with other children irrespective of their relationship with their father. The most likely explanation is an interaction between the two; that is, there are benefits for children of having a close relationship with their father, but this will depend, to some extent at least, on how responsive and sociable they are themselves.

*2.5. Conclusion*

So, do fathers really matter for children's psychological adjustment? It seems that they do. The more that fathers are actively involved in parenting, the better the outcome for children's social and emotional development. However, it is not simply their maleness that matters. Instead, it seems that fathers have a positive effect on their children's development through the same processes as do mothers. Fathers who are affectionate to their children, who play with them, who are sensitive and responsive to them, and who provide effective discipline, are more likely than distant fathers to have well-adjusted children. Nevertheless, this does not necessarily mean that the absence of a father, in itself, will have a negative influence on children's lives.

## 3. Children's gender development

Whether or not fathers matter for children's gender development depends on the extent to which it is possible for parents to influence the development of sex-typed behavior in their children. It is often assumed that parents play a key role in the development of masculinity and femininity in their daughters and sons [15]. This belief derives from the traditional psychoanalytic view that the successful resolution of the Oedipal conflict forms the basis for identification with the male or female role. Classic social learning theory also assumes that parents play a key role in the gender development of their children, both by differentially reinforcing their daughters and sons, and by acting as models of gender role behavior.

However, other theoretical approaches suggest a different conclusion. Over the past 25 years, there has been growing understanding of biological influences on gender development including genetic and hormonal influences that are thought to influence neural structures associated with sex-typed behavior [16]. It is now generally accepted that the prenatal hormonal environment has a part to play. The best evidence comes from studies of girls exposed to high levels of testosterone prenatally as a result of the genetic disorder Congenital Adrenal Hyperplasia. Girls with this disorder, compared with matched control groups, show more masculine gender role behavior. This includes greater preference for traditionally male toys such as cars and trucks, reduced preferences for traditionally feminine toys such as dolls, increased preferences for boys as playmates, and increased preferences for rough, active play. Insofar as gender development is determined prenatally through the action of prenatal hormones on the developing fetus, the behavior of fathers will make little difference to the femininity of their daughters or masculinity of their sons. Similarly, from the perspective of cognitive developmental and social cognitive theories, which emphasize the importance of cognitive processes and cultural stereotypes in the acquisition of gender role behavior, the role of parents is a minor one. In addition, it is increasingly being recognized that peers play a key role in children's gender development. According to Maccoby [17], children segregate by gender largely due to behavioral compatibility with children of the same sex as themselves, and in this way sex-typed behavior is established and maintained.

Thus, the different theoretical perspectives lead to different predictions about whether or not fathers matter for children's sex role development ranging from the view that fathers are essential to the position that fathers make no difference at all. Once again, fathers' influence on children's gender development can be examined empirically by studying children in different family types, the two most informative of which are father-absent families and lesbian mother families.

### 3.1. Father-absent families

If fathers matter for children's gender development then the absence of a father would be expected to result in atypical gender role behavior. Specifically, it has been argued that boys in fatherless families would be less masculine in their identity and behavior, and girls less feminine, than their counterparts from two-parent homes. Although early studies produced contradictory results, a metaanaylsis by Stevenson and Black [18] concluded that there were no effects for girls or boys when only the highest quality and best-controlled studies were examined. In a more recent study by Serbin et al. [19] of 5–12 year olds in the United States, no differences in gender-typed preferences were identified according to the presence or absence of a father in the home. And in a study in the United Kingdom of a large, general population sample, no difference in gender role behavior was found between father-present and father-absent families for either boys or girls [20]. Taken together, the findings of these investigations suggest that gender–role behavior is not affected by father absence.

*3.2. Lesbian mother families*

Lesbian mother families provide an even better paradigm for studying this issue. Children in this situation not only lack a father figure but also are raised by a mother, and often two mothers, who do not conform to the traditional female role. Studies of lesbian mother families have produced strikingly similar findings. Daughters are no less feminine, and sons are no less masculine, than the daughters and sons of heterosexual parents—this is in spite of lesbian mothers' encouragement of less sex-stereotyped behavior in their boys and girls [21]. Thus, it seems that fathers do not really matter for children's gender development. Children who have no father, or even no father and two mothers, are no less sex-typed than children raised in a traditional two-parent family. The determinants of sex-typed behavior, it seems, have more to do with prenatal hormones, cognitive processes and the peer group than with the presence or absence of a father in the home.

## 4. Solo mothers and their children

There has been a great deal of controversy in recent years about whether single heterosexual women should have access to assisted reproduction. The concerns that have been expressed center around the effects of growing up in a fatherless family and are based on the research described above that shows negative outcomes in terms of cognitive, social and emotional development for children raised by single mothers following parental separation or divorce. However, these outcomes cannot necessarily be generalized to children born to single mothers following donor insemination (DI) (solo mothers) because these children have not experienced parental separation and generally are raised without financial hardship. It is possible, however, that other pressures on solo mothers, such as social stigma and lack of social support, may interfere with their parenting role, and leave their children vulnerable to emotional and behavioral problems.

Little research has yet been carried out on the quality of parenting of single women who opt for donor insemination as a means of having a child. In an investigation of 27 solo mothers of 1-year-old DI children [22], the main reason for opting for DI was to avoid the need to have casual sex in order to become pregnant. There was a strong sense that time was running out to fulfil the lifelong dream of having a child and that there was no choice but to have a child in this way due to the lack of a partner. Solo DI mothers appeared to be more open towards disclosing the donor conception to the child than were a comparison group of married DI mothers; 93% of solo mothers reported that they planned to tell their child compared with 46% of the married DI mothers. With respect to parent–child relationships, solo DI mothers showed similar levels of warmth and bonding towards their infant as married DI mothers. However, solo mothers showed lower levels of interaction and sensitivity. A possible explanation for this finding is that the presence of a partner allowed married DI mothers more time with their child. In recent years, there has been a rise in the number of single professional women choosing to become single parents by means of donor insemination and going it alone right from the start. The outcome for these children in the years to come will not only be of interest in its own right but will also tell us more about the effects of father absence on children's psychological adjustment.

## References

[1] S. McLanahan, G. Sandefur, Growing Up with a Single Parent: What Hurts, What Helps, Harvard Univ. Press, Cambridge, MA, 1994.
[2] E. Ferri, Growing Up in a One Parent Family, NFER, Slough, 1976.
[3] J. Dunn, et al., and the ALSPAC Study Team, Children's adjustment and prosocial behaviour in step-, single-parent, and non-stepfamily settings: findings from a community study, Journal of Child Psychology and Psychiatry 39 (8) (1998) 1083–1095.
[4] M. Hetherington, M. Stanley-Hagan, Parenting in divorced and remarried families, in: M. Bornstein (Ed.), Handbook of Parenting, vol. 3, Lawrence Erlbaum Associates, Hove, UK, 1995, pp. 233–254.
[5] D. Flaks, et al., Lesbians choosing motherhood: a comparative study of lesbian and heterosexual parents and their children, Developmental Psychology 31 (1995) 105–114.
[6] R. Chan, B. Raboy, C. Patterson, Psychosocial adjustment among children conceived via donor insemination by lesbian and heterosexual mothers, Child Development 69 (2) (1998) 443–457.
[7] A. Brewaeys, et al., Donor insemination: child development and family functioning in lesbian mother families, Human Reproduction 12 (6) (1997) 1349–1359.
[8] S. Golombok, F. Tasker, C. Murray, Children raised in fatherless families from infancy: family relationships and the socioemotional development of children of lesbian and single heterosexual mothers, Journal of Child Psychology and Psychiatry 38 (7) (1997) 783–791.
[9] N. Radin, Primary caregiving fathers in intact families, in: A.E. Gottfried, A.W. Gottfried (Eds.), Redefining Families, Plenum, New York, 1994, pp. 11–54.
[10] M. Cox, et al., Prediction of infant–mother and infant–father attachment, Developmental Psychology 28 (1992) 474–483.
[11] M. van Ijzendoorn, M. De Wolff, In search of the absent father—meta analyses of infant–father attachment: a rejoinder to our discussants, Child Development 68 (4) (1997) 604–609.
[12] G. Suess, K. Grossmann, L. Sroufe, Effects of infant attachment to mother and father on quality of adaptation to preschool: from dynamic to individual organization of self, International Journal of Behavioural Development 15 (1992) 43–65.
[13] L. Youngblade, J. Belsky, Parent–child antecedents of 5-year-olds' close friendships: a longitudinal analysis, Developmental Psychology 28 (1992) 700–713.
[14] J. Mosley, E. Thomson, Fathering behavior and child outcomes: the role of race and poverty, in: W. Marsiglio (Ed.), Fatherhood: Contemporary Theory, Research and Social Policy, Sage, Thousand Oaks, CA, 1995, pp. 148–165.
[15] S. Golombok, R. Fivush, Gender Development, Cambridge Univ. Press, Cambridge, MA, 1994.
[16] M. Hines, Brain Gender, Oxford Univ. Press, Oxford, 2004.
[17] E. Maccoby, The Two Sexes: Growing Up Apart, Coming Together, Belknap Harvard, Cambridge, MA, 1998.
[18] M. Stevenson, K. Black, Parental absence and sex role development: a meta analysis, Child Development 59 (1988) 793–814.
[19] L. Serbin, K. Powlishta, J. Gulko, The development of sex typing in middle childhood, Monographs of the Society for Research in Child Development 58 (232) 1–99.
[20] M. Stevens, S. Golombok, J. Golding, and the ALSPAC Study Team, Does father absence influence children's gender development? Findings from a general population study of pre-school children, Parenting: Science and Practice 2 (2002) 49–62.
[21] S. Golombok, Lesbian and gay families, in: A. Bainham, S. Day Sclater, M. Richards (Eds.), What is a Parent? Hart, Oxford, 1999, pp. 161–180.
[22] C. Murray, S. Golombok, Going it alone: Solo mothers and their infants conceived by donor insemination. American Journal of Orthopsychiatry (in press).

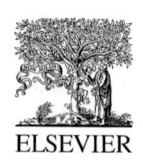

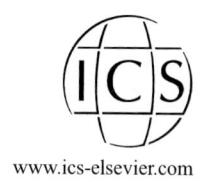

# Exit counseling

## Linda Hammer Burns*

*Counselling Services, Reproductive Medicine Center, University of Minnesota, Minneapolis, MA, USA*
*Department of Obstetrics and Gynecology, University of Minnesota Medical School, Minneapolis, MN 55410, USA*

**Abstract.** A referral for counseling—including *exit counseling*—is intended to improve the patient's quality of life, provide education, and improve couple and individual functioning. The patient must feel relaxed and trust the therapist—and so must the medical professional. Currently, the vast majority of counseling for infertile couples focuses on patients (1) entering treatment; (2) having difficulty coping with medical treatments; (3) with pre-existing mental health problems; and (4) considering third party reproduction. Exit counseling is not as common an arena of infertility counseling, but one that is receiving increasing attention. Patients should consider ending treatment when (1) their therapeutic options have been exhausted; (2) their resources have depleted (or near depleted); (3) other aspects of the couples life are adversely affected; (4) there is evidence of poor quality of life; (5) there is a serious illness and/or condition jeopardizing health of one or both partners; and/or (6) advancing age and increasing difficulty achieving pregnancy. Whether exit counseling is provided by medical caregivers or mental health professionals, the circumstances of the counseling are fundamental. Some clinics require exit counseling for all patients, thereby minimizing stigma and providing support and education regardless of whether the patient is pregnant or ending treatment without a successful pregnancy. By contrast, exit counseling may be the result of treatment failure or other patient circumstances, such as patient request for counseling to provide assistance with making the transition to non-treatment or decision-making. A summary of therapeutic interventions will be provided as well as an overview of To Whom, When, and How to refer for exit counseling. © 2004 Published by Elsevier B.V.

*Keywords:* Infertility counseling; Reproductive health counseling

Infertility is a multifaceted experience impacting health, reproduction, family life, social dynamics, and other intra- and interpsychic aspects of the infertile individual's life. It is an intergenerational developmental crisis that impacts religious beliefs, life plans, marital and sexual functioning, economic well-being, social relationships, and one's physical and mental health. In short, it is a life crisis of significant physical and emotional

---

* Department of Obstetrics and Gynecology, Reproductive Medicine Center, University of Minnesota, 606 24th Avenue South Suite 500, Minneapolis, MN 55410, USA. Tel.: +1-612-750-3368; fax: +1-612-926-7638.
 *E-mail address:* burns023@umn.edu (L. Hammer Burns).

magnitude requiring the attention and understanding of medical caregivers and mental health professionals alike.

Currently, the vast majority of counseling for infertile couples focuses on patients (1) entering treatment; (2) having difficulty coping with medical treatments; (3) with pre-existing mental health problems; and (4) considering third-party reproduction. *Exit counseling* is not as common an arena of infertility counseling, but one that is receiving increasing attention. Whether exit counseling is provided by medical caregivers or mental health professionals, the circumstances of the counseling are fundamental. Some clinics require exit counseling for all patients, thereby minimizing stigma and providing support and education regardless of whether the patient is pregnant or ending treatment without a successful pregnancy. By contrast, exit counseling may be the result of treatment failure—an occasion for examining other family building alternatives (e.g., adoption) or life goals (e.g., childfree lifestyle) or because of other patient circumstances. In fact, some patients request exit counseling themselves to provide assistance with making the transition to non-treatment or decision-making about future life plans or goals or if they are experiencing couple conflict.

A significant challenge or barrier to exit counseling is the patient's belief that counseling is unnecessary (in general) or they specifically do not need it. This is particularly the case for patients who are determined to pursue 'parenthood at any price'—financially, emotionally, relationally, or physically. This single-minded, even obsessive/compulsive pursuit of treatment, typically leads to repeated treatment cycles despite low odds of success, the inability to realistically assess alternatives, and ultimately, the inability to 'let go and move on' from the infertility experience. The emotional blow that what they have set their heart on will not be, or that their body is betraying them in such a cruel fashion, is so overpowering for some patients that it can prevent them from appropriate medical care and even create distress and/or conflict in the patient/caregiver relationship. The use of denial as a coping mechanism becomes not only problematic to the patient's ability to move on, but can become a significant relationship problem preventing the couple from being able to communicate and problem solve in a healthy fashion. Although each partner has his/her own coping style and each must respect these individual styles, it can be very challenging when one partner is able and willing to move on but the other is intractably invested in parenthood at any price and using denial and avoidance as a primary defense, particularly if parenthood is a means of meeting other needs. Typically, the perspective of these patients is that all of their problems will be solved if they can just get pregnant.

Understandably, differing coping mechanisms or definitions of the situation can be or become a source of marital conflict between partners. Differing levels of investment in parenthood may be an individual matter or it may reflect a difference between men and women in general [1]. While a couple may agree that they want to become parents, women have been found to be more identified with the maternal role and feel a greater loss when they are unable to achieve this role. This difference is common in cultures in which women's roles are limited to those involving home and hearth and in remarriage situations in which one partner already has children. For example, in the remarriage situation, partners may have different agendas but not realize it. The partner with children may feel that more children are fine if it is easy, while the partner without children may want 'children at any cost'. In such cases, covert or even overt coercion may arise as one partner pressures the other to continue treatment again, while the other wishes to quit. Conflict resolution becomes a significant part of exit counseling with these couples.

## 1. Basis for referral for exit counseling

Patients should consider ending treatment when (1) their therapeutic options have been exhausted; (2) their resources have depleted (or near depleted); (3) other aspects of the couple's life are adversely affected; (4) there is evidence of poor quality of life; (5) there is a serious illness and/or condition jeopardizing health of one or both partners; and/or (6) advancing age and increasing difficulty achieving pregnancy. Daniels [2] defined the indicators for referral to qualified infertility counselors on the basis of three areas: relationship, staff, and personal arenas. It should be stated that it is perhaps not frequent enough that the patient/staff arena is evaluated and a determination is made that exit counseling, with the purpose of terminating the patient's treatment, is made on the basis of the patient's interaction with staff. This is perhaps because clinics are reluctant to challenge or abandon patients and in part due to a belief that 'the customer is always right'—although this is not always in the patient's best interest. Staff problems that may highlight problems in the patient/medical caregiver relationship include situations in which the patient (1) does not like the doctor or vice versa; (2) is disruptive with staff and consistently demanding preferential and/or exceptional treatment; (3) has mental health problems that are disruptive to medical treatment and/or prevent the patient from grasping the issues and procedures involved; and/or (4) needs extensive support that is beyond the ability and expertise of medical staff. Relational and personal problems that may precipitate referral for exit counseling include (1) communication problems and conflicts about treatment; (2) partners at different stages in the grief process; (3) sexual difficulties or nonexistent sexual relations; (4) lack of or inadequate coping skills; and evidence of mental health problems, particularly anxiety and depression that are impacting health and medical treatment.

While staff may find these indications helpful in identifying patients to refer for counseling, patients may find the following helpful indicators for stopping treatment: (1) feeling 'stuck' or that treatment is futile; (2) feeling resentful about medical appointments or treatment; (3) feeling disappointed when the doctor offers new treatment; (4) feeling the need to move on with life versus continuing to invest one's time, energy, and money in infertility treatment; (5) feeling relieved when one's spouse or doctor suggests quitting or taking a treatment holiday; (6) fantasizing about a future date when one 'can' stop treatment; (7) feeling that one has already mourned the loss of one's biological child; and/or (8) feeling parenthood is more important than reproduction.

## 2. Therapeutic interventions

The achievement of a pregnancy may be the most common reason for exit counseling. Whether the pregnancy is achieved after minor interventions (a single clomid cycle or insemination) or after much more elaborate treatment (donor gametes and a gestational carrier), these are precious pregnancies. The pregnancy after infertility is typically fraught with a variety of anxieties and unique circumstances, including ambiguity, isolation, fear, and technological bewilderment [3]. If the pregnancy is achieved as the result of donor gametes, the patient may have difficulty bonding and may be experiencing significant feelings of ambiguity and ambivalence. Patients who have not had pre-treatment counseling may begin to have questions and concerns about the circumstances of the child's conception: Do they keep the issue private or opt for a more open approach? Are their educational materials that would be helpful? How will the child react to the information? Exit counseling provides an opportunity to explore these concerns for the first time, or again in greater depth, ensuring that the couple is comfortable with their decision and prepared for parenting.

Many infertile patients have difficulty separating from the staff at the infertility clinic and moving on to an obstetrical clinic where they feel (and perhaps are treated) like 'just another ob' rather than the unique and precious pregnancy that needs special care and attention. For many infertile patients, the circumstances of how their pregnancy was achieved or the cause of their infertility may require extensive obstetrical interventions—e.g., bed rest, hospitalization, creating even more technological bewilderment and invasiveness at a time when they want more than ever to feel 'normal'. Such concerns may heighten their fears about their baby being 'normal'—a fear of all expectant mothers, but a fear that is enhanced for the previously infertile, expectant mother.

For the infertile couple who is leaving the infertility clinic without a pregnancy, exit counseling should focus on helping the couple chart their future and adjust to an outcome that is not what they had originally hoped and planned. Very often simply giving the couple or infertile patient *permission* to stop treatment is the most helpful therapeutic intervention. A helpful way of framing this is presenting the question: "How would it feel if you were to give yourself permission or your spouse or physician were to give you permission to stop treatment?" While failure to give oneself permission to stop treatment can be a major obstruction, another is *assumptions* (either one's individual or one's assumptions about the physician's or one's partner's beliefs). Assuming that one's partner will never adopt or that one's doctor will be disappointed if one wants to quit treatment are the kinds of assumptions that are all too often unforeseen impediments to healthy communication and resolution of the infertility experience. Putting aside assumptions and proceeding with permission, couples find it is much easier to investigate and prioritize acceptable alternatives and plot out their future.

Fundamental to coming to terms with infertility for each couple is defining their goal, reproduction or parenthood. Whether their personal goal is reproduction or parenthood, each is fundamental to determining the alternatives that are acceptable for them and the direction their future will take. If their goal is reproduction and they have reached the limits of treatment that will allow them to achieve a pregnancy and transmit their own genes, they will have to consider a childfree lifestyle. Whereas, parenthood as a goal will leave far more alternatives, including prenatal adoption (donor gametes), traditional adoption, and/or surrogacy or gestational carrier.

One tool for helping couples is making a cost/benefit list in which they assess their recourses and the impact on the quality of their life of continuing /ending treatment. This should include extensive information gathering about their feelings, available alternatives and their medical situation. One suggestion is for couples to each separately write their *feelings* about ending treatment in which they organize them according to 'pros' and 'cons.' Many couples find that they are much closer to the same feelings and beliefs than they previously thought. Gathering information on the alternatives they are considering can be shared by the partners as a means of improving communication and sharing the experience. Getting a second medical opinion is another way of obtaining additional information for making sound decisions. Comparing notes on the information they have obtained and communicating about the alternatives can help the couple focus on the direction they wish to pursue or come to terms with the decision they have made.

Another technique for facilitating 'letting go' is to project into the future and ask the following questions: (1) what is most difficult about quitting? (2) what is preventing me/us from stopping treatment? and, (3) what should I/we do now to minimize regrets in the future? These questions not only help couples organize their thoughts and feelings, they also help crystallize their action plan and minimize regrets later in life by helping them project into the future and consider the present. Exit counseling can also be useful in helping couples define and set limits: how do they want to spend their resources, *all of their resources*? Couples should be encouraged to consider not simply their financial resources, but their physical, emotional, social, and spiritual resources. Spending all of their resources—a baby at any price—is too high a price and exit counseling is an excellent opportunity to encourage individuals and couples to set healthy limits in the process of coming to terms with the painful experience of involuntary childlessness. For some patients, decisions cannot be made quickly; in which case suggesting a 'treatment holiday' is a good idea. For some couples, this may be an open-ended time frame, while for others making the holiday a specific amount of time (e.g., 6 months) is more comfortable. It is also suggested that the couple use this time to put other parameters around the experience (e.g., when they return to treatment it will be for this number of cycles) and to truly refresh themselves during their break (e.g., take an actual holiday, limit conversations about infertility to specific times or days).

## 3. To whom, when, and how to refer for exit counseling

Physicians and nurses have always provided some measure of advice, guidance, and *support* to their infertile patients because emotional stakes are high and medical treatments are demanding and time-consuming. And, while medical caregivers continue to offer counsel, the field of infertility counseling or reproductive health counseling as a new specialty of mental health began to emerge about 30 years ago. By the late 1980s, this field was more clearly defined, in large part by the Warnock Report, which led to the Human Fertilisation and Embryology Authority in Great Britain, which required educational, supportive, implications, and decision-making counseling [4]. Professional organizations further defined the field of infertility. Some of the original infertility counseling organizations were the British Infertility Counseling Association, Australia/New Zealand Infertility Counseling Association, and what is now the Mental Health Professional Group of the American Society of Reproductive Medicine. Similar organizations have emerged in Europe, Germany, Japan, and are on the horizon in Canada, the Middle East, and Latin America. While in the past infertility counselors had some difficulty having the importance of their work and role on the treatment team being recognized, the challenge now is providing clinics trained and qualified infertility counselors. Infertility counselors offer advice, education, consultation, support, and analysis, and they are more likely to be patient advocates with caregivers or healthcare providers than in more traditional psychotherapies [5]. Therapeutic approaches that have been applied to infertility include psychodynamic therapy, cognitive-behavioral treatment, marriage and family therapy, group therapy, strategic/solution-focused brief therapy, psychopharmacological treatment, sex therapy, crisis intervention, and grief counseling [6]. Infertility counselors provide psychological assessment, screening, and therapy; diagnosing and treatment of mental disorders; psychometric testing (psychologist); decision-making counseling; bereavement therapy; crisis intervention; marriage and family therapy; and sex therapy.

For many medical caregivers, the dilemmas of *who, when, and how* of referring patients for counseling become significant barriers in the referral process. Patients should be referred for counseling to a licensed mental health professional (psychologist, psychiatrist, social worker, marriage and family therapist, or psychiatric nurse). They should be referred for counseling *when* (1) they are entering treatment; (2) undergoing assisted reproductive technology and/or third party reproduction; (3) have a pre-existing mental health problem that is affecting treatment; (4) when caregivers observe difficulties; (5) the patient asks for assistance; and finally, (6) there is evidence of difficulty ending treatment. *How to refer* can be challenging if counseling is not part of the treatment protocol, (e.g., everyone entering and/or ending treatment or using third-party reproduction must undergo therapy). This approach to counseling minimizes the stigma that is often (mistakenly) attached to counseling and psychotherapy. Other methods of referral are to write a letter to the therapist and patient specifying the issues to be addressed. It is particularly important to make the clinic's expectations of the outcome of counseling explicit, especially if counseling is a prerequisite to continuing medical treatment. Another helpful referral technique is to physically introduce the patient to the therapist or to connect them via email or telephone calls. Very often a call to or from the therapist is comforting and reassuring and decreases any patient apprehension. This also helps with determining if this therapeutic pair will be a 'good fit'—if not, it is better for both parties to make a referral to a different therapist immediately. Fundamentally, a referral for counseling—including exit counseling—is to improve the patient's quality of life, provide education, and improve couple and individual functioning. And finally, the patient must feel relaxed and trust the therapist—and so must the medical professional.

## References

[1] C.R. Newton, M. Houle, Gender differences in psychological response to infertility treatment, Infertil. Reprod. Med. Clin. North Am. 4 (1993) 545–558.
[2] K. Daniels, Infertility counseling—the need for a psychosocial perspective, Br. J. Soc. Work 23 (1993) 501–515.
[3] E.S. Glazer, The Long-Awaited Stork: A Guide to Parenting After Infertility, Lexington Books, New York, 1990.
[4] Human Fertilisation and Embryology Authority. London, HFEA, 1990, 1996 (See also: http://www.hfea.gov.uk).
[5] L.H. Burns, S.N. Covington (Eds.), Infertility Counseling: A Comprehensive Handbook for Clinicians, Parthenon Publishing, New York, 1999.
[6] L.D. Applegarth, Individual counseling and psychotherapy, in: L.H. Burns, S.N. Covington (Eds.), Infertility Counseling: A Comprehensive Handbook for Clinicians, Parthenon Publishing, New York, 1999, pp. 85–102.

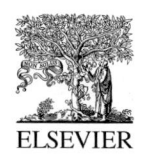

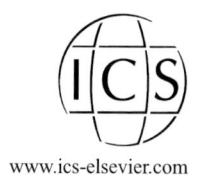

# Psychosocial aspects of infertility: sexual dysfunction

Andrea Mechanick Braverman[*]

*Pennsylvania Reproductive Associates, Psychological Services, Thomas Jefferson University, 5217 Militia Hill Road, Plymouth Meeting, PA 19462, USA*

**Abstract.** *Introduction*: Sexual dysfunction can be a silent partner of infertility treatment. Rarely is sexual dysfunction the cause of infertility. More often, sexual dysfunction is a consequence of the infertility experience and/or treatment. Sexual intimacy is profoundly affected by infertility sequelae, such as lowered self-esteem, depressive or anxiety feelings, and association of sexual intimacy with failure to procreate. *Methods*: The definition of primary sexual dysfunction is made by diagnosing a problem that has always existed. Secondary sexual dysfunction denotes situations in which a problem develops after an individual has had normal sexual function. Infertility, already a series of many losses for many couples, will create a loss of sexual intimacy and enjoyment. Treatment demands, e.g. producing semen specimens or timed intercourse, may also create disruption or dysfunction. *Results*: Sexual dysfunction can be treated to enhance both infertility treatments and dyadic adjustment. There are many treatment approaches that may include medical intervention, counseling and behavioral techniques. *Conclusion*: Clinicians practicing in the field of infertility need to bring heightened awareness to their patients' sexual function. Acknowledging that sexual function is a valued part of relationship, apart from the need to conceive, can give couples permission to address this sensitive area of their relationship. © 2004 Published by Elsevier B.V.

*Keywords:* Sexuality; Infertility; Intimacy; Function; Relationships

## 1. Introduction

Sexuality is a valued and special part of an intimate relationship. Sexual relations can express deep feelings, excite the imagination and the heart, add fun and excitement, and offer pleasure. Expectations of what constitute normal sexual relations and sexuality are subjective and can be distorted by images from television, film, and other popular sources. Separating function from fiction in the assessment of sexuality is not always easy. Sometimes this uncertainty can lead to concerns that the person is not performing adequately—sex researchers are still trying to get the ultimate answer to the question, "What is the average frequency for sexual intercourse per week for a couple?".

---

[*] Tel.: +1-610-834-1140; fax: +1-610-834-0962.
*E-mail address:* andrea@womensintitute.org (A.M. Braverman).

0531-5131/ © 2004 Published by Elsevier B.V.
doi:10.1016/j.ics.2004.01.085

Understanding loss of libido must be examined from both a medical and a psychological perspective.

When infertility is added to a relationship, it can cause significant disruption in an individual's or couple's sex life. This disruption can range from mild (with complaints of less enjoyment with sexual relations) to severe (in which sexual relations can cease or be associated with traumatic feelings). The majority of infertile individuals or couples are faced with exogenous causes for changes in their sexual function. The minority of couples will have entered infertility with endogenous organic dysfunctions.

This discussion will identify: (1) the causes and theories of both female and male sexual dysfunction, (2) the particular issues which intrude upon sexual function because of infertility, and (3) some of the common techniques used for assisting couples and individuals to overcome sexual problems.

## 2. What is sexual dysfunction?

There are four general categories for sexual dysfunction [1]:

1. Primary: refers to a sexual problem that has always been present
2. Secondary: refers to a sexual problem that has developed over time and after an individual has had adequate sexual functioning
3. Situational: refers to a sexual problem that only arises during certain situations, e.g. a particular activity or with a different partner
4. Global: refers to a sexual problem that occurs with all situations, sexual activities, and partners.

Different theories have been constructed to conceptualize the human sexual response. Masters and Johnson [2], the founders of American human sexuality research and theory, initially posited a linear progression theory. In this theory, both men and women moved through stages of excitement, plateau, orgasm, and resolution. In more recent theories, Basson [3–5] posits a feedback cycle, which is reactive to both psychological and biological influences and represents a more accepted status. Indeed, current understanding of sexual desire identifies multiple aspects of function and includes a tapestry of drive, expectations, beliefs, values, and motivation.

Reports of the incidence of sexual dysfunction in the general population vary greatly. In a 1990 study by Spector and Carey, the rates were estimated to be [6]:

| | |
|---|---|
| Inhibited female orgasm | 5–10% |
| Male erectile disorder | 4–9% |
| Inhibited male orgasm | 4–10% |
| Premature ejaculation | 36–38% |

However, age and other factors can greatly influence the rate of dysfunction in the population. Laumann et al. [7] found the rate of sexual dysfunction for women ages 18–59 to be 43% ($n=1749$); for the comparable group of men ($n=1410$), the rate of sexual dysfunction was reported at 31%.

## 3. Female sexual dysfunction

Female sexual dysfunction can be categorized into three areas [1]:

1. *Hypoactive sexual desire*: in which there can be a deficiency of sexual fantasies or thoughts and/or receptivity accompanied by feelings of personal distress, or a phobic aversion to or avoidance of sex.
2. *Sexual arousal disorder*: in which there is a persistent or recurrent inability to attain or maintain sufficient sexual excitement accompanied by personal distress.
3. *Orgasmic disorder*: in which attaining orgasm is met with persistent or recurrent difficulty, delay in or absence of response even following sexual stimulation and arousal and is accompanied by personal distress.
4. *Sexual pain disorders*: the two key areas are dyspareunia, or recurrent genital pain with sexual intercourse, and vaginismus, which involves involuntary spasm of the outer third of the vagina that interferes with penetration and causes personal distress.

Phillips [8] identified four different psychological causes of female sexual dysfunction:

1. Intrapersonal conflicts, which arise from religion, social or cultural influences.
2. Interpersonal conflicts, which involve relationship conflicts and communication problems.
3. Sexual history, which can involve past or current sexual abuse, date rape, or sexual harassment or simple inexperience.
4. Stressors, which can vary from problems of depression to illnesses within the family or financial or job-related problems.

## 4. Male sexual dysfunction

Similar to female sexual dysfunction, male sexual dysfunction can be categorized into areas that involve the human sexual response cycle of disorders of desire, arousal, orgasm, and sexual pain [1].

Erectile dysfunction (ED) is the most well known of male sexual disorders and is more accessible to public awareness, because of the introduction of sildenafil (Viagra) to the general population. ED is defined as "the persistent inability to achieve and maintain an erection sufficient to permit satisfactory sexual intercourse" [9]. ED is increasing, in part, due to an aging population and other factors, such as medications, that contribute to or are causative of the problem. Estimates are that ED affects up to 30 million men in the United States and that, among men in their 40s, nearly 40% report at least occasional difficulty and that, among men in their 70s, nearly 70% report difficulties.

ED is diagnosed through typical investigation: thorough history, which includes medical, sexual and psychosocial, and physical examinations, and blood work for identifying or ruling out organic causes of the disorder. Organic causes involve a wide range of pathologies that include neurogenic, hormonal, vascular, drug-induced, and penile-related etiologies [10]. Common medications that can contribute to or cause ED are antihypertensives, psychiatric medications (tricyclic antidepressants, MAO inhibitors, benzodiazepenes, antipsychotics, and selective serotonin reuptake inhibitors (SSRIs).

The most commonly prescribed drugs for ED are sildenafil, yohimbine, and alprostadil. Both sildenafil and yohimbine are oral medications; alprostadil can be injected or taken as a mini-suppository in the urethra. In addition to drug therapies, psychosexual counseling, androgen replacement therapy, vacuum constriction devices, and surgical treatment exist. As in all therapies, an evaluation of a partner's attitude and investment in the therapy contributes and is integral to the success of the therapy.

## 5. Infertility and sexuality

Studies have been conflicted about what aspects of sexuality are affected by infertility. In some studies, investigation has concentrated on the intrusiveness of the treatment and testing regimen, while other studies have examined the level of desire, activity, and sense of fulfillment experienced by men and women as they go through infertility investigations and treatment. A small number of studies have looked at the impact of an infertility diagnosis on sexual function. Specifically, a few early studies showed a correlation between the diagnosis of azoospermia and resulting temporary impotence [10, 11].

The major focus of most investigations has been on the impact of infertility on the marital relationship in general, not specifically on the impact on the couple's sex life. Salvatore et al. [12] showed that women undergoing in vitro fertilization had higher levels of anxiety and emotional tension than controls, as well as a different marital relationship pattern. In addition, the study examined the duration of infertility experiences as a factor affecting couple dynamics. In other earlier studies, women have been reported to have more marital difficulties and negative changes in sexual function [13–18].

When working with an infertile couple, a particular challenge to sexual relations may arise during treatment cycles, when intercourse is timed to ovulation or the male partner needs to produce a specimen on demand. Although not well studied, the anecdotal report of sexual difficulties, such as loss of erection during timed intercourse, inability to achieve an erection, or inability to masturbate to produce a specimen, is frequent. Clearly, the pressure and the embarrassment factor for many men to masturbate, when the medical team will be aware of it, is a major factor in these temporary sexual problems. A classic anecdotal report involves timed intercourse for a post-coital test. Many times a couple will fail to have intercourse for the test due to an argument or the male partner having erectile difficulties. These situations are reported to occur because of one or both partners' acute awareness that the doctor and the staff will know that intercourse has just occurred, and this awareness is accompanied by feelings of embarrassment or shame. At the very least, couples talk about their intimate life being intruded upon by the testing.

Overall, many individuals and couples will report less enjoyment of sexual intimacy as they go through treatment. This may be due to the association of sexual intimacy with failure to get pregnant and, in strictly behavioral terms, individuals and couples get conditioned to associate intimacy with failure rather than pleasure. Add to this the feelings that many women and men express about feeling less feminine or masculine as a result of their infertility, and the recipe for lowered sexual enjoyment is created.

## 6. Taking a sexual history

For many practitioners, both medical and mental health, an area that has received little training is in taking a sexual history. The very fact that a history is taken by a professional will affirm that the couple's sexual life has importance. Cultural and religious factors will figure prominently in the approach to the sexual history the professional takes.

When working with an infertility patient (as with any patient), sexual history should be taken directly and respectfully. Realistically, most medical professionals have very limited time with their patients, so it is important to develop a few critical questions that can be asked efficiently and comfortably. The key questions to ask are:

- On intake, any history of sexual trauma, which can include questions such as, "As a child or adolescent, did an older person ever approach you sexually?" or "Have you ever been forced into having sex against your will?"
- An assessment of current sexual function, which may include questions such as, "Are you having any problems or concerns in your sexual relations?" or "Have you noticed any changes in your sexual relationship with your partner?"

A general question of safety in a relationship should be asked of all women and can be asked as, "Are there are any problems in safety in your relationship—either physical, emotional or sexual abuse?". These questions can be difficult to ask at first, but with practice become routine. Furthermore, patients come to expect that both their safety and sexual function will be attended to at each visit with their medical professional or will be involved in their general care with a mental health professional.

## 7. Treatment

As mentioned earlier, no treatment can begin to be successful without taking into consideration both partners' attitudes and motivation for treatment. In addition to a medical assessment for both male and female sexual dysfunction, psychosexual counseling is available.

There are many different approaches to psychosexual counseling. In all approaches, a therapist will first try to understand the individual/couple's attitude and knowledge about sex. Sometimes lack of knowledge can be the largest impediment to sexual relations. Therapy cannot be successful if it violates the individual's religious, moral, or cultural proscriptions. In addition, a thorough exploration of the couple's level of function and communication skills is critical before starting any behavioral techniques.

Among the treatment strategies for sexual dysfunction, the most frequent approach is utilizing behavioral techniques in addition to, or in place of, an analytic approach. According to Burns [6], the six most frequent approaches are:

- Anxiety reduction techniques
- Directed masturbation
- Orgasmic reconditioning
- Imagery techniques
- Explicit homework assignments
- Sensate-focus techniques.

## 8. Same sex couples

There are many special considerations that can be overlooked when treating infertile individuals. One of the most prominent issues is acknowledging same sex couples; these couples are infrequently asked about the impact of infertility on their sexuality. Indeed, sexual health is rarely raised as part of the health history. Once again, it is important to inquire about the individual or couple's sexual function and whether there have been any changes as a result of the infertility.

## 9. Conclusion

Sexuality and intimacy are important and special parts of a couple's relationship. Sexual dysfunction exists for both men and women and is usually very treatable. When experiencing infertility, sexual dysfunction can emerge as an issue in preventing pregnancy, but more often presents itself as a concomitant of the feelings and tasks associated with treatment. Developing good skills at taking an initial sexual history and developing a comfort level with addressing an individual or couple's sexual health will promote better communication between professional and patient, as well as affirm sexuality as a valued part of the relationship. Referring patients to qualified sex therapists for further assistance can be very helpful in a team approach for treating men and women as they go through infertility treatment.

## References

[1] J.L. Carroll, P.R. Wolpe, Sexuality and Gender in Society, Harper Collins College Publishers, New York, 1996.
[2] W.H. Masters, V.E. Johnson, Human Sexual Response, Little Brown, Boston, 1996.
[3] R. Basson, Human sex-response cycles, J. Sex Marital Ther. 27 (2001) 33–43.
[4] R. Basson, S. Leiblum, L. Brotto, L. Derogatis, J. Fourcroy, K. Fugl-Meyer, A. Graziottin, J.R. Heiman, E. Laan, C. Meston, L. Schover, J. van Lankveld, W.W. Schultz, Definitions of women's sexual dysfunction reconsidered: advocating expansion and revision, J. Psychosom. Obstet. Gynaecol. 24 (2003) 221–229.
[5] R. Basson, The female sexual response: a different model, J. Sex Marital Ther. 28 (2002) 51–65.
[6] L.H. Burns, Sexual counseling and infertility, in: L.H. Burns, S.N. Covington (Eds.), Infertility Counseling: a Comprehensive Handbook for Clinicians, Parthenon Publishing, New York, 1999, pp. 149–176.
[7] E.O. Laumann, A. Paik, R.C. Rosen, Sexual dysfunction in the United States, JAMA 281 (1999) 537–544.
[8] N.A. Phillips, Female sexual dysfunction: evaluation and treatment. Am. Fam. Phys. 62 (2000) 127–36, 141–42.
[9] G. Matfin, New treatments for erectile dysfunction, Sex. Reprod. Menopause 1 (2003) 40–45.
[10] D.M. Berger, Impotence following the discovery of azoospermia, Fertil. Steril. 34 (1980) 154–156.
[11] T. Drake, G. Grunert, A cyclic pattern of sexual dysfunction in the infertility investigation, Fertil. Steril. 32 (1979) 542–545.

[12] P. Salvatore, S. Gariboldi, A. Offidani, F. Coppola, M. Amore, C. Maggini, Psychopathology, personality, and marital relationship in patients undergoing in vitro fertilization procedures, Fertil. Steril. 75 (2001) 1119–1125.
[13] G.J. Hynes, V.J. Callan, D.J. Terry, C. Gallois, The psychological well-being of infertile women after a failed IVF attempt: the effects of coping, Br. J. Med. Psychol. 65 (1992) 269–278.
[14] P. Thierring, J. Beaurepaire, M. Jones, D. Sauders, C. Tennat, Mood state as a predictor of treatment outcome after in vitro fertilization/embryo transfer technology (IVF/ET), J. Psychosom. Res. 37 (1993) 481–491.
[15] B.J. Oddens, I. Tonkelaar, H. Nieuwenhuyse, Psychosocial experiences in women facing fertility problems: a comparative survey, Hum. Reprod. 14 (1999) 255–261.
[16] A. Eugster, A.J. Vingerhoets, Psychological aspects of in vitro fertilization: a review, Soc. Sci. Med. 48 (1999) 575–589.
[17] M.P. Lukse, N.A. Vace, Grief, depression, and coping in women undergoing infertility treatment, Obstet. Gynecol. 93 (1999) 245–251.
[18] C.R. Newton, M.T. Heran, A.A. Yuzpe, Psychological assessment and follow-up after in vitro fertilization: assessing the impact of failure, Fertil. Steril. 54 (1990) 879–886.

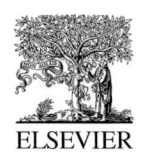

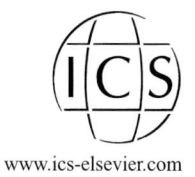

# Sexually transmitted chlamydial infections and subfertility

Jorma Paavonen*

*Department of Obstetrics and Gynecology, University of Helsinki, Haartmaninkatu 2, 00290 Helsinki, Finland*

**Abstract.** *Introduction:* Sexually transmitted infections (STI) are on the rise in Europe and the United States. The major cause is changing sexual behavior. The median age of sexual debut continues to decrease, and the time window between age of first sexual intercourse and marriage has lengthened extending the period of experimentation and changing partners. The resurgence of STIs among young people during the last decade may also reflect declining awareness and fear of HIV and AIDS. STIs, most notably infections caused by Chlamydia trachomatis, are the major threat to reproductive health among women. *Methods:* To review the role of C. trachomatis (CT) in subfertility among women and to review the current strategies of STI prevention. *Results:* CT is the leading cause of permanent tubal damage. Tubal factor infertility (TFI) is the only preventable type of infertility. However, secondary prevention of CT infections (and other STIs) by so-called opportunistic screening has largely failed. This is frustrating since CT infection fills the prerequisites for disease prevention by screening. Furthermore, results with primary prevention through sexual or reproductive health education have been disappointing. The pathogenesis of CT-associated tubal damage is not yet fully understood, and a number of heavily interconnected factors appear to play a role. Immune response to chlamydial HSP60 is associated with long-term sequelae of chlamydial infections. Because of the complexity of the host immune response to CT, development of CT vaccine is a huge challenge. Preventing or limiting the long-term sequelae of chlamydial infection such as PID, adverse pregnancy outcome, and TFI would be a realistic goal for the first generation CT vaccine. *Conclusions:* New emphasis on CT control strategies is needed to shorten the period of infectiousness and to reduce risk-taking behavior among young people. © 2004 Published by Elsevier B.V.

*Keywords:* Sexually transmitted infections; Chlamydia trachomatis; Subfertility; Infertility

## 1. Introduction

While it is healthy for individuals to enjoy active sex lives, it is important to realize that there are over 25 sexually transmitted infections (STIs) some which, if left untreated may cause serious and permanent health problems. STIs are among the most common causes of illness and a major public health problem. Many STIs favor the spread of HIV infection and can cause serious health problems in newborns, or may cause infertility. The past decade has seen a continuing and considerable deterioration in sexual health particularly among young

---

* Tel.: +358 50 4272060; fax: +358-94-7174902.
  E-mail address: Jorma.paavonen@hus.fi (J. Paavonen).

0531-5131/ © 2004 Published by Elsevier B.V.
doi:10.1016/j.ics.2004.01.114

people. Risk-taking sexual behavior is increasing, STIs have increased alarmingly, and teenage pregnancies are increasing. We are now facing a public health crisis in sexual health.

The basic reproductive number of STI, Ro, is defined as the average number of secondary infections generated by one infectious individual in an entirely susceptible population. For persistence of infection, the magnitude of Ro must be greater than or equal to unity in value. The immediate determinants of STI epidemics include three components, beta, $C$, and $D$. A simple formulation of the basic reproductive number for an STI spreading in a homogeneously mixing population is as follows:

$$Ro = \text{beta} \times C \times D.$$

Beta indicates the transmission probability or transmission efficiency per partnership, $C$ denotes the average rate of sexual partner change (contact rate), and $D$ is the mean duration of infectiousness [1]. The development of mathematical models of the transmission and control of STIs has proven useful, and can serve several purposes, such as testing well-defined STI hypotheses, designing and evaluating different STI interventions, and defining STI epidemiological patterns and trends.

## 2. Reasons for high rates of STIs

STIs have rapidly increased during the last decade in Europe and elsewhere [2–5]. The current high rates of STIs is surprising and unexpected since general awareness, diagnostic techniques, and management have all improved, and comprehensive STI guidelines have been developed and implemented. The rise has been associated with increasing risk-taking sexual behavior among young adults. Sex education among adolescents has deteriorated. There is a lack of high profile campaigns to highlight sexual health risks and encourage safe sex behavior. The decline in the number of STIs in the late 1980s and early 1990s in response to the HIV epidemic demonstrated the importance of awareness in the prevention of STIs. Change in attitudes and behavior has since then changed including decrease in age at first sexual intercourse, delay of first pregnancy, increased partner change, and concurrent multiple sexual partners.

In Finland, between 1995 and 2000, the incidence of Chlamydia trachomatis (CT) infections increased although there were no major changes in public STI services or screening practices [6]. National sentinel clinic surveillance network based on laboratory notification system documented rapidly increasing incidence rates especially among adolescents and young people, from 23.4 per 10,000 to 29.2 per 10,000. In the age group of less than 29 years, 19% reported five or more annual sex partners in 2000, compared with 8% in 1995. This risk group of young people living in metropolitan cities should remain the main target for screening and reproductive health education programs to control STIs.

## 3. Extent of subfertility

Subfertility is defined as a failure to conceive after 1 year of unprotected regular sexual intercourse [7]. One in six couples have an unwanted delay in conception. Roughly half of these couples will conceive either spontaneously or with relatively simple treatment. The other half will remain subfertile and need more complex treatment such as in vitro fertilization (IVF) and other assisted conception techniques; about half of these will have primary subfertility. Most couples presenting with a fertility problem do not have absolute infertility, but rather subfertility with a reduced chance of conception because of one or more relative subfertility factors in one or both partners. The likelihood of spontaneous conception is affected by age, previous pregnancy outcome, duration of subfertility, timing of intercourse during the natural cycle, body mass index, and gynecologic pathology present. Conception is most likely to occur in the first months (about 30% conception rate per month). The chance then falls steadily to about 5% by the end of first year. Cumulative conception rate is approximately 75% after 6 months, 90% after 1 year, and 95% after 2 years. Fecundity rates in developed countries may be declining. However, it is difficult to separate changes in social behavior and trends in delaying starting a family from other factors that might affect reproductive health and reduce the chance of conception, such as environmental factors.

## 4. Major causes of subfertility

The major causes of subfertility can be classified as ovulation disorders, male factor subfertility, tubal damage, unexplained subfertility, and other causes, such as endometriosis and fibroids [8]. The proportion of each type of subfertility varies in different populations. Tubal subfertility is more common in those with secondary subfertility and in populations with a higher prevalence of STIs. Patent Fallopian tubes are a prerequisite for normal fertility. However, patency alone is not enough—normal function is crucial. Fallopian tubes are highly specialized organs, having a critical role in picking up eggs and transporting eggs, sperm, and embryo. The Fallopian tubes are also needed for sperm capacitation and egg fertilization. Because the egg is fertilized in the Fallopian tubes and the first stages of development of the embryo occur during its 4-day journey to the uterine cavity, the tubes are also important in nutrition and development. The Fallopian tubes are vulnerable to infection and surgical damage, which may impair function by affecting the delicate fimbriae or endosalpinx. Fallopian tube obstruction occurs in up to one third of all infertile couples. It should be emphasized that tubal factor infertility (TFI) is the only preventable type of infertility.

## 5. Causes of tubal damage

Pelvic infection is a major cause of tubal subfertility. Infective tubal damage can be caused by STIs, or can occur after miscarriage, termination of pregnancy, puerperal sepsis, or insertion of an intrauterine contraceptive device (IUD) [8]. The severity of tubal subfertility after pelvic infection depends on the number and severity of episodes. Although a history of symptomatic PID may heighten suspicion of tubal damage, most women with TFI do not have such history of overt PID. Even in women with serological evidence of past chlamydial or gonococcal infections, most are unaware of the infection. CT accounts for around one third of the cases of PID in developed countries [9]. Both symptomatic and asymptomatic chlamydial infection can damage the reproductive tract. Delayed treatment increases the risk of permanent tubal damage and duration of infectiousness. CT is responsible for approximately 25–50% of ectopic pregnancies, and approximately 50% of TFI. Gonorrhoeae can also cause an infection of the upper genital tract. Coinfection with CT is present in 30–50% of patients with gonorrhoeae.

Other infectious causes of tubal damage are genital tuberculosis, post-abortion and puerperal infections.

Upper genital tract infection associated with IUD is temporally linked to the insertion of the device (first 3 weeks). The risk of infertility after the use of an IUD is not increased, nor is fertility impaired.

Complete tubal occlusion is rarely caused by pelvic endometriosis, but tubal distortion and limitation of fimbrial mobility can occur. Previous laparotomy is a recognized risk factor for tubal subfertility. History of perforated appendix can also have a negative long-term effect on fertility.

## 6. Chlamydia trachomatis: the ultimate intracellular pathogen

CT is the major threat of reproductive health in women [10]. The chlamydia epidemic during recent decades has led to a secondary epidemic of subfertility and adverse pregnancy outcome (APO). CT is an intracellular bacterial pathogen. Chlamydial serovars D-K cause nearly 4 million new STI cases annually in the United States and 90 million cases worldwide. Other serovars (A, B, Ba, and C) are responsible for trachoma, the leading cause of preventable blindness, afflicting some 500 million people worldwide. In part, because chlamydiae are true obligate intracellular pathogens, chlamydial diseases tend to be chronic in nature [11]. These bacteria survive and grow only after they invade mucosal epithelial cells. During this growth, or developmental cycle, the bacteria alternate between two structurally and physiologically distinct forms. In one, the elementary body (EB), the bacteria are infectious and make initial contact with susceptible target epithelial cells. Following attachment to such cells, endocytosis, the EB containing endosome travels on microtubules, moving away from the endocytic pathway and toward the exocytic pathway. The EB envelope changes, transforming the metabolically inert EB into the metabolically active reticulate body (RB). DNA, RNA, and protein are synthesized within the RB, leading to successive rounds of binary fission and increased numbers of progeny. To accommodate this growing RB population, the endosomal vacuole membrane expands, and this entity is called an inclusion. Next, metabolically active, noninfectious RBs are ready to complete the cycle by becoming infectious EBs. Following escape or release from the host cell, the compact, rigid EB can survive extracellularly for limited periods before finding new susceptible epithelial cells to invade and begin another infectious round of growth and amplification. Soon after chlamydiae infect a host cell, they induce anti-apoptotic signals and thus gain time to move through this developmental cycle. Late during each cycle host cells degrade liberating infectious EB. Under some circumstances intracellular environment may not be favorable for this cycle, and an aberrant, slowly metabolizing form of RB appears, which can persist for extended periods. This slowly metabolizing RB form may well be the predominant chlamydial form in vivo, and its behavior may explain the chronic nature of chlamydial diseases and the long-term sequelae.

## 7. Clinical manifestations of chlamydial infection

Mucopurulent cervicitis (MPC), endometritis, and PID are the major clinical manifestations of genital chlamydial infection in women. MPC represents the ignored counterpart of urethritis in males [12]. Clinical diagnosis of MPC is difficult, and no uniform or accurate criteria for the diagnosis of MPC exist. Endometritis as a clinical-pathologic syndrome represents the first step of a lower genital tract infection ascending to the upper genital tract [13]. Clinical and laboratory correlates suggest that endometritis is a distinct clinical entity. However, the natural history and long-term prognosis of endometritis alone (in the absence of laparoscopic signs of salpingitis) remain undefined. In particular, the frequency with which endometritis remains limited to the uterus or progresses into salpingitis has not been well understood. Risk factors for endometritis include chlamydial and gonococcal infection, current IUD use, recent douching, and being in days 1 to 7 of the menstrual cycle. The clinical spectrum of endometritis alone probably encompasses mostly asymptomatic women who may in fact outnumber women with symptoms and signs suggestive of acute PID. The potential for the progression to salpingitis warrants prompt antimicrobial therapy. The potential effects of endometritis on implantation and pregnancy outcome are not known. However, it is biologically plausible that subclinical endometritis increases the risk for subfertility and APO. PID comprises a spectrum of inflammatory disorders of the upper female genital tract, including any combination of endometritis, salpingitis, tubo-ovarian abscess, and pelvic peritonitis [14]. Bilateral lower abdominal pain is the most common presenting symptom of PID. Perihepatitis causes right quadrant upper abdominal pain mimicking acute cholecystitis. Other common symptoms are abnormal vaginal discharge, metrorrhagia, postcoital bleeding, dysuria and fever. However, symptomatic PID only represents the tip of the iceberg. Minimally symptomatic patients usually seek medical care late which increases the risk for tubal damage and long-term sequelae. After a single episode of PID, the risk for TFI is approximately 11%. Each repeat episode of PID doubles or triples the risk. Women with a history of PID have approximately 6- to 10-fold increased risk of tubal pregnancy compared with women with no history of PID. Chronic pelvic pain occurs in a large proportion of women crippled with past PID. Women with a history of PID are approximately 10 times more likely to be admitted for pelvic pain, and hysterectomy rates are eight times higher than in other women. Thus, women with PID suffer substantial long-term gynecological morbidity in later life.

## 8. Immunopathogenesis of chlamydial infection

Given the intracellular developmental cycle of chlamydia, there is strong evidence for the involvement of host immune response such as IFN-γ, in the natural history of chlamydial infection. Host response to chlamydial infection can result either in a protective or pathological immune response [15]. Tissue damage results more from immune recognition of specific antigens expressed by the organism. Given the primary protective role effected by the cell-mediated Th-1 response in resolving infection, inflammatory damage within the upper reproductive tract may be the result of a failed or weak Th-1 action resulting in chronic infection or as a result of an exaggerated or overstimulated Th-1 response. A balance, therefore, exists between the protective and deleterious effects of cell-mediated immunity. Carefully regulated cytokine production is central to successful immune responses to intracellular pathogens. Deficiencies in the production or activity of these proinflammatory cytokines can be associated with failure of protective immunity or harmful inflammation.

The model of pathogenesis by which CT progresses from acute to chronic infection remains to be fully understood. The pathways by which acute chlamydial infection achieves resolution or alternatively progresses to chronic infection appear to depend on a close interplay between host and pathogen. A number of interconnected factors appear to play significant roles—human genetics and endocrinology, cytokine profile, previous infections, pathogen load, chlamydial strain, the presence of other genital infections, among others.

## 9. The role of chlamydial heat shock protein 60 in tubal factor infertility

The major chlamydial component associated with permanent tubal damage and other long-term sequelae is chlamydial heat shock protein 60 (CHSP60) which has the unique capability to modulate host immune responses [16]. Evidence implicating CHSP60 as the critical antigen is extensive through studies reporting the increasing prevalence of CHSP60 antibodies among women with increasing severity of chlamydial disease. A number of studies investigating serological responses of infertile women to CHSP60 have demonstrated a correlation between antibodies and TFI. CHSP60 exhibits greater than 80% homology between Chlamydia species, 60% identify with bacteria, and 50% homology with eukaryotic HSP60. CHSP60 is involved in the assembly of the outer membrane of the elementary body during the developmental change from the large intracellular RB to the compact infective EB. The mechanism by which exposure to CHSP60 elicits pathology has been explained in many ways. CT enters a persistent state within human host cells during which expression of CHSP60 is enhanced whereas levels of the major outer membrane protein (MOMP) are minimized. This provides a continued source of antigenic stimulation. Repeated exposure to other bacteria carrying homologous HSPs or repeated chlamydial infections may result in a prolonged antibody response and with chronic inflammation. In addition, there is a possibility of autoimmune-mediated damage to tissue as a result of molecular mimicry between antigenic CHSP60 and self-HSP. Furthermore, human HSP60 is expressed during the early stages of pregnancy by the embryo and maternal decidua. These host HSP60s may, in the presence of a chronic chlamydial infection, cross-react with T cells previously sensitized to CHSP60. The activated lymphocytes release cytokines that can disturb the immune regulatory mechanisms necessary to implantation and maintenance of the embryo, and increase the risk for habitual abortion.

CHSP60 antigen is recognized by T cells present in the peripheral blood and in the inflamed fallopian tube tissue of TFI patients [17,18]. Most CHSP60 specific T cell clones produce predominantly IL-10 [19]. CHSP60 seems to induce Th2-type cytokine response in chlamydia-specific T cells and may thereby downregulate or replace an initial Th1 mediated immune response needed to eliminate Chlamydia. CHSP60 specific immune response is associated with specific HLA-DQ alleles and IL10 polymorphism in TFI patients [20]. Thus, in genetically predisposed individuals the induction of deleterious cytokine response can lead to a cycle of persistent infection associated with continuous antigenic stimulation and chronic inflammation the end result of which would then be scarring and structural damage of the fallopian tube. It is possible that CHSP60 associated genetic markers can be used as surrogate markers to identify individuals at risk for developing TFI.

## 10. Chlamydia trachomatis antibody testing in subfertility evaluation

CT is the leading cause of permanent tubal damage worldwide. Detecting evidence of past chlamydial infection using serology is noninvasive, simple, and quick to perform [21].

Chlamydial antibodies persist for years as a serologic scar consistent with past infection. Thus, chlamydial antibody titers (CAT) can be used as a screening test for distal tubal damage among subfertile women. A linear trend has been observed between serum CAT and the likelihood of tubal damage [21]. Chlamydia serology is useful as a screening test for tubal damage in subfertile women and can be used for tailoring further management of such women [22]. Specifically, CATs>1:32 or 1:64 by immunofluorescence test are sufficiently high to predict TFI, as demonstrated by receiver operating characteristic (ROC) curve analysis. However, the choice of cut-off level used for screening depends on the prevalence of chlamydial infection in the population and the antibody test used. In many infertility clinics, CAT screening has already been introduced in the initial work-up of subfertile couples.

## 11. Control strategies

Disease prevention can be primary, secondary, or tertiary. Clinicians and other health care providers have an important role in the primary prevention of STIs through lifestyle counseling and health education, and by asking questions about risk-taking sexual behavior, by encouraging screening tests for those at risk, by ensuring that sex partners are properly managed, and by counseling about safe sex practices. Unfortunately, primary STI prevention by health education has not proven very effective [23,24]. Partner notification, expedited partner care, and patient initiated partner treatment are important but often ignored steps in preventing the spread of STIs [25].

Secondary prevention by screening for CT is likely to have the most critical role in the prevention of subfertility. Because CT is the major cause of upper genital tract infection and tubal damage, it is logical to focus prevention efforts on chlamydia. Thus, screening for CT is of paramount importance in the prevention of upper genital tract infection. Chlamydial infection fills the prerequisites for disease prevention by screening because chlamydial infections are highly prevalent, are associated with significant morbidity, can be readily diagnosed, and are treatable [26]. Use of the first void urine (FVU) specimens (or vulvar or vaginal swabs) and NAA tests for diagnosis, and single dose of azithromycin for treatment should enhance these efforts. One recent randomized trial showed that intervention with selective screening effectively reduced the incidence of symptomatic PID by 64% during 1 year of follow-up [27]. High CT screening activity in Sweden resulted in a dramatic decrease of CT rates (which unfortunately has been recently increasing again), followed by a rapid decrease in the rates of hospitalizations for PID [28]. Even more important, 5–10 years later this was followed by a significant fall in the rate of ectopic pregnancies, especially in young age groups [29]. However, it is not yet known whether CT screening produces a corresponding fall in the incidence of TFI. Although CT screening seems to be a straightforward approach, many research questions need to be addressed before nationwide screening programs can be implemented [30,31]. Stochastic simulation model analysis of screening programs for CT in an age-structured heterosexual population with a sexually highly active core group showed that the prevalence of asymptomatic infections in women could be reduced from 4.2% to 1.4% in 10 years, through screening of men and women between ages 15 and 24 years [32]. Partner referral contributed substantially to prevalence reduction. The restriction of a screening program to younger age groups or women only is more cost-effective because CT prevalence is higher, and the probabilities of preventing adverse pregnancy outcome and subfertility are also higher.

Cost-effectiveness analyses heavily advocate CT screening [33]. A recent critical review of such studies concluded that screening is cost effective because future sequelae of untreated infection can be prevented. However, we do not know whether the natural history of nucleic acid amplification test (NAAT) detected infections is the same as culture detected infections. NAATs are at least 30–40% more sensitive than culture for detecting chlamydia. It is unknown whether NAAT positive (culture negative) infections are as likely to progress into upper genital tract infection and cause irreversible tubal damage [30]. The probability of upper genital tract infection subsequent to untreated infection is central to the cost-effectiveness of screening programs.

Tertiary prevention includes treatment that prevents upper-genital tract infection from leading to tubal obstruction. However, the damage may already be there. Partner notification and appropriate counseling are of paramount importance in order to prevent recurrent infections which double or triple the risk for permanent tubal damage.

## 12. STI vaccine development

The future of primary prevention of viral STIs through vaccination looks bright [34,35]. Virus-like particle-based prophylactic vaccines against high risk human papillomavirus (HPV) type 16 and 18 infection have already entered phase III efficacy trials, and the early results with HPV 16 vaccine are very promising [34]. The prospects for herpes simplex virus (HSV) type 2 subunit vaccine are also promising [35]. However, neither HPV nor HSV has been directly linked to subfertility. CT is a huge challenge for vaccine development [36]. Using the whole organism for vaccination has proved unattractive and no single subunit vaccine has yet produced sterilizing long-term immunity. Most of the chlamydia vaccines developed and tested so far in animal models only give temporary or partial protection. A protective antichlamydial immune response is mediated primarily by a T cell response involving induction and recruitment of Th1 cells and an IgG and IgA antibody response onto mucosal membranes. The potential CT vaccine will probably contain a cocktail of recombinant proteins to be able to deliver enough T cell epitopes. A partially protective vaccine effective against PID and tubal damage would be an acceptable goal of the first generation chlamydia vaccine.

## References

[1] R.M. Andersen, G.P. Garnett, Mathematical Models of the transmission and control of sexually transmitted diseases, Sex. Transm. Dis. 27 (2000) 636–643.
[2] M.W. Adler, Sexual health—health of the nation, Sex. Transm. Dis. 79 (2003) 84–85.
[3] A.C. Gerbase, J.T. Rowley, T.E. Mertens, Global epidemiology of sexually transmitted diseases, Lancet 351 (Suppl. III) (1998) S2–S4.
[4] L. Hansen, T. Wong, M. Perrin, Gonorrhoea resurgence in Canada, Int. J. STD AIDS 14 (2003) 727–731.
[5] A. Nicoll, F.F. Hamers, Are trends in HIV, gonorrhoea, and syphilis worsening in western Europe? BMJ 324 (2002) 1324–1327.
[6] E. Hiltunen-Back, et al., Nationwide increase of Chlamydia trachomatis infection in Finland, Sex. Transm. Dis. 30 (2003) 737–741.

[7]  A. Taylor, Subfertility. Extent of the problem, BMJ 327 (2003) 434–436.
[8]  Y. Khalaf, Tubal subfertility, BMJ 327 (2003) 610–613.
[9]  I. Simms, J.M. Stephenson, Pelvic inflammatory disease epidemiology: what do we know and what do we need to know? Sex. Transm. Infect. 76 (2000) 80–87.
[10] J. Paavonen, W. Eggert-Kruse, Chlamydia trachomatis: impact on human reproduction, Hum. Reprod. Updat. 5 (1999) 433–447.
[11] P.B. Wyrick, C. trachomatis: infection strategies of the ultimate intracellular pathogen, ASM News 68 (2002) 70–76.
[12] R.C. Brunham, et al., Mucopurulent cervicitis—the ignored counterpart in women of urethritis in men, N. Engl. J. Med. 311 (1984) 1–6.
[13] L.O. Eckert, et al., Endometritis: the clinical-pathologic syndrome, Am. J. Obstet. Gynecol. 186 (2002) 690–695.
[14] J. Paavonen, P. Molander, Pelvic inflammatory disease, in: R.W. Shaw, et al. (Eds.), Gynecology, 3rd ed., Churchill Livingstone, London, 2003, pp. 891–900.
[15] J. Debattista, et al., Immunopathogenesis of Chlamydia trachomatis infections in women, Fertil. Steril. 79 (2003) 1273–1287.
[16] A. Kinnunen, J. Paavonen, H.-M. Surcel, Heat shock protein 60 specific T-cell response in chlamydial infections, Scand. J. Immunol. 54 (2001) 2001.
[17] A. Kinnunen, et al., Chlamydia trachomatis reactive T lymphocytes from upper genital tract tissue specimens, Hum. Reprod. 15 (2000) 1484–1489.
[18] A. Kinnunen, et al., Chlamydial heat shock protein 60 specific T cells in inflamed salpingeal tissue, Fertil. Steril. 77 (2002) 162–166.
[19] A. Kinnunen, et al., Chlamydia trachomatis heat shock protein-60 induced interferon-γ and interleukin-10 production by peripheral blood lymphocytes in infertile women, Clin. Exp. Immunol. 131 (2003) 299–303.
[20] A. Kinnunen, et al., HLA DQ alleles and interleukin-10 polymorphism associated with Chlamydia trachomatis-related tubal factor infertility: a case-control study, Hum. Reprod. 17 (2002) 2073–2078.
[21] V.A. Akande, et al., Tubal damage in infertile women: prediction using chlamydia serology, Hum. Reprod. 18 (2003) 1841–1847.
[22] J.A. Land, J.L.H. Evers, V. Goossens, How to use Chlamydia antibody testing subfertility patients, Hum. Reprod. 13 (1998) 1094–1098.
[23] S.O. Aral, Determinants of STD epidemics: implications for phase appropriate intervention strategies, Sex. Transm. Infect. 78 (Suppl. I) (2002) i3–i13.
[24] D. Wight, et al., Limits of teacher delivered sex education: interim behavioural outcomes from randomized trial, BMJ 324 (2002) 1430–1433.
[25] M.R. Golden, et al., Partner management for gonococcal and chlamydial infection, Sex. Transm. Dis. 28 (2001) 658–665.
[26] J.S. Wilson, et al., Stray-Pedersen B for the EU Biomed Concerted Action Group. A systematic review of the prevalence of Chlamydia trachomatis among European women, Hum. Reprod. Updat 8 (2002) 385–394.
[27] D. Scholes, et al., Prevention of pelvic inflammatory disease by screening for cervical chlamydial infection, N. Engl. J. Med. 334 (1996) 1362–1366.
[28] F. Kamwendo, et al., Programmes to reduce pelvic inflammatory disease—the Swedish experience, Lancet 351 (1998) 25–28.
[29] M. Egger, et al., Screening for chlamydial infections and the risk of ectopic pregnancy in a county in Sweden: ecological analysis, BMJ 316 (1998) 1776–1780.
[30] S.D. Mehta, M. Shahmanesh, J.M. Zenilman, Spending money to save money, Sex. Transm. Infect. 79 (2003) 4–6.
[31] N. Low, M. Egger, What should we do about screening for genital chlamydia? Int. J. Epidemiol. 31 (2002) 891–893.
[32] M. Kretzschmar, et al., Comparative model-based analysis of screening programs for Chlamydia trachomatis infections, Am. J. Epidemiol. 153 (2001) 90–101.
[33] E. Honey, et al., Cost effectiveness of screening for Chlamydia trachomatis: a review of published studies, Sex. Transm. Infect. 78 (2002) 406–412.

[34] L.A. Koutsky, et al., Jansen KU for the proof of principle study investigators. A controlled trial of a human papillomavirus type 16 vaccine, N. Engl. J. Med. 347 (2002) 1645–1651.
[35] L.R. Stanberry, et al., for the GlaxoSmithKline Herpes Vaccine Efficacy Study Group, Glykoprotein-D-adjuvant vaccine to prevent genital herpes, N. Engl. J. Med. 347 (2002) 1652–1661.
[36] J.U. Igietseme, F.O. Eko, C.M. Black, Contemporary approaches to designing and evaluating vaccines against Chlamydia, Expert Rev. Vaccines 2 (2003) 129–146.

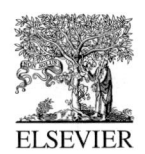

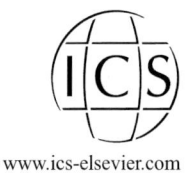

# Tuberculosis in assisted reproduction and infertility

Timur Gurgan[a,1], Aygül Demirol[b,*]

[a] Clinic Women Health, Infertility and IVF Center, Ankara, Turkey
[b] Reproductive Endocrinology and IVF Unit, Hacettepe University, Faculty of Medicine, Dept. of OB&Gyn, Ankara, Turkey

**Abstract.** The incidence of tuberculosis (TB) has declined in the developed countries; however, the disease continues to be an important cause of tubal factor infertility in the developing world. Tubal affliction is the rule, and fibrotic squeal of the infection result in tubal occlusion that is not amenable to reconstructive tubal surgery. Genital tuberculosis often exists without any symptoms or clinical signs. The most common initial symptom of genital tuberculosis is infertility; the other symptoms are lower abdominal and pelvic pain and menstrual abnormalities. Endometrial involvement is noted in 50% to 60% of subjects. In vitro fertilization (IVF) appears to be the only option for women suffering from infertility due to genital tuberculosis; however, endometrial involvement diminishes successful implantation. The success rates with IVF may be improved by adequate preoperative antituberculous chemotherapy and selection of patients without endometrial involvement, as shown by normal configuration of endometrial cavity at hysterosalpingography and a normal hysteroscopy. Patient selection for IVF should be performed carefully and the evaluation of each patient should be done fastidiously. © 2004 Published by Elsevier B.V.

*Keywords:* Tuberculosis; Infertility; Treatment

## 1. Introduction

Tuberculosis (TB) is one of the oldest diseases known to affect humans [1]. The reported prevalence of genital tuberculosis in infertility clinics varies widely with an incidence of 0.69% in Australia to 19% in India [2]. In the United States, genital tuberculosis is rarely encountered, but genital tuberculosis should be considered in infertile women with midtubal occlusion and characteristic hysterosalpingographic (HSG) signs. Case series were reported with biopsy-proved forms in 16 Canadian women with midtubal obstruction [3]. Genital tuberculosis often exists without any symptoms or clinical signs. The most common initial symptom of genital tuberculosis is infertility; the other symptoms are lower abdominal and pelvic pain and menstrual abnormalities [4]. Despite the advances in chemotherapeutic treatment, pregnancy after diagnosis of genital tuberculosis has been reported to be rare and when it did occur was more likely to be an ectopic

---

* Corresponding author. Tel.: +90-312-442-74-04; fax: +90-312-442-74-07.
*E-mail addresses:* tgurgan@gurganclinic.com (T. Gurgan), ademirol@gurganclinic.com (A. Demirol).
[1] Tel.: +90-312-442-74-04; fax: +90-312-422-74-07.

0531-5131/ © 2004 Published by Elsevier B.V.
doi:10.1016/j.ics.2004.01.119

pregnancy or resulted in a spontaneous abortion [5,6]. Incidence of infertility differs according to the pattern in the genital tract; for example in a series of 704 women reported by Sutherland, infertility was the presenting symptom in 307 (43.6%) [7].

Early diagnosis and medical treatment, with culture positive for acid-fast bacilli before the development of fulminating genital tuberculosis, has been associated with higher pregnancy rates. In vitro fertilization and embryo transfer (IVF-ET) offers the best chance of a successful pregnancy outcome in these patients, but the pregnancy rate depends on endometrial involvement. There are conflicting data regarding the success rate with IVF-ET because of the decreasing incidence. Patients' selection for IVF should be performed carefully and the evaluation of each patient should be done fastidiously.

## 2. Pathogenesis

Tuberculosis is caused by Mycobacterium tuberculosis. Pulmonary infection is generally the primary focus. The mycobacterium is transmitted by human contact. Following exposure, the mycobacterium lodges in the macrophage and multiplies slowly. In most cases primary TB is a self-limited, mild, pneumonic illness. The organism may lie dormant for many years or become reactivated and cause an inflammatory response that is marked by macrophages, lymphocyte infiltration, and granulomas with central 'Langhans' giant cells. The response to infection is often dependent on the patient's immune system.

Genitourinary TB is caused by M tuberculosis and it is the second most common form of extrapulmonary TB after peripheral lymphadenopathy. It is estimated that genitourinary TB comprises 30% of non-pulmonary TB [8]. Both fallopian tubes are invariably involved in all women with genital TB [9]. Infection of the endometrium, however, is encountered in 50–60% of cases. TB cervicitis afflicts only 5% of women with pelvic infection and the ovaries are involved in 20–25% of cases with pelvic TB [10]. TB infection of the ovary is usually in the form of perioophoritis without ovarian parenchimal involvement. Extension of the infection to the ovarian parenchyma may be prevented by the tunica albuginea.

## 3. Clinical presentation

Infertility is the most common initial symptom and it can be diagnosed in 40% to 50% of patients [11,12]. After all, 85% of women with genital TB have never been pregnant. Lower abdominal and pelvic pain is present in 25% to 50% of the subjects. The spectrum of pelvic pain is variable and may be chronic and low grade, but may also be intermittent and severe. Menorrhagia, menometrorragia, intermenstrual bleeding, postmenopausal bleeding, olgomenorrhea, amenorrhea, and dysmenorrhea are the menstrual irregularities encountered with genital TB. The amenorrhea cases in TB are mostly because of the total or near-total obliteration of the endometrial cavity with post-infection adhesions.

## 4. Diagnosis

Genital TB may be diagnosed during:

- The course of acute pelviperitoneal tuberculosis,
- The investigation of an adnexal mass,

- The investigation of menstrual irregularity, especially postmenopausal bleeding,
- The course of an infertility workup.

The diagnosis is usually done by HSG and laparoscopy.

In infertile patients, HSG is an important and easy tool for the diagnosis of TB but once genital TB is diagnosed, HSG should not be done as it may disseminate the disease.

However, the progression of TB is so slow and insidious with 1 to 10 years needed for diagnosis according to the HSG [13].

The diagnostic criteria for genital TB in HSG are:

- Uterine cavity shriveled, sometimes obliterated, irregular in outline,
- Calcified tube or ovary,
- Bilateral corneal block,
- Lead pipe appearance with distension of ampullary region,
- Distal tubal obstruction with jagged fluffiness of tubal outline.

There are specific findings in laparoscopy too and multiple-directed biopsies can be taken from suspicious areas.

In a great majority of cases, genital TB is latent, and the diagnosis is suspected when HSG is performed during the course of an infertility workup.

The characteristic HSG images related to TB are: golf club appearance (Fig. 1, left), tobacco pipe (Fig. 1, right), Maltese-cross appearance, rosette-type image at the tubal extremity, diverticular appearance indistinguishable from salpingitis istmica nodosa, speckled appearance, and intrauterine adhesions of varying degree.

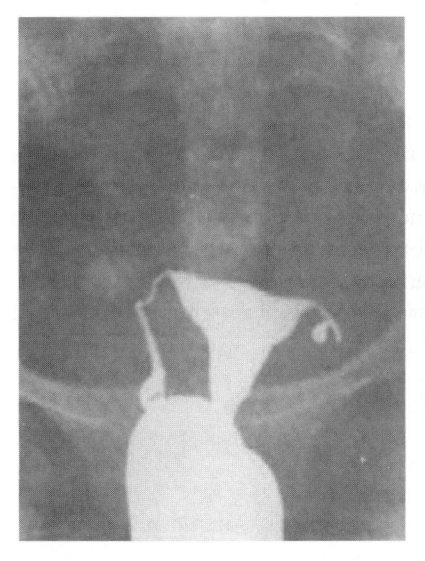

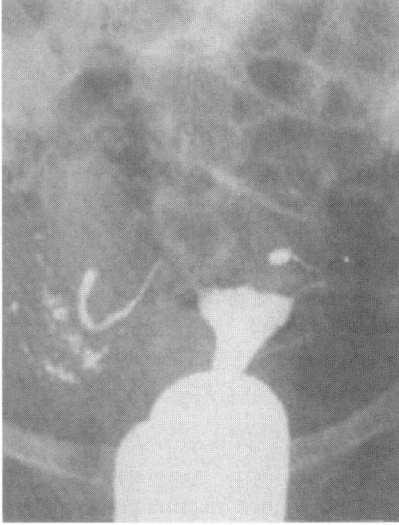

Fig. 1. Left: golf club appearance. Right: tobacco pipe.

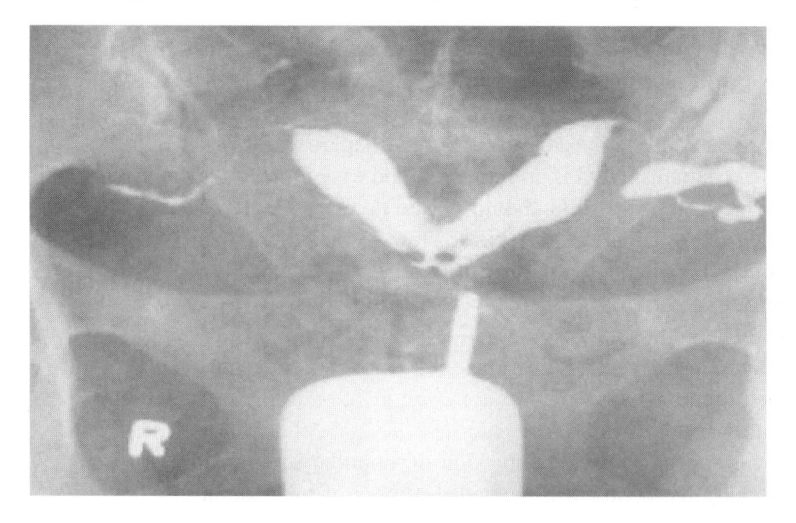

Fig. 2. Intrauterine synechiae giving the appearance of 'septate uterus' (pseudomalformative appearance) and hydrosalpinx in the left tube, beaded appearance in the right tube.

Hysterosalpingographic images of intrauterine adhesions and intravasation are most characteristic of endometrial involvement, and intrauterine adhesions increase with progression of the disease. Intrauterine adhesions may result in a glove finger appearance or mimic different Müllerian anomalies, most commonly unicornous and septate uterus (Fig. 2). HSG is accurate in revealing the fibrotic consequences of TB salpingitis. TB causes sclerosis of the connective tissue, and this sclerosis results in rigidity of the fallopian tube and loss of function. In some cases calcification in the pelvic region can be seen (Fig. 2). Tubal rigidity leads to dilatation and with distal obstruction of the tube may cause hydrosalpinx and some typical appearance (Fig. 2) [14,15].

Endometrium is involved in over half of cases with genital TB, and endometrial biopsy may be useful for histological diagnosis. Endometrial biopsy is best performed in the early menstrual phase, and special attention should be directed to the corneal areas when obtaining the specimen. Endometrial biopsy may be performed during the hysteroscopy and multiple biopsies may be taken from the chronic endometritic areas.

There are some other tools but they were not used for routine diagnosis. For example, detection of M. tuberculosis antigens using monoclonal antibody-based sandwich enzyme-linked immunosorbent assay (ELISA) in infertile patients has been reported [16]. In our genital tuberculosis cases, we reported the elevation of serum and peritoneal fluid CA-125 levels in two patients [17].

## 5. Treatment

### 5.1. Treatment of tuberculous infection

Treatment includes treatment of the infection and squeals. Antituberculous chemotherapy is the mainstay of treatment for acute and chronic infection. Isoniazid, rifempicin, ethambutol, and pyrazinamide are the main antituberculous agents. Two or more of them are given in combination for 9 to 12 months. Over 95% of patients who follow the treatment are expected to be cured. After treatment, the patient should be followed by X-ray, urine cultures, and endometrial sampling.

Surgical treatment is indicated for those cases:

- Persistent or recurrent disease after chemotherapy,
- Persistent or recurrent pelvic masses,
- Lack of healing fistulas,
- Multiple-drug-resistant disease,
- Other associated conditions, such as benign or malignant tumors.

Surgery should be performed after a 2- to 4-week period of chemotherapy, and usually consists of total abdominal hysterectomy and bilateral salpingo-oophorectomy.

### 5.2. Treatment of infertility associated with genital tuberculosis

#### 5.2.1. Medical treatment and reconstructive tubal surgery

IVF-ET offers the only realistic chance of conception in infertile women with genital TB. Medical treatment eradicates the infection, but post-infectious fibrotic sequels of the disease prevent the occurrence of the intrauterine pregnancy. Extensive tubal destruction associated with tuberculous salpingitis does not lend itself to reconstructive tubal surgery. Palmer and Dalsace [18] reported only two ectopic pregnancies in 50 women with tuberculous salpingitis who underwent reconstructive tubal surgery after chemotherapy. Furthermore, reactivation of silent pelvic tuberculosis has been reported subsequent to reconstructive tubal surgery [19].

#### 5.2.2. Hysteroscopic synechialysis

Endometrial involvement may be noted in over half of the cases and the uterine cavity may be partially or totally obliterated with intrauterine synechiae [10]. Despite the lack of supporting data, hysteroscopic lysis of intrauterine synechiae is indicated to restore the uterine cavity before IVF-ET treatment. In our series [20], 12 consecutive patients with total corporal synechiae (American Society for Reproductive Medicine Stage III) (American Fertility Society, 1988) due to TB were analyzed. All patients had secondary amenorrhea and infertility. Hysteroscopic synechialysis was performed under general anesthesia and with laparoscopic assistance. Intrauterine re-formation was assessed by postoperative HSG performed 3–4 months after the procedure. The 12 patients underwent 15 attempts, three perforations occurred and all were managed with laparoscopic extracorporal suturing. Total intracorporal synechiae recurred in all patients at control HSG, and we concluded that surrogacy was an option for such couples. In another case of our team [21], a nulligravid woman with genital TB and partial dense intrauterine adhesions underwent hysteroscopic adhesiolysis, a fundal perforation of 1 cm occurred and no suturing was performed. A postoperative HSG performed 3 months after the procedure revealed a normal intrauterine cavity and that woman conceived with the IVF-ET procedure. Uterine rupture occurred at 36 weeks gestation and immediate caesarean section and repair of the ruptured uterus were performed. Uterine rupture was in the fundal area that previously ruptured in the procedure. We concluded that women with a history of uterine perforation should be counseled regarding the risk of uterine rupture during their subsequent pregnancies.

### 5.2.3. Treatment of infertility associated with genital tuberculosis with assisted reproductive techniques

The most common presentation of genital TB is infertility that is due to extensive tubal destruction not amenable to reconstructive tubal surgery [22,23]. Treatment with IVF-ET remains the only therapeutic option in these patients. However, there are conflicting data related to the efficacy of IVF-ET. Frydman and associates [24] have reported six intrauterine pregnancies in 49 IVF-ET cycles in 20 women with genital TB. Of the 20 patients, five had endometrial involvement; the extent of cavity deformation and whether there is intrauterine synechiae were not specified. Failure of stimulation was encountered in seven cycles (16.3%). Oocyte retrieval was successful in 81.6% of the cycles, fertilization rate was 69% and ET was performed in 66.6% of the cases. Pregnancy was achieved in eight of the cases. Clinical pregnancy rates per initiated cycles; oocyte pick-up and ET were 16.3%, 16.3%, and 25%, respectively. The authors concluded that these figures were comparable with the IVF performance of nontuberculosis tubal factor patients, but the pregnancy rate was directly related to the endometrial involvement. In patients having a history of tuberculosis endometritis, the prognosis was very poor (only one pregnancy in five patients with 11 cycles), in contrast to five deliveries in 15 patients (38 cycles) occurring without endometrial involvement.

Tavmergen et al. [25] reported 61 patients with genital TB who were treated with a single cycle of IVF-ET. Five cycles were cancelled because of poor ovarian response (8%) and 10 clinical pregnancies were achieved (16% per cycle).

Marcus et al. [26] reported their experience with IVF in 10 patients having genital TB (27 treatment cycles). In that study, endometrium was graded according to the echogenecity in response to estrogen levels (Grade I: endometrium was less echogenic than the myometrium, Grade II: the endometrial echogenecity was similar to the myometrial echogenecity, Grade III: endometrium was more echogenic than the myometrium). Ten patients underwent 22 IVF cycles and 9 cryopreserved-thawed ET. Six clinical pregnancies were achieved, with clinical pregnancies per patient 40%. The patients who had trophic endometrium achieved pregnancy at a rate of 42.9% (six of 14) per embryo transfer compared with 0% (one of 14) if the endometrium was atrophic. Interestingly, the atrophic endometrium failed to respond to a repeated course of hormone replacement therapy, probably because of permanent damage inflicted by TB infection. These findings concluded that endometrial response appears to be the primary factor closely related with the pregnancy outcome.

In the report of Soussis et al. [27], they treated 13 women with genital TB who had an hysteroscopically proven normal uterine cavity and functional ovaries. Six clinical pregnancies were achieved (28.6% success rate) after 21 IVF-ET cycles in 13 patients. In that study the patients were selected carefully before committing them to IVF treatment.

In the former report of our team [28,29], a retrospective case control study was performed. Forty-four cycles of IVF-ET were undertaken in 24 women with genital TB

Table 1
Various characteristics of patients with genital tuberculosis undergoing IVF-ET compared with tubal factor patients

| Characteristic | Genital TB | Other tubal factor | p value |
| --- | --- | --- | --- |
| No. of patients | 24 | 274 | – |
| No. of cycles | 44 | 366 | – |
| No. of transfers | 34 | 311 | – |
| Mean age (years) | 33.7 | 33.2 | NS |
| Duration of stimulation (days) | 10.3 | 7.5 | <0.01 |
| Ampules of HMG | 27.3 | 18.4 | <0.05 |
| $E_2$ on the day of HCG (pg/ml) | 852 | 1141 | <0.05 |
| No. of oocytes | 5.8 | 7.7 | <0.05 |
| No. of embryos | 2 | 2.9 | <0.05 |
| Clinical pregnancies (%) | 4 (9.1) | 78 (21.3) | <0.05 |
| Implantation rate per embryo(%) | 5.8 | 8.6 | NS |

Gurgan et al.
NS: not significant.

and the results were compared with 366 cycles in 274 nontuberculous tubal factor couples. All patients were evaluated by hysteroscopy. Hysteroscopic evaluation was normal in 18, whereas varying degrees of intrauterine synechiae was observed in six patients, and synechialysis was performed for these patients. They were evaluated 1 month later by HSG and the uterine cavity was accepted as sufficient for ET in all subjects. Patients' characteristics in the two groups are shown in Table 1. Subjects with genital TB had higher basal FSH levels, required more gonadotropins, reached lower peak $E_2$ levels, and yielded fewer oocytes and embryos when compared with tubal factor patients. Furthermore, in genital TB cases the clinical pregnancy rate per cycle was lower and the abortion rate was higher. In our study, genital TB cases represented a less favorable outcome in comparison to other tubal factor cases.

## 6. Discussion

Infertility is one of the leading features of genital TB [7]. Despite the success in eradicating active infection in almost all subjects, subsequent intrauterine pregnancy is a rare occurrence, with most conceptions ending in spontaneous abortion or ectopic pregnancy [10]. Tubal reconstructive surgery has no place in the treatment of infertility due to genital TB [23]. IVF-ET has been proposed as the only realistic treatment option. Endometrial involvement is noted in 50–60% of the subjects and diminishes the implantation rate. The success rates with IVF may be improved by adequate preoperative antituberculous chemotherapy and selection of patients without endometrial involvement, as shown by normal configuration of the endometrial cavity at HSG and a normal hysteroscopy [24–29].

## Acknowledgements

We thank Professor Mulazım Yıldırım for providing us with hysterosalpingographic pictures from his own archives.

## References

[1] M.C. Raviglione, R.J. O'Brien, Tuberculosis, in: A.S. Fauci, E. Braunwal, K.J. Isselbacher, J.D. Wilson, J.B. Martin, D.L. Kasper, et al. (Eds.), Harrisons' Principles of Internal Medicine, McGraw-Hill, New York, 2001, pp. 1024–1035.
[2] A.M. Sutherland, The treatment of tuberculosis of female genital tract, Tubercle 57 (1963) 137.
[3] B. Urman, et al., Midtubal occlusion: etiology, management and outcome, Fertil. Steril. 57 (1992) 747–750.
[4] M.G. Martens, Pelvic inflammatory disease, in: J.A. Rock, J.D. Thompson (Eds.), Telind's Operative Gynecology, Lippincott-Raven, New York, 1997, pp. 678–685.
[5] G. Schaefer, Full term pregnancy following genital tuberculosis, Obstet. Gynecol. Surv. 19 (1964) 81–124.
[6] V. Falk, K. Ludviksson, G. Agten, Genital tuberculosis in women, analysis of 187 newly diagnosed cases from 47 Swedish hospitals during the ten year period 1968–1977, Am. J. Obstet. Gynecol. 138 (1980) 974–977.
[7] A. Sutherland, The changing pattern of tuberculosis of the female genital tract: a thirty year survey, Arch. Gynecol. Obstet. 234 (1993) 95–101.
[8] A.C. Weinberg, S.D. Boyd, Short-course chemotherapy and role of surgery in adult and pediatric genitourinary tuberculosis, Urology 31 (1988) 95.
[9] G. Schaefer, Female genital tuberculosis, Clin. Obstet. Gynecol. 19 (1976) 223–239.
[10] T. Varma, Genital tuberculosis and subsequent fertility, Int. J. Gynaecol. Obstet. 35 (1991) 1–11.
[11] A. Sutherland, The changing pattern of tuberculosis of the female tract: a thirty-year survey, Arch. Gynecol. Obstet. 234 (1983) 95–101.
[12] A.M. Siegler, V. Kontopoulos, Female genital tuberculosis and the role of HSG, Semin. Roentgenol. 14 (1979) 295–304.
[13] G.R.G. Monif, Infectious Diseases in Obstetrics and Gynecology, Second edition, 1982, pp. 301–316.
[14] M. Yıldırım, Tubal Infertility in New Trend (1995) 72, by Broer Hc, Turanlı I.
[15] M. Yıldırım (Ed.), Clinical Infertility, Second edition, 2000, pp. 227–243.
[16] A. Rattan, et al., Detection of antigens of M Tuberculosis in patients of infertility by monoclonal antibody based sandwich enzyme linked immunosorbent assay (ELISA), Tuber. Lung Dis. 74 (1993) 200–203.
[17] T. Gurgan, et al., Pelvic peritoneal tuberculosis with elevated serum and peritoneal fuluid CA-125 evels: a report of two cases, Gynecol. Obstet. Investig. 35 (1993) 60–61.
[18] R. Palmer, J. Delsace, Le treitment chirurgical des sterilites tubaires, Bull. Fed. Soc. Gynecol. Obstet. 20 (1968) 139–142.
[19] S. Ballon, Reactivation of silent pelvic tuberculosis by reconstructive tubal surgery, Am. J. Obstet. Gynecol. 122 (1975) 991–993.
[20] O. Bukulmez, H. Yarali, T. Gurgan, Total corporal synechiae due to tuberculosis carry a very poor prognosis following hysteroscopic synechialysis, Hum. Reprod. 14 (1999) 1960–1961.
[21] T. Gurgan, et al., Uterine rupture following hysteroscopic lysis of synechiae due to tuberculosis and uterine perforation, Hum. Reprod. 11 (1996) 291–293.
[22] G. Schaefer, Female genital tuberculosis, Clin. Obstet. Gynecol. 19 (1976) 223–239.
[23] V. Gomel, Microsurgery in Female Infertility, Little Brown and Co., Boston, 1983, pp. 129–130.
[24] R. Frydman, et al., In vitro fertilization in tuberculous infertility, J. Assist. Reprod. Genet. 2 (1985) 184–189.
[25] E.N. Tavmergen, E. Tavmergen, R. Capanoglu, The outcome of in vitro fertilization and embryo transfer in genital tuberculosis, J. Assist. Reprod. Genet. 12 (1995) 190S.
[26] S.F. Marcus, et al., Tuberculous infertility and in vitro fertilization, Am. J. Obstet. Gynecol. 171 (1994) 1593–1596.
[27] I. Soussis, et al., In vitro fertilization treatment in genital tuberculosis, J. Assist. Reprod. Genet. 15 (1998) 378–379.
[28] T. Gurgan, B. Urman, H. Yarali, Results of in vitro fertilization and embryo transfer in women with infertility due to genital tuberculosis, Fertil. Steril. 65 (1996) 367–370.
[29] T. Gurgan, B. Urman, H. Yarali, Genital tuberculosis-associated infertility: treatment with assisted reproduction techniques, Assist. Reprod. Rev. 6 (1996) 6–10.

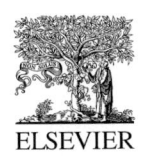

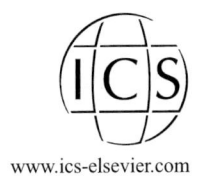

# Ethical challenges in reproductive medicine: posthumous reproduction

## G. Bahadur*

*Fertility and Reproductive Medicine Laboratories, Department of Obstetrics and Gynaecology, Royal Free and University College Medical School, 25 Grafton Way, London WC1E 6DB, UK*

**Abstract.** *Introduction*: New technologies in the field of reproductive medicine have given rise to new possibilities for the application of this technology. These possibilities have in turn led to new ethical and policy dilemmas. This paper discusses the complex moral, ethical and legal concerns that posthumous assisted reproduction (PAR) gives rise to: questions such as what constitutes informed consent, and whether it is ethical to retrieve spermatozoa from patients who are in a coma. It considers legal issues, such as whether gametes can be considered as property and the need to clarify the legal definition of paternity in cases of children born in such circumstances. It outlines the various considerations that need to be taken into account in deciding on the advisability of PAR, including respect for the wishes of the deceased donor and the imperative need to protect the interests of the unborn child. It examines the motives of gestating women, and discusses the effects on the children born by means of this process. *Methods*: The paper makes use of legal studies of cases of posthumous reproduction, and draws on the experiences of fertility clinics to consider the motives of gestating women and mistakes that can be made in fertility treatments. It refers to philosophical discussions of the ethical considerations involved, and considers the legal and regulatory framework around assisted reproduction in the UK and in other countries. *Conclusions*: The paper helps to raise the awareness of policy makers and clinicians in the field of assisted reproduction of the complex legal, ethical and moral issues that PAR involves. It urges policy makers to evaluate the issues at stake, particularly regarding the need for consent and for the children concerned to have a legally recognisable father and inheritance rights, and to formulate a suitable legislative response. It argues that caution should be exercised in encouraging PAR, and market forces should not influence decisions on the practice. It asserts the need for responsible accounting on the part of fertility clinics, calling on them to help the bereaved to reach an unbiased but informed decision on PAR. Finally, the welfare of unborn children must be taken into account by both clinicians and policy makers. © 2004 Published by Elsevier B.V.

*Keywords:* Conception; Consent; Cryopreservation; Embryo; Gamete; Oocyte; Ovarian tissue; Posthumous; Insemination; Reproduction; Sperm

---

\* Tel.: +44-207-380-9436; fax: +44-207-380-9143.
*E-mail addresses:* g.bahadur@ucl.ac.uk, gulam.bahadur@uclh.org (G. Bahadur).

0531-5131/ © 2004 Published by Elsevier B.V.
doi:10.1016/j.ics.2004.01.105

## 1. Introduction

Rapid innovations in reproductive technology, gamete retrieval and cryopreservation have created new possibilities in human procreation, as a result of which, new ethical and policy dilemmas have arisen. The issues raised by the topic of posthumous reproduction are some of the most challenging, difficult and sensitive one is likely to encounter in any field of medicine, entailing complex moral, ethical and legal concerns.

It has become possible to retrieve, freeze and store sperm, embryos, and even oocytes or ovarian tissue, thereby creating new uses for this technology. Men and women who receive cancer therapy that will leave them sterile now have the option of storing gametes for use later in life. The rapid rate of technological advances means that new treatments are being rushed into use before they are proven safe or effective, potentially putting some women and children at risk of physical and psychological harm.

The death of a husband is a difficult time for a widow to make a rational decision about whether she wants the sperm of a dead husband to be harvested [1–3]. Because illnesses in the deceased partner are often unanticipated, the patient typically has not given prior consent for sperm retrieval. In these situations, physicians who are asked to perform sperm retrieval and storage face an array of difficult ethical issues. These include the question of whether posthumous reproduction is ethically justifiable, and whether it is ethical to retrieve spermatozoa from patients who are dead or in a persistent vegetative state (PVS). If retrieved spermatozoa are frozen, what should be the terms of the sperm storage agreement? Should there be time limits on storage? Should there be restrictions on the person who can be inseminated, or should the use of a surrogate be permitted? Additional dilemmas lie in the form of the legal requirements to have effective consent from the deceased, as well as the medico-legal implication for the clinician performing the procedure, since theoretically assault charges could be levelled at the clinician.

All of these issues also apply to cases in which a husband or partner conceives a child with the frozen ova of a dead wife or partner. The advent of intracytoplasmic sperm injection technique (ICSI) and the potential for cryopreservation of ova may extend the options for posthumous reproduction, with the added requirement of a surrogate uterus. Surrogates can now in principle be used to create grandchildren, which adds considerable social and legal complexity to the status of the child [4].

## 2. Legal status of gametes

To date courts in England and Wales have not addressed the issue of the legal status of human reproductive material outside the human body. Although we know there is no property status in corpses and, since the abolition of slavery, living persons cannot be the subject of property, the status of tissue is undefined in cases of accidental damage, modification or destruction.

Recognition of proprietary interests in reproductive material would not be incompatible with the UK law as it stands. Several cases have stated that an embryo is not a legal person; this judgement was reiterated by the Warnock Committee in the report of their enquiry into fertilisation and embryology. If not a person, the embryo risks being classified a chattel. Public opinion is opposed to the idea, since it threatens the value of potential human beings through commercialisation. It may only be a matter of time, however, before the property status of sperm, egg and embryos will become a subject of court application or clarification, especially if inheritance disputes arise.

In the case of Hecht v. Superior Court, the children of William Kane battled with Kane's lover over possession of sperm that Kane deposited in a sperm bank with the express intention that Hecht, his girlfriend, would use the sperm to conceive children after Kane committed suicide. The court was faced with the question of whether sperm was something a person could leave to another through a will [5]. In deciding whether sperm, eggs and embryos should be treated as property, Steinbock and McClamrock [6] analyse the question accordingly:

(1) First, they find that property rights exist whenever a person has the ability to sell or transfer control of something.
(2) Second, they find that protection of unborn children from potential harm is an inadequate basis for a morally based legal ban on posthumous reproduction.
(3) Third, they examine the arguments against commercial traffic in body parts and reproductive capacities, concluding that the transfer of sperm by will does not involve similar concerns.
(4) Finally, they conclude that concerns for individual autonomy in matters of reproduction justify allowing the transfer of sperm by will.

## 3. The donor

Decisions concerning whether or not to have a child have been considered a private matter and a fundamental human right, but there are limited precedents regarding how this might be respected after one's death. In the UK, it is imperative that the donor has given written, informed consent, and it is illegal to store sperm, oocyte or embryos without the written consent of the genetic provider(s) under the HFEAct 1990 [7].

Most people do not expect that their gametes will be used for procreation after death, so generally do not make their views regarding this practice explicit. However, it is both unfair and undesirable to place the onus upon individuals to state their opposition to posthumous conception.

A landmark UK case involved Mrs. Blood [8], whose comatose husband's sperm was retrieved surgically and frozen upon her request, after which the patient died. It was deemed that effective consent, which must be in written form, was not in place before the taking and freezing of gametes. It was even felt that there may have been a case for pressing assault charges against the clinician who undertook the retrieval procedure. Had the sperm been retrieved and not frozen but used immediately, then the provisions of the HFEAct 1990, s4(1)(b) would not have applied.

Recently, Israel has issued formal regulations allowing the removal of sperm from a man's body at the request of his wife or common law wife. This follows a series of eight cases in which bereaved widows filed urgent requests in the courts to allow their husband's sperm to be retrieved within hours of death [9]. One important reason given by the attorney was that having children has high importance in Judaism and Israeli society, and that most people, especially men, wished their genes and name to be passed on. The decisions further indicated that parents of soldiers could not automatically gain access to the sperm to create grandchildren, although it appeared that good reasons could be offered to enable further consideration.

Many international programs for assisted reproduction have consent forms that stipulate the disposition of gametes and embryos after the death of one or both gamete donors, or after a certain period of time. If the use of a gamete or embryo after death is declined, this should be honoured. In the UK this would also mean the destruction of an embryo irrespective of the surviving genetic contributor's wishes. It is still open to debate whether a time limit should be imposed on how long after death such gametes or embryos might still be used. It is not clear how the interval between death and use would affect the outcome, but the general presumption is that such use should occur within an interval of no more than a few years.

In the UK, and to some extent Europe, there are added dimensions about the increased power individual patients possess thanks to the HRAct [10]. This declares that public bodies should not interfere with privacy or family life unless they can justify it in terms of protecting public health or morals, or protecting the rights of others.

## 4. The need for consent

Any coherent ethical framework in the area of posthumous assisted reproduction (PAR) must be sensitive to the many interests at stake. It is all too easy to overlook the interests of the dead, as the dead have no voice. Some may claim that we cannot speak sensibly of the dead as having interests, who can be harmed by the conduct of surviving parties because, once a person dies, concepts of harm or benefit are redundant. Certain acts committed after a person's death can, however, affect that individual's interests; for example, a posthumous event that destroys a deceased person's reputation harms his or her interests.

Posthumous conception redefines the content and outlines of the deceased's life. When it occurs without the person's consent, it deprives an individual of the opportunity to be the author of a highly significant event in his or her life. This is one of the reasons why an analogy between posthumous conception and organ donation fails; procreation is central to an individual's identity in a way that organ donation is not. Respect for autonomy requires that this procedure should not be permitted unless the deceased's consent is clear.

Our society has developed procedures that allow us to control certain matters after death, such as the transfer of property, or the transplantation of organs. It is important that individuals have the assurance that their bodies will not be used in a manner inconsistent with their expectations. Even if there is evidence that the deceased desired parenthood in life, it is a considerable leap to assume that he or she would have wished to become a parent posthumously.

If the deceased person's wishes are to be safeguarded adequately, clear evidence of intent to reproduce after death should be required. The potential for a serious conflict of interest justifies a limited decision-making role for the family. Difficulties could arise in estate distribution after PAR, although no cases are yet documented.

Policymakers must identify and evaluate important interests, and codify them in a workable policy. The UK HFEAct 1990 provides exemplary directions as to the need for a written and informed consent prior to any storage and use of gametes or embryos. Contentious areas remain, however, such as the non-recognition inheritance rights, although the genetic father may now be included on the birth certificate if he had previously consented [11].

## 5. The gestating woman

A bereaved, grieving woman might wish to use the sperm of the deceased as a means of prolonging and affirming the value of their relationship, by having the deceased's genes contribute to the genetic makeup of her child. In Mrs. Blood's case (UK), she made it amply clear that she could, if she wanted, use an unknown donor's sperm, but it was her late husband's sperm that mattered to her, since they had taken marriage vows and spoken of having babies. The experience associated with pregnancy and child rearing might serve as a significant part of the mourning process and a way for a woman in this position to resume a normal life.

In our clinic, among requests by 21 new widows to keep frozen sperm, there has been no evidence of its subsequent use, which reflects just how strong the psychological bond was with the deceased, and the complex process of mourning that ensues [12]. After 7 years, even those 11 widows who stated their intention to use frozen sperm did not resort to PAR. Their desire to continue to maintain the sperm without use is another important aspect of the grieving process. We are aware of two widows who, once in a newly found stable relationship, requested disposal of the deceased's sperm sample. It is therefore important to formulate a mourning period of 1–1.5 years when no insemination should occur, during which counselling should be provided.

In the case of a husband wanting to use frozen embryos or ova for posthumous reproduction after his wife has died, a gestational carrier is required. The woman would not be considered a traditional surrogate if she were planning to be a rearing parent as well; for example, if she married the man after his wife died. In other instances, all of the concerns that arise with the use of gestational carriers also would apply. In the UK, the gestating mother would be the legal mother and parental rights would need to be gained by the commissioning parent(s) or person(s). In some countries, embryos could be donated to infertile couples, and in these cases, the recipient couple ought to know of the unusual circumstances before receiving the gift.

## 6. Legal and social status of the child

The effects on a child of being the product of posthumous reproduction are not completely known. Little is known about the psychological effects on a child who eventually learns that one or both parents were dead long before that child's own gestation began. Some experts complain that, in the modern conception industry, the rights and privileges of potential parents have precedence over the welfare of children.

The concern with PAR is that bringing the child into a single-parent household would be harmful to the child. However, a serious problem with this objection is that the act that supposedly harms the child is the very process that brings it into being [13–15]. Persons are harmed only if they are caused to be worse off than they otherwise would have been [16].

If pregnancy and birth occur within the context of marriage in which one partner has died, the effects on the child might not be very different to those which occur in the much more common case of posthumous birth, in terms of legitimacy and inheritance. The psychological impact on the child should be minimal and probably within the range of experiences seen in some parallel studies on, for example, single parent families [17,18].

The legal and social status of a child born using frozen gametes raises complex issues even if the insemination and pregnancy occurs with the wife of the dead man. A child born from conception and pregnancy after a man's death may not always be attributed to him for purposes of inheritance and legitimacy. In the UK, the child that is the product of PAR does not have a legally recognisable father on its birth certificate and may not automatically qualify for inheritance rights. This may disadvantage the child by, for example, requiring him or her repeatedly to explain to schools or public authorities why the father does not exist. These dilemmas may extend to emergency health care where history of the genetic parents may be needed. Representations were made by Mrs. Blood through the HRAct 1998 [10] in order to address this anomaly. As a result, a new UK law has been formulated to enable fathers to be named in cases of posthumous conception, providing consent was in place, although the law falls short of securing inheritance rights [11].

The issues for a child born through PAR attracted debate in 1983 when Mario and Elsa Rios died in a plane crash, leaving behind two frozen pre-embryos in an IVF clinic in Melbourne, Australia. The question of when life began was considered by the courts in deciding on whether the embryos could inherit the couple's $8 million. The Tasmanian judge felt that embryos had the potential to become human beings and therefore could inherit. An independent group set up to look at the case, however, concluded that the embryos would better serve the interests of science. They were donated for research instead of being made available to another infertile couple [19].

Some states in the USA have adopted the Uniform Parentage Act, according to which the deceased man would be presumed to be the father of the child provided the couple had been married and the birth occurred within 300 days of the man's death [20]. If birth occurs after 300 days in those states, or if birth occurs in states without statutes addressing posthumous conception, then current law provides no basis for presuming that the deceased is the legal father [20].

Future developments in the field of in vitro maturation of gametes have recognised the potential for using foetal ovaries as an unlimited source of oocytes. The ethical, social and legal issues would be profound if such oocytes were used, since the donor would never have given consent. The psychological well being of children born to an unborn genetic mother could be profoundly affected by such a situation. Society as a whole needs to face up to a bizarre fact that the genetic mother, the donor, was never born.

## 7. Obligations of clinics

Unfortunately, fertility clinics around the world have a history of lost, damaged or misappropriated sperm, eggs and embryos. In the UK, there is an ongoing case against an embryologist and gynaecologist from a Hampshire clinic in relation to false accounting and misappropriated embryos. Such situations highlight the need for better accountability, record-keeping, auditing, and other aspects of quality control. Regulation, too, may be deficient here, since the UK's HFEA gave the Hampshire clinic clearance weeks before the problems surfaced. People given the responsibility of looking after and using frozen gametes and embryos and counselling women considering PAR should be of a high calibre.

## 8. Conclusions

The practice of PAR raises complex legal, ethical and moral issues that need to be taken into account by clinicians. Whilst it is preferable to have explicit consent, cases around the world are likely to occur where the wishes of the dead and the living will have to be deciphered either through local hospital committees or by courts. Caution must be exercised in encouraging PAR, and market forces must not be allowed to decide the outcome. Prolonged counselling and delays have shown that widows who have 'attached' themselves to their late husbands' sperm have eventually not utilised them. Fertility clinics need to display transparency, fairness, and patience, to help the bereaved to reach an informed decision about PAR through a process of unbiased and supportive counselling. Finally, the welfare of unborn children needs to be taken into account in a balanced, pragmatic and sensible manner.

## References

[1] E. Aziza-Shuster, A child at all costs: posthumous reproduction and the meaning of parenthood, Hum. Reprod. 9 (1994) 2182–2185.
[2] G. Bahadur, Death and conception, Hum. Reprod. 17 (10) (2002) 2769–2775.
[3] C. Strong, J.R. Gingrich, W.H. Kutteh, Ethics of sperm retrieval after death or persistent vegetative state, Hum. Reprod. 15 (4) (2000) 739–745.
[4] L. Fraser, Our son is dead, but his sperm survives and we must give him the baby he wanted so much, Mail on Sunday (1999 December 19).
[5] Hecht v Superior Court, 16 Cal.App.4th 836, 20 Cal. Rptr.2d 275 (1993 June).
[6] B. Steinbock, R. McClamrock, When is birth unfair to the child? Hastings Cent. Rep. 24 (1994) 15–21.
[7] HFEAct, Human Fertilisation and Embryology Act 1990, HMSO, London, 1990, ISBN 0-10-543790-0, 1990.
[8] R v Human Fertilisation and Embryology Authority, exp Blood, 1997. 2 All ER 687 (1997) 35 *BMLR* 1, CA.
[9] J. Siegel-Itzkovich, Isreal allows removal of sperm from dead men at wifes' request, BMJ 327 (2003) 1187.
[10] G. Bahadur, The Human Rights Act (1998) and its impact on human reproductive issues, Hum. Reprod. 16 (4) (2001) 785–789.
[11] Human Fertilisation and Embryology (Deceased Father) Act 2003, Customer Service, London UK. The Parliamentary Bookshop, London, ISBN 0-10-562403-9.
[12] G. Bahadur, Posthumous assisted reproduction (PAR): cancer patients, potential cases, counselling and consent, Hum. Reprod. 11 (12) (1996) 2573–2575.
[13] J.A. Robertson, Children of Choice: Freedom and the New Reproductive Technologies, Princeton Univ. Press, Princeton, USA, 1994.
[14] J.A. Robertson, Posthumous reproduction, in: R.D. Kempers, J. Cohen, A.F. Haney, et al (Eds.), Fertility and Reproductive Medicine, Elsevier, New York, USA, 1998, pp. 255–259.
[15] C. Strong, Ethics in Reproductive and Perinatal Medicine: A New Framework, Yale Univ. Press, New Haven, CT, USA, 1997.
[16] J. Feinberg, Harm to Others, Oxford Univ. Press, New York, USA, 1984.
[17] S. Golombok, New families, old values: considerations regarding the welfare of the child, Hum. Reprod. 13 (1998) 2342–2347.

[18] G. Pennings, Measuring the welfare of the child: in search of the appropriate evaluation principle, Hum. Reprod. 14 (1999) 1146–1150.
[19] G.P. Smith III, Australia's frozen 'orphan' embryos: a medical, legal, and ethical dilemma, J. Fam. Law 24 (1985–1986) 27–41.
[20] J.A. Gibbons, Who's your daddy?: a constitutional analysis of post-mortem insemination, J. Contemp. Health Law Policy 14 (1997) 187–210.

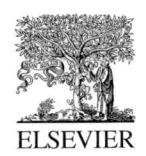

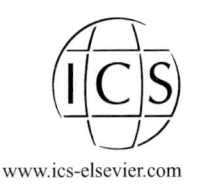

# Sperm and oocyte donation: gamete donor issues

Yvon Englert*, Emiliani Serena, Revelard Philippe,
Devreker Fabienne, Laruelle Chantal, Delbaere Anne

*Fertility Clinic, Department of Obstetrics/Gynecology and Laboratory for Research on Human Reproduction,
Hopital Erasme, Faculty of Medicine, Free University of Brussels (U.L.B.),
Route de Lennik 808, B-1070 Brussels, Belgium*

**Abstract.** Between the many ethical questions that are still in debate around gamete donation, the authors analyse some of them including why oocyte and sperm donation are experienced very differently by couples, despite their apparent similarity, and stress the ethical impact of the difficulties of donor recruitment in all oocyte donation programs. The various types of donors (occasional, relational, IVF patient, and professional) are described with their motivations, resistances, advantages and disadvantages. The contradictory consequences with free or paid donation and the particular risks of oocyte donation (in comparison to sperm donation), both for the donor as for the recipient, are highlighted. The paper also examines the actual debate of gamete donors' CMV serology status, as well as the question of eventual quarantine of donated oocytes. The problem of maintaining anonymity is then analysed in ethical terms but also in terms of technical efficacy. A strategy which, due to the decision of retaining anonymity, increases treatment efficacy by avoiding wastage of oocytes offered as a donation, is described. The pregnancy rate per donor oocyte pickup rises from 35% to 99% using this strategy, significantly reducing shortage. © 2004 Published by Elsevier B.V.

*Keywords:* Anonymity; Ethics; Oocyte donation; Sperm donation

## 1. Introduction

Medically performed artificial insemination with donor semen (AID) appears in the medical literature at the end of the 19th century when Pr Pancoast in Philadelphia performed, in 1894, an AID in a medical lecture room. Nevertheless, AID remains a more or less clandestine activity up to the end of 1940 when, with a change in dominant ethical values in the west European Christian cultures, slowly, AID became a subject of scientific research.

Dependent of IVF technology, oocyte donation is a much more recent activity, successfully described for the first time by the Australian team of Trounson and Wood in 1983 [1]. Since then, the procedure has spread around the world, although in a limited way when compared with in vitro fertilization (3867 cycles of oocyte donations for 220,591 IVF

---

\* Corresponding author. Tel.: +32-2-5554570; fax: +32-2-5556841.
*E-mail address:* yenglert@ulb.ac.be (E. Englert).

and ICSI cycles in 1993) [2]. This modest activity is probably due more to the difficulties in donor recruitment than to the lack of medical indications, since it is estimated that >100,000 women in the USA present with premature ovarian failure [3]. The difficulty of donor recruitment plays a crucial role in ethically questionable practices under the pressure arising from shortage.

## 2. Oocyte and sperm donation: similarities and differences

From a purely rational point of view, oocyte donation is the mirror of sperm donation. It consists of introducing, in the couple, half of the genetic material from a third party.

However, the similarity is much more limited than it seems. Symbolically, sperm and oocyte donation are experienced very differently by couples. A study showed that 86% of the women and 66% of their partners in recipient couples were favourable to the possibility of recruiting a sister for oocyte donation, but 9% of the women and 14% of the men expressed the same preference for a brother in sperm donation [4]. This illustrates the different perception of feminine and masculine sterility, both by couples and society [5].

A couple confronted with the possibility of a sperm donation must overcome a symbolic barrier of medical adultery [6]. Also, the donation of spermatozoa deprives the male partner of his only biological participation in filiation.

It is altogether different in the oocyte donation: If the social and affective mother of the child is not its biological mother, then she is the gestational mother. From the legal viewpoint, the mother is almost always the woman who gives birth. Symbolically, a woman will declare herself to be the mother of a child "because she carried it and brought it into the world" and nobody would ever think of saying "it's my child because it's my egg." This symbolic reality explains the lack of interest from candidate oocyte recipients for the distinctive character of oocyte donation we observed in Erasme Hospital, in contrast with the attitude of couples towards sperm donation. In addition, maternity by oocyte donation repairs a double major wound in women not only confronted by the failure to become a mother, but also perturbed in their female identification (absence of a cycle) and even in their sexual identity (Turner's syndrome, gonadic dysgenesis). All these reasons explain the massive denial observed in pregnant women or having given birth after an oocyte donation, which can go as far as "forgetting" the distinctive character of their filiation ties [7,8].

As well as these symbolic differences, there are equal distinctions concerning the material aspects of oocyte donation in comparison to sperm donation. If it is "biblically" simple to donate sperm, the same is not true for oocytes: It is necessary for the female donor to undergo a full IVF procedure, which represents a significant effort and is not entirely without risks even though complications are rare [9,10]. This can explain the difficulty in recruiting oocyte donors, which is reported by all the oocyte donation programmes.

## 3. Donor recruitment, counselling, payment, and free and informed consent

### 3.1. Donor recruitment

Since the first donor insemination made by Pancoast with the sperm of "the best looking member of the class," rules for sperm donor recruitment have largely changed. In Europe, most of the clinics are recruiting by word of mouth. In the United States, advertising by private banks is allowed. Most of the banks recruit single men, frequently students from University. Shortage of semen donors is not usual except for ethnic minority groups.

Oocyte donors are recruited in four distinct situations. *Occasional donors* are women who, without any ties to a recipient, donate oocytes without payment either spontaneously or when undergoing surgical procedure unrelated to a sterility problem. Spontaneous initiatives are rare, and according to our experience, are very often taken by women with a particularly fragile personality and psychological disturbance, looking for recognition or a massive repair. For these reasons, they are generally not considered able to give a free and informed consent and their use as donors involves risks of disrupting an extremely unstable psychological balance.

*Patients undergoing IVF treatment and agreeing to share oocytes* implies asking patients who are undergoing oocyte retrieval for their own needs to donate some oocytes to an anonymous recipient, provided they have "a sufficient number." Although the unquestionable advantage of this approach is that the donor does not have to suffer any additional medical aggression [11], it does involve some ethical objections because patients agreeing to share oocytes receive advantages in terms of either speedy treatment or free or heavily subsidised treatments. It has been described in 1987–1988 [12,13] and is still current mainly in countries where no social security refund of IVF cost is offered [14]. This is why a large debate exists on these practices considered to be a sign of inequality of access to health care system [15] or a hidden trading of eggs discussed in major medical journals [16–18] and strongly supported by different teams practicing egg sharing, especially in England where it is now accepted by the HFEA [14,19,20]. The fact that pregnancy chances are higher in recipients than in donors increases the uneasy feeling [21]. It should be considered as a form of payment discussed later in this section. *Related donors* are women recruited as donors by the couples themselves within their family circle or friends. Many oocyte donation programmes in Western Europe operate in this way. The donors have a close relationship, often using intra-family donations in the broadest sense. These donations, even if they come from very close relatives, are valued as much by the requesting couples [4] as by the public at large [21]. On the other hand, authorities occasionally oppose them invoking the fear of psychological consequences for the children involved in family relations which are too complicated [22]. *Professional donors* are women who accept to give their oocytes in return for payment. These programmes exist openly in the United States, the candidates being recruited by way of classified advertisements [23] and escalating fees paid to young women seem to be aggressively advertised [24]. If such practices are not within European traditions, it is true that some compensation is often anticipated and that private arrangements are possible in the case of related oocyte donors [25].

Counselling and free and informed consent has been largely stressed elsewhere [26]. It is obvious and largely accepted that written consent must be obtained from putative donors and that extended information should be given about the use of donated samples.

## 3.2. Free, reward, expenses, or payment?

Reimbursement of expenses or payment is usually offered to sperm donors, but it is in oocyte donors that a lot of money is offered [24].

In most states in the United States, the recourse to professional oocyte donors is legitimized as much by the moral requirement of compensating the effort and time of the oocyte donor as by "the desire of the recipient to receive good genes in placing a premium on women who are in good health and who appear to be a good investment" [22].

Such an approach, which restricts the medical techniques to well-off people, is not specific to oocyte donation. Typically, according to Robertson [22], oocyte donors come from the middle and poorer classes of American society. This approach is reprehensible, as much from the commercial aspect (using products of the human body) as from the risks for both donors and recipients in the nonobservance of sanitary norms, and the oocyte donors being interested in hiding possible health problems, as described in blood donation [27]. Subtler is the practice, which consists of sharing the expenses of a patient in an in vitro fertilization cycle in exchange for oocytes [22,25] (see above).

The other extreme, which consists of demanding the absence of all financial transactions, is also barely tenable. The oocyte donor gives up her time, undergoes a procedure, and engages in costs, which, if they are not compensated, could be considered, as exploitation. It could also be considered necessary to provide a reward for the oocyte donor, which symbolizes the recognition of her act, but our experience is that it is often considered as an offence by related donors. This is very different for sperm donors for which social recognition does not exist.

This is an important aspect, which is often neglected; a blood donor benefits from a social reward in the form of recognition and unquestionable self-enhancement. Such a reward does not exist when sperm is concerned. In a psychological study of sperm donors, neither financial compensation nor altruism was found to be the main motive for taking the step. Behind the announced motivation other motives are found, principally motives of reparation [28], which are found even amongst American professional oocyte donors [23]. The financial compensation, provided it is not exaggerated, plays a facilitating role of reward and of compensation for expenses incurred. Positions, which are too dogmatic because of the shortage, which they entail, can generate negative effects, encouraging the development of an underground traffic in oocyte, which makes the cure worse than the pain.

## 4. Donor selection

Donor selection on medical grounds has been largely discussed and well summarized in papers [29] and in a recent seminar [26] where guidelines were published [30] confirming numerous national recommendations in Europe and the USA.

### 4.1. Particular aspects of oocyte donation

Unlike sperm donation, oocyte retrieval is not without risks. Information to the potential donor on the non-exceptional risks of treatment is therefore all-important, especially when it concerns non-anonymous donations where the medical risks often appear to be minimized [31]. Since this consent is only of value if it is freely given, the discussion, in the case of a related donor, must aim at detecting the candidates who may be pressurised by the recipient couple.

The present impossibility of freezing oocytes in a satisfactory way and the significant embryonic loss involved in the freezing of the embryo makes it difficult to apply the generally recommended quarantine for HIV detection in sperm donation. The residual risk, if it exists, is extremely small (estimated risk in blood transfusion for HIV transmission between 1/500,000 and 1/1,000,000) and it seems unethical, in view of reducing the risk, to transfer burdens and risks on donors by using a freezing procedure that, in decreasing the pregnancy chances, will lead to repetitive oocyte retrieval in donors for equal pregnancy chances [32]. The almost uniformly preferred strategy consists of a single detection, as practised in blood donation. The increase in genetic risk with increasing age also implies more restrictive age limits than for sperm donors. It is generally accepted that no special precautions are required when the donor is aged <35 years. After this, the genetic risk increases and the efficacy of the procedure diminishes [33,34]. However, it seems acceptable to tolerate the admission of donors between 35 and 39 years (particularly for recipients in the same age group), as long as the recipient couples have been informed of the implications of genetic risks in such a situation.

*4.2. What to do with CMV Igg-positive gamete donors?*

Recently, the British Andrology Society recommended excluding all CMV seropositive semen donors to prevent the risk of congenital CMV infection. The recommendation is based on the results of recent studies that identified a high percentage of symptomatic congenital CMV infections in newborns of women with CMV seropositivity preexisting to pregnancy, and on the fact that CMV can be detected in semen of CMV seropositive men. CMV seropositive women can infect their fetuses with their own latent CMV strain that can reactivate or with an exogeneous strain that can be transmitted to them by a sexual partner, but also by contacts, for example, with an excreting child. The efficiency of these various ways of transmission to the fetus and the factors that could influence this transmission are for the moment completely unknown. Exclusion of a large population of donors on the sole criteria of a positive CMV serology introduces the message that this part of the male population is not suitable as possible partners to a couple who has no fertility problems. Alternatives to the drastic BAS recommendation exist and should be investigated [35].

## 5. Anonymous, partially anonymous and known donors. Who should decide?

Traditionally anonymous, AID has in recent years moved towards more openness in two ways: either by building systems where the child would have access, when adult, to his genitor's identity either by laws (in Sweden) or by agreement (in some AID clinics in Holland, where it is largely oriented by homosexual couples' demand) or, in some very specific cases, where known direct donation occurs between friends or relatives, but where medical intervention is seeking either for medical security or for desexualisation. We experienced rare cases in Brussels (where some were performed) and a few publications exist in the literature [36].

In oocyte donation, the fundamental debate is to a large extent parallel to that of sperm donation, but the greater openness which now exists with oocytes has two consequences: the de facto existence of a known donation when this remains rather an academic assumption in sperm donation and, in addition, a known donation that really opens the way to contact between the donor and the child's family, as a majority of these non-anonymous donations are close or within the family [31]. Issues of anonymity (which implies that no secrecy about donation has been kept) generate many questions and passionate debates, even recently [37,38].

We do not intend to reopen the debate on anonymity, but to recall that, currently there were no data which could demonstrate the superiority of one approach or the other [39]. A fact is that non-anonymity is gaining grounds, mainly because (true or not), in a society that gives more and more space to genetics, it is believed that knowing your genetic origin is an important part of knowing who you are, and that knowing the identity of her or his donor is part of your wellbeing. It is also true that people who are still considering that gamete donation is morally wrong uses "the interest of the child" to try to promote a disposition they think would make donation more difficult.

Another sign of this growing belief for genetic origin is illustrated by the practice of "non-identifying data" as social class, education, hobbies of donors to be given to recipient couples or future children.

One question, rarely addressed in these debates, is "who should decide" rather than "what to do." The author position is more to promote autonomy for couples, as well as for donors, to decide to enter one or another donation programme (anonymous, non-anonymous or with late disclosed anonymity). Indeed, this freedom of choice of an anonymous or non-anonymous treatment restores to the future parents a choice, which, in fact should belong only to them, to decide, for their child, to reveal or not the secret of the donation, to guard or not the anonymity, to allow him or not to meet the oocyte donor. Studies show that there are candidates for both procedures [4,31]. This freedom has the merit of taking from the medical professionals, as from society, a power which they have wrongly assumed and a responsibility, which must in priority fall to the parents who in our societies are the persons responsible for the children's future and who moreover, in the end, are those who will have to face the consequences of this choice.

However, the organisation of a programme of anonymous or non-anonymous oocyte donation has an impact, which goes far beyond the problem of the management of anonymity. In a system of related donation practised in the Erasmus hospital since 1989, the maintenance of anonymity by a permutation of oocyte donors (usually family members or close friends), has led to a very considerable reduction in oocyte shortage. Firstly, the anonymous permutation offers to the family of the recipient's partner the possibility of recruiting a donor (since in any case the oocytes will go to another recipient), which already represents a considerable advantage. Secondly, this permutation permits avoiding, to a large extent, supernumerary embryos. The retrieved oocytes are shared between several recipients following a pre-established sharing key and each recipient can benefit from part of the oocytes of several donors. Retrieval from each donor is carried out one after the other to

Table 1
Direct and anonymous donation: the Hospital Erasmus oocyte donation programme in Brussels

|  | Direct donation | Anonymous donation | $P$ |
|---|---|---|---|
| Donation cycles ($n$) | 31 | 84 |  |
| Receivers cycles | 31 | 289 |  |
| Number of oocytes received for each recipient | 8.8±5.4 | 4.7±2.3 | <0.001 |
| Number of transferred embryos (fresh) | 2.4±0.7 | 2.2±0.7 |  |
| Pregnancy rate per operated donor | 11 (35%) | 83 (99%) | <0.001 |

enable recipients to be synchronized with different donors in successive cycles. The result of such an approach is avoiding freezing or having to destroy supernumerary embryos.

In our experience (Table 1), while the pregnancy rate per transfer (35%) is very similar to other effective programmes of directed donation, this approach made it possible to obtain in the anonymous donation program, a pregnancy rate of 99% by oocyte retrieval, i.e., avoiding wastage of this rare and precious commodity [32,40,41]. Of course, technical efficacy is not an ethical argument in itself, but it becomes so to some extent when it reduces the shortage, a phenomenon that most threatens the ethical aspects of this medical procedure.

## 6. Conclusions

This too short review stresses the number of ethical issues still in debate around gamete donors, a field at the border between medicine and social sciences, at the limit between science and passion. Nevertheless, to produce as strong data as possible makes the social debate well informed and well documented. The authors hope to have contributed not to solving these questions, but to have clarified some aspects of the debate.

## Acknowledgements

This work was supported by a grant from the Belgian "Fonds National pour la Recherche Scientifique".

## References

[1] A. Trounson, et al., Pregnancy established in an infertile patient after transfer of a donated embryo fertilized in vitro, Br. Med. J. 286 (1983) 835–836.
[2] K.G. Nygren, A.N. Andersen, Assisted reproductive technology in Europe, 1999. Results generated from European registers by ESHRE, Hum. Reprod. 17 (2002) 3260–3274.
[3] Z.O. Rozenwaks, Donor eggs: the applications in modern reproductive technology, Fertil. Steril. 47 (1987) 895.
[4] M.V. Sauer, et al., Survey of attitudes regarding the use of siblings for gamete donation, Fertil. Steril. 49 (1988) 721–722.
[5] D. David, M. Soulé, M.J. Mayaux, IAD: enquête psychologique sur 830 couples, J. Gynecol. Obstet. Biol. Reprod. 17 (1988) 47–74.
[6] J.C. Czyba, Aspects psychologiques des procréations médicalement assistées pour indication masculine, in: Y. Englert, J.F. Guerin, P. Jouannet (Eds.), Sterilité Masculine et Procréations Médicalement Assistées, 1989, pp. 213–223, Doin, Paris.
[7] E. Weil, L'abord psychologique des couples receveuses de dons d'ovocytes anonymes, Contracept. Fertil. Sex. 7 (8) (1987) 690–691.
[8] A. Raoul-Duval, H. Letur-Konirsch, R. Frydman, Les enfants du don d'ovocytes anonyme personnalisé, J. Gynecol. Obstet. Biol. Reprod. 20 (1991) 317–320.
[9] I. Govaerts, et al., Short-term medical complications of 1500 oocyte retrievals for in vitro fertilization and embryo transfer, Eur. J. Obstet., Gynecol., Reprod. Biol. 77 (1998) 239–243.
[10] M.V. Sauer, Defining the incidence of serious complications experienced by oocyte donors: a review of 1000 cases, Am. J. Obstet. Gynecol. 184 (2001) 277–278.
[11] K.K. Ahuja, et al., Minimizing risk in anonymous egg donation, Reprod. Biomed. Online 7 (2003) 504–505.
[12] P. Kemeter, W. Frichtinger, E. Bernat, The willingness of infertile women to donate eggs, in: W. Frichtingen, P. Kemeter (Eds.), Future Aspects in Human in vitro Fertilization, Springer-Verlag, Berlin, 1987, pp. 145–153.
[13] A.M. Junca, et al., Anonymous and non anonymous oocyte donation. Preliminary results, Hum. Reprod. 3 (1988) 121–123.
[14] F. Rapport, Exploring the beliefs and experiences of potential egg share donors, J. Adv. Nurs. 43 (2003) 28–42.

[15] Y. Englert, Ethics of oocyte donation are challenged by the health care system, Hum. Reprod. 11 (1996) 2353–2355.
[16] [No authors listed], Eggs shared, given, and sold, Lancet 362 (9382) (2003 Aug. 9) 413.
[17] J. McMillan, T. Hope, Gametes, money, and egg sharing, Lancet 16 (2003) 362–584.
[18] P.A. West, "Egg giving" is trading, not one way process of giving, BMJ 11 (2003) 872.
[19] M.R. Rimington, et al., Should non-patient volunteers donate eggs? Reprod. Biomed. Online 6 (2003) 277–280.
[20] K.K. Ahuja, One hundred and three concurrent IVF successes for donors and recipients who shared eggs :ethical and practical benefits of egg sharing to society, Reprod. Biomed. Online 1 (2000) 101–105.
[21] J.H. Check, et al., Evaluation of the mechanism for higher pregnancy rates in donor oocyte recipients by comparison of fresh with frozen embryo transfer pregnancy rates in a shared oocyte programme, Hum. Reprod. 10 (1995) 3022–3027;
R. Lessor, et al., A survey of public attitudes toward oocyte donation between sisters, Hum. Reprod. 5 (1990) 889–892.
[22] J.A. Robertson, Ethical and legal issues in human egg donation, Fertil. Steril. 52 (1980) 353–363.
[23] L.R. Schover, et al., The psychological evaluation of oocytes donors, J. Psychosom. Obstet. Gynaecol. 11 (1990) 299–309.
[24] M.V. Sauer, Indecent proposal: $5000 is not "reasonable compensation" for oocyte donors, Fertil. Steril. 71 (1999) 7–10.
[25] F. Shenfield, S.J. Steele, Why gamete donors should not be paid, Hum. Reprod. 10 (1994) 253–255.
[26] Y. Englert (Ed.), Gamete Donation: Current Ethics in the European Union, Hum. Reprod., vol. 13, Suppl. 2, 1998, 137 pp.
[27] P. Rodriguez del Pezo, Paying donors and ethics of blood supply, J. Med. Ethics 20 (1994) 31–35.
[28] Ch. Laruelle, Y. Englert, Don de sperme: retribution ou reparation, Contracept. Fertil. Sex 17 (1989) 667–668.
[29] N. Garrido, et al., Sperm and oocyte donor selection and management: experience of a 10 year follow-up of more than 2100 candidates, Hum. Reprod. 17 (2002) 3142–3148.
[30] C. Barratt, et al., Gamete donation guidelines. The Corsendonk consensus document for the European Union, Hum. Reprod. 13 (1998) 500–501.
[31] E. Weil, et al., Psychological aspects in anonymous and non anonymous oocyte donation, Hum. Reprod. 9 (1994) 1344–1347.
[32] A. Delbaere, I. Govaerts, Y. Englert, Don d'ovocytes: synchronisation et cycles différés: expérience de la clinique de fertilité de l'hôpital Erasme (Belgique), Reprod. Hum. Horm. XIV (7) (2001) 466–468.
[33] H. Leridon, Demographic aspect of human fertility, in: C. Thibault, M.C. Levasseur, R.H.F. Hunter (Eds.), Reproduction in Mammals and Man, Ellipse, Paris, 1993, pp. 643–651.
[34] M.A. Cohen, S.R. Lindheim, M.V. Sauer, Donor age is paramount to success in oocyte donation, Hum. Reprod. 14 (1999) 2755–2758.
[35] C. Liesnard, E. Strebelle, Y. Englert, Is the British Andrology Society recommendation to recruit cytomegalovirus negative semen donors only, a reasonable one? Hum. Reprod. 16 (2001) 1789–1791.
[36] N. Nikolettos, et al., Father-to-son sperm donation. A report of three cases, Clin. Exp. Obstet. Gynecol. 30 (2003) 226–228.
[37] E. Fortescue, Gamete donation. Where is the evidence that there are benefits in removing the anonymity of donors? A patient's viewpoint, Reprod. Biomed. Online 7 (2003) 139–144.
[38] C. Murray, S. Golombok, To tell or not to tell: the decision-making process of egg-donation parents, Hum. Fertil. (Camb.) 6 (2003) 89–95.
[39] P.P. Mahlstedt, D.A. Greenfeld, Assisted reproductive technology with donor gametes: the needs for patients preparartion, Fertil. Steril. 52 (1989) 908–914.
[40] Y. Englert, et al., Oocyte shortage for donation may be overcome in a programme of anonymous permutation of related donors, Hum. Reprod. 11 (1996) 101–104.
[41] A. Delbaere, S. Emiliani, Y. Englert, Don d'ovocyte direct ou don croisé anonyme? L'expérience de l'hôpital Erasme, Reprod. Hum. Horm. 6 (2002) 487–490.

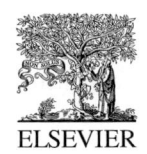

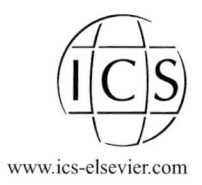

# Saviour siblings: using preimplantation genetic diagnosis for tissue typing

Guido Pennings*

*Department of Philosophy, Centre for Environmental Philosophy and Bioethics, Ghent University, Blandijnberg 2B-9000, Ghent, Belgium*

**Abstract.** The major ethical arguments for and against the use of preimplantation genetic diagnosis (PGD) for human leukocyte antigen (HLA) tissue typing are analysed. It is concluded that conceiving a child to save a sibling is a morally defensible decision on the condition that the use that will be made of the future child would be acceptable if the child would already exist. There are no indications that parents who ask medical assistance to have an HLA compatible sibling do not intend to love and care for the new child. In general, it is argued that too much importance is attributed to the motives underlying the decision to conceive. The morally relevant point is the way the child is treated by its parents once it is born rather than their reasons for having it. A number of new variations to the standard case are discussed: the donation of hard organs, a parent as tissue recipient, the child as backup, health risks for the donating child and miscellaneous factors. © 2004 Published by Elsevier B.V.

*Keywords:* Ethics; HLA; Parenthood; Preimplantation genetic diagnosis; Transplantation

## 1. Introduction

Preimplantation genetic diagnosis (PGD) is a relatively new technology to obtain genetic information about embryos before implantation into the uterus. Originally, it was offered to couples at high risk of transmitting a genetic disease as an alternative to conventional prenatal diagnosis, possibly followed by a termination of pregnancy. Very soon, however, it became clear that the specific technical characteristics of the technology offered new possibilities and led to deviations from the standard guidelines applied to prenatal diagnosis. The most important difference is the availability of several embryos. According to the opponents, this fact is responsible for lowering the indication threshold for selection of the embryos [1]. Also, the fact that no termination of pregnancy is needed would lead to the selection of embryos for less serious reasons [2]. This idea starts from the rather surprising idea that undergoing one or more in vitro fertilization (IVF) cycles (ovarian stimulation, oocyte pick-up) and PGD amounts to almost nothing. Infertility treatment is, arguably, as high a barrier against trivial indications as a termination of

---

* Tel./fax: +32-16-620-767.
  *E-mail address:* Guido.Pennings@UGent.be (G. Pennings).

pregnancy. Nevertheless, as far as the selection of the embryos is concerned, the opponents correctly analysed the situation but are mistaken in their evaluation. The availability of several embryos allows the application of the maximisation principle: when there is an embryo A with a minor handicap or deficit and an embryo B without a handicap, one should replace embryo B (all other things being equal). This evolution is not regrettable or pernicious; the decision is fully rational and ethically permissible. However, PGD for tissue typing is a completely different story: the embryos are selected on the basis of a characteristic that does not improve the health of the child that will be born, but on a characteristic that serves the interests of somebody else.

## 2. Tissue typing

Different methods can be used to obtain a child whose haematopoietic stem cells could be donated to a sibling: the parents can go on having children the natural way until a match is found, they can opt for prenatal diagnosis, or they can try for PGD. All methods have pros and cons, both medically and ethically. As mentioned in the introduction, the main advantage of PGD, compared with the other methods, is the availability of a large number of embryos. The age of the mother is the main determining factor for the number of embryos that will be obtained. The probability of finding an HLA-matched embryo is one in four. The chance of finding a matched non-affected embryo (for recessive diseases like Fanconi anaemia) is 3 out of 16. This relatively low chance should then be combined with the probability of implantation and later transplantation. The first successful case required four IVF cycles and the replacement of five HLA-compatible embryos (out of 30 embryos tested) before a pregnancy was obtained [3]. The low success rate caused some geneticists to argue that the couples should not be offered the possibility. Several remarks can be made regarding this point. Depending on their position regarding patient autonomy, some will leave the decision to the parents. They have to decide, after being informed about all aspects of the procedure, whether or not to proceed. However, patient autonomy also has its limits. Below a certain point, the procedure should be considered futile or out of proportion. Although a threshold is always arbitrary to some extent, it is possible to decide when the chance of success is so low that the effort is no longer justified. However, it should be kept in mind that we are not just talking of the chance of having a child, but of the chance of saving the life of the sick sibling. Especially when transplantation is the only chance of saving the child's life, the threshold should be low. Nevertheless, it is not unreasonable to restrict the application to women below a certain age. Finally, it is early days yet. As for other techniques, one should not judge the acceptability of the technique as a whole on the basis of the few attempts up till now. As for IVF, the success rate may improve in the future when technical problems with PGD have been solved.

## 3. The instrumentalization of the future person

The uneasiness of a number of people about the application of tissue typing is caused by the instrumentalization of the future child. Using another person, especially a person who is unable to consent to the use, always has a connotation of exploitation. We should respect the person as a person and not reduce him or her to a thing or a means to an end. This idea is deeply ingrained in Western thinking and explains the general acceptance of Kant's categorical imperative: 'Act so that you treat humanity, whether in your own person or in that of another, always as an end and never as a means only' [4]. However, the imperative should be read carefully: it does not say that it is wrong to treat another person as a means (in fact, we do that quite often in everyday life), but only that we should not treat another *solely* as a means. A major problem with this rule is that it is far from clear when the rule is violated [5]. Every wanted child can be considered as a means for the fulfilment of the parental desire. According to Heyd [6], the decision to procreate 'is the only one in which the child is treated purely as a means (usually to the parents' satisfaction, wishes, and ideals)!'. Even if that statement is mitigated, it can be argued that, to a certain extent, all parents have children to fulfil their own wishes. This is not considered a problem as long as the parents intend to love the child as it is.

## 4. The 'preceding wish' condition

Several participants in the discussion stated that a request from the parents is only acceptable if they planned to have another child anyway. This condition is rather peculiar. It presupposes that changes in a person's life or family should not influence his or her family planning. In fact, the same concerns underlie the creation of a 'replacement' child after the death of an older sibling.

The main purpose of the 'preceding wish' condition is to sever the reasons to conceive and the later use. As such, it is based on the separation principle, which is applied in a multitude of situations [7]. This principle states, for instance, that there should be a complete separation between the decision to abort and the later use that is made of the fetal material. The principle also underlies the opposition against the creation of embryos for research. In the present context, the condition that the parents should have wanted or planned another child before the need for a donor arose separates the motives for conception, to some extent, from the later use of the child. The principle wants to guarantee that the child will be respected, regardless of or beside its suitability as a donor. This seems a perfectly reasonable demand. However, the 'preceding wish' condition is erroneous, because it presupposes that the postnatal attitude of the parents toward the child depends on the preconceptional desire for a child. This would mean that most children who were conceived 'by accident' would not be loved. Luckily, the attitude of the parents towards their child after birth is not determined by the presence of a child wish before conception.

In a similar way, people seem to believe that the motives underlying the conception have a tremendous influence on the self-esteem and self-concept of the child. According to the opponents of the technology, children who are told that they were conceived in order to save their sibling's life will feel used and diminished. They will perceive themselves as not valued for themselves, as instrumental and subordinate to someone else. But then what should a child think when it is informed that it was an 'accident'? If the same reasoning applies, this information about its conception would take away the meaning and value of its life. It seems highly unlikely that this fact will have such an impact, unless the child does not feel loved during its upbringing. But even then, we condemn the attitude of the parents toward the child regardless of the motive preceding its conception or birth. The clearest demonstration the parents could give of considering the child as an 'organ bank' is if they abandon it after taking the tissue. That behaviour would be a blatant demonstration of disrespect.

One way to remove all doubts about respect for future persons would be to avoid the coming into existence of a person. If the body material can be harvested before viability or birth (e.g., embryonic stem cells or organs by aborting the fetus at a stage when the needed organ is sufficiently developed), problems of commodification and instrumentalization of persons are avoided.

## 5. Alternative scenarios

When the successive requests by patients are analysed, one already notices a number of variations which may be morally relevant. As a form of prospective ethics, we should prepare for such variations. A number of these variations run against fairly strong moral intuitions. The main question is whether we should consider these intuitions as sufficient to reject the requests or whether we should treat them as alarm bells, which point us at possible dangers that have to be taken seriously in the decision-making process.

### 5.1. Hard organs

Several committees have stated that harvesting hard or non-regenerating organs is morally unacceptable [8,9]. There has already been one report of a family that conceived a child to provide a kidney for a sibling with chronic kidney failure [10]. In general, parity for donation is restricted to cord blood or bone marrow. This position is defended by referring to the fact that the risks and inconveniences of donating an organ are more than minimal and that the donating child's best interests are not served. However, such a blanket prohibition on conception for organ donation might not be justified. In the past, the court has decided that minors and incompetent persons can serve as organ donors for siblings [11]. If the best interests of an existing child may be served by donating an organ to a sibling, it can also be argued that it is in the best interest of a future child to be able to serve as a donor. This position would be based on the close psychological relationship the donor will develop (or will have developed) with the recipient while growing up in the same family.

In order to know whether or not the geneticists should collaborate in the project of the parents to conceive a matched sibling, the postnatal test can be used: 'it is ethically acceptable to conceive a child for a certain reason if it is acceptable to use an existing child for the same reason' [12]. This test serves two purposes. (1) It clarifies the relationship between intending and doing. The general principle is that it can only be wrong to intend to do something if it is wrong to do that something. It can only be wrong to intend to use the future child as a donor if it is wrong to use an existing child as a donor. (2) It anticipates and respects the future rights of the child. Once it is born, its interests are protected to the same extent and evaluated according to the same standards as any other child's interests. The moral intuition about the unacceptability of organ donation points at the fact that the more serious the harm (pain, risk of the intervention, non-regenerating tissue, etc.) to the donating child, the more difficult it is to justify the decision.

## 5.2. Backup

While most procedures are started to obtain haematopoietic stem cells for a sick child that needs a transplantation as quickly as possible or in the near future, new cases turn up where tissue matching is directed at providing a backup for when the current therapy fails, the child relapses, or a second transplantation is needed in the future. For some diseases, such as adrenoleucodystrophy, there is a large variation in the expression of the disease. The affected person may need a transplantation in the near future, in 20 years, or maybe never. Is it justified to demand that all other possibilities and sources of tissue have been explored before parity for donation can be started? In other words, why cannot parents demand a matched sibling as a backup for when things go wrong?

The evaluation of the application of the procedure in these cases largely depends on the need to perform PGD to prevent the next child being born with the same disease. If PGD is performed solely to obtain a backup or a possible donor, the effort in terms of money, personnel, etc. may be disproportional. Other morally relevant elements of the situation will change as well. If the transplantation is only needed after 15 years, the candidate donor will be competent. He or she may not be happy with the additional choice. One could argue that, compared with a sibling who is HLA-compatible by coincidence, this person is not really free to donate. On the other hand, the situation resembles much more the family in which an existing sibling is a match. The 'instrumentalization' of the future child is considerably diminished: this child surely is also wanted for itself, since its use as a donor is only conditional.

## 5.3. A parent as recipient

Even the opponents of parity for donation express their understanding for the tragic position of the parents. However, a similar solution could be adopted to cure one of the parents. There are some reports of cases where a father was cured with the cord blood of his child [13]. Although these cases will be rare, it is predictable that they will arise again in the future. A parent who intends to have a child to save his or her own life cannot expect much goodwill from the social environment. Our moral intuitions condemn these applications, because of the considerable self-interest of the decision maker. The parent should declare him or herself incompetent due to a conflict of interest. Nevertheless, the same justification can be offered as for the donation to a sibling. The HLA-matched child will be better off, since it will have two healthy parents, while its incompatible possible sibling will experience parental death or will grow up in a family with a chronically ill parent. The conception of a child as a donor for a parent would also be acceptable according to the postnatal test; if an existing child in the family would be a suitable donor, it would be judged acceptable to use it as a donor of haematopoietic stem cells for a parent. However, we should take our moral intuitions into account by appointing an independent guardian who should, even more than in other cases, carefully scrutinise parental decision making.

## 5.4. Health risks for the donating child

Certain HLA antigens show striking associations with certain diseases, such as ankylosing spondylitis, insulin-dependent diabetes mellitus, multiple sclerosis, and rheumatoid arthritis. The best-known association is ankylosing spondylitis with HLA B27.

Persons with B27 have a markedly increased risk (relative risk=90.0) to develop this disease. At present, when the embryo is matched for HLA, one does not verify whether the selected HLA type is associated with a certain disease. Without this check, HLA matching may hold increased health risks for the future donor. Still, since the increase of risk will be relatively small in most cases, it is not clear whether this should be an obligatory part of testing.

### 5.5. Miscellaneous factors

One can easily imagine new cases complicated by a multitude of different factors. For instance, since the mean age of the mothers is relatively high (around 35 years), one should take into account the possibility that the HLA-compatible embryo is aneuploid. What should be done when the matched embryo has trisomy 21? Would it be acceptable to replace this embryo when other non-affected embryos are available? Another factor is linked to the strictness of the criteria. Should an IVF-PGD cycle be started when the success rate of the transplantation is around 50% or below? It is recommendable that, in this preliminary phase, we keep an open mind and evaluate each situation on its own merits. It is not because the application of PGD for tissue typing is accepted in principle that all new requests should be accepted. Some variations may be sufficient to refuse collaboration in the parental project.

## 6. Conclusion

The motives or reasons parents have for conceiving the child do not determine the relationship they will have with the child. The morally relevant point is not that parents have the right motive for conceiving the child, but that they love and care for the donating child and protect its best interests once it is born. The few instances in which parents have asked for medical assistance to obtain a compatible sibling strongly indicate that they intend to do so. The use or instrumentalization of the donating child does not demonstrate disrespect for his or her autonomy and intrinsic value.

### Acknowledgements

The author wishes to thank Prof. Dr. I. Liebaers and the team of the Centre for Medical Genetics at the Free University Brussels for the possibility of discussing these cases and for their courage in considering difficult and controversial requests.

### References

[1] J. Testart, B. Sèle, Towards an efficient medical eugenics: is the desirable always the feasible? Hum. Reprod. 10 (1995) 3086–3090.
[2] D.S. King, Preimplantation genetic diagnosis and the 'new' genetics, J. Med. Ethics 25 (1999) 176–182.
[3] Y. Verlinsky, S. Rechitsky, W. Schoolcraft, C. Strom, A. Kuliev, Preimplantation diagnosis for Fanconi anemia combined with HLA matching, JAMA 285 (2001) 3130–3133.
[4] I. Kant, Groundwork of the Metaphysics of Morals, Harper and Row, New York, 1964.
[5] D.W. Drebushenko, Creating children to save siblings' lives: a case study for Kantian ethics, in: J. Humber, R. Almeder (Eds.), Biomedical ethics reviews 1991, Humana Press, Totowa, NJ, 1991, pp. 89–101.
[6] D. Heyd, Genethics: Moral Issues in the Creation of People, University of California Press, Berkeley, 1992.

[7] G.J. Boer, Ethical issues in neurografting of human embryonic cells, Theor. Med. Bioethics 20 (1999) 461–475.
[8] Ethics Committee of the Human Fertilisation and Embryology Authority, Ethical issues in the creation and selection of preimplantation embryos to produce tissue donors. http://www.hfea.gov.uk/PressOffice/Press-Releasesbysubject/PGDandtissuetyping/Ethics Cttee PGD November 2001.pdf..
[9] Infertility Treatment Authority, Tissue typing in conjunction with preimplantation genetic diagnosis. http://www.ita.org.au/ documents/policies/Policy PGD HLA Matching.pdf, 2003..
[10] V.G. Norton, Unnatural selection: nontherapeutic preimplantation genetic screening and proposed regulation, UCLA Law Rev. 41 (1994) 1581–1650.
[11] M.P. Aulisio, T. May, G.D. Block, Procreation for donation: the moral and political permissibility of "having a child to save a child", Camb. Q. Healthc. Ethics 10 (2001) 408–419.
[12] G. Pennings, R. Schots, I. Liebaers, Ethical considerations on preimplantation genetic diagnosis for HLA typing to match a future child as a donor of haematopoietic stem cells to a sibling, Hum. Reprod. 17 (2002) 534–538.
[13] P. De Greef, Baby Redt Leven Vader Met Bloed Uit Navelstreng [Baby Saves Life of Father by Cord Blood], October 29, 2001, De Volkskrant, 2001, p. 1.

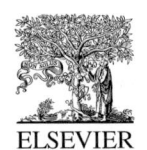

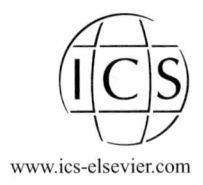

# Evidence-based management of recurrent miscarriage: optimal diagnostic protocol

Salim Daya*

*Departments of Obstetrics and Gynecology, and Clinical Epidemiology and Biostatistics, McMaster University, 1200 Main Street West, Hamilton, Ontario, Canada L8N 3Z5*

**Abstract.** Recurrent miscarriage is a relatively frequent but poorly understood disorder because of clinical heterogeneity arising from the lack of standardization of definitions and diagnostic evaluation. The diagnostic approach varies from clinic to clinic and, in a significant proportion of couples, no cause can be identified. In others, multiple causes are present. Thus, the approach of offering treatment for the first abnormal test may not be prudent. Ideally, a comprehensive approach to evaluation is required to identify factor(s) associated with recurrent miscarriage. The current approach should be to identify chromosomal abnormalities, uterine anomalies, cervical incompetence, endocrine dysfunction, thrombophilias, and alloimmune abnormality. Agreement among investigators on the definitions and evaluation process will improve the understanding of this disorder so that more valid and useful studies on treatment efficacy can be undertaken to improve the outcome for couples with recurrent miscarriage. © 2004 Published by Elsevier B.V.

*Keywords:* Recurrent miscarriage; Habitual abortion; Pregnancy loss; Diagnosis

## 1. Introduction

Miscarriage is the most common complication of pregnancy, occurring in 10–15% of pregnant women. Some women (prevalence estimated at 2–5%) will have three or more miscarriages. In women with recurrent miscarriage, it is necessary to conduct a comprehensive diagnostic evaluation so that a plan of care can be outlined based on the findings. Unfortunately, the paucity of good-quality evidence limits the ability to make confident recommendations regarding management, and has raised several issues that require discussion.

a) *Definition of miscarriage.* The term miscarriage is used to describe a pregnancy that fails to progress, resulting in death and expulsion of the embryo or fetus (weighing 500 g or less) [1], a stage that corresponds to a gestational age of up to 20 weeks.

---

* Tel.: +1-905-525-9140x22566; fax: +1-905-524-2911.
  *E-mail address:* dayas@mcmaster.ca (S. Daya).

Unfortunately, this definition is not used consistently or universally. Additionally, the term miscarriage has become synonymous with pregnancy loss, the definition of which has been expanded to include pregnancies that have ended in stillbirth and preterm neonatal death. Thus, the literature is replete with reports in which variable criteria have been used to characterize the population being studied. Consequently, the external validity of such studies and the inferences that can be drawn are limited when it comes to evaluating couples with recurrent miscarriage.

b) *Subgroups of recurrent miscarriage.* Based on the pregnancy history, three different groups of women with recurrent miscarriage can be identified, and the risk of subsequent miscarriage among these groups varies [2]:

   (i) *Primary recurrent miscarriage group.* This group consists of women with three or more consecutive miscarriages with no pregnancy progressing beyond 20 weeks' gestation.

   (ii) *Secondary recurrent miscarriage group.* This group consists of women who have had three or more miscarriages following at least one pregnancy that has gone beyond 20 weeks' gestation, and may have ended in live birth, stillbirth, or neonatal death.

   (iii) *Tertiary recurrent miscarriage group.* This group has not been well studied and consists of women who have had at least three miscarriages that are not consecutive but are interspersed with pregnancies that have progressed beyond 20 weeks' gestation (and may have ended in live birth, stillbirth, or neonatal death).

The current approach of lumping all three groups together makes it difficult to make recommendations regarding optimal evaluation and management.

c) *Effect of male partner.* It is well known that some women may have recurrent miscarriages with one male partner and not with another. The diagnostic evaluation should take this factor into account before a management plan can be outlined, particularly in situations where the miscarriages have preceded the relationship with a new partner.

d) *Effect of female age.* The perceived increased risk of miscarriage with gravidity may, in part, be related to the effect of maternal age; women with previous pregnancies tend to be older. The risk of miscarriage resulting from trisomic conception increases with maternal age, especially after the age of 35 years. However, after correcting for the effect of maternal age, the increased risk of miscarriages as a result of previous miscarriages is still present [3]. Thus, the number of previous miscarriages is an important factor in evaluating the efficacy of therapeutic interventions. Ideally, clinical trials of treatment in recurrent miscarriage should have stratification for the number of previous miscarriages, with randomization between control and experimental interventions taking place within each stratum.

e) *Karyotypic analysis of products of conception.* The possibility that a miscarriage following treatment is the result of a de novo aneuploidy must be investigated by subjecting all products of conception from women with recurrent miscarriages to karyotype analysis. The improvements in ultrasonography and cytogenetic techniques have permitted earlier access and more accurate and reliable assessment of the products of conception. Thus, every effort should be taken to obtain this information, which is necessary to ascertain whether the pregnancy loss is the result of treatment failure or a chromosomal anomaly.

## 2. Diagnostic testing for couples with recurrent miscarriage

Despite testing, which varies from clinic to clinic, the presumed cause of recurrent miscarriage may not be identified in a significant number of couples. Furthermore, there may be more than one abnormal test indicating the presence of a multifactorial problem. Thus, the approach of offering treatment for the first abnormal test may not be prudent and, ideally, a comprehensive evaluation should be undertaken before a plan of care can be outlined. A major problem with many of the diagnostic tests is that evaluation is performed in the nonpregnant state from which inferences are drawn regarding the cause(s) of the miscarriages that have already occurred, and the approach to management for the next pregnancy. Furthermore, for many diagnostic tests, a reliable gold standard does not exist, rendering the test incompletely evaluated for accuracy. Finally, the untreated prognosis in women in whom the diagnostic testing is positive has not been established confidently. Despite these methodological concerns, there are many tests available that can be offered to couples with recurrent miscarriage so that a management plan can be outlined when the testing has been completed.

### 2.1. Karyotype analysis

Chromosomal anomalies can be identified in either the male or female partner; the prevalence is very low but is higher in females than in males. The prevalence of anomalies from an analysis of data from a computerized database, generated from 200 publications on cytogenetics studies recording information from over 20,000 couples ascertained through recurrent miscarriages, is as follows: reciprocal translocation (1.3%), Robertsonian translocation (0.6%), inversion (0.2%), sex chromosome aneuploidy (0.1%), and supernumerary chromosome (0.003%) [4]. Thus, balanced translocation (including reciprocal and Robertsonian types) is the most common abnormality, the prevalence of which increases with the number of previous miscarriages.

The lack of chromosomal analysis in previous abortus material makes it difficult to attribute the etiology to chromosomal anomalies. However, it is now possible to study material archived in pathology laboratories using in situ hybridization methods combined with cytochemical staining. Studies of such material will provide very useful information to assist in the understanding of the etiology of recurrent miscarriage.

### 2.2. Uterine anomaly evaluation

Four major categories of uterine anomaly have been reported to be associated with recurrent miscarriage.

#### 2.2.1. Congenital uterine anomalies

Lack of agreement over nomenclature and diagnostic strategies has made it difficult to establish accurate incidence figures. The major evidence supporting a causal role for congenital uterine anomalies is the higher prevalence observed in women with recurrent miscarriage. Among the various congenital uterine anomalies (i.e., unicornuate, didelphys, bicornuate, septate, arcuate, and DES drug-related), the septate and arcuate anomalies are the most common. The hypothesis is that the septum (in a septate uterus), being relatively avascular, prevents adequate implantation, resulting in pregnancy loss. However, this theory has not been validated. Furthermore, the high rate of pregnancy loss associated with the arcuate anomaly [5] raises the question of whether other mechanisms are operative.

The problem with establishing a diagnosis of a uterine anomaly is the subjectivity associated with interpreting the findings on diagnostic testing. The hysterosalpingogram (HSG) has been the most frequently employed test, but it is limited to the delineation of cavities that communicate externally. It is important that the HSG be performed with appropriate positioning so that the longitudinal axis of the uterus is in the same plane as the X-ray film to avoid taking tangential views that would occur with anteversion or retroversion of the uterus. Tangential views are inadequate for the evaluation of the uterine fundus and may provide misleading reassurance that the uterine cavity is normal.

Hysteroscopy has improved the evaluation of the uterine cavity and also allows surgical correction of the anomaly.

Transvaginal ultrasonography has become a very useful screening tool. Clear visualization of the endometrium is necessary for a proper evaluation of the uterine cavity. Consequently, the examination should be performed during the luteal phase of the cycle because the endometrium is strongly echogenic at this time and provides a nice contrast against the relatively hypoechoic myometrium. More recently, the introduction of three-dimensional untrasonography has improved the diagnostic accuracy for detecting uterine anomalies and has enabled the assessment to be more objective with low interobserver variability [6]. Using this imaging technique, distortion of the uterine cavity can be observed in women with recurrent miscarriage [7].

Magnetic resonance imaging is also a useful method for distinguishing the different anomalies and identifying noncommunicating uterine horns [8].

### 2.2.2. Cervical incompetence

Cervical incompetence is the inability of the cervix to maintain an intrauterine pregnancy until term. Its incidence among women with recurrent miscarriage varies from 8% to 15% [9]. There are no universally accepted criteria for its diagnosis, which is based on clinical history and signs in the nonpregnant and pregnant states. The typical history is of second trimester pregnancy loss, often preceded by painless dilatation of the cervix and bulging membranes. The fetus usually appears normally developed and may be alive at birth.

The history of expulsion of a dead or macerated fetus generally argues against the diagnosis of cervical incompetence. Predisposing factors include previous pregnancy, procedures such as D&C and cone biopsy, and therapeutic abortion. It may also be associated with congenital uterine anomalies.

In the nonpregnant state, inspection of the cervix may reveal congenital anomalies or evidence of previous cervical laceration. The resistance of the cervix can be gauged by the ease with which a dilator (minimum diameter of 6 mm) can be passed through the internal os. Hysterosalpingography is also useful particularly if a wide cervical canal (6 mm or greater) with a funnel-like appearance is noted [2].

In the pregnant patient, effacement and/or dilatation of the internal os demonstrated on transvaginal ultrasonography (especially if the scanning is performed serially during the second trimester of pregnancy) is suggestive of cervical incompetence, as is the length of the cervix less than 2.5 cm [2]. Abdominal pressure or the Valsalva maneuver can often assist in demonstrating cervical incompetence on ultrasonography.

### 2.2.3. Intrauterine adhesions

Intrauterine adhesions should be suspected especially if the clinical history includes curettage in the pregnancy or puerperium followed by amenorrhea or hypomenorrhea. Hysterosalpingography is useful for the diagnosis by demonstrating single or multiple lacuna-shaped filling defects of variable size in the uterine cavity. These filling defects are characterized by their irregularity, angulated form, very sharp contours, homogeneous opacity, and persistent appearance on several exposures taken at various intervals [10]. Hysteroscopy is used to confirm the HSG findings and permits surgical correction.

### 2.2.4. Uterine fibroids

Uterine fibroids are common tumours, may be single or multiple, and may be of various sizes. They have been reported to be associated with miscarriage and implantation failure. The evidence from observational studies of a reduction in miscarriage rate after removal of fibroids suggests that fibroids may be implicated in causing miscarriages. It has been suggested that the miscarriages occur because of distortion of the uterine cavity, distortion of the vascular supply to the pregnancy, and uterine irritability from rapid growth of the fibroids during pregnancy. The diagnosis is made by clinical examination, ultrasonography, and magnetic resonance imaging (MRI). Laparoscopy and hysteroscopy provide useful additional information on the extent and location of the fibroids.

## 2.3. Endocrine abnormalities

Various types of endocrine dysfunction have been reported to be associated with recurrent miscarriage.

### 2.3.1. Luteal phase deficiency (LPD)

Progesterone production by the corpus luteum is necessary to promote secretory transformation of the endometrium and to support early pregnancy until the placenta can assume this function. Suboptimal corpus luteal function produces a clinical entity known as LPD. The current testing methods involve serum progesterone measurement in the late luteal phase and endometrial biopsy. Low progesterone levels (less than 21 nmol/l on days 25 and 26) and a lag of greater than 2 days between the histological dating of the endometrium and the chronological dating (from the LH surge or from the next menses) are the currently used criteria for detection of LPD. However, the accuracy of these tests is poor because of within-patient variability in progesterone measurement and interobserver variability in assessing the endometrial biopsies. Furthermore, the utility of the biopsy is now being questioned in light of recent evidence that demonstrates a higher prevalence of LPD in fertile women compared to infertile women.

Preliminary results using immunohistochemistry suggest that steroid receptor abnormalities may be present in some women with recurrent miscarriage. This area is the subject of further research.

### 2.3.2. Hypersecretion of LH

Elevated LH levels ($\geq 10$ IU/L) in the follicular phase have been observed to be more prevalent in women with recurrent miscarriage. However, this finding has not been observed consistently and may, in part, have to do with the assay systems depending on whether the radioimmunoassay or immunometric assay is used. Based on the more precise immunometric assay, hypersecretion of LH in the mid- to late-follicular phase has been observed in 8% of women with recurrent miscarriage [11]. The relevance of this finding is still questionable in light of the inefficacy of gonadotropin-releasing hormone agonists when used to reduce the elevated LH levels in such women.

### 2.3.3. High androgen levels

Androgen levels in the follicular phase have been observed to be higher in women with recurrent miscarriage compared to normal fertile controls [12,13]. The relevance of this information in clinical management awaits further study.

### 2.3.4. Thyroid function

Both hypothyroidism and hyperthyroidism have been associated with adverse effects on fertility and pregnancy. Reports in the literature acknowledge the association between thyroid disease and spontaneous or recurrent miscarriage, but the frequency is very small. Measurement of thyroid-stimulating hormone is a useful screening test.

### 2.3.5. Diabetes mellitus

An association between miscarriage and diabetes has been observed, but few studies have examined the role of maternal diabetes in recurrent miscarriage. From the available data, there is no evidence to support an association between gestational insulin-dependent diabetes under good control and spontaneous or recurrent miscarriage. Blood sugar assessment may be useful as a screening tool.

### 2.3.6. Hyperprolactinemia

There is no firm evidence for an association between hyperprolactinemia and recurrent miscarriage [11]. However, given the relationship between stress and hyperprolactinemia, it is good clinical practice to measure prolactin levels in women with recurrent miscarriage because of the high levels of stress associated with this disorder.

## 2.4. Prothrombolytic state

Several studies have observed an association between thrombotic predisposition and recurrent pregnancy loss. Proposed mechanisms for fetal loss include inhibition of thrombolytic system, placental thrombosis, placental infarction, abnormal prostacyclin metabolism, and direct cytotoxic effects [14]. The problem with many of the studies is the inclusion of miscarriages and late fetal loss together under the category of recurrent pregnancy loss. Thus, trying to evaluate the role of thrombotic predisposition only in recurrent miscarriage is a difficult task.

Thrombophilia is either an inherited or an acquired thrombotic tendency. The most common acquired thrombophilias are lupus anticoagulant (LAC) and anticardiolipin antibody (ACA). The number of inherited thrombophilias keeps increasing and includes factor V Leiden, prothrombin G20210A mutation, and the thermolabile variant of methylene tetrahydrofolate reductase (C677T MTHFR)—the most common cause of hyperhomocystenemia [14]. More rare thrombophilias include antithrombin, protein C, and protein S.

### 2.4.1. Antiphospholipid syndrome (APS)

APS is defined by at least one clinical and one laboratory criterion. The clinical criteria include three or more spontaneous miscarriages or unexplained second or third trimester fetal loss. The laboratory criteria include persistent abnormality of one of the following tests measured at least twice, more than 8 weeks apart: LAC or ACA (IgG greater than 15–20 GPL, i.e., medium to high positive). The testing for LAC can be done using a number of coagulation-based assays, such as the dilute Russell Viper venom test. Testing for ACA is done using the enzyme-linked immunosorbent assay technique.

### 2.4.2. Heritable thrombophilic deficiencies

There are five currently recognized heritable thrombophilic deficiencies: antithrombin, protein C, protein S, factor V Leiden, and prothrombin 20210A variant. The factor V Leiden mutation can be detected using a coagulation-based assay (activated protein C resistance) and is now the most common known genetic predisposition to thrombosis. There is much discrepancy in the literature regarding the association of the factor V Leiden mutation and recurrent pregnancy loss, particularly early loss [14].

Prothrombin 20210A mutation is responsible for thromboembolism in pregnancy. Although the evidence for its role in recurrent miscarriage is controversial, there may be a weak association, but not enough to warrant a recommendation for routine testing.

Homocysteine levels can be increased because of deficiencies in either the transsulfuration or remethylation pathways for its catabolism. A recent meta-analysis demonstrated a weak association between hyperhomocysteinemia and recurrent early pregnancy loss [15]. The mechanism of fetal loss is believed to be by interference with chorionic villous vascularization [16]. Although measurement of homocysteine levels should be undertaken in the fasting state, there is currently insufficient evidence to support its routine testing in women with recurrent miscarriage.

Deficiencies of antithrombin, protein C, and protein S are quite rare and, although associated with fetal loss, the relationship with recurrent miscarriage has not been demonstrated convincingly.

## 2.5. Immunological testing

There is increasing evidence to support the hypothesis that inappropriate humoral or cellular immunological responses may be involved in recurrent miscarriage.

### 2.5.1. Humoral response abnormalities

Several autoantibodies have been shown to be more commonly detected in women with recurrent miscarriage compared to controls. The role of antiphospholipid antibodies has already been discussed. Conflicting reports have appeared in the literature regarding thyroid antibodies. The prognostic value of thyroid antibodies was recently reviewed in a prospective study in which the presence of thyroid antibodies did not affect the outcome of subsequent pregnancies in women with recurrent miscarriage [17]. Thus, routine testing for thyroid antibodies is not necessary in women with recurrent miscarriage.

### 2.5.2. Cellular response abnormalities

Women with miscarriages of euploid pregnancies have been found to have elevated levels of natural killer (NK) cells in the blood [18]. In addition, increased levels of NK cells in normal nonpregnant women seem to be associated with a higher probability of miscarriage in a subsequent pregnancy [19]. Alterations in cellular immunity have also been examined in the endometrium and decidua. Women with recurrent miscarriage and a subsequent miscarriage had higher levels of NK cells of the CD $56^+$ type in the endometrium than those whose pregnancies ended in live birth [20]. Several mechanisms (including immunologic effect of progesterone, immunotrophism, helper cells, natural suppressor cells, and suppressor proteins) have been proposed to interact at the maternal–fetal interface to allow the pregnancy to be successful [3]. Women at risk of miscarriage from alloimmune dysfunction have been shown to benefit from treatment with allogeneic leukocyte administration, provided there is no evidence of antipaternal cytotoxic antibodies in the female [3,21]. Unfortunately, currently, there is no universally accepted diagnostic test that will identify women with alloimmune dysfunction.

### 2.6. Infection

Although several organisms have been associated with sporadic miscarriage, the role of infectious agents in recurrent miscarriage remains controversial. Nevertheless, *Ureaplasma urealyticum* (a genital mycoplasma) has been observed more frequently in the genital tract of couples with recurrent miscarriage [2]. Until definitive evidence is available, cervical and semen cultures for this organism may be advisable because treatment with antibiotics may be beneficial [2].

### 2.7. Endometriosis

A high prevalence of first trimester miscarriage has been reported in observational studies in women with endometriosis, which, when surgically treated, is associated with a marked reduction in the miscarriage rate [22]. Evidence from small controlled studies have shown a trend towards higher miscarriage rates in women with endometriosis [2]. However, in a randomized study of surgical ablation of minimal or mild endometriosis, the subsequent miscarriage rates in the treated and untreated groups were similar [23]. The difficulty in establishing a causal association between endometriosis and miscarriage is further complicated by the observation of an inverse relationship between severity of disease and miscarriage rate [22]. Thus, it is presently unclear whether endometriosis plays a role in predisposing women to having miscarriage.

## 3. Summary

Recurrent miscarriage represents a significant clinical problem, the evaluation and management of which leave a lot to be desired. The lack of universally accepted diagnostic criteria makes it difficult to study this problem because of the heterogeneity in the samples selected for study. Agreement on the definitions is a first step in this process of creating

Table 1
Diagnostic testing for couples with recurrent miscarriage

| | |
|---|---|
| Genetic testing | Karyotype both partners |
| Uterine evaluation | Hysterosalpingogram |
| | Transvaginal ultrasonography (preferably with three-dimensional scanning) |
| | Hysteroscopy and laparoscopy |
| Cervical competence testing | 6-mm dilator test |
| | Hysterosalpingogram looking for funneling |
| | Transvaginal ultrasonography of cervix in pregnancy |
| Endocrine testing | Late luteal phase serum progesterone and endometrial biopsy |
| | LH in mid- to late-follicular phase |
| | Androgen in follicular phase |
| | Thyroid-stimulating hormone |
| | Fasting and 2-h postprandial blood sugar |
| | Prolactin |
| Thrombophilia testing | Lupus anticoagulant |
| | Anticardiolipin antibody |
| | Factor V Leiden |
| Alloimmune testing | Antipaternal cytotoxic antibody in females |

homogeneous groups for study. Couples should then undergo comprehensive evaluation, as outlined in Table 1, before decisions regarding treatment can be made. Agreement on this process among investigators will improve the understanding of this disorder and will pave the way for more valid and useful studies on treatment efficacy.

## References

[1] World Health Organization, Recommended definitions; terminology and format for statistical tables related to the perinatal period, Acta Obstet. Gynaecol. Scand. 56 (1977) 247.
[2] S. Daya, Habitual abortion, in: L.J. Copeland, J.F. Jarrell (Eds.), Textbook of Gynecology, 2nd ed., Saunders, Philadelphia, 2000, pp. 227–271.
[3] S. Daya, Immunotherapy for unexplained recurrent spontaneous abortion, Infertil. Reprod. Med. Clin. North Am. 8 (1997) 65–77.
[4] M. DeBraekeleer, T.-N. Dao, Cytogenetic studies in couples experiencing repeated pregnancy losses, Hum. Reprod. 5 (1990) 519–528.
[5] P. Acien, Reproductive performance of women with uterine malformations, Hum. Reprod. 8 (1993) 122–126.
[6] R. Salim, et al., Reproducibility of three-dimensional ultrasound diagnosis of congenital uterine anomalies, Ultrasound Obstet. Gynecol. 21 (2003) 578–582.
[7] R. Salim, et al., A comparative study of the morphology of congenital uterine anomalies in women with and without a history of recurrent first trimester miscarriage, Hum. Reprod. 18 (2003) 162–166.
[8] V.H. Patel, et al., The role of magnetic resonance imaging in the evaluation of congenital uterine anomalies: a comprehensive review, J. Soc. Gynaecol. Can. 19 (1997) 235–244.
[9] B.E. Shortle, R. Jewelewicz, Clinical Aspects of Cervical Incompetence, Year Book Medical Publishers, Chicago, 1989.
[10] J.G. Schenker, E.J. Margalioth, Intrauterine adhesions: an updated appraisal, Fertil. Steril. 37 (1982) 593–610.
[11] T.C. Li, et al., Endocrinological and endometrial factors in recurrent miscarriage, Br. J. Obstet. Gynaecol. 107 (2000) 1471–1479.
[12] M.A. Okon, et al., Serum androgen levels in women who suffer recurrent miscarriage and their correlation with markers of endometrial function, Fertil. Steril. 69 (1998) 682–690.
[13] S. Bussen, M. Sutterlin, T. Steck, Endocrine abnormalities during the follicular phase in women with recurrent spontaneous abortions, Hum. Reprod. 14 (1999) 18–20.

[14] A.M. Adelberg, J.A. Kuller, Thrombophilias and recurrent miscarriage, Obstet. Gynecol. Surv. 57 (2002) 703–709.
[15] W.L.D.M. Nelen, et al., Hyperhomocysteinemia and recurrent early pregnancy loss: a meta-analysis, Fertil. Steril. 74 (2000) 1196–1199.
[16] W.L.D.M. Nelen, et al., Maternal homocysteine and chorionic vascularization in recurrent early pregnancy loss, Hum. Reprod. 15 (2000) 954–960.
[17] F.H. Rushworth, et al., Prospective pregnancy outcome in untreated recurrent miscarriages with thyroid autoantibodies, Hum. Reprod. 15 (2000) 1637–1639.
[18] D.A. Clark, C.B. Coulam, Is there an immunological cause of repeated pregnancy wastage?, Adv. Obstet. Gynecol. 3 (1995) 321.
[19] K. Aoki, S. Kajura, Y. Matsumoto, Preconceptual natural killer cell activities as a predictor of miscarriage, Lancet 345 (1995) 1340–1342.
[20] K. Clifford, A.M. Flanagan, L. Regan, Endometrial CD 56+ natural killer cells in women with recurrent miscarriage: a histomorphometric study, Hum. Reprod. 14 (1999) 2727–2730.
[21] S. Daya, J. Gunby, J. Recurrent Miscarriage Trialists Group, The effectiveness of allogeneic leukocyte immunization in unexplained primary recurrent spontaneous abortion, Am. J. Reprod. Immunol. 32 (1994) 294–302.
[22] S. Daya, Endometriosis and spontaneous abortion, Infertil. Reprod. Med. Clin. North Am. 7 (1996) 759–773.
[23] S. Marcoux, R. Maheux, S. Berube, S. Canadian Collaborative Group on Endometriosis, Laparoscopic surgery in infertile women with minimal or mild endometriosis, N. Engl. J. Med. 337 (1997) 217–222.

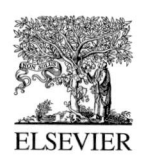

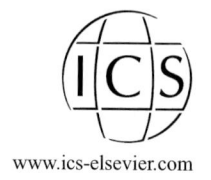

## Medical management of recurrent miscarriage—evidence-based approach

H.J.A. Carp*

*Department of Obstetrics and Gynecology, Sheba Medical Center, Tel Hashomer 52621, Israel*

**Abstract.** Various medical interventions have been used to improve the live birth rate in recurrent miscarriage. However, most often the indication for intervention was 3 or more miscarriages up to 20 weeks. Although this is a heterogeneous group of patients with many causes of miscarriage, randomized trials and meta-analyses have tried to provide evidence of efficacy. In this presentation, the efficacy of hormone supplements, paternal leucocyte immunization and intravenous immunoglobulin are assessed. The efficacy of anticoagulants for antiphospholipid syndrome and hereditary thrombophilias are also discussed. There is Grade I evidence for the efficacy of all of these, but there is also Grade I evidence against some of these interventions. Pregnancy loss can have maternal or fetal causes, such as chromosomal aberrations. If the cause is unknown, the results are confounded. If treatment for a maternal cause is tested on a patient losing a chromosomally abnormal embryo, it will be ineffective. Similarly, there are patients with good and poor prognoses. If treatment is given to a patient with a good prognosis, it will be ineffective. Hence, it is necessary to define a cohort of patients with a poor prognosis, and to reach an accurate diagnosis. At that point, a valid randomized control trial can be performed. At present, evidence-based medicine can only determine that a treatment is effective within the cohort of patients studied. It cannot provide information of efficacy in subgroups. Even if there is no evidence of efficacy, present trials cannot show evidence of inefficacy. © 2004 Published by Elsevier B.V.

*Keywords:* Recurrent miscarriage; Habitual abortion; Pregnancy loss; Evidence-based medicine

## 1. Introduction

In recurrent pregnancy loss, most medical interventions have assessed whether treatment raises the live birth rate in patients with three or more miscarriages up to 20 weeks. Two sets of circumstances may prevent trials from showing a "true" result; the cause of the pregnancy loss, and the prognosis for a live birth with no intervention. Fetal chromosomal aberrations, which account for 29–60% of recurrent miscarriages [1–3], are not usually investigated and can confound the results of any trial. After three miscarriages, the prognosis for a fourth miscarriage is approximately 40% [4]. If 60% of these 40% (24%) are chromosomally

---

* Tel.: +972-9-9557075; fax: +972-9-9574779.
*E-mail address:* carp@netvision.net.il (H.J.A. Carp).

0531-5131/ © 2004 Published by Elsevier B.V.
doi:10.1016/j.ics.2004.01.110

abnormal, any treatment of maternal causes of miscarriage can only raise the live birth rate from 60% to 76%. Therefore, any treatment effect will be small and a trial will need large numbers to reach statistical significance. After four miscarriages, the prognosis for a fifth miscarriage is 54% [4]. After five pregnancy losses, the chance of a live birth is only 29% [4]. If 50% are chromosomally abnormal, treatment could raise the live birth rate by 35%, making it easier to show a treatment effect. There are also other factors that can affect the prognosis for a live birth, viz. primary, secondary or tertiary aborter status, karyotype of previous miscarriage, time taken to conceive and maternal age [5].

As 20% of patients with three miscarriages will have two further miscarriages, accurate diagnosis and effective treatment are required. However, most trials have not accounted for the predictive factors above, or fetal chromosomal aberrations, but have relied on randomization to ensure equal distribution between test and placebo arms. Randomization can be designed to ensure that the different subgroups of patients are equally distributed, but few trials have done so as a larger number of patients are required for subgroup analysis. It is customary to grade the evidence of treatment effect according to a hierarchy in which the double-blind, randomized trial or metaanalysis is considered to be the highest level of evidence (Grade I), and well-designed, controlled studies are the next level (Grade II). Descriptive and comparative studies are the next level (Grade III), and the opinions of expert authorities are said to be Grade IV evidence. However, a trial of intervention can only assess the effect within the question asked. There may be no evidence of effect if patients with three or more pregnancy losses prior to 20 weeks are treated as a whole, but treatment may be effective in a subgroup, e.g. patients losing chromosomally normal embryos but fetal chromosome aberrations may have skewed the results. Hence, the term "no evidence of effect" cannot be construed to mean evidence of no effect.

This review examines the evidence that various medical treatments affect the subsequent live birth rate and the pitfalls in interpreting the effects of treatment. The evidence for some interventions and some of the problems encountered are summarised below.

## 2. Progesterone supplementation

Daya [6] has assessed 34 studies on progesterone supplementation. Only three trials from the 1950s and 1960s met the criteria of recurrent miscarriage, randomization and no threatened abortion at the start of treatment. Although none of these trials showed evidence of treatment effect, pooling the results in a meta-analysis, showed a 23% improvement in the live birth rate (Grade I evidence). However, there is no reliable laboratory test to diagnose luteal deficiency. Plasma progesterone levels are not helpful, as a low level may be the mechanism of abortion rather than the cause. If a pregnancy is chromosomally abnormal leading to fetal demise, there will be no fetal blood supply to the placenta and trophoblastic failure will follow with falling hCG levels [7]. Hence, the low progesterone levels will be the mechanism of abortion rather than its cause. Progesterone supplements can only be beneficial if progesterone deficiency is the cause of miscarriage rather than the mechanism.

## 3. HCG supplementation

HCG supplementation has been reported to be beneficial in three controlled studies [8–10]. However, Harrison [11] multi-centre trial failed to show a beneficial effect. Again, there was no correction for the predictive factors listed above, or confounding factors. Additionally, treatment was started after viability had been confirmed by ultrasound. After detection of a fetal heartbeat, 98% of pregnancies terminate in a live birth [12]. Combining the four trials in a meta-analysis showed hCG to have a beneficial effect [13]. However, the conclusions must be treated with caution as two trials assessed were not randomised and included patients with only two prior miscarriagss. Hence, the evidence is at best Grade II.

Quenby and Farquharson [14] have claimed hCG to be beneficial in women with recurrent miscarriage and oligomenorrhea, but not when all patients with recurrent miscarriage were treated as a whole. However, Quenby and Farquharson's [14] trial included patients with two miscarriages and did not correct for predictive factors. Hence, another trial is necessary using the criteria described above.

## 4. Leukocyte immunization

The "Recurrent Miscarriage Immunotherapy Trialists Group" (RMITG) performed a meta-analysis on 449 patients from eight double-blind, randomized studies [15]. After immunization, the live birth rate was 10% higher (RR=1.21) (Grade I). However, the other conclusions of the RMITG trial are probably more important than the overall benefit, viz: (1) When corrected for the predictive factors, the benefit was 24%; (2) Immunotherapy improved the live birth rate in 1° but not 2° aborters; (3) In control patients with pretreatment anti-paternal complement dependant antibody (APCA), the live birth rate was 70%; and (4) The live birth rate was 37% higher in patients who seroconverted to APCA positive after immunization. Since the RMITG trial, there have been two trends, to narrow the indications for treatment to a subgroup that is more likely to respond, and to widen the indications to include as many patients as possible. Both approaches have given different results. Daya and Gunby [16] have reanalysed the results of the RMITG register for 1° aborters who were APCA negative. Immunization increased the relative risk for a live birth to 1.46 (95% CI 1.19–1.69) (Grade I). However, they did not assess post-immunization seroconversion to APCA positive. The author has [5] published results of immunization in patients with five or more abortions who were APCA negative, and seroconverted after immunization. In 1° and 3° aborters, the benefit was 21% (RR=1.73, 95% CI=1.24–3.58) (Grade II evidence). There was no beneficial effect in 2° aborters. Therefore, the patients most likely to respond to immunotherapy are 1° or 3° aborters with a poor prognosis who are APCA negative.

Ober et al. [17] have performed a double-blind, randomized study which claims that immunization is ineffective in preventing miscarriage. However, this team used dead, refrigerated, stored cells (ineffective in the CBA/J×DBA/2J mouse model of resorbed pregnancies). All other teams had used fresh cells. Patients with pregnancy losses as late as 28 weeks were treated as abortions. In the 2° secondary aborters, the losses were not necessarily consecutive, which may have skewed the results. The effect of confounding factors was not addressed. There were seven patients in the immunized arm who subsequently aborted embryos with chromosomal anomalies. These patients were not excluded from the trial or accounted for by logistic regression analysis, but counted as failures of treatment. In the 1° aborters the numbers were too small to show statistical significance.

Clark et al. [18] has reported that if figures are corrected for karyotypic anomalies, immunization is highly effective, possibly saving almost all the pregnancies that can be saved. However, due to Ober et al.'s [17] report, the FDA has stopped the routine use of paternal leucocyte immunization in the U.S. until another trial is performed that shows efficacy. It must also be borne in mind that there is no mechanism to explain immunologically mediated abortion, or explanation as to why immunization should work. However, there is Grade I evidence of effect.

## 5. Intravenous immunoglobulin (IVIG)

Seven randomized, double-blind trials have been reported comparing IVIG with placebo [19–25]. Four reported no apparent benefit, three showed a benefit. Daya et al. [26] have published a meta-analysis of four of these trials. The 10% benefit in IVIG-treated patients did not reach statistical significance (Grade I). The author has carried out a trial on patients with five or more miscarriages [27]; 35 of 72 (49%) of pregnancies in treated women resulted in live births compared with 23 of 74 pregnancies (31%) in control patients ($p$=0.04) (Grade II evidence).

Christiansen et al. [21,25] have carried out two placebo-controlled, randomized studies of IVIG in recurrent miscarriage. Although the IVIG-treated patients had a higher live birth rate than placebo-treated patients in both trials, neither trial showed a statistically significant benefit. However, when the data from both trials were combined, 15/26 (58%) of secondary aborters had live births in the treatment group compared with 6/26 (24%) in the placebo group (RR=2.01, 95% CI=1.17–3.48). However, in order to confirm the effect in secondary aborters, another trial is necessary, which restricts itself to secondary aborters only.

## 6. Treatment of antiphospholipid antibody syndrome (APS)

There is confusion about the natural history of APS with figures for a subsequent live birth ranging from 10% [28] to 85% [29]. Pathologic antiphospholipid antibodies (aPL) are thought to bind to β2GP1 and the complex binds to phospholipids [30]. Antibodies binding directly to phospholipids may not be pathologic, but a response to infection. [30]. As no trial has assessed β2GP1-dependent aPL, β2GP1 is a confounding factor. Additionally, the presence of abnormal antibodies does not guarantee normal chromosomes. Chromosomally abnormal embryos can also be miscarried by women with APS [3,31].

Most physicians treat APS with low molecular weight heparin (LMWH) and aspirin [32]. However, this regimen has never been tested in a placebo-controlled trial. The previously used regimen of prednisone and aspirin had always been based on observational, rather than placebo-controlled, trials (Grade III). When prednisone and aspirin were compared with heparin and aspirin in a randomized trial of 20 women, the live birth rate was identical (75%) in both groups [33]. When aspirin was compared to aspirin with the addition of prednisone, the live birth rate was 100% in both groups [34]. Hence, steroids have no aparent beneficial action over aspirin alone or aspirin and heparin.

Aspirin has been assessed in placebo-controlled trials [35–37] and summarized in a meta-analysis [40]. No trial or metaanalysis showed aspirin to have a beneficial effect

(Grade I). None of these trials corrects for predictive factors, β2GP1-dependent antibodies or chromosomal aberrations. There are three trials comparing aspirin with aspirin with the addition of heparin [38–40]. Two trials found heparin or low molecular weight heparin to significantly increase the live birth rate. If the three trials are combined, heparin or LMWH raises the live birth rate by 67% (RR=1.67, 95% CI 1.21–2.30). Heparin or LMWH have not been assessed without aspirin.

Heparin and aspirin do not reduce the obstetric complications associated with APS. A recent editorial [41] assessed whether IVIG may reduce obstetric complications. Although descriptive and observational studies were included in that editorial, it seems that IVIG may reduce the incidence of obstetric complications (Grade IV), but a trial is necessary before conclusions can be drawn.

## 7. Hereditary thrombophilias

Recently, hereditary thrombophilias have been linked to recurrent pregnancy loss [42], and the evidence has been sufficient to indicate that treatment with anticoagulants may improve the subsequent live birth rate [43]. The author [44] has published a controlled trial on the effect of the LMWH enoxaparin. Treatment was associated with a 25% increase in the live birth rate. Patients were matched for age and number of miscarriages. The treatment effect was also apparent in patients with 5 or more miscarriages (Grade II). Chromosomal aberrations were equally distributed in the abortions of both arms of the trial (enoxaparin arm: unbalanced translocation and 16 trisomy, control arm: 13 trisomy and 45XO). A double-blind, randomized trial is now necessary to confirm the results.

## 8. Conclusions

There is evidence of the highest grades that interventions are effective in improving the live birth rate in recurrent miscarriage. However, the evidence so far only indicates if treatment is effective in a large and heterogeneous group of patients. Additionally, all the interventions discussed are for maternal causes of pregnancy loss. It is clear that the clinical features must be much more closely defined. In addition, confounding factors must be taken into account. Patients with a good prognosis may need nothing more than dedicated, tender loving care and reassurance. However, patients with a poor prognosis do require accurate diagnosis and effective treatment. Patients with a fetal cause for pregnancy loss should not be confused with those with a maternal cause. Embryo biopsy and replacement of normal embryos might be an option for women recurrently aborting aneuploid fetuses. However, this treatment is inappropriate for women aborting normal embryos. In these cases, the medical interventions described above still have much to offer.

## References

[1] J.J. Stern, A.D. Dorfman, M.D. Gutierez-Najar, Frequency of abnormal karyotype among abortuses from women with and without a history of recurrent spontaneous abortion, Fertil. Steril. 65 (1996) 250–253.
[2] H.J.A. Carp, et al., Karyotype of the abortus in recurrent miscarriage, Fertil. Steril. 5 (2001) 678–682.
[3] M. Ogasawara, et al., Embryonic karyotype of abortuses in relation to the number of previous miscarriages, Fertil. Steril. 73 (2000) 300–304.

[4] H.J.A. Carp, Investigation and treatment for recurrent pregnancy loss, in: P. Rainsbury, D. Vinniker (Eds.), A Practical Guide to Reproductive Medicine, Parthenon, Carnforth, Lancs. U.K, 1997, pp. 337–362.
[5] H.J.A. Carp, et al., Allogeneic leucocyte immunization in women with five or more recurrent abortions, Hum. Reprod. 12 (1997) 250–255.
[6] S. Daya, Efficacy of progesterone support for pregnancy in women with recurrent miscarriage. A meta-analysis of controlled trials, Br. J. Obstet. Gynaecol. 96 (1989) 275–280.
[7] D.I. Rushton, The classlification and mechanisms of spontaneous abortion, Perspect. Pediatr. Pathol. 8 (1984) 269–287.
[8] S.W. Sandler, P. Baillie, The use of human chorionic gonadotropin in recurrent abortion, S. Afr. Med. J. 19 (1979) 832–835.
[9] J. Svigos, Preliminary experience with the use of human chorionic gonadotrophin therapy in women with repeated abortion, Clin. Reprod. Fertil. 1 (1982) 131–135.
[10] R.F. Harrison, Treatment of habitual abortion with human chorionic gonadotropin: results of open and placebo-controlled studies, Eur. J. Obstet. Gynecol. Reprod. Biol. 20 (1985) 159–168.
[11] R.F. Harrison, Human chorionic gonadotrophin (hCG) in the management of recurrent abortion; results of a multi-centre placebo-controlled study, Eur. J. Obstet. Gynecol. Reprod. Biol. 47 (1992) 175–179.
[12] R. Achiron, O. Tadmor, S. Mashiach, Heart rate as a predictor of first trimester spontaneous abortion after ultrasound proven viability, Obstet. Gynecol. 78 (1991) 330–334.
[13] J.R. Scott, N. Pattison, Human chorionic gonadotrophin for recurrent miscarriage, Cochrane Database Syst. Rev. 2 (2000) (CD000101).
[14] S. Quenby, R.G. Farquharson, Human chorionic gonadotropin supplementation in recurring pregnancy loss: a controlled trial, Fertil. Steril. 62 (1994) 708–710.
[15] Recurrent Miscarriage Immunotherapy Trialists Group, Worldwide collaborative observational study and meta-analysis on allogenic leukocyte immunotherapy for recurrent spontaneous abortion, Am. J. Reprod. Immunol. 32 (1994) 55–72.
[16] S. Daya, J. Gunby, The effectiveness of allogeneic leucocyte immunization in unexplained primary recurrent spontaneous abortion, Am. J. Reprod. Immunol. 32 (1994) 294–302.
[17] C. Ober, et al., Mononuclear-cell immunisation in prevention of recurrent miscarriages: a randomised trial, Lancet 354 (1999) 365–369.
[18] D.A. Clark, et al., The Recurrent Miscarriage Immunotherapy Trialists Group, Implication of abnormal human trophoblast karyotype for the evidence-based approach to the understanding, investigation and treatment of recurrent spontaneous abortion, Am. J. Reprod. Immunol. 35 (1996) 495–498.
[19] B. Jablonowska, et al., Prevention of recurrent spontaneous abortion by intravenous immunoglobulin: a double-blind placebo-controlled study, Hum. Reprod. 14 (1999) 838–841.
[20] M.D. Stephenson, et al., Prevention of unexplained recurrent spontaneous abortion using intravenous immunoglobulin: a prospective, randomized, double-blinded, placebo-controlled trial, Am. J. Reprod. Immunol. 39 (1998) 82–88.
[21] O.B. Christiansen, et al., Placebo-controlled trial of treatment of unexplained secondary recurrent spontaneous abortions and recurrent late spontaneous abortions with IV immunoglobulin, Hum. Reprod. 10 (1995) 2690–2695.
[22] The German RSA/IVIG Group, Intravenous immunoglobulin in the prevention of recurrent miscarriage, Br. J. Obstet. Gynaecol. 101 (1994) 1072–1077.
[23] C.B. Coulam, et al., Intravenous immunoglobulin for treatment of recurrent pregnancy loss, Am. J. Reprod. Immunol. 34 (1995) 333–337.
[24] A. Perino, et al., Short-term therapy for recurrent abortion using intravenous immunoglobulins: results of a double-blind placebo-controlled Italian study, Hum. Reprod. 12 (1997) 2388–2392.
[25] O.B. Christiansen, et al., A randomized, double-blind, placebo-controlled trial of intravenous immunoglobulin in the prevention of recurrent miscarriage: evidence for a therapeutic effect in women with secondary recurrent miscarriage, Hum. Reprod. 17 (2002) 809–816.
[26] S. Daya, J. Gunby, D.A. Clark, Intravenous immunoglobulin therapy for recurrent spontaneous abortion: a meta-analysis, Am. J. Reprod. Immunol. 39 (1998) 69–76.
[27] H.J.A Carp, et al., Further experience with intravenous immunoglobulin in women with recurrent miscarriage and a poor prognosis, Am. J. Reprod. Immunol. 46 (2001) 268–273.

[28] R.S. Rai, et al., High prospective fetasl loss rate in untreated pregnancies of women with recurrent miscarriage and antiphosspholipid antibodies, Hum. Reprod. 10 (1995) 3301–3304.
[29] M. Empson, et al., Recurrent pregnancy loss with antiphospholipid antibody: a systematic review of therapeutic trials, Obstet. Gynecol. 99 (2002) 135–144.
[30] M. Ogasawara, et al., Anti-beta(2)-glycoprotein I antibodies and lupus anticoagulant in patients with recurrent pregnancy loss: prevalence and clinical significance, Schweiz. Med. Wochenschr. 126 (1996) 2136–2140.
[31] K. Takakuwa, et al., Chromosome analysis of aborted conceptuses of recurrent aborters positive for anticardiolipin antibody, Fertil. Steril. 68 (1997) 54–58.
[32] A. Tincani, et al., Treatment of pregnant patients with antiphospholipid syndrome, Lupus 12 (2003) 524–529.
[33] F.S. Cowchock, et al., Repeated fetal losses associated with antiphospholipid antibodies: a collaborative randomised trial comparing prednisone with low-dose heparin, Am. J. Obstet. Gynecol. 166 (1992) 1318–1323.
[34] R.K. Silver, et al., Comparative trial of prednisone plus aspirin vs. aspirin alone in the treatment of anticardiolipin antibody-positive obstetric patients, Am. J. Obstet. Gynecol. 169 (1993) 1411–1417.
[35] S. Cowchock, E.A. Reece, Organizing Group of the Antiphospholipid Antibody Treatment Trial, Do low-risk pregnant women with antiphospholipid antibodies need to be treated? Am. J. Obstet. Gynecol. 176 (1997) 1099–1100.
[36] N.S. Pattison, et al., Does aspirin have a role in improving pregnancy outcome for women with the antiphospholipid syndrome? A randomized controlled trial, Am. J. Obstet. Gynecol. 183 (2000) 1008–1012.
[37] M. Tulppala, et al., Low-dose aspirin in prevention of miscarriage in women with unexplained or autoimmune related recurrent miscarriage: effect on prostacyclin and thromboxane A2 production, Hum. Reprod. 12 (1997) 1567–1572.
[38] W.H. Kutteh, Antiphospholipid antibody-associated recurrent pregnancy loss: treatment with heparin and low-dose aspirin is superior to low-dose aspirin alone, Am. J. Obstet. Gynecol. 174 (1996) 1584–1589.
[39] R. Rai, et al., Randomised controlled trial of aspirin and aspirin plus heparin in pregnant women with recurrent miscarriage associated with phospholipid antibodies (or antiphospholipid antibodies), Br. Med. J. 314 (1997) 253–257.
[40] R.G. Farquharson, S. Quenby, M. Greaves, Antiphospholipid syndrome in pregnancy: a randomized, controlled trial of treatment, Lupus 100 (2002) 408–413.
[41] H.J.A. Carp, Y. Shonfeld, The role of intravenous immunoglobulin in pregnancies complicated by the antiphospholipid syndrome, J. Clin. Rheumatol. 7 (2001) 291–294.
[42] E. Rey, et al., Thrombophilic disorders and fetal loss: a meta-analysis, Lancet 15 (361) (2003) 901–908.
[43] J.S. Younis, et al., Familial thrombophilia, the scientific rationale for thrombophylaxis in recurrent pregnancy loss, Hum. Reprod. 12 (1997) 1389–1390.
[44] H.J.A. Carp, M. Dolitzky, A. Inbal, Thromboprophylaxis improves the live birth rate in women with consecutive recurrent miscarriages and hereditary thrombophilia, J. Thromb. Hemostas. 1 (2003) 433–438.

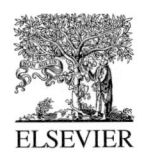

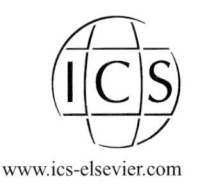

# Evidence-based management of recurrent miscarriage. Surgical management

## Pedro Acién*, Maribel Acién

*Department/Division of Gynecology, Miguel Hernández University,
School of Medicine and San Juan University Hospital, Campus de San Juan, Alicante, Spain*

**Abstract.** *Objectives*: (1) To analyse the anatomic-physiological bases, which justify that uterine anomalies could cause recurrent miscarriage; and (2) to study each one of these causes with regards to the evidence of their relationship with the recurrent miscarriage, as well as the evidence that surgical treatment also corrects the reproductive losses. *Methods*: Revision of the literature and our own investigations on uterine malformations and recurrent miscarriage. *Results*: *Synechiae*. The evidence for synechiae causing recurrent miscarriage is scarce. More probably, they are the result of repeated curettages and cause infertility. *Leiomyomas*. In up to 7% of women with recurrent miscarriage, the cause could lie in the presence of myomas. Present evidence suggests a beneficial effect of myomectomy as treatment, but there are no prospective studies that adequately confirm this. *Cervical incompetence*. It is defined as the incapacity to support or take a pregnancy to its full term due to a functional or structural defect of the cervix. Cervical cerclage is recommended at about 12–14 weeks of pregnancy after diagnosis made before pregnancy, but this operation is a controversial subject. The Cochrane revision concluded that cervical cerclage should not be offered to women at low or medium risk of mid-trimester loss, regardless of cervical length by ultrasound. However, none of the studies included in the meta-analysis based the randomization for carrying out prophylactic cerclage or not on a correct pre-gestational diagnosis, but only on history or on ultrasound. *Congenital uterine anomalies*. Many authors think that septate uterus is the anomaly with the worst reproductive results and propose metroplasty as soon as it is diagnosed. However, we find more reproductive losses in arcuate and bicornuate uteri and we have similar results to metroplasty when only carrying out a cerclage if there is cervical insufficiency. There is no randomized and prospective study, which analyses the necessity of metroplasty. Except in specific cases (20%), metroplasty is not necessary. *Hypoplastic uterus-DES syndrome*. The usefulness of hysteroscopic metroplasty in these cases is still to be demonstrated. There are no randomized studies. *Conclusions*: Surgical management is indicated only in a few cases of recurrent miscarriage: useful myomectomy, cervical cerclage if the incompetence is well diagnosed, metroplasty in some cases of recurrent miscarriage and septate or bicornuate uterus, and hysteroscopic metroplasty in septate and a Strassman operation for a bicornuate uterus. © 2004 Published by Elsevier B.V.

*Keywords:* Miscarriage; Surgical treatment; Uterine anomalies

---

\* Corresponding author. Tel.: +34965919524; fax: +34965203943.
*E-mail address:* paciena@meditex.es (P. Acién).

0531-5131/ © 2004 Published by Elsevier B.V.
doi:10.1016/j.ics.2004.02.003

The majority of causes of recurrent miscarriage are susceptible to medical advice and treatment, but in other cases *surgical treatment* may be advisable. The causes that could require surgical treatment are precisely those included among *uterine causes* (synechiae, leiomyomas, cervical insufficiency and congenital uterine anomalies), which are probably the most important etiological factor in recurrent miscarriage. But we will also quote, although we doubt that it is a cause of recurrent miscarriage, endometriosis. We will briefly analyse the anatomic-physiological bases, which will justify that the mentioned uterine anomalies were the causes for recurrent miscarriage. Then we will study each one of these causes with regards to the evidence of their relationship to the cause of recurrent miscarriage, as well as the evidence that their surgical treatment also corrects recurrent miscarriage at a higher percentage than that of spontaneous observation without treatment (68% children alive in our material [1]).

## 1. Anatomic-physiological bases

The implantation of the egg takes place 6–7 days after fertilization in the functional layer of the endometrium, which is transformed by the action of progesterone after adequate estrogenic preparation. Other very different substances proceeding from the egg and the endometrium (decidua), and the interaction between both, enable a successful implantation and continuation of the pregnancy. So, it is apparent that such an endometrium should have an appropriate structure and vascularization, because some present substances have to reach the endometrium via the blood or they are produced there under the effect of different hormonal actions. Therefore, the presence of any infection or substance, which is toxic for embryo development, or any anatomic change which distorts the structure and functional transformation of all or part of the endometrium could provoke changes in the peri-implantative phase, which will lead to miscarriage. Congenital uterine anomalies with bad septal vascularization, or in any case with inadequate terminal vascularization of the intrauterine area coming from the defective fusion or reabsorption of the müllerian ducts, could lead to miscarriage. The same thing happens with the endometrium, which lines submucous leiomyomas, due to the distortioning and irritative effect it has on the rest of the endometrial cavity; or with the endometrium absent to a greater or lesser degree in the case of synechiae (intrauterine adhesions). On the other hand, especially after the first term of gestation, the following factors are involved: (1) capacity of growth, distention and conformation of the uterus, as well as the later conversion from a spherical form into a cylindrical form; and (2) the adaptation of the structures to cervical closure. Both factors become affected in many uterine anomalies, and for this reason there is a greater frequency of late miscarriages and pre- or immature births. Some authors [2] have not observed deficiency in septal vascularization of malformed uteri, but they have noted a decrease in connective tissue and an increase in muscular tissue, which could be the cause of miscarriage because of the high and uncoordinated contractility of these muscular areas.

## 2. Analysis of the causes of recurrent miscarriages susceptible to surgical treatment

### 2.1. Synechiae

Synechiae, or intrauterine adhesions in the uterine cavity, are frequently quoted as contributing to miscarriage. However, the evidence is not clear and these synechiae are more likely the result of repeated curettages. In any case, although evidence is scarce, the absence of the endometrium to a greater or lesser degree and the deformation of the useful cavity could in theory be contributing factors in recurrent miscarriage. Valli et al. [3] observed them among the hysteroscopic findings of 344 women, 4% with recurrent miscarriage against 2% in the control group, without any significant differences.

## 2.2. Leiomyomas

Leiomyomas are also frequently mentioned among the causes of recurrent miscarriage. However, it is not very likely that myomas are the cause of miscarriage. At least, that is what should happen with subserous myomas. In other cases, to the contrary, myomas could be the cause because: First, submucous myomas and others, which affect the endometrium and its vascularization, clearly seem to be a justifiable cause. Second, after myomectomy normal pregnancy has been observed. Therefore, intramural myomas, and especially those that are submucous, could evidently be the cause of miscarriage and recurrent miscarriage in certain patients. In our material [4], myomas were present in 18% of the cases of recurrent miscarriage. However, in several of these cases, myomas were subserous and/or they were small intramural myomas, along with other associated causal factors, and so we do not believe they were a well-defined cause of miscarriage. Nevertheless, in other studies [5] we have observed a certain relationship; although the myomas were not frequently related to recurrent miscarriage, when they were, myomectomy corrected such a recurrent miscarriage. In more recent publications [6], 14% of women with recurrent miscarriage had myomas and 50% of them did not have any other detectable cause of recurrent miscarriage. Therefore, for up to 7% of women with recurrent miscarriage, the cause could lie in myomas.

Vollenhoven et al. [7] observed high rates of miscarriage if the implantation took place on submucous myomas, and in other publications [8,9], they also highlight the controversial association between intramural and subserous myomas with pregnancy loss. There is no prospective data that suggests whether these myomas increase the rate of miscarriage, nor up to what point they cause recurrent miscarriage. But in the mentioned studies, there was a high rate of pregnancy losses (60% and 19% in cases of recurrent miscarriage), which was reduced after myomectomy (to 33%), especially through the decrease in late miscarriages [8] and without differences between abdominal or laparascopic myomectomy [9]. A higher rate of late miscarriage related to myomas was also demonstrated by Salvador et al. [10]; 7% in cases with myomas with or without genetic amniocentesis versus <1% in cases with genetic amniocentesis without the presence of myomas.

With regards to *myomectomy*, although myomas are not symptomatic (apart from infertility or recurrent miscarriage), we recommend myomectomy, preferably abdominal myomectomy following a careful technique [5] as long as the myoma or myomas are larger than 3–4 cm and before trying for pregnancy. Our recommendation is based on: (1) Although myomas do not make difficulties for the pregnancy, they grow during gestation and occasionally provoke serious problems, especially painful symptoms at the beginning of the second term, apart from delivery-related problems; (2) If there is a need to operate during gestation, myomectomy (although it can be done) is a complicated and risky technique; and (3) As the possibilities of implantation and pregnancy in assisted reproduction sometimes decrease, we always recommend myomectomy before these techniques.

Present evidence suggests the beneficial effect of myomectomy as a treatment for cases of recurrent miscarriage without other causes, but there are no prospective studies that adequately confirm this.

## 2.3. Cervical insufficiency or incompetence

Cervical incompetence is generally defined as the incapacity to support or take a pregnancy to its full term due to a functional or structural defect of the cervix. The problem is its diagnosis before pregnancy or at the beginning of gestation in order to evaluate the need for cerclage. Of course, the congenital form (frequently related with uterine malformations), as well as the acquired form (generally in relation to a traumatic obstetric history), is well known as a cause of late miscarriages and immature births. In our earlier studies [1], cervical incompetence was diagnosed in 39 patients (22%), but it was associated with a uterine anomaly in 22 cases (56%) and in 11 patients (6.4%) it was found as the only detected cause possibly related. In any case, the repercussion of uterine anomalies on the structures of cervical closure should be considered. But besides this, it is necessary to also investigate the clinical history for previous traumatic obstetric and gynecological problems (cervical laceration, fetal extractions, forced cervical dilatation in previous curettages, conization with cold knife, etc). The existence of late miscarriages, a cervical channel which is too wide in the hysterosalpingography (HSG) and a Hegar test showing permeability without force to dilator No. 7 or higher in the second half of the cycle (always beginning with higher numbers and decreasing), will permit a diagnosis of cervical insufficiency outside of pregnancy. Therefore, for the next pregnancy a prophylactic cerclage is carried out at about 12–14 weeks of amenorrhea, and not before, because the general principle is that early miscarriages (before 12 weeks) should not be attributed to cervical insufficiency, although it also exists.

However, such cervical cerclage has been a controversial subject during the last few years and these controversies refer to the effectiveness, safety and risk/benefit as much for the mother as for the foetus. It is said that avoiding cervical trauma could be as effective as the operation. There have been many randomized and non-randomized studies on the effectiveness of cerclage. The latest studies are meta-analyses [11,12], revisions about therapeutic or emergency cerclage [13] and the meta-analysis-revision of Cochrane [14]. The only effectiveness shown was a small reduction in premature births before 33 weeks (RR 0.75, 95% CI 0.58–0.98), and the conclusion by the Cochrane reviewers is that cervical cerclage should not be offered to women at low or medium risk of mid-trimester loss, regardless of cervical length by ultrasound. However, we would like to analyse this revision of Cochrane a little further, because we do not share the same diagnostic and randomized criteria for the studies included, nor for the meta-analysis results. None of the studies included in the meta-analysis based the randomization for carrying out prophylactic cerclage or not on the mentioned pre-gestational tests (HSG and Hegar test), but only on the obstetric record. Therefore, many cerclages have been carried out unnecessarily. History alone is not an indication for prophylactic cerclage [15]. We believe when there is a suggestive history and in any case with recurrent miscarriage, an HSG should be carried out to evaluate the morphology of the uterine cavity (frequently associated with uterine malformation) and the width of the cervical channel. Likewise, a Hegar test is necessary. In these cases, we believe that not carrying out prophylactic cerclage between 12 and 14 weeks is to run a great risk of another miscarriage.

At present, a short cervical length by ultrasound (<25 or<30 mm) is highly appreciated in women with a high risk of late miscarriage, in order to then apply cerclage instead of the early elective or prophylactic form [16–19]. But the conclusions of the Cochrane revision and those of other meta-analyses are that the role of cerclage in women with a shortened cervix by ultrasound studies (therapeutical cerclage) remains uncertain as the numbers of randomised women are too few to draw firm conclusions. Short cervical length is not an indication for a therapeutic cerclage [15], and the comparison of its results with that from the cerclage carried out only from the history data does not seem appropriate to us either (see Ref. [16]). Neither are there conclusions about emergency cerclage, nor about the technique or via vaginal or abdominal for elective cerclage. We recommend prophylactic cerclage in the presence of suggestive antecedents of cervical incompetence and after HSG and Hegar tests, which also indicate this, but especially if there is some associated uterine malformation.

## 2.4. Congenital uterine anomalies

Here we will underline several aspects.

### 2.4.1. Controversies about the cataloguing of uterine malformations and the importance of each type of uterine anomaly in miscarriage

The main controversies arise because of: (1) Cases that should be included as uterine malformation: inclusion or not of the hypoplastic uterus, of the arcuate uterus, etc., that is to say the minor uterine anomalies, or only the uterine malformations which are clinically well recognised (subseptate, septate, bicornuate, unicornuate or didelphys uterus). We believe that, in any case, they should be analysed separately, since, for example, early miscarriages are more frequent among these minor anomalies and perhaps they are not related directly to the malformation or anomaly whereas the major malformations are related to late miscarriage and immature birth, also in relation to the associated cervical insufficiency. (2) The criteria for cataloguing these clinically well-recognised anomalies. Such criteria are in general well established, but because the diagnostic investigation is incomplete or because there are many transitional cases among septate and bicornuate uterus, the differences observed in fertility problems between these two anomalies in different published series are enormous. We have informed about worse fertility results in the arcuate and bicornuate uterus in different publications. However, other authors have observed worse reproductive results in the septate uterus in such a way that this malformation has miscarriage percentages, which oscillate between 21–26% and 85–94% (see Ref. [20]). It is even said that "recurrent first trimester pregnancy loss is associated with uterine septum but not with bicornuate uterus" [21], but when we analyse the HSG figures included in this publication or the hysteroscopic observation of septate uterus, we do not share the diagnostic criteria of the authors. And this is also related to the systematic recommendation or not for metroplasty (previously done through laparatomy and now through hysteroscopy) in order to correct the malformation, very often even in the absence of a history of obstetric problems.

### 2.4.2. The role of uterine anomalies in miscarriage and recurrent miscarriage

Uterine malformations are observed in 30% of patients with recurrent miscarriage, but it depends on the inclusion criteria in the recurrent miscarriage and in such anomalies [22]. In the series of 189 patients with recurrent miscarriage analysed by Acién [1], 7.5% had hypoplastic uterus, 9% arcuate, 12% bicornuate and 8% presented with other malformations, which included septate uterus. That is to say, there were uterine anomalies in 37% of women with recurrent miscarriage if we include hypoplastic uterus. Inversely, congenital uterine anomalies are associated with pregnancy losses in 40–50% of women who suffer from them, although this also depends on the type of anomaly and in 17% of the cases there is a recurrent miscarriage. In our studies [23], 36% of the gestations ended in early (29%) or late (17%) miscarriage in the cases with malformation versus 15% of women with normal uteri. And this incidence is much higher for the bicornuate uterus, and lower in the septate uterus. We also observed that if among the recurrent miscarriages there are cases of late miscarriage or immature birth, then uterine anomalies are observed with even more frequency (49% against 33% if there are only early miscarriages). The clinically well-recognised uterine anomalies are present in 3% of all women, the same percentage in infertile women, while these major anomalies were observed in more than 5% of cases with recurrent miscarriage [24].

The termination of pregnancy, following the study of all the patients with recurrent miscarriages, showed that *20%* of them have an early (15%) or late (5%) miscarriage again (increasing significantly with the number of miscarriages). But, if the recurrent miscarriage is related to or the women also have a uterine anomaly, then miscarriage would happen again in *30%* of the cases (20% early and 10% late).

In short, uterine anomalies are an evident cause of miscarriage and recurrent miscarriage (the latter, in at least 20% of the cases) as much in one sense or the other. If minor anomalies are included, there will logically be many more uterine malformations among miscarriages, and if there are more recurrent miscarriages, and especially, if late miscarriages and immature deliveries are included, then the uterine malformation is also much more likely.

### 2.4.3. Management and reproductive results for each type of uterine anomaly

Management differs according to the type of genital anomaly and we have analysed them in relation to therapeutic approach. In this sense, although some authors are in favour of correcting the malformation as soon as it is diagnosed, a conservative approach, in general, is recommended for uterine anomalies. Thereby, we can rule out and eventually treat other possible, associated etiological factors and carry out only one cerclage, even prophylactic, in the 12th week of pregnancy if there is cervical insufficiency, which we would recommend.

#### 2.4.3.1. Hypoplastic uterus-DES syndrome.
This is particularly related to early miscarriage, but frequently other associated causes exist that could justify recurrent miscarriage. For this reason, some authors do not include it, although it can be observed in 12% of recurrent cases. The approach in the case of this anomaly could be to carry out a hysteroscopic metroplasty, although cervical cerclage, even prophylactic, seems to be preferred if there is a history of late miscarriage or immature delivery. The usefulness of hysteroscopic metroplasty is still to be demonstrated. However, Barranger et al. [25] have observed an increase in the rate of births from 3.8% to 63.2% after metroplasty, and indicate that for malformed-hypoplastic uteri, it is the operation of choice. There are no randomized studies and in any case, this percentage can be obtained without treatment.

#### 2.4.3.2. Bicornuate uterus.
In our material, it is the genital anomaly that is most frequently associated with miscarriage and recurrent miscarriage. The controversy exists because of the problems of differential diagnosis with the septate uterus; however, many authors assign this latter anomaly to the worst reproductive development. The fact that the possibilities and

means of surgical correction are totally different should also be considered. In the case of the bicornuate uterus, Strassman metroplasty by laparotomy can be carried out, but as cervical incompetence is frequent in these patients, many authors recommend cervical cerclage, even prophylactic, as primary treatment. If this fails or miscarriage occurs again, then the Strassman operation should be carried out.

*2.4.3.3. Didelphys uterus.* This is rarely related to recurrent miscarriage and does not require specific treatment, although in some cases cerclage may be necessary.

*2.4.3.4. Unicornuate uterus.* Practices are similar to those for didelphys uterus.

*2.4.3.5. Septate uterus.* We have already indicated that for many authors it is the anomaly with the worst reproductive result, although in our material it is not the case with regards to recurrent miscarriage. It is true we have frequently observed premature births and the cause of this could be in the increase of intrauterine pressure, with a greater probability of associated cervical incompetence [26]. Because of the risk of miscarriage, many authors recommend hysteroscopic resection of the septate as soon as it is diagnosed; however, the finding of a septate uterus per se is not an indication for surgical intervention because it is not always associated with poor obstetric performance [20]. Operation should be considered when there is adverse reproductive outcome, and other authors only recommend cerclage if there is cervical insufficiency, or in a prophylactic form. The results in this case, with regard to live births, are also 80% in our material, which is similar or higher to those given by other authors [27–29] after conventional or hysteroscopic metroplasty. However, we think that the hysteroscopic metroplasty should be carried out if miscarriages are repeated.

Several studies present the positive outcome of surgery, and in particular hysteroscopic metroplasty, if there are uterine malformations and recurrent miscarriage. They also indicate the spectacular improvement in percentages for the consecution of viable pregnancies. But as we have commented, this can also be achieved by expectation only (we already mentioned 68%) or by only carrying out cerclage if there is cervical insufficiency (about 80%). There is not one randomized and prospective study, which analyses this matter. For this reason, we have indicated that except in specific cases (20% of septate or bicornuate uterus with recurrent miscarriages), abdominal or hysteroscopic metroplasty is not necessary. And although the simplicity and low risk of the hysteroscopic technique permits its liberal use at present, it does not exclude a higher risk of uterine rupture in a future pregnancy, and it does not mean that we should exclude the convenience of carrying out prophylactic cerclage during the following pregnancy.

*2.5. Endometriosis*

This pathology has also been referred to as among the causes of recurrent miscarriage. But on the basis of controlled, prospective studies, there is no evidence that endometriosis is associated with (recurrent) pregnancy loss or that medical or surgical treatment of endometriosis reduces the spontaneous abortion rate [30], and this is also our opinion.

## References

[1] P. Acién, Uterine anomalies and recurrent miscarriage, Infertil. Reprod. Med. Clin. North Am. 7 (1996) 689–719.

[2] H. Dabirashrafi, et al., Septate uterus: New idea on the histologic features of the septum in this abnormal uterus, Am. J. Obstet. Gynecol. 172 (1995) 105–107.
[3] E. Valli, et al., Hysteroscopic findings in 344 women with recurrent spontaneous abortion, J. Am. Assoc. Gynecol. Laparosc. 8 (2001) 398–401.
[4] P. Acién, Miomas: clínica y diagnóstico. Mioma y embarazo, Cuad. Med. Reprod. 5 (1999) 51–73.
[5] P. Acién, F. Quereda, Abdominal myomectomy: results of a simple operative technique, Fertil. Steril. 65 (1996) 41–51.
[6] P. Acién, Miomas y reproducción, in: J. En Remohí, A. Pellicer, C. Simón, J. Navarro (Eds.), Reproducción Humana, 2nd ed., McGraw-Hill. Interamericana, Madrid, 2002, pp. 245–262.
[7] B.J. Vollenhoven, A.S. Lawrence, D. Healy, Uterine fibroids: a clinical review, Br. J. Obstet. Gynaecol. 97 (1990) 285–298.
[8] T.C. Li, R. Mortimer, I.D. Cooke, Myomectomy: a retrospective study to examine reproductive performance before and after surgery, Hum. Reprod. 14 (1999) 1735–1740.
[9] S. Campo, V. Campo, P. Gambadauro, Reproductive outcome before and after laparoscopic or abdominal myomectomy for subserous or intramural myomas, Eur. J. Obstet., Gynecol., Reprod. Biol. 110 (2003) 215–219.
[10] E. Salvador, et al., Leiomyomata uteri, genetic amniocentesis, and the risk of second-trimester spontaneous abortion, Am. J. Obstet. Gynecol. 186 (2002) 913–915.
[11] L.M. Bachmann, et al., Elective cervical cerclage for prevention of preterm birth: a systematic review, Acta Obstet. Gynecol. Scand. 82 (2003) 398–404.
[12] A.O. Odibo, et al., Prevention of preterm birth by cervical cerclage compared with expectant management: a systematic review, Obstet. Gynecol. Surv. 58 (2003) 130–136.
[13] J.H. Harger, Cerclage and cervical insufficiency: an evidence-based analysis, Obstet. Gynecol. 100 (2002) 1313–1327.
[14] A.J. Drakeley, D. Roberts, Z. Afirevic, Cervical stitch (cerclage) for preventing pregnancy loss in women (Cochrane Review). The Cochrane Library, Issue 4, Wiley, Chichester, UK, 2003.
[15] S.M. Althuisius, G.A. Dekker, H.P. van Geijn, Cervical incompetence: a reappraisal of an obstetric controversy, Obstet. Gynecol. Surv. 57 (2002) 377–387.
[16] S. Kelly, et al., Early transvaginal ultrasonography versus early cerclage in women with an unclear history of incompetent cervix, Am. J. Obstet. Gynecol. 184 (2001) 1097–1099.
[17] D. Kassanos, et al., The value of transvaginal ultrasonography in diagnosis and management of cervical incompetence, Clin. Exp. Obstet. Gynecol. 28 (2001) 266–268.
[18] M.S. To, et al., Elective cerclage vs. ultrasound-indicated cerclage in high-risk pregnancies, Ultrasound Obstet. Gynecol. 19 (2002) 475–477.
[19] J. Owen, J.D. Iams, J.C. Hauth, Vaginal sonography and cervical incompetence, Am. J. Obstet. Gynecol. 188 (2003) 586–596.
[20] H.A. Homer, T.C. Li, I.D. Cooke, The septate uterus: a review of management and reproductive outcome, Fertil. Steril. 73 (2000) 1–14.
[21] J.A. Proctor, A.F. Haney, Recurrent first trimester pregnancy loss is associated with uterine septum but not with bicornuate uterus, Fertil. Steril. 80 (2003) 1212–1215.
[22] P. Acién, Alteraciones del aparato genital como causa de aborto, Rev. Iber. Fertil. 1 (2000) 41–54.
[23] P. Acién, Reproductive performance of women with uterine malformations, Hum. Reprod. 8 (1993) 122–126.
[24] P. Acién, Incidence of Müllerian defects in fertile and infertile women, Hum. Reprod. 12 (1997) 1372–1376.
[25] E. Barranger, et al., Reproductive performance after hysteroscopic metroplasty in the hypoplastic uterus: a study of 29 cases, BJOG 109 (2002) 1331–1334.
[26] J.A. Rock, A.A. Murphy, Anatomic abnormalities, Clin. Obstet. Gynecol. 29 (1986) 886–911.
[27] A. Ayhan, et al., Reproductive performance after conventional metroplasty: an evaluation of 102 cases, Fertil. Steril. 57 (1992) 1194–1196.
[28] N. Colarcurci, et al., Reproductive outcome after hysteroscopic metroplasty, Eur. J. Obstet. Gynecol. Reprod. Biol. 66 (1996) 147–150.
[29] G. Porcu, et al., Hysteroscopic metroplasty for septate uterus and repetitive abortions: reproductive outcome, Eur. J. Obstet. Gynecol. Reprod. Biol. 88 (2000) 81–84.
[30] E.E. Vercammen, T.M. D'Hooghe, Endometriosis and recurrent pregnancy loss, Semin. Reprod. Med. 18 (2000) 363–368.

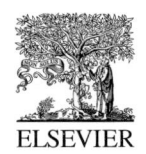

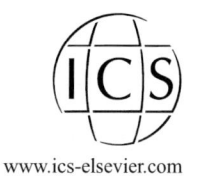

# Paediatric outcome following infertility management/genetic outcome

Maryse Bonduelle*

*Centre for Medical Genetics, University Hospital—Dutch-speaking Free University of Brussels, AZ VUB, Laarbeeklaan, 101, B 1090 Brussels, Belgium*

**Abstract.** *Introduction*: A higher number of genetic problems in children born after ART can be expected due to the ART procedures themselves and due to parental characteristics of the population needing these procedures. *Materials and results*: Most of the recent IVF and ICSI studies indicate that there is a slightly higher risk of congenital malformations in children born after ART in comparison to children in the general population. This risk seems to be mostly related to parental background, more specifically to factors such as a higher maternal age, a longer period of infertility prior to conception, pre-existing parental diseases or genetic conditions, etc. However, a procedure-related risk cannot be ruled out completely either. An increase in malformations of specific organ systems was reported in a few studies but not confirmed by others. No increase in major malformations was found to be associated with the use of sperm from different sperm sources such as testicular sperm or with the use of very poor sperm quality. If a major malformation is estimated (following a clearly defined definition and methodology) to be present in approximately 2.5% of newborns, then a risk of 3.5% is to be given in ICSI or IVF children. A higher rate of non-balanced inherited chromosomal anomalies was reported (1.4%), mainly due to paternal structural chromosomal anomalies, as well as a higher rate of de novo chromosomal anomalies (1.6%), related to paternal sperm characteristics. Animal research and recent reports in literature warn that there could be a low risk of epigenetic defects and rare diseases (such as the Beckwith–Wiedemann syndrome) related to imprinting disorders, but this has to be further elucidated. *Conclusion*: Parents should be told that a possible effect of the ART techniques on the outcome of the children (in terms of chromosomal anomalies and malformations) cannot be excluded, but that it is probably far less important than the underlying parental background. Extensive counselling and a search for individual risk factors can help to modify the individual risk for each couple. A systematic survey aimed at those syndromes and at defined phenotypes linked to imprinted genes may clarify whether epigenetic anomalies play a role in ART more often than in the general population. © 2004 Published by Elsevier B.V.

*Keywords:* Congenital malformation; Follow-up study; Intracytoplasmatic sperm injection; In vitro fertilisation; Children; Prenatal diagnosis

---

* Tel.: +32-2-4776071; fax: +32-2-4776860.
  *E-mail address:* maryse.bonduelle@az.vub.ac.be (M. Bonduelle).

0531-5131/ © 2004 Published by Elsevier B.V.
doi:10.1016/j.ics.2004.02.001

## 1. Introduction

### 1.1. Risk of IVF and ICSI

Even though great concern was voiced in 1978 at the introduction of IVF, no formal and systematic evaluation of the outcome of this high-tech procedure was carried out and relatively few studies on the children were undertaken. Gradually, IVF became accepted as a safe technique, mostly on the basis of the information in registries with retrospectively collected data. When ICSI was introduced it was considered a risky procedure from the start [1]. ICSI is indeed a more invasive procedure than classic IVF, since one spermatozoon is injected through the oocyte membrane and fertilisation can ensue from sperm which would otherwise not have been fit or mature enough to achieve fertilisation [2].

Since its introduction ICSI has spread over the world and various initiatives to collect data on the children have been undertaken. Much more attention was given to possible adverse effects for the children born after ICSI and controlled studies on the outcome of the children were prospectively initiated [3–5].

#### 1.1.1. Reasons for concern in IVF and ICSI: genetic and epigenetic risk

At the introduction of IVF in 1978 a number of concerns were raised and animal data suggested a possible risk due to in vitro culture techniques. These concerns included: an altered hormonal environment, the loss of a selective mechanism against morphologically abnormal sperm in vivo, and point mutations due to various chemical exposures in the in vitro procedure. Since 1993 it was clear from animal research that culture of preimplantation embryos can affect foetal development and expression of imprinted genes [6].

At the introduction of the ICSI procedure two types of risks were mentioned by several authors: ICSI procedure-dependent and ICSI procedure-independent risk factors.

Concerning the ICSI-independent risk factor, there is no doubt that spermatozoa used for ICSI have higher levels of defects (chromosomal or monogenic), which are in turn likely to have an adverse effect on embryo development, e.g. increased levels of aneuploidy in the spermatozoa and higher risks of transmitting an already existing genetic disease or transmitting gene defects related to the fertility problem. A major concern was also the bypassing of the natural selection process since ICSI circumvents several steps necessary in the natural fertilisation process. However, other researchers argue that even in spontaneous conceptions, there is no natural selection of spermatozoa [7].

Microinjection of sperm carrying a chromosomal anomaly is probably the major cause of finding the higher rate of chromosomal anomalies in the foetuses. The ICSI-dependent risk, related to the procedure itself, which involves the penetration of the zona pellucida and oocyte cytoplasm, may result in a number of problems such as damage to the internal structure of the oocyte leading to aneuploidisation and an increased risk of chromosomal anomalies. Other risk factors include the injection of biochemicals of foreign, sperm-associated exogenous DNA and the injection of paternal mitochondrial DNA.

### 1.2. Detection of the genetic and epigenetic risk

In order to detect a possible increase of the above mentioned mechanisms a systematic examination of the children searching for congenital anomalies, for malformative syndromes, for karyotype anomalies and for infertility problems should be established. In order to evaluate the whole range of possible genetic or epigenetic mechanisms, a further evaluation of the long-term health status, of the incidence of childhood cancer and of mental development should be carried out.

## 2. Registration of congenital anomalies

Congenital malformations arise from three major mechanisms: genetic, responsible for 15–25%, environmental for approximately 10% (including maternal infections, uteroplacental problems and maternal exposure to drugs and other toxins) and multifactorial diseases (combined effect of genetic and environmental factors) responsible for 20–25%. Within the genetic diseases a majority is related to chromosome anomalies (10–15%) whereas a minority is related to single gene defects (2–10%). Other mechanisms such as imprinting problems are a minor cause of multiple congenital anomaly syndromes such as Beckwith–Wiedemann.

Observing major congenital anomalies is not a straightforward task. Very variable malformation rates have been reported in ART children. These malformation rates have been compared with children born after natural conception, for whom data were recorded in a registry. For a number of reasons, however, it is not possible to compare these data sets [9]. In the following remarks we shall try to give an overview of the possible problems encountered when interpreting different studies.

### 2.1. Different type of risk factors

If children born after ART are compared with children in the general population or to a selected control group out of the general population we must be aware that different types of risk factors can be present in the two populations. Under these risk factors demographic variables (such as maternal age, numbers of years of unwanted childlessness, parity, exposure to environmental agents, smoking and drinking habits, social class, multiplicity) and general health can be different.

Genetic background can also differ in both populations and can be expressed by the number of miscarriages, pregnancy losses, number of malformed foetuses or children, pregnancy complications and premature delivery. Genetic diseases in the parents or their relatives can also vary [10].

Moreover, ART treatment in itself can influence pregnancy outcome. Controlled ovarian stimulation in itself (without other fertility treatment) has been claimed to be responsible for a higher malformation rate [11], but this was not confirmed by other studies [12].

### 2.2. Pitfalls in registration of congenital anomalies

Different pitfalls such as observation bias can occur when ART children who stay more often in neonatal units and tend to be examined more exhaustively and by specialised physicians. In this way, overestimation of the rate of anomalies can occur. Several definitions and classification systems can be used to classify a malformation as a major or a minor type (or not as a malformation) and even if standardised coding systems are used such as the International Classification of Diseases (ICD) [13], additional guidelines or definitions necessary to classify the malformations listed into major and minor conditions can differ from one study to another. Minor malformations can be taken into account or not [14]. If results from ART are compared with those in the general population, it would be better to separate the prenatally detected anomalies (in stillborn infants or in terminations for a foetal anomaly) from malformations detected at birth, since otherwise detection bias can be present. Duration of follow-up period in which the malformations are observed will influence malformation rate since approximately 30% of the congenital anomalies up to one year are registered after 1 month of age. Time period during which study and control group are examined should be simultaneous in order to limit a number of minor changes due to time related variables. Sample size has to be adequate to allow for meaningful conclusions. The proportion of children lost for follow-up should remain minimal otherwise a skewing of the observed anomaly rate can occur. Control groups must be comparable and selected for similar characteristics of a number of maternal demographic and health characteristics.

## 3. Evaluation of the major published studies

### 3.1. IVF compared with the general population evaluation of major studies

Different extensive studies based on register data analysis have yielded contradictory results. After confounders were taken into account the difference disappeared in the studies of Westergaard, Ericson and Anthony but remained in the Hansen study even after adjusting for maternal age, parity, sex and sibling correlation (OR 2.0; 95% CI: 1.5–2.9) [15–18]. This study did not, however, control for a number of variables (as explained in the next paragraph), which could have been different in the two populations and could have led to different results.

### 3.2. ICSI compared with the general population evaluation of major studies

#### 3.2.1. Retrospective studies comparing ICSI children with registers

Two Swedish studies based on register-based data analysis have shown an increase in major malformations in ICSI (OR 1.75; CI: 1.19–2.58) [19] as well as in IVF (OR 1.47; CI: 1.34–1.61) [16]. However, after adjustment for maternal age, year of birth and multiple births [19], as well as time of unwarranted childlessness [16], the difference disappeared.

In the Australian study [18], congenital malformations at the age of one year the odds ratio for malformations in ICSI compared with the general population remained 2.0 (95% CI: 1.3–3.2) even after adjustment for maternal age, parity, sex and sibling correlation. The authors could not, however, adjust for number of years of infertility or other sociodemographic factors such as ethnic background, which could have been different in the two populations.

#### 3.2.2. Prospective studies comparing ICSI children with control groups

Only one study on ICSI children was designed with a prospective protocol on a group of ICSI children ($n=3372$) compared with a selected control group out of the general population ($n$=8016) [5]. This prospective standardised cohort study in Germany compared major malformation rate in ICSI children with the malformation rates in a population-based control cohort. This resulted in a crude relative risk (RR) of 1.44 (95% CI: 1.25–1.65) After adjustment for different risk factors the risk declined to 1.24 (95% CI: 1.02–1.50) showing that parental background played a role in the increase of congenital malformations in ICSI.

### 3.3. ICSI compared with IVF

Major malformations in ICSI compared to IVF were studied in a prospective study on a cohort of 2995 IVF and 2889 ICSI children (liveborn and stillborn) by Bonduelle et al. [3]. No difference in malformation rate was found between ICSI and IVF children with 3.4% major malformation in ICSI and 3.8% in IVF. When total malformation rate was considered including terminations for foetal anomaly and stillbirths, similar results were obtained with 4.2% total major malformations in ICSI and 4.7% in IVF.

### 3.4. Malformations in different organ systems

Differences in malformation frequency per organ system were reported by several authors in IVF as well as in ICSI. None of these reports were consistent, apart from the fact that if a difference was found it was always larger in the ART group than in the control group. An increase of uro-genital malformations in ICSI [4,16,19] was reported in several studies, but only in IVF in others [18]. Comparison of all uro-genital malformations in ICSI compared with IVF by Bonduelle et al. [3] led to the conclusion that no difference could be recorded on 2840 liveborn ICSI and 2955 IVF children. Information on the uro-genital status of the parents is lacking in all these studies and this parental genetic background could be the key factor responsible for this relatively small increase of uro-genital malformations.

### 3.5. ART and chromosomal anomalies

In the series of 1586 prenatal tests described by Bonduelle et al. [20], statistically more de novo chromosomal anomalies (1.6%) (mainly due to a 2- to 3-fold increase of sex chromosomal anomalies) as well as inherited (1.4%) anomalies were found in ICSI compared with the general population. Other literature data show similar results on very limited numbers.

### 3.6. ICSI in relation to sperm quality and sperm source

There is increasing evidence that in severe oligo- and azospermic patients with serious testicular failure a higher chromosomal aneuploidy rate is present in the sperm. Several studies also support an association between morphological aberration or abnormal motility and sperm chromosome aneuploidy. More chromosomal anomalies (2.1%) were found in foetuses when spermatozoa from men with a sperm count of less than $<20.10^6$/ml were used in comparison to higher concentrations (1.6%) [20]. However, this difference was not reflected in a higher percentage of congenital anomalies in the children born from fathers with more abnormal sperm parameters; neither was a difference observed when spermatozoa from other sources than ejaculate were used [4,19,21]. However, all these results have to be considered with caution since the numbers of children born in these subgroups are still very limited.

### 3.7. Rare imprinting disorders

Genomic imprinting describes the exclusive expression of a gene from only one of the parental alleles. Many imprinted genes play a key role in embryonic development and foetal growth.

Imprinted genes are functionally haploid and may therefore be more vulnerable to inducing diseases when subjected to mutations or to epi-mutations, if these occur during the early exposure of gametes and embryo to artificial conditions. The imprinting process itself may be disturbed by in vitro culture leading to aberrantly imprinted genes which was already shown in animal studies. Only recently, evidence for a higher risk of these imprinting anomalies has been documented in IVF and ICSI children, since multiple reports on imprinting syndromes have been published [22,23,24,25,26]. DeBaun et al. [23], Maher et al. [25] and Giquel et al. [24] report evidence that ART is associated with BWS on the basis of a higher frequency (3- to 6-fold) of history of ART in a BWS registry than in the general population. This risk has however not yet been established in prospective follow-up studies. On the basis of all these findings, sufficient evidence exists to suggest that some aspects of the ICSI procedure may increase the frequency of epigenetic anomalies leading to congenital malformation syndromes. As all imprinting disorders are rare disorders a large sample size is needed to detect minor increases.

## 4. Conclusions

Most of the recent IVF and ICSI studies indicate that there is a slightly higher risk of congenital malformations in the ART population in comparison with a control group out of the general population. This risk seems to be related to the parental background, more specifically to influencing factors such as a higher maternal age, a lower parity, a longer period of infertility prior to conception, parental pre-existing disease or genetic condition, etc. There is also evidence that these influencing factors determine the differences found in literature between ICSI, IVF and naturally conceived children. Parents should be told that a possible effect of the ART techniques cannot be excluded, but that it is probably far less important than the underlying parental background. If a major malformation is estimated (following a certain definition and methodology) to be present in approximately 2.5% of the newborns, then in ICSI or IVF children a risk of 3.5% is to be given. Moreover, there could be a very low risk of rare diseases related to imprinting disorders that has to be further elucidated. Extensive counselling and searching for individual risk factors can help to modify the individual risk for each couple. More research is also needed in order to evaluate the importance of the different influencing factors.

Only a systematic survey aimed at those syndromes/diseases which have a known, defined phenotype linked to imprinted genes may clarify whether epigenetic anomalies play a role in ART more often than in the general population. Further biological studies are required in order to understand the pathogenesis of these events and to find out whether precautions can be taken to prevent their occurrence.

## Acknowledgements

Vera Van Beneden is kindly acknowledged for helping with the references.

## References

[1] G.P. Palermo, et al., Pregnancies after intracytoplasmic sperm injection of single spermatozoon into an oocyte, Lancet 340 (1992) 17–18.
[2] A. Van Steirteghem, et al., Higher success rate by intracytoplasmic sperm injection than by subzonal insemination. Report of a second series of 300 consecutive treatment cycles, Hum. Reprod. 8 (1993) 1055–1060.
[3] M. Bonduelle, et al., Neonatal data on a cohort of 2889 infants born after intracytoplasmic sperm injection (ICSI) (1991–1999) and of 2995 infants born after in vitro fertilization (IVF) (1983–1999), Hum. Reprod. 17 (2002) 671–694.
[4] M. Ludwig, A. Katalinic, Malformation rate in fetuses and children conceived after intracytoplasmic sperm injection (ICSI): results of a prospective cohort study, RBM Online 5 (2002) 171–178.
[5] A. Katalinic, C. Rösch, M. Ludwig, Pregnancy course and outcome after intracytoplasmic sperm injection (ICSI)—a controlled prospective cohort study, Fertil. Steril. (2004) (in press).
[6] L.E. Young, et al., Epigenetic change in IGF2R is associated with fetal overgrowth after sheep embryo culture, Nat. Genet. 27 (2001) 153–154.
[7] D. Sakkas, et al., Nature of DNA damage in ejaculated human spermatozoa and the possible involvement of apoptosis, Biol. Reprod. 66 (2002) 1061–1067.
[9] W. Engel, D. Murphy, M. Schmid, Are there genetic risks associated with microassisted reproduction? Hum. Reprod. 11 (1996) 2359–2370.
[10] D. Meschede, et al., Non-reproductive heritable disorders in infertile couples and their first degree relatives, Hum. Reprod. 15 (7) (2000) 1609–1612.
[11] P.A.L. Lancaster, Congenital malformations after in vitro fertilization, Lancet 1392 (1987) 3 (ii).
[12] J.L. Mills, et al., Risk of neural tube defects in relation to maternal fertility and fertility drug use, Lancet 336 (8707) (1990) 103–104.
[13] Manual of the International Statistical Classification of Diseases, Injuries and Causes of Death (ICD). Based on the 10th Revision Conference. World Health Organization, Geneva, 1992, ISBN:92 4 154419 8 (v.1).
[14] K.A. Leppig, et al., Predictive value of minor anomalies, association with major anomalies, J. Pediatr. 110 (1987) 531–537.
[15] H. Westergaard, et al., Danish National In-Vitro Fertilization Registry 1994 and 1995: a controlled study of births, malformations and cytogenetic findings, Hum. Reprod. 14 (1999) 1896–1902.
[16] A. Ericson, B. Kallen, Congenital malformations in infants born after IVF: a population based study, Hum. Reprod. 16 (2001) 504–509.
[17] S. Anthony, et al., Congenital malformations in 4224 children conceived after IVF, Hum. Reprod. 17 (8) (2002) 2089–2095.
[18] M. Hansen, et al., The risk of major birth defects after intracytoplasmic sperm injection and in vitro fertilization, NEJM 345 (10) (2002) 725–730.
[19] U.B. Wennerholm, et al., Incidence of congenital malformations in children born after ICSI, Hum. Reprod. 15 (2000) 944–948.
[20] M. Bonduelle, et al., Prenatal testing in ICSI pregnancies: incidence of chromosomal anomalies in 1586 karyotypes and relation to sperm parameters, Hum. Reprod. 17 (2002) 2600–2614.
[21] V. Vernaeve, et al., Pregnancy outcome and neonatal data of children born after ICSI using testicular sperm in obstructive and non-obstructive aoospermia, Hum. Reprod. 18 (2003) 1–5.
[22] G.F. Cox, et al., Intracytoplasmic sperm injection may increase the risk of imprinting defects, Am. J. Hum. Genet. 71 (2002) 162–164.
[23] M.R. DeBaun, E.L. Niemitz, A.P. Feinberg, Association of in vitro fertilization with Beckwith–Wiedemann syndrome and epigenetic alterations of LIT1 and H19, Am. J. Hum. Genet. 72 (2003) 156–160.

[24] C. Gicquel, et al., In vitro fertilisation may increase the risk of Beckwith Wiedemann syndrome related to the abnormal imprinting of KCNQ1OT gene, Am. J. Hum. Genet. 72 (2003) 1338–1341.
[25] E.R. Maher, et al., Beckwith–Wiedemann syndrome and assisted reproduction technology (ART), J. Med. Genet. 40 (2003) 62–64.
[26] A.C. Moll, et al., Incidence of retinoblastoma in children born after in-vitro fertilisation, Lancet 361 (2003) 273–274.

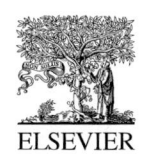

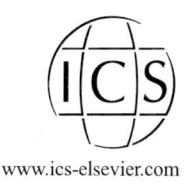

# Parenting and child psychosocial development after infertility management

Frances Gibson[a,*], Catherine McMahon[b]

[a] Department of Newborn Care, Royal North Shore Hospital, Pacific Highway, St Leonards, 2065 NSW, Australia
[b] Department of Psychology, Macquarie University, Sydney, 2109 NSW, Australia

**Abstract.** Infertility management through assisted reproductive technology (ART) has increased over several decades. Concerns have been expressed that the distress associated with infertility, together with the medical and psychosocial demands of ART, may impact adversely on subsequent family functioning. A review of current research, however, revealed few differences in parenting after ART, relative to natural conception families. The parenting characteristics identified (e.g. early, child-focused concerns, more protective attitudes and warmth in parenting) are best understood contextually, and do not appear to translate into differences in ART-conceived children's psychosocial development compared with naturally conceived peers. While cultural factors differentiate some aspects of ART parent adjustment, the findings indicate that protective social factors combined with an investment in parenthood mitigate adverse outcomes. Further targeted research is required as little is known of family adjustment beyond childhood or following conception through newer and less traditional ART procedures. © 2004 Published by Elsevier B.V.

*Keywords:* Parenting; Child; Psychosocial; Infertility; Assisted reproduction

## 1. Introduction

Medical intervention for infertility problems has increased over the past few decades, and in some developed countries up to 2% of children are conceived through assisted reproductive technology (ART). Infertility can be seen as a public, as well as a private problem, as treatment draws on public resources, requires policy to regulate it and poses psychological, sociological and ethical dilemmas for the community [1]. This paper provides an overview of what is currently known about parenting and child psychosocial development following ART. Background and salient research issues are introduced, and the findings are summarised from pregnancy to childhood and beyond with reference to theoretical constructs that assist our understanding of the special path to parenthood following ART.

\* Corresponding author. Tel.: +61-2-94134389 (alt. +61-2-99267509); fax: +61-2-94134574.
  *E-mail address:* frgibson@laurel.ocs.mq.edu.au (F. Gibson).

0531-5131/ © 2004 Published by Elsevier B.V.
doi:10.1016/j.ics.2004.01.116

## 2. Background

Assisted reproduction broadly encompasses ovulation induction (OI), artificial insemination (AI) and more invasive procedures such as in vitro fertilisation (IVF) or intracytoplasmic sperm injection (ICSI). Third party reproduction, including donor insemination (DI), conception using donor eggs or embryos or a gestational/surrogate mother, introduces more complex social issues in the process of conception and challenges the usual boundaries of relatedness.

Concern has been expressed that the psychosocial distress of infertility experienced by couples might impact negatively on subsequent parent–child relations [2]. There are also biological risks for ART pregnancies and children, since the chances of premature birth, lower birth weight and neonatal nursery admission are increased, although more so for multiple births [3,4]. Some uses of assisted conception are more controversial than others and potentially involve increased issues around secrecy or stigma for ART families, while other challenges to ART families include older parental age, family completion and frozen embryo dilemmas [2,4–6].

Despite the documented stresses associated with infertility and treatment, research has generally indicated that infertile families are no more vulnerable to psychological disturbance than non-infertile parents, and some studies concerning the parent–child relationship and child adjustment following ART have demonstrated more positive results [2,7]. Thus, the research has been reassuring, although not conclusive, in part due to the rapidly evolving nature of ART.

## 3. Research issues

A recent comprehensive review of parenting and the psychosocial development of children conceived through IVF confirmed a growing body of literature concerned with IVF family adjustment [7]. Several papers related to adjustment among a broader group of ART families have since been published [5,8–11]. Factors limiting integration of research findings include: more focus on obstetric and child development outcomes than on parenting, differences between samples, control groups, the salience of cultural factors and varied research instruments [2,7]. Availability of less traditional ART is not uniform cross-culturally and more likely to be socially and politically determined, further limiting the application of research findings. Finally, few studies have been embedded in theory that can assist differentiation of experiences, such as ART on parenting and child adjustment, or have used multiple methods (e.g. self-report, interview, observation) and cross-informants (e.g. mother, father, teacher) to increase reliability and validity [1,7]. Examples of theoretical constructs used to guide research to date include attachment theory and the importance of early parent–child relationships [1], parental warmth, responsiveness and sensitivity in relation to child development [5,8], specific aspects of parenting related to mode of conception (e.g. overprotectiveness) [1,12,13] and the role of contextual factors [7].

Belsky's [14] model of the determinants of parenting noted that the quality of parenting was related to an interaction between characteristics of the parents, characteristics of the child and contextual factors (e.g. social support). The current paper used this model, together with the notions of both risk and vulnerability leading to poorer outcome, and protection and resilience that might buffer against poorer outcome, to summarise the findings primarily from recent published reviews and studies concerned with ART parenting and child psychosocial development.

## 4. Current findings

### 4.1. Pregnancy

#### 4.1.1. Parental wellbeing and parenting

In the first study to recruit families conceiving through ART during pregnancy, IVF mothers revealed no differences compared with naturally conceiving mothers on general measures of mood state, personality and marital satisfaction, although they reported lower self-esteem and a more external locus of control [1]. In contrast, IVF fathers reported higher trait anxiety, lower marital satisfaction and self-esteem than controls [1]. While treatment effects differentiated certain aspects of the IVF pregnancy experience, IVF mothers reported a higher level of anxiety concerning health defects in their child and damage to their babies during childbirth and they engaged in less preparation for childbirth and parenthood. Despite these concerns, they did not differ from comparison mothers in self-report of attachment with the unborn baby [15].

Whereas McMahon et al. [1,15] investigated adjustment from 28 weeks of pregnancy, a recent study conducted more frequent assessments on couples during pregnancy at 13, 26 and 36 weeks [16]. Consistent with McMahon et al. [15], IVF mothers reported higher levels of anxiety over pregnancy loss compared with naturally conceiving mothers, although in contrast IVF fathers, not mothers, were concerned about injury to the baby during childbirth [16]. Possibly not surprisingly, IVF mothers and fathers with high recalled infertility distress were more anxious and concerned about the pregnancy than those with low recalled distress. Again, similarly to McMahon et al. [15], IVF mothers also differed from comparison mothers in that they experienced the pregnancy in a less negative way despite their concerns [16].

Both studies enrolled primiparous mothers with singleton IVF pregnancies [15,16]. Findings concerning quality of life issues for multiple birth families indicated the potential for some unique concerns during pregnancy [6]. Themes to emerge were the social stigma of a multiple pregnancy/birth, now viewed as infertility per se, and compounded pregnancy losses, including selective reduction [6]. These findings may well apply more powerfully to cultures where fertility treatment is provided in a "market-driven medical environment that is marked by competition for success rates" [6]. Nonetheless, there is a tension between risk reduction and both the physician and patient's desire for a live birth in ART pregnancies.

Women's attempts to become pregnant can be lengthy and typically accelerate from OI into more invasive, "hi-tech" procedures [6]. Thus, these findings may have some application to parents conceiving through the less traditional third party procedures, although more complex relationship issues are likely to be present.

### 4.2. Infancy

#### 4.2.1. Parent wellbeing and parenting

An observational study using small groups compared IVF, regular infertility treatment and naturally conceiving mothers in play with their infants from 4 to 21 weeks of age and found that non-infertile "maternal caretaking" (analogous to parental warmth and involvement) decreased over time relative to infertile and IVF mothers [17].

Colpin et al. [18] compared parenting stress and psychosocial wellbeing among three groups of parents with 1-year-old twins who conceived following hormonal treatment, through AI/IVF or without assistance. No group differences were found overall, however, first-time mothers with a history of infertility reported higher parenting stress and lower wellbeing than naturally conceiving first-time mothers and those with a history of infertility who had older children.

During the first year postpartum, no differences were found between IVF mothers and fathers and naturally conceiving parents on measures of mood, reported attachment to their child or in social support [1]. IVF mothers, however, reported lower self-esteem and sense of parenting competency at 4 months and saw their 1-year-old infant as more vulnerable and special while IVF fathers reported lower marital satisfaction at 12 months [1]. Despite these minor differences in parental adjustment, observational measures revealed no differences between IVF and naturally conceiving mothers' behaviour in interaction with their child.

*4.2.2. Child psychosocial development*

Differences have not been found in parenting stress, due to child factors between 1-year-old ART twins compared with naturally conceived twins [18], or between IVF singletons and controls [1]. Nonetheless, IVF mothers of singletons reported more difficult infant temperament (mean scores in community range), and were more concerned about child behaviour during the first year [1]. Observational measures of child interaction with their mothers have led to slightly mixed findings with young IVF infants demonstrating more "fussy" behaviour and AI/IVF infants exhibiting more "play" behaviour relative to comparison groups [1,17]. This discrepancy may reflect differences in sampling (size, selection biases, neonatal factors) and observational methodologies. Regardless, at 12 months IVF singletons demonstrated predominantly secure attachment relationships and appropriate responsiveness in play with their mothers and did not differ from controls [1].

Golombok and MacCullum [5] concluded, from two controlled studies that included infants conceived following egg donation and children born following surrogacy, respectively, that there were no indications of detrimental outcome on parenting and child social emotional development.

*4.3. Childhood*

*4.3.1. Parent wellbeing and parenting*

Past research for this period has generally indicated parental psychological adjustment (depression, anxiety) and marital satisfaction to be within the community range and no different to comparison groups. Studies have indicated, compared with naturally conceiving parents, more favourable adjustment among IVF mothers (lower anxiety), cultural differences in IVF parenting stress and satisfaction, a higher sense of parental competence for both IVF and previously infertile mothers, and more maternal "emotional involvement" with their IVF children [5,7,12]. Hahn and DiPietro [12] also found IVF mothers reported higher levels of protectiveness towards their 3- to 7-year-old children, concurrent with teacher's ratings of higher maternal warmth, but not overprotective or intrusive parenting behaviour.

Recent research has also indicated overall, positive parent adjustment. Similar to Hahn and DiPietro [12], IVF and ICSI mothers of 5-year-old children reported more protective attitudes, although they did not differ in parenting stress from naturally conceiving mothers [13]. McMahon et al. [19] examined parenting stress, with respect to subsequent IVF treatment for parents of 5-year-olds, and found higher levels of treatment predicted lower maternal stress but more defensive responding, which may reflect a positive responding bias among IVF mothers or that they were highly motivated, competent parents.

A large Danish study found that parents of both ICSI/IVF and non-ICSI/IVF 3- to 4-year-old twins experienced more marital stress and a greater impact on the mother's life than for families of singletons [10]. Consistent with this finding of a twin rather than ART effect, Tully et al. [11] found no difference in maternal adjustment and parenting between mothers of 5-year-old twins conceived after IVF/OI and mothers who conceived naturally. Surprisingly, ISCI/IVF treatment predicted low separation/divorce in the Danish study and multiple births have also been reported to potentially improve marital stability as it threw couples into teamwork [6,11]. Thus, while concerns have been raised about the impact of multiple births on parental adjustment for ART families (reasonably so for higher order multiples), the desire to have a child may mitigate some of the difficulties.

Golombok and Murray [20] addressed the issue of social versus biological parenting through a study of families who had adopted children or conceived through IVF, DI, or egg donation. Although there was greater psychological wellbeing among parents in families where there was no genetic link between the mother and the child, there were no differences between groups in quality of parenting.

### 4.3.2. Child psychosocial development

Comprehensive investigations of ART children's functioning, including twins and those conceived through DI and egg donation, have examined behaviour (parent and teacher report), child perceptions of family relations, perceived competence and acceptance and self-reports of emotion [5,11–13,21,22]. The majority of studies have found behavioural and emotional adjustment in the community range and no difference between children conceived through various forms of ART and natural conception controls, however, some mixed findings have emerged. Whereas IVF 3- to 7-year-old children were rated with fewer behavioural problems than naturally conceived controls [12], 9- to 10-year-old children were more poorly adjusted at school and reported poorer emotional wellbeing [21]. IVF mothers of children under 4 years of age, compared with mothers who conceived through egg donation and IVF mothers of 5-year-olds in comparison to ICSI and naturally conceiving mothers, expressed more concern about child behaviour, even though in the latter study there were no group differences in behavioural adjustment based on parent and teacher completed questionnaires [13,22].

## 4.4. Beyond childhood

### 4.4.1. Parent wellbeing and parenting

Very few published studies have investigated families who conceived through ART beyond childhood. While DI has been in use for some time, non-disclosure of mode of conception and a lack of donor information has prevailed. Ideas of identity and origin are most salient in adolescence. Issues around mode of conception may arise and some parents might also begin to reflect upon their child's growing independence and autonomy, as well as their future fertility status.

Notwithstanding these potential concerns, Golombok et al. [23] used a standardised interview to examine parent–child relationships (child age 11–12 years) and, once again, found few differences in parenting, with those evident more related to the experience of infertility than ART. Mothers who experienced a period of infertility (IVF and adoptive mothers) received lower ratings of sensitive responding towards their child, although both mothers and fathers of IVF children demonstrated higher levels of warmth than adoptive parents and there were no differences in ratings of parental control. In a related study, no differences were identified between DI and IVF families for any variables relating to quality of relationship between parents and children [8].

### 4.4.2. Child psychosocial development

Standardised interviews were also used to gather perceptions of 11- to 12-year-old children concerning parent–child relationships in IVF, adoptive and naturally conceiving families [23]. Few differences were revealed, apart from mothers who experienced infertility being perceived as more dependable and both mothers and fathers being perceived as using less reasoning in regard to control. There was a low level of child "psychiatric" disorder across the three groups and no difference in maternal and teacher ratings of child prosocial and deviant behaviour [23]. Children conceived through DI were also reported as well adjusted in terms of their social emotional development at adolescence [5,9]. While these findings at adolescence are reassuring, anecdotal reports from adults who are aware of their DI conception have revealed more mixed feelings concerning relationships with parents [5].

## 5. Discussion

### 5.1. Parenting

Assisted conception following infertility appears to have little adverse impact on parent wellbeing and parenting. The differences identified have not indicated clinical problems, but more likely reflect realistic concerns and attitudes in the context of a long and sometimes high-risk path to achieving parenthood. During pregnancy, and to a lesser extent infancy, evidence of more concern over child wellbeing in the context of parental perceptions of child "specialness" was apparent. In childhood, parental expressions of more protective attitudes, but not overprotectiveness towards the child, and greater warmth have been shown. The evidence supports the notion that protective social factors (e.g. older, educated, financially stable) and parental qualities (e.g. satisfying relationships, adaptive problem solving, desire to have a child) may buffer against adverse parental outcomes.

### 5.2. Child psychosocial development

Fewer differences in child psychosocial adjustment following ART conception were evident than in parenting. The children appear to have secure attachment relationships with their parents in childhood and behavioural adjustment is mostly comparable with naturally conceived peers. Thus, overall differences in parental adjustment following infertility management do not appear to translate into differences in child psychosocial function.

As assisted reproductive technologies continue to evolve, so too will the challenges confronting families and practitioners. It is inevitable that some families will pioneer the way in dealing with new issues in parenting and relatedness as they arise. While there is a need for clinical audit and population-based studies to monitor potential high-risk outcomes, targeted research, particularly on parenting and developmental issues, can inform families and professionals alike. In conclusion, despite the fact that these families have "complex biogenetic origins"[2], their family relationships are more like those of naturally conceiving families than not.

## References

[1] C. McMahon, F. Gibson, A special path to parenthood: parent child relationships in families giving birth to singleton infants through IVF, Reprod. Biomed. Online 5 (2002) 179–186.
[2] L.H. Burns, Parenting after infertility, in: L.H. Burns, S.N. Covington (Eds.), Infertility Counselling: A Comprehensive Handbook for Clinicians, Parthenon Publishing Group, Pearl River NY, 1999, pp. 449–472.
[3] S. Koivurova, et al., Growth, psychomotor development and morbidity up to 3 years of age in children born after IVF, Hum. Reprod. 18 (2003) 2328–2336.
[4] F. Olivennes, et al., Perinatal outcome and developmental studies on children born after IVF, Hum. Reprod. 8 (2002) 117–128.
[5] S. Golombok, F. MacCallum, Practitioner review: outcomes for parents and children following non-traditional conception: what do clinicians need to know, J. Child Psychol. Psychiatry 44 (2003) 303–315.
[6] M. Ellison, J. Hall, Social stigma and compounded losses: quality-of-life issues for multiple-birth families, Fertil. Steril. 80 (2003) 405–414.
[7] H. Colpin, Parenting and psychosocial development of IVF children: review of the research literature, Dev. Rev. 22 (2002) 644–673.
[8] S. Golombok, et al., The European study of assisted reproduction families: the transition to adolescence, Hum. Reprod. 17 (2002) 830–840.
[9] S. Golombok, F. MacCallum, E. Goodman, Families with children conceived by DI: a follow-up at age 12, Child Dev. 73 (2002) 952–968.
[10] A. Pinborg, et al., Morbidity in a Danish national cohort of 472 IVF/ICSI twins, 1132 non-IVF/ICSI twins and 634 IVF/ICSI singletons: health-related and social implications for the children and their families, Hum. Reprod. 18 (2003) 1234–1243.
[11] L.A. Tully, T.E. Moffitt, A. Caspi, Maternal adjustment, parenting and child behaviour in families of school-aged twins conceived after IVF and ovulation induction, J. Child Psychol. Psychiatry 44 (2003) 316–325.
[12] C.-S. Hahn, J.A. DiPietro, In vitro fertilization and the family: quality of parenting, family functioning and child psychological adjustment, Dev. Psychol. 37 (2001) 37–48.
[13] F. Gibson, et al., Children conceived through ICSI and IVF at 5 years of age: behavioural adjustment, parenting stress and attitudes: a comparative study, Fertil. Steril. 78 (Supp. 1) (2002) S28–S29.
[14] J. Belsky, The determinants of parenting: a process model, Child Dev. 55 (1984) 83–96.
[15] C.A. McMahon, et al., "Don't count your chickens': a comparative study of the experience of pregnancy after IVF conception, J. Reprod. Infant Psychol. 17 (1999) 345–356.
[16] A. Hjelmstedt, et al., Patterns of emotional responses to pregnancy, experience of pregnancy and attitudes to parenthood among IVF couples: a longitudinal study, J. Psychosom. Obstet. Gynaecol. 24 (2003) 153–162.
[17] Z. Papaligoura, C. Trevarthen, Mother–infant communication can be enhanced after conception by in-vitro-fertilization, Infant Ment. Health J. 22 (2001) 591–610.
[18] H. Colpin, et al., Parenting stress and psychosocial wellbeing among parents with twins conceived naturally or by reproductive technology, Hum. Reprod. 14 (1999) 3133–3137.
[19] C. McMahon, et al., Parents of 5-year-old in vitro fertilisation children: psychological adjustment, parenting stress, and the influence of subsequent in vitro fertilisation treatment, J. Fam. Psychol. 17 (2003) 361–369.

[20] S. Golombok, C. Murray, Social versus biological parenting: family functioning and the socioemotional development of children conceived by egg and sperm donation, J. Child Psychol. Psychiatry 40 (1999) 519–527.
[21] R. Levy-Shiff, et al., Medical, cognitive, emotional and behavioural outcomes in school-age children conceived by in-vitro-fertilization, J. Child Psychol. Psychiatry 27 (1998) 320–329.
[22] V. Soderstrom-Anttila, et al., Health and development of children born after oocyte donation compared with that of those children born after in-vitro-fertilization, and parents' attitudes regarding secrecy, Hum. Reprod. 13 (1998) 2009–2015.
[23] S. Golombok, F. MacCallum, E. Goodman, The "test-tube" generation: parent–child relationships and the psychological wellbeing of in vitro children at adolescence, Child Dev. 72 (2001) 599–608.

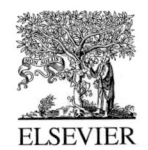

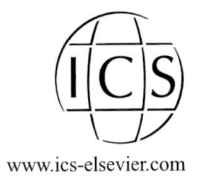

# The long-term paediatric outcomes of assisted reproductive therapies

Alastair G. Sutcliffe*

*University College London, London, UK*
*Academic Department of Child Health, Royal Free Campus, Royal Free and University College Medical School, Rowland Hill Street, London NW3 2PF, UK*

**Abstract.** *Introduction*: In vitro fertilisation has just celebrated its 25th anniversary and there have been a number of further advances since then such as intracytoplasmic sperm injection (ICSI). Few centres have established systematic outcome follow-up of children thus conceived. Herein is a review of what is known about the longer-term outcomes of assisted reproductive therapies (ART). *Methods*: In essence, the main, and most important, cause of longer-term problems after assisted reproductive therapies remains preventable. This is a result of twin and higher-order births and prematurity. Longer-term outcomes can be considered in terms of neurodevelopmental well being, physical development and growth and in terms of emerging concerns about these children. In addition, the literature is described in summary form taking into account categories of ART-conceived children, such as those conceived after standard in vitro fertilisation, embryo cryopreservation and intracytoplasmic sperm injection. *Results*: The balance of evidence shows that when born mature, children born after ART are no different neurodevelopmentally than their naturally conceived peers. In physical terms, they appear to be healthy apart from their risks of congenital anomalies, which are described elsewhere. However, there is early evidence to suggest there may be more unusually tall children and this topic needs to be carefully investigated. In addition, there are long-term further concerns about these children, which can be described, in essence, their future fertility, their long-term risk of cancer and imprintable disorders. Future fertility will be an extremely difficult question to answer because of the confidential nature of this. There are emerging reports that suggest there is a higher risk of imprintable disorders in these children, such as Beckwith–Weidemann syndrome. This may also have implications for childhood cancer and there is one report suggesting a higher risk of retinoblastoma. *Conclusions*: These matters need to be fully investigated with a robust study. When these children grow up, they will

---

* Corresponding author. Academic Department of Child Health, Royal Free Campus, Royal Free and University College Medical School, Rowland Hill Street, London NW3 2PF, UK. Tel.: +44-20-7830-2049 (direct), +44-20-7830-2540 (dept.); fax: +44-20-7472-6709.
 *E-mail address:* icsi@rfc.ucl.ac.uk (A.G. Sutcliffe).

0531-5131/ © 2004 Published by Elsevier B.V.
doi:10.1016/j.ics.2004.01.101

become a significant group and will have a different view of the justification for using fertility methods for them to be conceived than those who were involved in the treatment process in the first place. We all need to be attentive to supporting studies, which try to follow these children into adult life. © 2004 Published by Elsevier B.V.

*Keywords:* Paediatric; Outcome; Assisted reproductive therapies; Childhood

## 1. Introduction

There is clear evidence that there are higher rates of prematurity and subsequent morbidity from assisted reproductive therapy (ART) conception, largely but not entirely, as a consequence of twin or higher-order births. These represent the *largest cause of longer-term problems after ART* and are largely preventable. Rates of twinning are rising in developed nations, e.g., in the United States from 1.8% of births in 1971–1977 to 2.8% in 1998; in Denmark, observed twin birth rates were 0.91/100 births in 1972 and 1.84/100 in 1996, (other figures are similar throughout Europe). Twins are associated with an increased frequency of obstetric complications and higher perinatal morbidity and mortality. Fifty percent of twin births weigh less than 2500 g, one-third are born <37 weeks gestation and mortality/morbidity is 5× singletons. The outcome for triplets is much worse.

## 2. Developmental outcome studies of IVF and ICSI children

(See Tables 1 and 2 for an overview of some earlier studies). ICSI-CFO—an international collaborative study of intracytoplasmic sperm injection (ICSI) child and family outcomes—is by far the largest (and most recent) study on IVF/ICSI children performed in five European countries. Approximately 500 singleton ICSI, 500 IVF and 500 NC (naturally conceived) children aged 5 years are placed in groups and each assessed with observer blinding to conception status. Confounders were avoided by ensuring that all children were >32 weeks gestation, singleton, matched for sex, social class and Caucasian. This study showed no effect whatsoever of conception status on neuro-development [1–3]. Although there was greater use of health service resources by ICSI and IVF children in relation to NC children, when examined comprehensively 'top to toe', these children were found to be physically no different from NC children with the exception of congenital anomalies (see chapter by Dr. Bonduelle) and possibly their growth (see below.)

Developmental differences in an ICSI-conceived group of children when compared with conventional IVF and naturally conceived controls were reported in 1998 [10]. They found an increase in mild developmental delay using the Bayley Scales of Infant Development to derive a mental development index. However, the study used comparison groups of IVF and naturally conceived children that were already enrolled in a separate study and had differing demographics to the ICSI group. There was also no blinding of the assessors and the number of participants in the study was small with 89 ICSI-conceived children.

Table 1
Developmental outcome studies for conventional IVF children (modified from unpublished thesis of C. Peters with kind permission)

| Authors | Study group | Study type | Outcome | Key results | Comments |
|---|---|---|---|---|---|
| D'Souza et al. [4] | 278 IVF and 278 naturally conceived UK children. IVF singletons mean 25.5 months (S.D. 7.9). IVF multiple births mean 24.8 months (S.D. 5.1) | Prospective case-control study. Matched for sex and social class. | Results of Griffiths scales of development | Mean developmental quotient (DQ): IVF singletons 116.9 (S.D. 12.6). IVF multiple births 106.9 (S.D. 10.9). Not stated for controls*. Developmental delay (DQ<70) noted in two multiple birth IVF children only. | 46% IVF children from multiple births. All controls were singleton. No matching for prematurity, birth weight or gestation. |
| Cederblad et al. [5] | 99 Swedish IVF children (age 33–85 months) | Single cohort compared with Swedish and American norms | Results of Griffiths scales of development | Developmental quotient (DQ) above Swedish norm | No matched control group. High numbers of multiple births and prematurity |
| Brandes et al. [6] | 116 Israeli (Hebrew speaking) IVF children and 116 matched non-IVF children (age 12–45 months) | Case-control study. Matched for birth weight, gestational age, birth order, order in multiple births, mode of delivery, sex, age, maternal age and education. | Bayley scales for infants up to 30 months. Stanford–Binet scales for children>30 months. Scales mean 100±16 | MDI Bayley scores: IVF 106±19.6, Non-IVF 110.6±19.3, Composite Index for Stanford–Binet IVF 106.2±8, Non-IVF 104.4±10.2 | No correction for prematurity because children all > 12 months. |
| Morin et al. [7] | 83 IVF children from Norfolk, USA and 93 matched non-IVF children (age 12–30 months) | Case-control study. Matched for age, sex, race, multiple births and maternal age. | Results of Bayley scales: mean developmental index (MDI) and physical developmental index (PDI). Mean score 100 | MDI scores: IVF 115±13, Non-IVF 111±13, PDI scores: IVF 114±14, Non-IVF 108±15 | Study had power of 99% to detect difference. Strongly suggests no difference. However, scores corrected for prematurity. |
| Mushin et al. [8] | 33 Australian children (age 12–37 months) | Single cohort from first 52 infants conceived at Monash IVF centre. No matched controls. | Results of Bayley scales. One child (37 months) assessed using McCarthy scales | Overall MDI of 111 (S.D.=15) and PDI of 105 (S.D.=23). 4 children with physical and developmental problems had lower scores. | High numbers of multiple births and prematurity. Of four children with poor scores, two were VLBW, one severe CHD. |
| Yovich et al. [9] | 20 Australian children (age 12–13 months) | Single cohort of first 20 infants conceived after IVF in Western Australia | Results of Griffiths scales of development | General developmental quotient (GQ) was greater than mean of 100 in 19/20 children after correction for gestational age. | No matched control group. Increased rate of multiple births, IUGR, prematurity and caesarean section. |

Bonduelle et al. [11–16] have published several papers investigating congenital malformation rates and physical development of ICSI children. Several of these papers allude to the fact that developmental milestones were assessed, but formal assessments of these children, undertaken between 1995 and 1998, were published in a research letter to

Table 2
Developmental outcome studies for ICSI children (modified from unpublished thesis of C. Peters with kind permission)

| Authors | Study group | Study type | Outcome | Key results | Comments |
|---|---|---|---|---|---|
| Bonduelle, Wennerholm Loft Tarlatzis and Sutcliffe et al. [19] | 1515 children, 538 natural (NC) 437 IVF 540 ICSI, aged 5 years | Population control study Singleton, >32 weeks, Caucasian | Results of WPPSI, McCarthy Motor scales, Laterality Full physical check Growth, Audiometry Ophthalmic checks | Normal IQ, Normal Laterality, Normal motor skills, Taller than NC peers, Higher anomalies | The most important study in the medical literature. In press. Ability at 5 is predictive of ability at adult life. |
| Sutcliffe et al. [20] | 208 UK children conceived after ICSI compared with 221 naturally conceived controls. Age 12–24 months. | Case-control study. Matched for social class, maternal educational level, region, sex and race. | Results of Griffiths scales of infant development. | Griffiths quotients: ICSI 98.08 (SD 10.93), Controls 98.69 (SD 9.99) | No correction for gestational age in Griffiths scales. Single observer. 90% follow-up. |
| Bowen et al. [10] | 89 Australian ICSI children compared with 84 conventional IVF children and 80 naturally conceived. Assessed at birth and at corrected age of 12 months. | Prospective case-control study. Matched for parental age, parity and multiplicity of the pregnancy. Conventional and IVF children were recruited through separate study. | Results of Bayley scales of infant development | 98% follow up at one year. MDI Bayley scores: ICSI 95.9 (SD 10.7), IVF 101.8 (SD 8.5), Non-IVF 102.5 (SD 7.6) | Included frozen embryos (39% ICSI, 31% IVF). Lack of blinding and differences in sociodemographic factors, particularly between the parents of the ICSI group and other groups. |
| Bonduelle et al. [13] | 201 Belgian (Dutch-speaking) ICSI children compared with 131 conventional IVF children. Assessment age 22–26 months | Blinded prospective case-control trial. | Results of Bayley scales. Test results scored by subtracting chronological age from test age. Test age calculated from subset of 1283 Dutch children aged 2–30 months | Scored mean age differences: ICSI singleton+2.11 (SD 3.12), IVF singleton+2.30 (SD 2.63), ICSI twin+1.67 (SD 3.06), IVF twin+0.31 (SD 3.75), Lower scores for triplets with males scoring lower than females. | No correction for gestational age. Higher scores for singletons. Matching not discussed in this letter. Single observer. 60% follow-up |

the Lancet in 1998 [13]. This article reported 201 ICSI children and 131 IVF children who were assessed using Bayley, and the results were compared with a subset of children representing the Dutch population. The age of the children was not corrected for gestational age, but the ICSI and IVF children were found to have similar scores to the general population. The twins scored slightly lower than the singletons.

Sutcliffe et al. [17,18] studied 208 singletons, ICSI-conceived children at around 18 months and compared them with a matched, naturally conceived control group. The children were assessed by a single observer using the Griffiths scales of mental development. No differences in developmental outcome were found between the two groups.

## 3. Embryo cryopreservation

The limited literature here shows [19–21] that these children are not any different in any areas from ART-conceived children as a whole. They will not be discussed separately any further in this brief overview.

## 4. Physical assessments other than for congenital anomalies

### 4.1. Use of medical services

IVF children are more likely to need neonatal care, primarily because of the prematurity related to multiple pregnancies. Initial reports suggested that IVF children did not require extra medical attention after the neonatal period [22,23]. Leslie studied 95 IVF children and compared them with 79 naturally conceived children matched for maternal age and parity. IVF children were also less likely to be breastfed by the time of discharge. However ICSI-CFO has disagreed with these findings and clearly shown higher use of medical resources amongst IVF/ICSI children, including surgery. The point to emphasise here is that the ICSI-CFO study was performed with older children and was $10\times$ as large as any of these early studies and thus far more likely to detect a difference.

### 4.2. Growth

Saunders et al. [23] published a case-matched control study of children conceived after assisted reproduction and found that the physical outcomes (weight, head circumference and malformation rates) were no different between groups. The IVF group had a greater mean length percentile and the twins in each group had poorer physical outcomes with an increase in prematurity and lower birth weights, and reduced height and weight at age 2 when compared with singletons in each group. Here the ICSI-CFO study concurs in showing that the growth SDS scores (standard deviation scores) for both IVF and ICSI are higher than for NC. This latter finding needs verification, but is somewhat alarming as, so far, nobody has accurately charted the growth of ART children and, so far, larger children have been 'buried' in the effects of prematurity and higher order births.

### 4.3. Childhood cancer

There have been case reports of children conceived after assisted conception developing neuroectodermal tumours [24,25], but no large study has confirmed this finding. Bruinsma et al. [26] used a record linkage cohort design linking assisted reproduction births to a population-based cancer registry in Australia. This study included 5249 births and found no increase in the incidence of cancers in the assisted reproduction groups. However, these groups were relatively small and underpowered for the outcomes measured. The mean length of follow up was only 3 years 9 months, although neuroblastomas tend to occur within the first year of life. These findings were supported by a smaller, similar Israeli study [27].

More recently, Klip et al. [28] examined a large, population-based historical cohort, established to investigate gynaecological disorders in women undergoing IVF. This cohort included 9484 children whose mothers had been given IVF or related fertility treatments and 7532 children whose mothers were subfertile, but had conceived naturally. The mothers were mailed questionnaires enquiring about cancer in their children. There was a 67% response rate and no difference between the groups was noted, implying that IVF and related treatments do not increase the cancer risk to the child.

The cancer incidence in IVF children studied for the UK MRC working party [29] and a Swedish national cohort study of IVF children [30] also found no increase in cancer rates, but the power of these studies was limited by too small a number of children studied. Doyle et al. [29] estimated that 20,000 children would be required to observe a doubling or halving of the risk of childhood cancer in children conceived after assisted reproduction compared with the general population. This would provide 95% significance and 90% power if children were followed up for 5 years [30].

### 4.4. Neurological outcomes

There has been some suggestion from a Swedish study that children born after IVF have an increased risk of developing neurological problems, particularly cerebral palsy [31]. They found a fourfold increase in the risk of cerebral palsy in children born after IVF compared with matched controls—OR 3.7 (95% CI 2.0–6.6). The risk in singletons was nearly 3×—OR 2.8 (95% CI 1.3–5.8). After adjusting for birth weight and a gestation of >37 weeks, the risk remained with an OR of 2.5 (95% CI 1.1–5.2). The authors admitted that the frequency of cerebral palsy in controls was lower than the Swedish norm. In a commentary by Sutcliffe, it was noted that the study used proxy measures for disability and that it was unexplained why the rate of problems seemed higher in the singleton group than the IVF group in contradiction to the entire twin literature!

### 4.5. Genomic imprinting

Genomic imprinting is the mechanism that determines the expression or repression of genes from maternal or paternal chromosomes. This modification of genetic material is epigenetic, i.e., reversible between generations and is not a mutation. Maternal and paternal germ lines confer an imprint or sex-specific mark on certain chromosome regions. Therefore, although the sequence of the genes on these chromosomes could be identical, they are not functionally equivalent.

There is evidence that several syndromes are also caused by imprinting disorders such as Prader–Willi, Angelmans, Russell–Silver, transient neonatal diabetes, Beckwith–Weidemann, Pseudohypoparathyroidism and McCune–Albright syndrome.

Two recent studies have suggested that there may an increased incidence of Beckwith–Weidemann syndrome after assisted conception [32,33]. Although small, these studies support previous findings. Olivennes et al. [34] reported a boy with Beckwith–Weidemann in a cohort of 73 children conceived after IVF. An earlier study by Sutcliffe et al. [35] in 1995 also reported a child with Beckwith–Weidemann in a cohort of 91 children born after replacement of frozen embryos.

Angelmans syndrome is caused by a loss of the maternal allele function secondary to uniparental disomy of the paternal allele, a mutation of the maternal allele, or a sporadic genetic imprinting error causing a paternal imprint on a maternal chromosome [36]. A report of two children with Angelmans syndrome, conceived after ICSI, suggested an inherited defect was unlikely in these cases and therefore the defect was possibly caused at a postzygotic stage.

## 5. In conclusion

Generally, ART-conceived children who are born singleton and at term are similar in most long-term outcomes to naturally conceived children (with the exception of congenital anomalies.) They do, however, appear to use more health service resources. There is earlier evidence that they may be taller than their naturally conceived peers. There are questions, which are unresolved, concerning their progress into adult life [37].

These are as follows. Are there longer-term risks of imprintable disorders and cancer? Will these children be fertile when they are sexually mature?

ART-conceived children will be a significant client group as they grow up (at least 1% of the population in rich countries.) If their ART conception has exposed them to undue risk because these factors were not studied, when the techniques were introduced, they may well take a very different view of the justifications for ART than the readers of this chapter. Further studies need to be performed. The ideal one has yet to be done.

## References

[1] A.G. Sutcliffe, et al., Follow-up of children ICSI: international collaborative study of ICSI-child and family outcomes-physical development at 5 years. Abstract O-281, Hum. Reprod 19th Annual Meeting of ESHRE, Madrid, 2003.
[2] I. Ponjaert-Kristiffersen, Follow-up of children ICSI: abstract O-282, Hum. Reprod 19th Annual Meeting of ESHRE, Madrid, 2003.
[3] J. Barnes, et al., Follow-up of children ICSI: family functioning and socio-emotional development. Abstract O-283, Hum. Reprod 19th Annual Meeting of ESHRE, Madrid, 2003.
[4] S.W. D'Souza, et al., Children conceived by in vitro fertilisation after fresh embryo transfer, Arch. Dis. Child., Fetal Neonatal Ed. 76 (2) (1997 Mar.) F70–F74.
[5] M. Cederblad, et al., Intelligence and behaviour in children born after in-vitro fertilization treatment, Hum. Reprod. 11 (1996) 2052–2057.
[6] J.M. Brandes, et al., Growth and development of children conceived by in vitro fertilization, Pediatrics 90 (1992) 424–429.
[7] N.C. Morin, et al., Congenital malformations and psychosocial development in children conceived by in vitro fertilization, J. Pediatr. 115 (1989) 222–227.
[8] D.N. Mushin, M.C. Barreda-Hanson, J.C. Spensley, In vitro fertilization children: early psychosocial development, J. In Vitro Fertil. Embryo Transf. 3 (1986) 247–252.
[9] J.L. Yovich, et al., Developmental assessment of twenty in vitro fertilization (IVF) infants at their first birthday, J. In Vitro Fertil. Embryo Transf. 3 (1986) 253–257.
[10] J.R. Bowen, et al., Medical and developmental outcome at 1 year for children conceived by intracytoplasmic sperm injection, Lancet 351 (1998) 1529–1534.
[11] M. Bonduelle, et al., Prospective follow-up study of 423 children born after intracytoplasmic sperm injection, Hum. Reprod. 11 (1996) 1558–1564.
[12] M. Bonduelle, et al., Prospective follow-up study of 877 children born after intracytoplasmic sperm injection (ICSI), with ejaculated epididymal and testicular spermatozoa and after replacement of cryopreserved embryos obtained after ICSI, Hum. Reprod. 11 (Suppl. 4) (1996) 131–155.
[13] M. Bonduelle, et al., Prospective follow-up study of 1987 children born after intracytoplasmic sperm injection (ICSI), Treatment of Infertility: The New Frontiers, Communications Media for Education, Inc., 1998, pp. 445–461.
[14] M. Bonduelle, et al., Mental development of 201 ICSI children at 2 years of age, Lancet (North Am. Ed.) 351 (1998) 1553.

[15] M. Bonduelle, et al., Seven years of intracytoplasmic sperm injection and follow-up of 1987 subsequent children, Hum. Reprod. 14 (Suppl. 1) (1999) 243–264.
[16] M. Bonduelle, et al., Neonatal data on a cohort of 2889 infants born after ICSI (1991–1999) and of 2995 infants born after IVF (1983–1999), Hum. Reprod. 17 (2002) 671–694.
[17] A.G. Sutcliffe, et al., Children born after intracytoplasmic sperm injection: population control study, BMJ 318 (1999) 704–705.
[18] A.G. Sutcliffe, et al., Outcome in the second year of life after in-vitro fertilisation by intracytoplasmic sperm injection: a UK case-control study, Lancet 357 (2001) 2080–2084.
[19] A.G. Sutcliffe, et al., Minor congenital anomalies, major congenital malformations and development in children conceived from cryopreserved embryos, Hum. Reprod. 10 (12) (1995 Dec.) 3332–3337.
[20] A.G. Sutcliffe, et al., Outcome in children from cryopreserved embryos, Arch. Dis. Child. 72 (4) (1995 Apr.) 290–293.
[21] U.B. Wennerholm, et al., Obstetric and perinatal outcome of children conceived from cryopreserved embryos, Hum. Reprod. 12 (8) (1997 Aug.) 1819–1825.
[22] G.I. Leslie, et al., Infants conceived using in-vitro fertilization do not over-utilize health care resources after the neonatal period, Hum. Reprod. 13 (1998) 2055–2059.
[23] K. Saunders, et al., Growth and physical outcome of children conceived by in vitro fertilization, Pediatrics 97 (1996) 688–692.
[24] L. White, et al., Neuroectodermal tumours in children born after assisted conception, Lancet 336 (1990) 1577.
[25] N. Kobayashi, et al., Childhood neuroectodermal tumours and malignant lymphoma after maternal ovulation induction, Lancet 338 (1991) 955.
[26] F. Bruinsma, et al., Incidence of cancer in children born after in-vitro fertilization, Hum. Reprod. 15 (2000) 604–607.
[27] L. Lerner-Geva, et al., The risk for cancer among children of women who underwent in vitro fertilization, Cancer 88 (2000) 2845–2847.
[28] H. Klip, et al., Risk of cancer in the offspring of women who underwent ovarian stimulation for IVF, Hum. Reprod. 16 (2001) 2451–2458.
[29] P. Doyle, et al., Cancer incidence in children conceived with assisted reproduction technology, Lancet 352 (1998) 452–453.
[30] T. Bergh, et al., Deliveries and children born after in-vitro fertilisation in Sweden 1982–1995: a retrospective cohort study, Lancet 354 (1999) 1579–1585.
[31] B. Stromberg, et al., Neurological sequelae in children born after in-vitro fertilisation: a population-based study, Lancet 359 (2002) 461–465.
[32] M.R. DeBaun, E.L. Niemitz, A.P. Feinberg, Association of in vitro fertilization with Beckwith–Wiedemann syndrome and epigenetic alterations of LIT1 and H19, Am. J. Hum. Genet. 72 (2003) 156–160.
[33] E.R. Maher, M. Afnan, C.L. Barratt, Epigenetic risks related to assisted reproductive technologies: epigenetics, imprinting, ART and icebergs? Hum. Reprod. 18 (2) (2003) 508–511.
[34] F. Olivennes, et al., Perinatal outcome of pregnancy after GnRH antagonist (ganirelix) treatment during ovarian stimulation for conventional IVF or ICSI: a preliminary report, Hum. Reprod. 16 (2001) 1588–1591.
[35] A.G. Sutcliffe, et al., Outcome in children from cryopreserved embryos, Arch. Dis. Child. 72 (1995) 290–293.
[36] G.F. Cox, et al., Intracytoplasmic sperm injection may increase the risk of imprinting defects, Am. J. Hum. Genet. 71 (2002) 162–164.
[37] A.G. Sutcliffe, IVF Children: The First Generation, CRC Press, London, UK, 2002.

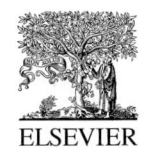

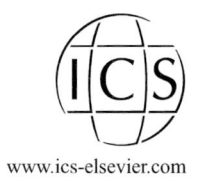

# An introduction to genomics in reproduction

Gareth C. Weston*

*Department of Obstetrics and Gynaecology, Monash University, Melbourne, Australia*

**Abstract.** Genomics is a vast and rapidly progressing field of study. This article aims to provide a brief introduction to the key concepts of genomics and in particular microarray studies of the genome. The emphasis of this article is on the role of genomics in reproductive health, and a review of the existing literature on microarray studies in the field is included. © 2004 Published by Elsevier B.V.

*Keywords:* Genomics; Reproduction; Microarrays; Review

## 1. Introduction

On 15 February 2001, two groups simultaneously announced the completion of the first draft of the entire human genetic sequence [1,2]. The total number of genes to be found in the human genome has been estimated at between 32,000 and 39,000 [3]. Traditionally, molecular biology studied genes singly or in small groups. 'Genomics' is the study of genes in context within their genetic system, rather than as individual genes. Activity or structure of all, or large numbers, of genes is carried out simultaneously. Study of genes as larger groups within a broader molecular context has been limited in the past by lack of complete genetic information, and lack of technological tools capable of interrogating large numbers of genes concurrently. The former obstacle to genomics has been largely dealt with by the completion of the Human Genome Project, while the latter is being addressed by the platform of emerging 'microarray' technologies. Recent advances in genomics and microarray technology, as well as their specific applications to the reproductive field, will be considered in this review.

## 2. Microarrays

Microarrays are one of the tools available for the study of genomes. They consist of a pattern (array) of spots on a 'micro' scale designed to interrogate thousands of components of the genome simultaneously. The two aspects of the genome most commonly studied are variations in genetic sequence or structure (e.g. single nucleotide polymorphisms, or SNPs) and changes in gene expression or function (via measurement in differences in message RNA abundance).

---

\* Tel.: +61-3-9594-6666; fax: +61-3-9594-6389.
*E-mail address:* gareth.weston@med.monash.edu.au (G.C. Weston).

0531-5131/ © 2004 Published by Elsevier B.V.
doi:10.1016/j.ics.2004.01.083

It must be remembered that the genome consists not only of DNA coding for a protein product (genes), but non-coding DNA as well. Non-coding DNA has functional importance in the activation of gene expression via transcription factors as well as gene silencing through DNA methylation. These non-coding but functionally relevant parts of the genome are also being studied with the aid of microarray technology, with spots consisting of non-coding DNA such as transcription binding sites [4], and CpG island methylation sites. 'Intergenic' arrays are being successfully employed to identify gene targets for transcription factors [5], while methylation microarray analysis is being used to identify genes 'switched off' in some tissues and disease states by methylation [6].

The predominant use of microarrays has been to analyze differences in gene expression, either between diseased and normal tissue, or between stimulated and unstimulated cells in vitro. However, microarrays can be used to investigate differences in mRNA abundance between any two samples of RNA. The 'probe' used to assess the amount of gene product (mRNA) in the sample can be either a cDNA or an oligonucleotide [7]. A cDNA probe is usually cloned, amplified by PCR, and spotted on the array surface with the aid of an arrayer (an XYZ axis robot with multiple printing pins). Oligonucleotide probes, on the other hand, are shorter probes which can therefore be arrayed in greater density (down to 20

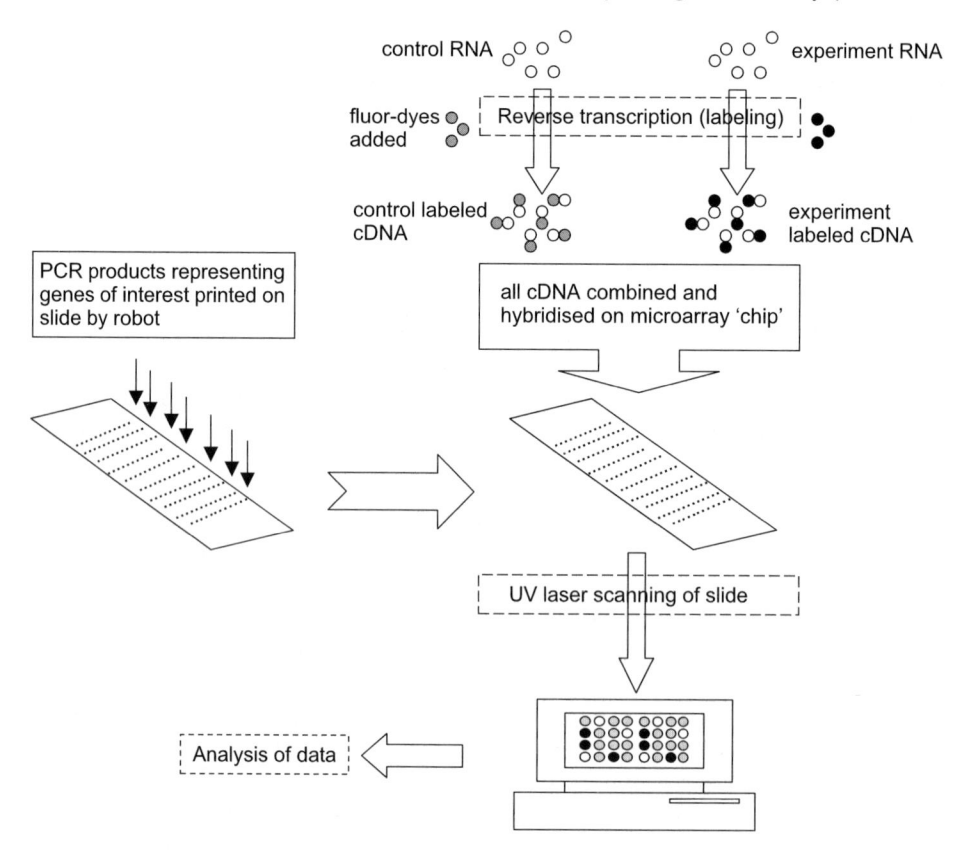

Fig. 1. Technical steps of a gene expression microarray experiment.

μm diameter). They are either spotted onto the array, or synthesized in situ [8]. The solid support on which the spots are printed can be either glass (often called 'chips'), or nylon filter papers. The process of creating fluorescently labelled cDNA probes from the mRNA followed by competitive hybridization, scanning and data analysis is outlined in Fig. 1.

Vast amounts of data are obtained with each microarray performed, with the capacity for tens of thousands of genes to be represented on each chip. Relative fluorescent intensity at each spot gives information about relative gene activity by providing an estimate of transcript abundance in each of two samples competitively hybridized on the slide. As the technology has progressed, the lab-bench components of microarray experimentation have become more efficient and more available. It has long been recognized that the real challenge of microarrays is in the analysis of the data produced [9,10].

Without appropriate use of computational biology it is difficult to obtain meaningful information about the biological process under examination. Data from microarray experiments need to be normalized, or scaled, so that the fluorescent signals from the two separate samples can be directly compared [11]. Once the two signals at each spot (control signal and experiment signal) are able to be compared, the genes with the greatest and most consistent change in expression are identified. Simple fold-change analysis, while easy to perform, can result in unacceptable, high false positive results. Statistical methods for obtaining a set of candidate genes with a lower false positive rate include $t$-tests with multiple $t$-test correction, and Bayesian statistical methods such as GeneRaVE™ which generates a 'league table' of genes most to least-likely to explain the differences in gene expression between two samples in a set of microarray experiments [12].

## 3. Validating gene targets

It is generally accepted that genes identified to have interesting expression patterns via microarray experiments still require further investigation. False positive rates for genes vary markedly with microarray quality, biological variation, RNA sample quality, experimental design, scanner quality, and statistical analysis used. As a result, conventional single-gene techniques such as quantitative PCR methods and Northern blots are used by most investigators to confirm changes in expression in genes of interest. If working on whole tissue, spatial localization of cellular source of mRNA production necessitates the use of techniques such as in-situ hybridization [13]. For example, a change in gene expression found in human endometrium during the menstrual phase of the cycle could be from the influx of white blood cells, or from a change in expression of the endometrial stroma. A temporal analysis, such as a time course microarray experiment [14], is necessary to determine whether gene expression changes are primary to the stimulus in question, or downstream secondary effects. Determination of these molecular pathways is of primary importance in unraveling the function of genes.

Given that proteins are the ultimate arbiters of cell function, changes in protein levels are arguably more important in inferring alteration in function in two different tissues or conditions. Since changes in mRNA are not always reflected in changes in protein levels [15], techniques such as Western blot and ELISA are required to confirm that the changes in transcription are also causing a change in translation. Unlike a negative result in confirmation of mRNA changes, however, a negative result for protein does not mean a false positive microarray result—changes in mRNA levels may be due to an increased turnover, or translation may be interfered with by an alternative mechanism. Equally, a change in protein level may occur without a change in mRNA expression. Proteomics promises to solve much of this confusion, but detection mechanisms for proteins such as antibodies are not always available.

## 4. Microarrays and reproduction

There are many excited claims in the scientific literature that microarrays will soon become routine in diagnosis of disease, selecting optimal drug treatment, avoiding adverse drug reactions, monitoring success of treatment, and selecting and assessing drugs for pharmaceutical development. Just how many of these claims are realized is uncertain. Whether microarrays have sufficient sensitivity and specificity to help clinicians make diagnostic and therapeutic decisions is not clear at present. Currently, the main area of impact for microarrays in all areas of medicine, including reproductive medicine, is in early drug discovery and in hypothesis generation research—and that impact has been phenomenal. It has been estimated that by the year 2000, 60% of new drugs were based on genomics-based technology [16]. As for basic research publications, there were about 3000 publications per year in 2002–2003 with 'DNA microarray' as a search term.

Where does reproduction stand in the genomics revolution? Predictably, research in the reproductive field has lagged behind better funded areas such as cancer and cardiovascular disease [17]. However, there have still been a large and rapidly increasing number of genomic microarray studies published in the reproductive field. A brief overview of the existing literature follows, with all experiments being the more common gene expression microarrays unless otherwise mentioned. Studies can be divided into four main categories (with considerable overlap), depending on whether they are concerning physiological processes, diseases, drugs, or individuals.

### 4.1. Physiological processes

There have been many microarray studies of physiological reproductive processes. Gene expression changes in the endometrium [18] and whole uterus [19] at the time of implantation have been profiled in the mouse, as well as of endometrium in the human [20, 21]. Implantation-associated gene expression changes in the mouse uterus [22] and in human endometrial explants [23] have also been identified by administering the progesterone receptor antagonist RU486 to block progesterone-mediated changes in endometrial receptivity. In an ambitious project, our department is attempting to profile gene expression profiles in the human endometrium via a seven-phase time-course analysis throughout the menstrual cycle [24]. Profiling gene expression changes in normal physiological processes such as implantation allows identification of abnormal gene expression in disease states. For example a recent study of implantation-phase endometrium from women with and without endometriosis revealed 206 genes with differential expression, many with potential roles in mediating reduced implantation in women with endometriosis [25].

Gene expression microarray studies have been published of endometrial decidualisation [26], ovarian follicle development [27], gonad differentiation in embryogenesis [28], parturition [29, 30] and normal placentation [31]. Oestrogen [32] and progesterone [33] responses in the uterus have also been reported, as well as genomic studies of gene expression secondary to FSH stimulation [34]. In our own laboratory, an in vitro model of human myometrial endothelial cells has been used to elucidate gene expression responses to VEGF (vascular endothelial growth factor) [35].

## 4.2. Diseases

There have been a large number of microarray studies of reproductive diseases reported in the literature. Studies of diseases can have a variety of aims, including identification of therapeutic targets, diagnostic markers (either single genes, or molecular 'signatures' due to change in expression or sequence in a number of genes), unraveling disease aetiology, and determining prognosis by linking gene expression or gene sequence data with clinical outcome data.

Ovarian, cervical and endometrial cancer, as well as gestational trophoblastic disease, have all been studies using gene expression microarrays [17]. Benign obstetric and gynaecological conditions as diverse as pre-eclampsia [36], fibroids [12], trisomy-21 pregnancies [37], endometriosis [38], and uterine prolapse [39] have been studied. All of these studies identified by the author to date seek to identify therapeutic targets or diagnostic markers.

## 4.3. Drugs

Potential applications for microarrays to contribute to drug development and utilization exist at virtually every stage from initial development to optimal use of existing drugs in clinical practice. Target tissue gene expression can be analyzed to elucidate previously unknown actions of drugs [40]. Broad-scale mRNA screening of in vitro studies, animal testing, and clinical trials can be used to anticipate potential adverse effects, and it is predicted by some that in the future individual susceptibility to rare adverse drug reactions will be able to be screened for before the drug is administered through gene mutation screening [41].

At present, the author is aware of no studies in the reproductive field linking genomic data with clinical pharmacological responses. However, studies are in progress, in particular for ovarian cancer responses to chemotherapy [42], and ovarian stimulation regimes for infertility treatment, both to optimize ovarian response, and reduce the incidence of ovarian hyperstimulation syndrome, is another area deserving attention.

## 4.4. Individuals

Most of the discussion of arrays to examine genomic-scale genetic variation in individuals is theoretical, as there have been no published studies to date. It is possible in the future that our genetic structure on a genomic scale will be examined from as early as the first stages of embryo development prior to embryo transfer in IVF. Given that 61% of first trimester miscarriages have been reported to have chromosomal abnormalities by comparative genomic hybridization (CGH) [43], it is not surprising that preimplantation CGH has been turned to as a way of reducing miscarriage rates in IVF recipients, with a live healthy birth reported in 2001 after use of the technique [44]. Array CGH may be employed in the future to screen for chromosomal defects in embryos prior to selection for transfer.

As mutations become linked with development of reproductive clinical diseases, it is inevitable that genomic testing will be marketed to look for them. Just what role these tests should play, and how useful testing will be in patient management will be in part up to reproductive clinicians to evaluate. This is a space to watch for future development, as genetic mutations linked to the development of diseases as diverse as premature rupture of the membranes [45] and polycystic ovarian syndrome [46] are beginning to be reported.

## 5. Conclusion

It is clear that microarray studies in the reproductive field have already permeated almost every field of study. Although at present most studies are at the level of basic research and hypothesis generation, it is clear that in the next few years, there will be the emergence of genomic studies in our field seeking to link genomic data with clinical outcomes. Genomics has an enormous potential to improve the reproductive health outcomes in our patients. Improving access to the appropriate technical platforms for reproductive health researchers must be a top priority for this potential to be realized.

## References

[1] J.C. Venter, et al., The sequence of the human genome, Science 291 (2001) 1304–1351.
[2] International Human Genome Sequencing Consortium, Initial sequencing and analysis of the human genome, Nature 409 (2001) 860–921.
[3] P. Bork, R. Copley, Filling in the gaps, Nature 409 (2001) 818–820.
[4] J.R. Pollack, V.R. Iyer, Characterizing the physical genome, Nat. Genet. 32 (2002) 515–521.
[5] S.K. Kurdistani, et al., Genome-wide binding map of the histone deacetylase Rpd3 in yeast, Nat. Genet. 31 (2002) 248–254.
[6] T.H. Huang, M.R. Perry, D.E. Laux, Methylation profiling of CpG islands in human breast cancer cells, Hum. Mol. Genet. 8 (1999) 459–470.
[7] A.J. Holloway, et al., Options available—from start to finish—for obtaining data from DNA microarrays II, Nat. Genet. 32 (2002) 481–489.
[8] E. Southern, K. Mir, M. Shchepinov, Molecular interactions on microarrays, Nat. Genet. 32 (1999) 5–9.
[9] Y.X. Zhou, et al., Information processing issues and solutions associated with microarray technology, in: M. Schena (Ed.), Microarray Biochip Technology, Eaton Publishing, Natick, MA, 2000, pp. 167–200.
[10] S.K. Smith, S. Charnock-Jones, Principles of molecular biology and the application of the human genome project, in: R.W. Shaw, W.P. Soutter, S.L. Stanton (Eds.), Gynaecology, third ed., Churchill Livingstone, China, 2003, pp. 179–185.
[11] S. Knudsen, A Biologist's Guide to Analysis of DNA Microarray Data, Wiley, New York, 2002.
[12] G.C. Weston, et al., Fibroids display an anti-angiogenic gene expression profile when compared with adjacent myometrium, Mol. Hum. Reprod. 9 (2003) 541–549.
[13] S.K. Smith, Functional genomics in reproductive medicine, in: D.L. Healy, G.T. Kovacs, R. McLachlan, O. Rodriguez-Armas (Eds.), Reproductive Medicine in the Twenty-First Century, Parthenon, New York, 2002, pp. 49–56.
[14] J.L. DeRisi, V.R. Iyer, P.O. Brown, Exploring the metabolic and genetic control of gene expression on a genomic scale, Science 278 (1997) 680–686.
[15] S.P. Gygi, et al., Correlation between protein and mRNA abundance in yeast, Mol. Cell. Biol. 19 (1999) 1720–1730.

[16] N.M. Gough, The impact of genomics on drug discovery, Proceedings of the Australian Health and Medical Research Congress 2002, Melbourne, Abstract vol. 503, 2003.
[17] G.C. Weston, et al., Genomics in obstetrics and gynaecology, Aust. N. Z. J. Obstet. Gynaecol. 43 (2003) 264–272.
[18] J. Reese, et al., Global gene expression analysis to identify molecular markers of uterine receptivity and embryo implantation, J. Biol. Chem. 276 (2001) 44137–44145.
[19] K. Yoshioka, et al., Determination of genes involved in the process of implantation: application of GeneChip to scan 6500 genes, Biochem. Biophys. Res. Commun. 272 (2000) 531–538.
[20] L.C. Kao, et al., Global gene profiling in human endometrium during the window of implantation, Endocrinology 143 (2002) 2119–2138.
[21] J.M. Borthwick, et al., Determination of the transcript profile of human endometrium, Mol. Hum. Reprod. 9 (2003) 19–33.
[22] Y. Cheon, et al., A genomic approach to identify novel progesterone receptor regulated pathways in the uterus during implantation, Mol. Endocrinol. 16 (2002) 2853–2871.
[23] R.D. Catalano, et al., The effect of RU486 on the gene expression profile in an endometrial explant model, Mol. Hum. Reprod. 9 (2003) 465–473.
[24] A.P. Ponnampalam, G.C. Weston, P.A.W. Rogers, Microarray analysis of human endometrial gene expression during menstrual cycle, Proceedings of the Australian Health and Medical Research Congress 2002, Melbourne, Abstract, vol. 2684, 2003.
[25] L.C. Kao, et al., Expression profiling of endometrium from women with endometriosis reveal candidate genes for disease-based implantation failure and infertility, Endocrinology 144 (2003) 2870–2881.
[26] R.M. Popovici, L.C. Kao, L.C. Guidice, Discovery of new inducible genes in in vitro decidualized human endometrial stromal cells using microarray technology, Endocrinology 141 (2000) 3510–3513.
[27] Z. Bryant, et al., Characterization of differentially expressed genes in purified Drosophila follicle cells: toward a general strategy for cell type-specific developmental analysis, Proc. Natl. Acad. Sci. 96 (2003) 5559–5564.
[28] S. Grimmond, et al., Sexually dimorphic expression of protease nexin-1 and vanin-1 in the developing mouse gonad prior to overt differentiation suggests a role in mammalian sexual development, Hum. Mol. Genet. 9 (2000) 1553–1560.
[29] R.A. Muhle, et al., A high-throughput study of gene expression in preterm labor with a subtractive microarray approach, Am. J. Obstet. Gynecol. 185 (2001) 716–724.
[30] M. Girotti, H.H. Zingg, Gene expression profiling of rat uterus at different stages of parturition, Endocrinology 144 (2003) 2254–2265.
[31] T.S. Tanaka, et al., Genome-wide expression profiling of mid-gestation placenta and embryo using a 15,000 mouse developmental cDNA microarray, Proc. Natl. Acad. Sci. 97 (2000) 9127–9132.
[32] H. Watanabe, et al., Genome-wide analysis of changes in early gene expression induced by estrogen, Genes Cells 7 (2002) 497–507.
[33] N. Takamoto, et al., Identification of Indian hedgehog as a progesterone-responsive gene in the murine uterus, Mol. Endocrinol. 16 (2002) 2338–2348.
[34] R. Sasson, et al., Novel genes modulated by FSH in normal and immortalized FSH-responsive cells: new insights into the mechanism of FSH action, FASEB J. 17 (2003) 1256–1266.
[35] G.C. Weston, I. Haviv, P.A.W. Rogers, Microarray analysis of VEGF-responsive genes in myometrial endothelial cells, Mol. Hum. Reprod. 8 (2002) 855–863.
[36] T. Reimer, et al., Microarray analysis of differentially expressed genes in placental tissue of pre-eclampsia: up-regulation of obesity-related genes, Mol. Hum. Reprod. 8 (2002) 674–680.
[37] S.J. Gross, et al., Gene expression profile of trisomy 21 placentas: a potential approach fro designing noninvasive techniques of prenatal diagnosis, Am. J. Obstet. Gynecol. 187 (2002) 457–462.
[38] K.M. Eyster, et al., DNA microarray analysis of gene expression markers of endometriosis, Fertil. Steril. 77 (2002) 38–42.
[39] A.G. Visco, L. Yuan, Differential gene expression in pubococcygeus muscle from patients with pelvic organ prolapse, Am. J. Obstet. Gynecol. 189 (2003) 102–112.
[40] D.L. Gerhold, R.V. Jensen, S.R. Gullans, Better therapeutics through microarrays, Nat. Genet. 32 (2002) 547–552.

[41] U.A. Meyer, Pharmacogenetics and adverse drug reactions, Lancet 356 (2000) 1667–1671.
[42] R. Mirhashemi, et al., Candidate gene in predicting in vivo ovarian cancer response t combination therapy with paraplatin and paclitaxel, Sci. World J. 2 (2002) 19–20.
[43] Y.Q. Tan, et al., Genetic changes in human fetuses from spontaneous abortion after in vitro fertilization detected by comparative genomic hybridization, Biol. Reprod. 70 (2003) 1495–1499.
[44] L. Wilton, et al., Birth of a healthy infant after preimplantation confirmation of euploidy by comparative genomic hybridization, N. Engl. J. Med. 345 (2001) 1537–1541.
[45] P.E. Ferrand, et al., A polymorphism in the matrix metalloproteinase-9 promoter is associated with increased risk of premature rupture of membranes in African Americans, Mol. Hum. Reprod. 8 (2002) 494–501.
[46] S. Korhonen, et al., Two exonic single nucleotide polymorphisms in the microsomal epoxide hydrolase gene are associated with polycystic ovarian syndrome, Fertil. Steril. 79 (2003) 1353–1357.

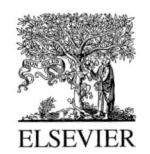

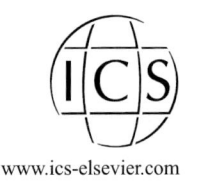

# Mass spectrometry-based proteomics

Brian L. Hood, Timothy D. Veenstra, Thomas P. Conrads*

*Laboratory of Proteomics and Analytical Technologies, Mass Spectrometry Center, SAIC-Frederick, Inc., National Cancer Institute at Frederick, P.O. Box B, Frederick, MD 21702, USA*

**Abstract.** Advances in genomic analysis, including improvements in DNA sequencing, bioinformatics and the routine application of microarray technology to characterize gene expression profiles, have set the stage for understanding how genes are organized and regulated. However, the genetic blueprint cannot accurately predict which proteins are expressed, where they are localized in a cell, and in what quantity and form they are present. Proteomics is a field of study that addresses these important and varied issues. Rapid innovations in core technologies such as separations and mass spectrometry (MS) required to characterize proteins on a global scale are poised to bring about a comprehensive understanding of how changes in protein expression and function affect complex signaling and regulatory networks. These advances have significant implications for understanding how the myriad activities carried out in a cell are regulated in health and disease. This review discusses basic proteomics advances including specific examples that utilize such methodologies as two-dimensional polyacrylamide gel electrophoresis (2D PAGE), solution-based "shotgun" proteomics utilizing multidimensional separations of complex mixtures and the use of stable-isotope labeling for conducting global protein abundance profiles.
© 2004 Published by Elsevier B.V.

*Keywords:* Proteomics; Mass spectrometry; Multidimensional separation; 2D PAGE; ICAT

## 1. Introduction

The rapidly evolving field of proteomics is directed toward providing a comprehensive view of the characteristics and activity of every cellular protein. Proteomics aims to supplement analytical techniques designed to study proteins by "one species-at-a-time" with methodologies that enable thousands of proteins to be studied concomitantly. Rather than being hypothesis-driven where subsequent studies are directed based on previous findings and specific results are anticipated, proteomics is largely discovery-driven where newly acquired data provide details about the system under study, largely without inclination of predictable results. The goals of conducting such discovery-driven measurements is to characterize thousands of proteins in a single experiment. With these large

---

* Corresponding author. Tel.: +301-846-7353; fax: 301-846-6037.
  *E-mail address:* conrads@ncifcrf.gov (T.P. Conrads).

0531-5131/ © 2004 Published by Elsevier B.V.
doi:10.1016/j.ics.2004.02.087

datasets in hand, the goal is to further understand how cells function under conditions of function and malfunction.

Sequencing of an entire genome (genomics) or analysis of tens of thousands of gene transcripts using mRNA array technologies (transcriptomics) has become very efficient [1–3]. Like genomics and transcriptomics, current state-of-the-art proteomic techniques depend strongly on the development of specific new methodologies and instrumentation that have occurred over the past half-century, which include mass spectrometry (MS), protein/peptide fractionation techniques, and bioinformatics to name a few [4–7]. While impressive in its overall capability, proteomics is not yet capable of providing the depth and breadth at the level of throughput of transcriptomics and genomics.

Before going into a further analysis of MS-based proteomics, it is essential to understand how proteins are identified using this technology. In the analysis of complex proteomes, proteins per se are rarely used for identification, rather, they are more typically digested by chemical or enzymatic means into their constituent peptides and it is these species that are identified using either MS or tandem MS. In the MS mode, the mass spectrum of a protein's peptide fragments produces a "peptide map" or a "peptide fingerprint" [8]. These measured masses can be used to compare with theoretical peptide maps derived from in silico translated genomic database sequences to identify the protein that would most likely give rise to this ensemble of peptide masses. In tandem MS, an individual peptide can be dynamically isolated by the mass spectrometer and fragmented by collision-induced dissociation by an inert gas such as argon. The tandem MS spectrum that results is a measure of the various fragment ions produced from CID of the molecular peptide ion from which the partial or complete amino acid sequence information can be obtained. Since peptides typically fragment across the amide bond, ensembles of y and b ion series are produced that contain varying lengths of residues originating from the parent peptide. The measured tandem mass spectrum is then compared with theoretical tandem mass spectra calculated from the protein sequences in an in silico translated genomic database or de novo sequenced to obtain the identity of the intact peptide [9].

## 2. Two-dimensional polyacrylamide gel electrophoresis

Presently, numerous hyphenated front-end protein and peptide separation methods are utilized to increase the depth and breadth of proteomic measurements, but in the earliest applications of proteomics, two-dimensional polyacrylamide gel electrophoresis (2D PAGE) was utilized to resolve, visualize and compare protein abundances between two samples. The principle procedure is based on isoelectric focusing (IEF), which separates the proteins based on their isoelectric points (p$I$), followed by electrophoresis in the presence of sodium dodecyl sulphate (SDS) to separate the proteins based on their molecular weight. These separation parameters allow for the resolution of proteins differing by a single charge, thereby allowing such in vivo modifications such as phosphorylation and certain mutations to be detected. The high resolving power of 2D PAGE and the development of various staining procedures to visualize these protein "spots" have resulted in a very robust methodology for identifying protein abundance changes between two proteome samples. In conducting such studies, proteome samples from a control and treated (or generically different) cell (or organism or tissue) are extracted and separated on distinct gels. The proteins can be visualized by colorimetric staining and the spots resolved on both gels are aligned to enable the relative staining intensities of each protein on the distinct gels to be compared. Protein spots that show a difference in staining intensity can be excised from the gel and digested within the gel plug [10]. The resulting peptides can be extracted from the gel and analyzed by either MS or tandem MS. The MS or tandem MS data are bioinformatically compared with an appropriate database (i.e., species from which the proteome was extracted) to identify their protein of origin. While there are many ongoing efforts to identified solution-based fractionation methods to circumvent 2D PAGE, it is still the most commonly used separation technique used in proteomics [12]. Advances have been made in 2D PAGE technology that allow thousands of species to be resolved on a single gel, which can be combined with better protein staining methods that allow for more accurate and precise quantitation of proteins [12].

Unfortunately, there are other disadvantages inherent to 2D PAGE that limits its overall proteome coverage. Very large or small molecular weight proteins are not resolved within the gel, neither are proteins with extreme p*I* values (both highly basic and acidic). In addition, the ability to quantify and subsequently identify very low abundance proteins is lacking. While increasingly sensitive staining techniques are being made available, they still do not affect the ability to identify the protein spot once it is excised from the gel. Comparative quantitation can also be extremely difficult since multiple proteins may migrate to the same position within a gel. For example, six proteins within a single silver-stained spot in the analysis of a yeast cell extract fractionated by 2D PAGE were identified using MS [11].

## 3. Solution-based proteomics

Due to the recognized limitations of 2D PAGE, a significant amount of effort has been focused on the development of alternative, non-gel methods of resolving proteome samples prior to MS analysis. An early example showing the utility of solution-based fractionation techniques was developed by Yates and co-workers [12]. Their 2D separation method, called MudPit, is a hyphenated strong cation exchange/reversed-phase liquid chromatography (i.e., SCX/RPLC) separation method coupled online with MS detection, and was initially demonstrated using a *Saccharomyces cerevisiae* proteome digest. In this MudPIT experiment, the entire proteome sample was digested with trypsin and the tryptic peptides were systematically resolved based on charge in the first dimension (i.e., SCX) and hydrophobicity (i.e., RPLC) in the second. The peptide mixture is loaded onto a SCX column and discrete fractions are displaced directly onto the RPLC column, and are then separated and eluted from the RP column and directly analyzed by MS/MS to identify the eluting peptides. To maximize sample transfer from the stationary phases, the SCX and RP stationary phases are sequentially packed into a single capillary column. The tryptically digested yeast proteome was analyzed using 15 iterations of the MudPit separation cycle. In this early demonstration, a total of 5540 unique peptides originating from 1484 proteins were identified. Fifty-three percent of the proteins identified had codon adaptation index (CAI) values less than 0.2. This ability to detect low abundance proteins is in stark contrast to studies that have shown that 2D PAGE analysis makes it very difficult to detect yeast proteins with CAI values less than 0.2.

## 4. Solution-based quantitative proteomics

While much of the development in MS-based proteomics has focused on methods to identify thousands of proteins in a high throughput manner, significant effort has been invested in developing methods to quantitate the relative abundances of proteins from two distinct proteome samples. A key aspect to remember is that a vast majority of high throughput quantitative proteomic studies measure relative abundances of proteins between two proteomes, they are not designed to measure absolute abundance of these proteins. The use of differential isotopic labeling is performed either by metabolic incorporation of an isotope as the cells of interest are cultured or chemically after the proteome is extracted from the cell.

Metabolic labeling of proteins of microorganisms or in tissue cultured cells is effected by growth in medium containing either the natural abundance of the isotopes of nitrogen or in $^{15}$N-enriched media [13]. The two populations of cells are then harvested and pooled. The combined sample is digested with trypsin and analyzed by multidimensional chromatography coupled with tandem MS. Mass spectrometry is well suited to distinguish between the two separate pools of proteins since one set contains the natural abundance of nitrogen whereas proteins from the other set will be substituted with the $^{15}$N isotope. The result of this substitution will increase the mass of $^{15}$N-labeled peptides by 1 Da/nitrogen atom and as a result, the resulting mass spectrum will contain pairs of peptide peaks. The ratio of the pairs of peptide peaks is used for relative quantitation between the two samples. Therefore, MS analysis is used to compare the relative amounts of each protein in the two different samples and also to identify the protein.

While stable isotope labeling can be accomplished at the metabolic level during protein translation, it is necessarily so in cases where the system is amenable to growth in a medium enriched for a given isotope or is able to survive on a diet containing the heavy isotope being targeted. As mentioned above, methods exist to differently label proteins on a global level after they have been extracted from the cell via chemical modification. While many different types of labeling technologies have been proposed, the most popular methodology utilizes isotope-coded affinity tag (ICAT) reagents, which allow for conducting global measurements of peptide relative abundances from virtually any source, including tissues [14–16].

The key aspect of ICAT reagents is that they posses three key features: an iodoacetyl functionality that is used to covalently modify sulfhydryls of reduced cysteinyl residues, a linker region that can be synthesized to possess either complete carbon atoms ($^{13}C_0$) or nine heavy isotopes of carbon ($^{13}C_9$) and a biotin moiety that allows ICAT-labeled peptides to be specifically extracted using avidin affinity chromatography. In the use of ICAT reagents for quantitation of protein abundances, two cell extracts to be compared are labeled either with the $^{13}C_0$ or the $^{13}C_9$-ICAT isotopomer. The labeled proteins are combined into a single complex mixture that is digested with trypsin and the modified peptides isolated by avidin affinity chromatography. The enriched mixture of ICAT-labeled peptides can then be fractionated by SCX chromatography into a series of fractions, which are individually analyzed by LC-tandem MS to identify the peptides while concomitantly providing a measure of their relative abundances. Within the MS spectra, a series of differential, stable-isotope labeled cysteinyl peptides will be observed, whose masses are separated exactly by the mass of the heavy ICAT label, or approximately 9 Da. The relative abundance of the peptide in the different samples is measured by measuring the signal intensities of each of the "sister" cysteinyl peptides.

## 5. The future

While many groups ranging from small academic laboratories to large pharmaceutical companies are actively utilizing proteomic technologies, the science is still in its infancy. Indeed, while the gel separation of proteins has been around for decades, and the foundation of modern 2D PAGE for almost 30 years, it has been only recently that the proteomic capability of this separation tool was realized with the development of MS approaches to identify the separated proteins. Only very recently has active research focused on methods to obviate 2D PAGE, however, it still remains a foundation of proteomics. Will it someday become obsolete? It is unlikely as the ongoing efforts into improving both the resolution and sensitivity of 2D PAGE suggest that it will remain a very viable tool for many years to come.

Even with the exceptional developments being made in proteomics, the full realization of the power of this science is still not in sight. How can we be certain of this? When any cellular proteome is considered under a single condition of environment and time, it is clear that we are only beginning to understand the complexity of biological systems' intricate details. Protein identification and quantitation is only the tip of what proteomics offers. How proteins interact with other biological molecules, their modifications, their subcellular localization, their stability, and their activity and are only a few of the other characteristics that need to be determined before we can fully grasp the complexity of the cell.

## Acknowledgements

This project has been funded in whole or in part with Federal funds from the National Cancer Institute, National Institutes of Health, under Contract No. NO1-CO-12400.

The content of this publication does not necessarily reflect the views or policies of the Department of Health and Human Services, nor does mention of trade names, commercial products, or organization imply endorsement by the U.S. Government.

## References

[1] R. Simon, Diagnostic and prognostic prediction using gene expression profiles in high-dimensional microarray data, Br. J. Cancer 89 (2003) 1599–1604.
[2] C. Mundy, The human genome project: a historical perspective, Pharmacogenomics 2 (2001) 37–49.
[3] G. Jenkins, Unfolding large-scale maps, Genome 46 (2003) 947–952.
[4] T.A. Nyman, The role of mass spectrometry in proteome studies, Biomol. Eng. 18 (2001) 221–227.
[5] H.J. Issaq, The role of separation science in proteomics research, Electrophoresis 22 (2001) 3629–3638.
[6] S.A. Carr, et al., Integration of mass spectrometry in analytical biotechnology, Anal. Chem. 63 (1991) 2802–2824.

[7] E.T. Maggio, K. Ramnarayan, Recent developments in computational proteomics, Trends Biotechnol. 19 (2001) 266–272.
[8] D. Fenyo, Identifying the proteome: software tools, Curr. Opin. Biotechnol. 11 (2000) 391–395.
[9] W.H. McDonald, J.R. Yates III, Shotgun proteomics and biomarker discovery, Dis. Markers 18 (2002) 99–105.
[10] T. Rabilloud, Two-dimensional gel electrophoresis in proteomics: old, old fashioned, but it still climbs up the mountains, Proteomics 2 (2002) 3–10.
[11] S.P. Gygi, et al., Evaluation of two-dimensional gel electrophoresis based proteome analysis technology, Proc. Natl. Acad. Sci. U. S. A. 9 (2000) 9390–9395.
[12] M.P. Washburn, D. Wolters, J.R. Yates III, Large-scale analysis of the yeast proteome by multidimensional protein identification technology, Nat. Biotechnol. 19 (2001) 242–247.
[13] T.P. Conrads, et al., Quantitative analysis of bacterial and mammalian proteomes using a combination of cysteine affinity tags and 15N-metabolic labeling, Anal. Chem. 73 (2001) 2132–2139.
[14] S.P. Gygi, et al., Quantitative analysis of complex protein mixtures using isotope-coded affinity tags, Nat. Biotechnol. 17 (1999) 994–999.
[15] L.R. Yu, et al., Proteome analysis of camptothecin-treated cortical neurons using isotope-coded affinity tags, Electrophoresis 23 (2002) 1591–1598.
[16] T. Guina, et al., Proteomic analysis of *Pseudomonas aeruginosa* grown under magnesium limitation, J. Am. Soc. Mass Spectrom. 14 (2003) 742–751.

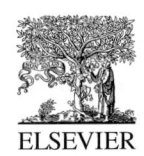

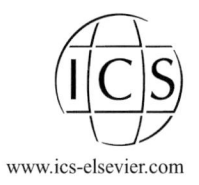

# Office operative endoscopy in infertility

Hugo Christian Verhoeven*

*Center for Reproductive Medicine and Endocrinology, Voelklinger Strasse 4, Düsseldorf 40219, Germany*

**Abstract.** The implementation of ambulatory surgical procedures in endoscopic surgery has been inspired by several coincidental factors. First, there is a necessity to reduce the cost of interventions because of government restrictions on payments, and second, there is a general trend to reduce the invasiveness of endoscopic procedures, thus pushing companies to develop smaller endoscopes without loss of optical quality. At present, however, confusion exists between the concepts of minimal invasive surgery and minimal access surgery. As accuracy of smaller-diameter endoscopes with very high optical quality is comparable with that of larger endoscopes, surgeons were inspired to use less-invasive surgery and to use smaller instruments. As a result, performing diagnostic procedures and minor interventions under local anaesthesia became possible and was widely accepted. Despite these advances, ambulatory surgery must not diminish the quality of care for patients. In particular, the use of the term 'office laparoscopy' can create some confusion in countries outside the US. Many so-called "office settings" in the US have fully equipped operating theaters and, although located outside a hospital setting, they tend to be situated closely to a hospital. For the patient's benefit and also for medico-legal reasons, full laparoscopies have to be performed in a fully equipped operating theater. Ambulatory surgical procedures must offer patients the requirements of classical surgery in terms of safety and quality. A 1-day clinic setting reduces the costs of hospitalization while, at the same time, minimal invasiveness will result in a low morbidity with a faster resumption of normal professional or home activities. Certainly in reproductive surgery, these are important issues, as we are dealing with healthy patients who dislike frequent interruptions to their daily activities. As such, patients are trying to conceive as soon as possible, a minimal invasive approach with a maximal conservation of their reproductive potential is mandatory. Ambulatory reproductive surgery involves both uterine and tubo-ovarian interventions. © 2004 Published by Elsevier B.V.

*Keywords:* Office endoscopy; Hysteroscopy; Transvaginal endoscopy; Endometriosis; Ovarian drilling

## 1. Intrauterine interventions

### 1.1. Technique

In general, the interventions are performed under sedation or general anesthesia with the patient in the normal lithotomy position. After cervical dilatation, if necessary, a 3.5- or

---

* Tel.: +49-211-9019797; fax: +49-211-9019750.
 E-mail address: H.C.Verhoeven@t-online.de (H.C. Verhoeven).

0531-5131/ © 2004 Published by Elsevier B.V.
doi:10.1016/j.ics.2004.01.111

5-mm operative hysteroscope is introduced under visual control into the uterine cavity. A continuous flow instrument with separate in- and out-flow channels is used and is connected to a video camera system. This ensures continuous irrigation of the uterine cavity with optimal visualization. As distension medium, Purisole (sorbitol+mannitol) or Glykokol® (glycine 1.5%) are preferred, keeping the distension pressure between 90 and 120 mm Hg. Duration of the procedure should be kept as short as possible, with continuous surveillance of the fluid balance. In case of a negative fluid balance of more than 1200 ml, the procedure should be interrupted and further treatment should be performed at a later stage.

## 1.2. Complications

Operative hysteroscopic procedures are frequently proposed and explained to the patients as minor operative interventions. Nevertheless, some of these operations can cause severe and sometimes life-threatening complications. Knowledge of these complications and how to avoid them is mandatory. Complications are caused by the instrumentation and/or the distension medium, and can occur during or after the operation.

The most common complication is uterine perforation, which occurs mainly in the fundal region. In different studies, the rate of uterine perforation varies between 0.8% and 3.0% [1,2]. Significant bleeding is unlikely in this area. On the other hand, if the perforation is lateral in the area of the uterine artery or one of its branches a life-threatening hemorrhage can occur. Where perforation is due to the use of monopolar current or a laser, a laparoscopy or laparotomy is advisable to exclude intraabdominal damage, and the patient should be monitored carefully for several days to exclude intestinal injury and delayed perforation. Such monitoring includes warning the patient that unexpected and increasing abdominal pain is a cause to return immediately for further evaluation. The concomitant use of abdominal sonography can be helpful in the prevention of uterine perforation. The energy source should only be activated when the position of the working instrument is carefully checked for its safety.

Distension medium fluid may enter into the patient's circulation via the uterine vessels and the lymphatic system. The height of the intrauterine pressure and the duration of the procedure are the determining factors. A status of hypotonic hyperhydration may occur as a consequence. This is known in urologic surgery as the TURP-Syndrome (transurethral resection of the prostate). The frequency of this complication is reported to be between 0.14% and 16% [3]. Careful monitoring of the patient's fluid and electrolyte balance is mandatory, and, in the case of severe overload, a central venous catheter should be installed and diuresis started.

## 1.3. Procedures

All intrauterine pathology related to reproduction can be treated in a 1-day clinical setting. As mentioned above, utmost care should be taken to avoid any complications. Pathology can be divided into congenital and acquired. In ambulatory pre-IVF diagnostic hysteroscopies, the incidence of abnormal findings is reported as 28.5%, with 13.2% congenital disorders and 15.3% acquired disorders [4]. In the latter, the frequency of intracavitary polyps and myoma is 26%, Asherman 0.1% and intrauterine synechiae

17.5%. With adequate experience, myomas and polyps can easily be removed using a resectoscope. Although more expensive, the Nd–YAG laser is an alternative tool for treatment. In cases of larger myomata, the preoperative use of gonadotropin-releasing hormone analogues can be considered in an attempt to reduce the size of the myoma and thus facilitate the intervention.

The restoration of the normal contours of the uterine cavity becomes more difficult in cases of complete or incomplete Asherman. For subfertility, the incidence in the literature is reported to range from 0.1% to 2% [4–6]. When the basal layer of the endometrium is destroyed as a result of manipulation of the endometrial cavity following a pregnancy, reformation of adhesions tend to reoccur after treatment and restoration is sometimes only achieved after several procedures. The Versapoint®, which vaporizes the cells, probably has a beneficial effect in the prevention of recurrence.

Amongst congenital malformations, septate uterus is the most frequent, with a frequency of 63% of the congenital malformations [4]. Diagnosis must be confirmed by laparoscopy to distinguish it from a bicornual uterus. Several instruments can be used for resection of the septum: semi-rigid scissors, Nd–YAG laser or the resectoscope, the latter being the most inexpensive and readily available. Continuous irrigation is applied during the procedure with careful inspection of the right and left tubal ostia. Concurrent application of transabdominal sonography can be helpful to decide where to stop the dissection in order to avoid perforation or, during later pregnancy, uterine rupture. In some cases, a double cervical canal may be present in association with a complete septum. Whereas some authors tend to conserve the double cervical channel to avoid eventual cervical incompetence [7], others advise a resection of the intracervical septum followed by further resection of the total uterine septum. No cervical incompetence has been observed by Donnez and Nisolle [8].

Implantation can also be impaired in the case of a T-shaped uterus. Enlargement of the uterine cavity is obtained by symmetrical incision of the uterine sidewalls using a bipolar cutting needle or the Versapoint.

*1.4. Discussion*

In the hands of experienced hysteroscopists, intrauterine pathology can easily be treated in an ambulatory, same-day clinic setting. Surgeons must be aware of the risks of complications and the necessary precautions must be taken to avoid them. Special care should be given to the fluid balance during the intervention, and the procedure must be interrupted at a negative balance of 1200–1500 ml. The use of a watery distension medium is preferred over the use of $CO_2$, as the former increases diagnostic accuracy and decreases morbidity.

## 2. Tubo-ovarian interventions via transvaginal endoscopy

*2.1. Introduction*

For many years, standard laparoscopy was considered the gold standard for the exploration of the female genital tract. With the introduction of mini-endoscopes to decrease patient discomfort, the umbilical approach remains the same, along with the blind insertion of a Veress needle and trocar. Complications in major vessels have been described as frequently from the insertion of the Veress needle as from the trocar [9,10]. Initial interest in the transvaginal approach by culdoscopy was abandoned in the 1970s, as laparoscopy provides a more panoramic view and lower risk when performing tubal ligations. However, sepsis in culdoscopy was found to be due to the exteriorization of tubes [11].

Gordts et al. [12] described the technique of transvaginal hydrolaparoscopy (THL) based on a needle puncture technique of the pouch of Douglas. The technique demonstrated in Fig. 1 differs from culdoscopy by the use of the lithotomy position for the patient and warm saline as a distension medium. As the endoscope is in the same axis as the tubo-ovarian structures, easy access is provided to the fossa ovarica and the anterolateral site of the ovary without the need for extra manipulation (Fig. 2). This creates excellent exposure for ovarian and tubal surgery under direct vision. The use of a saline solution keeps the organs afloat, prevents collapse of microvascularization and filmy adhesions, and is helpful for atraumatic manipulation of the different structures and for a better delineation of the surfaces. Recently, new instruments were developed and manufactured by the Storz and transvaginal hydrolaparoscopy was renamed into transvaginal endoscopy (TVE).

## 2.2. Technique

The access to the pouch of Douglas is performed in the same way described for diagnostic THL [13] and is based on a needle puncture technique of the pouch of Douglas familiar to many as the technique of culdocentesis. For this purpose, initially a specially developed Veress needle was used in which there is progressive dilatation from the diameter of the Veress needle to the outer diameter of the external trocar sheet (5 mm). A rigid mini-endoscope with a 30° optical angle is used and is attached to a video camera

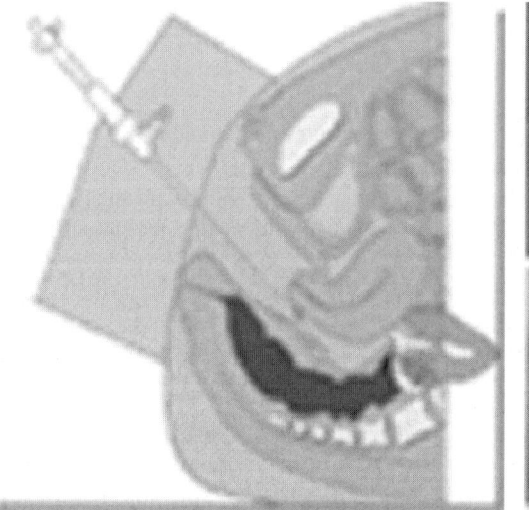

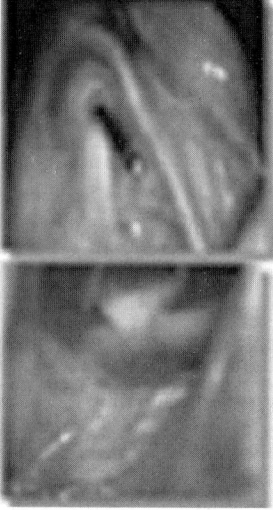

Fig. 1. Technique of TVE.

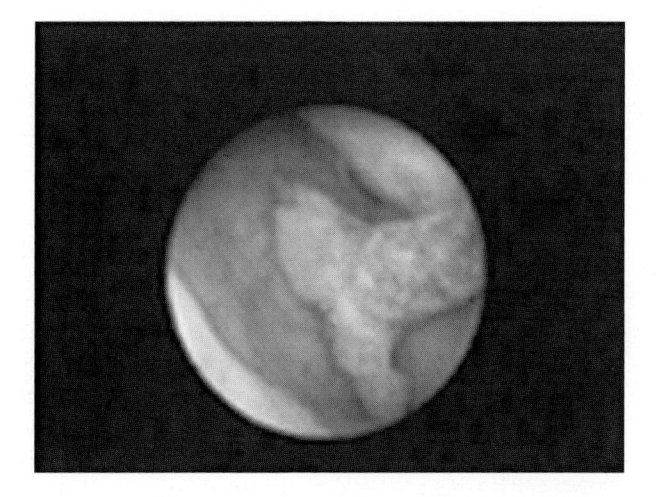

Fig. 2. Ampulla during TVE.

system. Once access to the pouch of Douglas is obtained, the Veress needle and the dilating obturator are removed and replaced by the operative endoscope. The operative channel allows the insertion of five French scissors and forceps and a thin bipolar coagulating probe (Bicap®, Circon ACMI) or a bipolar coagulating and cutting needle (Storz, Tuettlingen, Germany). Before starting the procedure, about 100-ml warm saline is instilled in the pouch of Douglas to obtain adequate distension (Figs. 3–5).

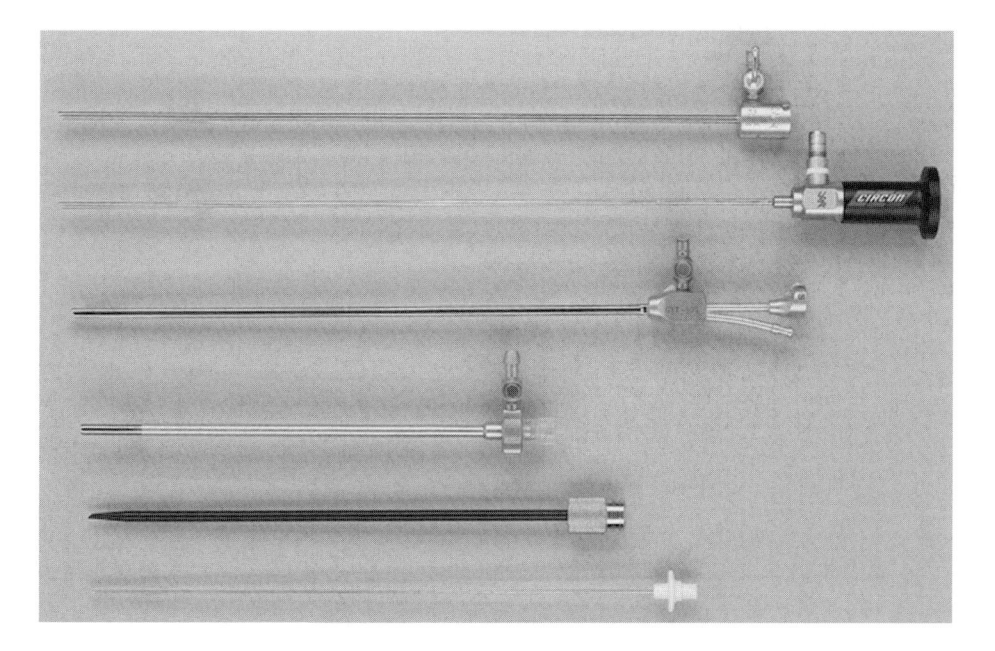

Fig. 3. Operative TVE instrumentation.

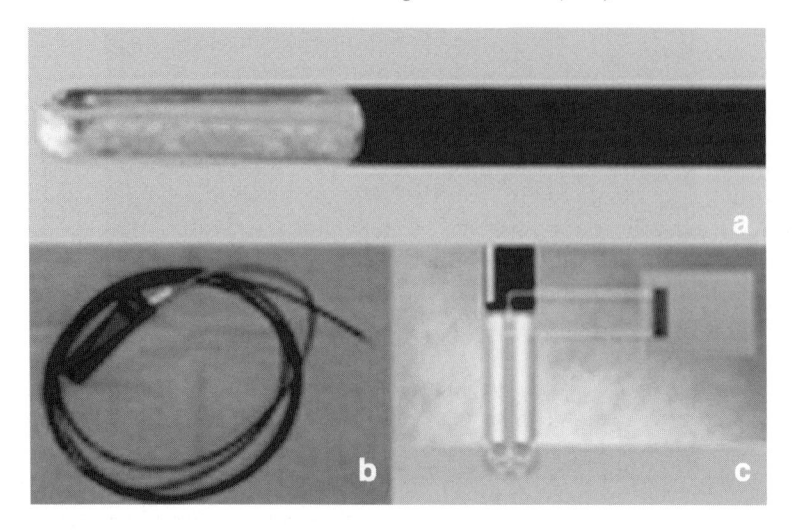

Fig. 4. BICAP probe.

As one is working in a saline distension medium, preventive hemostasis is mandatory in order to avoid insufficient or disturbed visualization. All procedures are performed under general anesthesia or conscious sedation.

## 2.3. Procedures

Gordts et al. carried out an operative procedure in 78 patients and included treatment of endometriosis ($n=51$), ovarian capsule drilling ($n=14$), adhesiolysis after pelvic inflammatory disease or surgery ($n=10$), resection of a functional cyst ($n=2$) and salpingoneostomy ($n=1$). No conversion to laparoscopy was necessary and no complications occurred. Patients resumed their professional or other activities after 2 days. All patients gave informed consent and they were informed that conversion to laparoscopy could be possible.

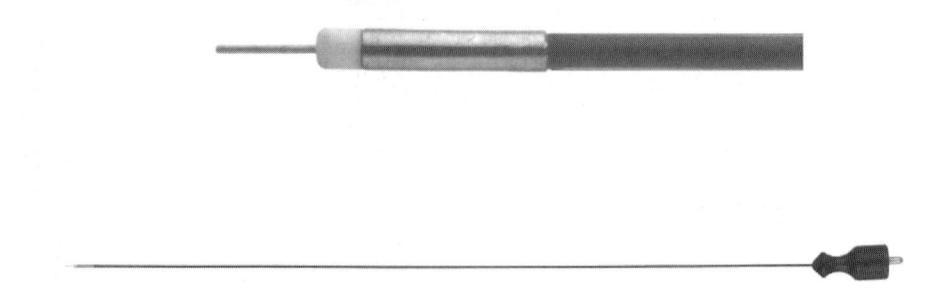

Fig. 5. Bipolar needle used during transvaginal endoscopy.

## 2.3.1. Endometriosis

*2.3.1.1. Selection of patients.* Selection of patients was based upon findings at diagnostic TVE or the presence of an endometrioma at transvaginal ultrasound. They were only referred for an operative TVE if vaginal examination revealed absence of any significant induration in the posterior fornix. Patients were classified using the revised American Fertility Society (rAFS) scoring system [14]: rAFS I, $n=34$; rAFS II, $n=11$; rAFS III, $n=6$.

It is interesting to note that in a comparative study the presence of subtle ovarian adhesions in patients with minimal or mild endometriosis was observed in 40% of the patients at standard laparoscopy and in 70% at transvaginal endoscopy [15].

*2.3.1.2. Reconstruction of large endometrioma.* Similar to standard laparoscopy, treatment of an endometrioma larger than 5 cm is performed in two steps. The technique differs from fenestration and coagulation in the first step [16]. The ovary is carefully dissected and fully mobilized and the site of inversion is identified. The cyst is opened at the site of inversion and rinsed. After aspiration, the site of retraction or inversion is opened widely. Using this technique, there is no collapse of the wall. The absence of high intra-abdominal pressure and the hydroflotation technique maintain the micro-neoangiogenesis and therefore the identification of the implants and keeps the adhesions floating. The fibrotic area at the site of inversion and the visible vascularized endometriotic implants are coagulated (Figs. 6 and 7). The second step is performed 2–3 months later and includes adhesiolysis, whenever necessary, and the complete coagulation of suspected implants in the involuted pseudocyst.

*2.3.1.3. Results.* The endometrioma was larger than 5 cm in four patients and the procedure was performed in two steps, reducing the severity of the disease from rAFS III to rAFS II in two patients and to rAFS I in the other two. In the first two patients, the size of the endometrioma was reduced from 7 to 4 cm, with the presence of small adhesions in the fossa ovarica involving about 1 cm of the ovarian surface. In the latter two patients, the endometriomas were reduced from 5 to 1 cm without adhesions. At second intervention,

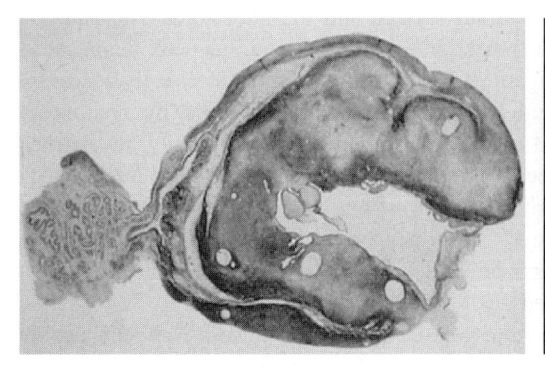

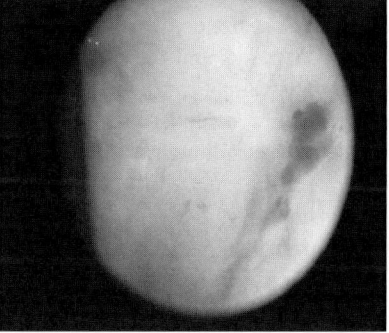

Fig. 6. An endometrioma is formed by the inversion of the ovarian capsule and is lined by fibroreactive tissue, free endometriotic implants and adhesions.

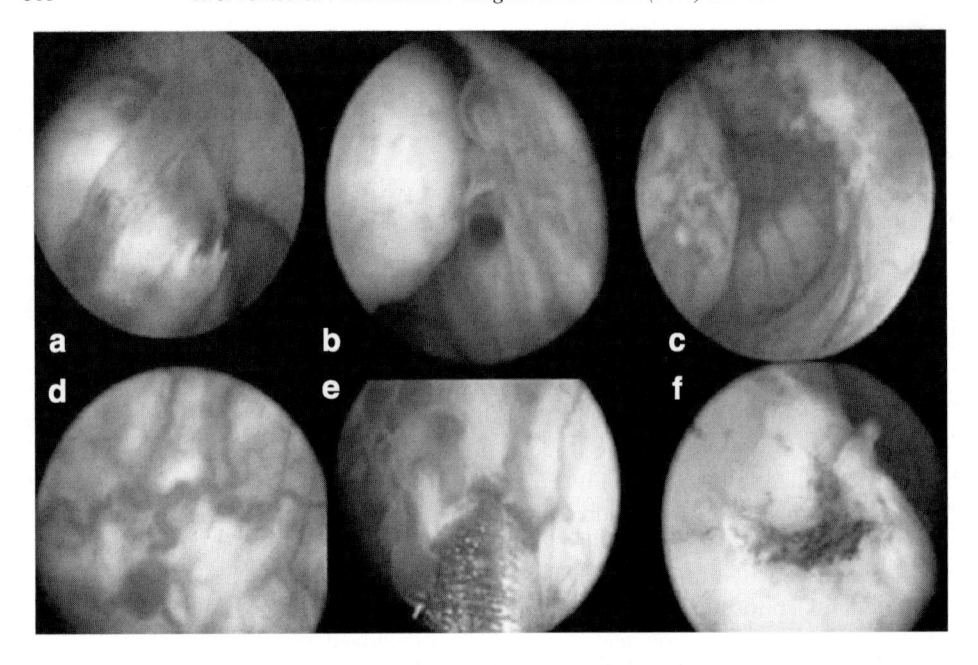

Fig. 7. Treatment of endometrioma during TVE. (a) Endometrioma with adhesions. (b) Complete adhesiolysis. (c) Enlargement of the opening of the endometriotic cyst at the site of inversion. (d) Biopsy of endometriotic tissue. (e) Coagulation of vascularised areas. (f) Final view after coagulation.

the invaginating edges of the reduced cyst could easily be identified in all cases and remaining adhesions were easily removed. In this way, the reduced chocolate cyst was widely opened allowing adequate visualization and complete ablation of the remaining endometriotic implants [17]. Thirty-three patients have a follow-up period up to 2 years and no recurrence of endometriosis at ultrasound has been detected.

*2.3.1.4. Benefits.* The transvaginal approach using the hydroflotation technique provides a remarkable delineation between the ovarian surface and the adhesions. The endometrioma is most frequently adherent to the posterior leaf of the broad ligament, the posterior side of the uterus and the uterosacral ligament. All these structures are directly accessible by the transvaginal route. In contrast with transabdominal access, whether by laparoscopy or laparotomy, a meticulous dissection can be performed and, surprisingly, in this way rupture of the endometriotic cyst can be avoided in most cases. Access to the endometriotic cyst at the site of inversion minimizes ovarian trauma and bleeding. After aspiration and rinsing of the cyst, the pseudocyst is further opened and, on close inspection underwater, the vascularized endometriotic implants and neoangiogenesis are clearly visible and can be selectively cauterized.

In contrast to standard laparoscopy, transvaginal endoscopy allows inspection of the ovaries and, particularly, the antero-lateral site and the fossa ovarica without supplementary manipulation. Manipulation of the ovary with standard laparoscopy to expose the posterior leaf of the broad ligament and the antero-lateral site of the ovary frequently causes traumatic bleeding, with rupturing of the adhesions and rupture of the endometriotic cyst.

### 2.3.2. Ovarian capsule drilling

Transvaginal endoscopy is quite suitable for drilling of the ovarian capsule in patients with polycystic ovarian syndrome (PCOS) that is resistant to medical therapy. For this purpose, the Versapoint probe and a bipolar needle (Storz, Tuettlingen) can be used (Fig. 8).

The arguments against surgical treatment of PCOS are the risk of adhesion formation and morbidity as well as the cost of a standard laparoscopy. At laparoscopy, the exposure to carbon dioxide has been shown to have adverse effects on the peritoneal microcirculation and cell protective systems, such as free radical scavengers, which may be the mechanism involved in adhesion recurrences [18]. Although reduction of adhesion formation occurs after reduced exposure to $CO_2$ [18], further evaluation is needed to prove an eventual reduction of adhesion formation after drilling of the ovarian capsule using warm saline as the distension medium. The data of Fernandez et al. [19] show the feasibility of the transvaginal approach with results comparable with those obtained after standard laparoscopic procedures.

As the procedure is easy to perform and permits at the same time, a complete exploration of the female pelvis, with low morbidity, this approach may be preferable to a prolonged low-dose step-up protocol with gonadotropins. It is certainly recommendable before referring patients to an in vitro fertilization (IVF) program. Restoration of monofollicular cycles, reduction of multiple pregnancies and lower rates of miscarriages are factors in favor of surgical treatment of PCOS.

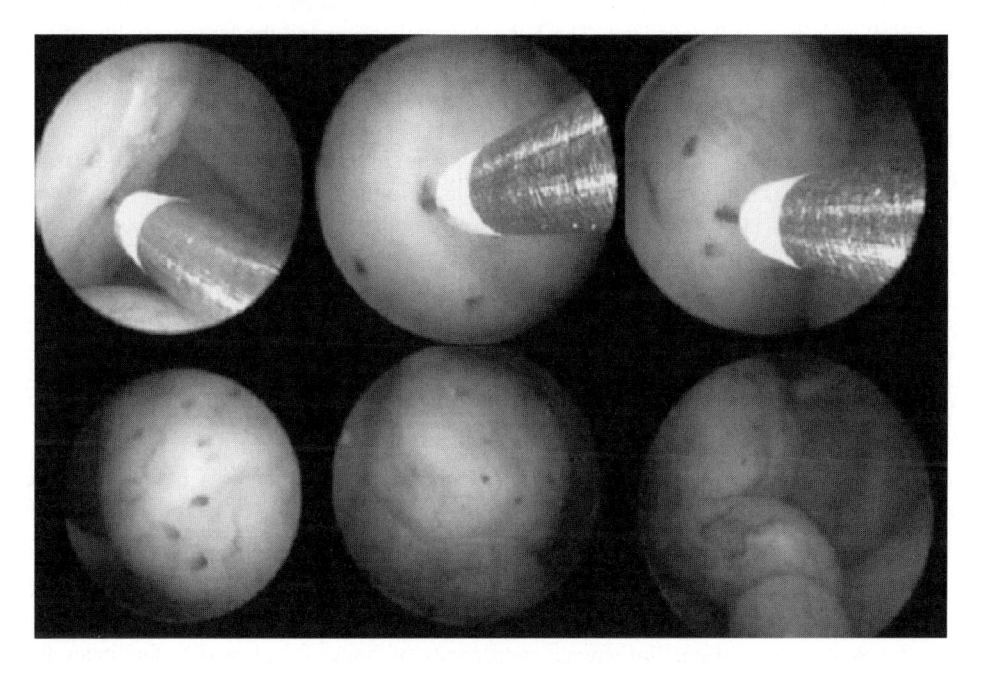

Fig. 8. Ovarian drilling during TVE.

## 2.3.3. Sequellae of pelvic inflammatory disease

In pelvic inflammatory disease, the patient's fertility outcome is compromised by the presence and extension of peri-ovarian and particular tubal mucosal adhesions. This interferes with fimbrial capture and transport of the oocyte, but may also impair ovulatory function and oocyte release at the moment of ovulation [20]. The physiological position of the tubo-ovarian structures and the use of saline distension medium during transvaginal endoscopy allow easier performance of a salpingoscopy when required [21]. In hydrosalpinx, the site of occlusion can clearly be recognized. Using the bipolar cutting needle, the hydrosalpinx is opened at this site and staging of the tubal mucosa is performed [22]. Salpingostomy is indicated in stages I and II of the salpingoscopic classification. The salpingoneostomy is performed via transvaginal endoscopy or by a conversion to laparoscopy. In cases of severely damaged tubes (stage III and IV), the patient is referred to an IVF program.

## 2.4. Discussion

This series of operative procedures confirms the feasibility of the transvaginal approach, as was previously reported [13]. In contrast to the transabdominal technique, the transvaginal route offers excellent visualization of the tubo-ovarian structures with direct access and without additional manipulation.

During operative TVE procedures, conversion to laparoscopy is seldom required. In comparison to a standard laparoscopy, morbidity after the transvaginal procedures is very low, most of the patients have no sensation of pain afterwards and, at most, complain of a slight tenderness in the lower abdomen. All patients return home the same day and resume their full activity 1 or 2 days later. The 1-day hospitalization and the low morbidity of the procedure make a second-step procedure, when indicated, more acceptable for the patient. The transvaginal approach and hydroflotation technique also allow study of the pathophysiology of endometriosis. The inspection of small endometriomas or early implants in ovaries with in situ endometriomas confirms the inversion origin of most ovarian endometriomas, as suggested by Sampson [23] and Hughesdon [24], and recently restated by Brosens et al. [17], using in situ ovarioscopy and selective biopsies. What initially appears as small brown or black vesicles upon the ovarian surface are, on closer inspection, small invaginated areas of the ovarian cortex, covered by small adhesions and filled with typical endometriotic fluid. At the base of these invaginations, endometriotic implants with their neoangiogenesis can be clearly identified. The use of TVE facilitates a close inspection of lesions, which might be difficult in laparoscopy and impossible at laparotomy.

In conclusion, it can be stated that the transvaginal approach for reconstructive tubo-ovarian endoscopic surgery is feasible. The direct access to the fossa ovarica and the ovaries, the use of hydroflotation and close inspection are of major benefits to achieve reconstructive tubo-ovarian surgery.

## 3. Conclusions

The introduction of small-diameter endoscopes of high optical quality facilitates the success of minimal access surgery in an ambulatory setting. However, the final invasiveness of the procedure is in the hands of the reproductive surgeon. As for microsurgery, a minimal invasive approach is not only a matter of technique, but also and essentially of philosophical and personal attitude.

The use of a fluid distension medium is very helpful, not only in intrauterine interventions but also in exploration of the female pelvis and for operative procedures in transvaginal hydrolaparoscopy. It improves accuracy in visualization of small lesions and provides a better distinction between different tissue layers, with a clear delineation between adhesions and organs and conservation of the microvascularization. In contrast to intrauterine and mild pelvic pathology, which can always be treated on an ambulatory basis, severe pelvic pathology necessitates hospitalisation. Because transvaginal endoscopy is still limited due to the absence of the panoramic view of standard laparoscopy, the latter cannot be abandoned as operative procedure. However, for limited interventions, the transvaginal approach diminishes the patient's morbidity drastically, shortens the hospitalization and reduces the final costs. In this way, standard laparoscopy, with higher morbidity and cost, can be reserved for more severe pathology.

## References

[1] P.G. Brooks, Complications of operative hysteroscopy: how safe is it? Clin. Obstet. Gynecol. 35 (1992) 256.
[2] F.D. Loffer, Contraindications and complications of hysteroscopy, Obstet. Gynecol. Clin. North Am. 22 (1995) 445.
[3] C.A. Witz, et al., Complications associated with the absorption of hysteroscopic fluid media, Fertil. Steril. 60 (1993) 745.
[4] R. Campo, et al., Office mini-hysteroscopy, Hum. Reprod. Updat. 5 (1999) 73–81.
[5] J. Hucke, R. Campo, Intrauterine synechien, in: J. Keckstein, J. Hucke (Eds.), Die endoskopischen Operationen in der Gynakologie, Urban and Fisher, Munchen, 2000, pp. 394–399.
[6] J.G. Schenker, E.J. Margalioth, Intrauterine adhesions: an updated appraisal, Fertil. Steril. 37 (1992) 593.
[7] J.A. Rock, A.A. Murphy, W.H. Cooper, Resectoscopic technique for the lysis of a class V complete uterine septum, Fertil. Steril. 48 (1987) 495.
[8] J. Donnez, M. Nisolle, Operative laser hysteroscopy in Mullerian fusion defects and uterine adhesions, in: J. Donnez (Ed.), Laser Operative Laparoscopy and Hysteroscopy, Nauwelaerts Printing, Leuven, 1994, pp. 295–304.
[9] C. Chapron, D. Querleu, M.A. Bruhat, Surgical complications of diagnostic and operative gynecological laparoscopy: a series of 29 966 cases, Hum. Reprod. 13 (1998) 867–872.
[10] F.W. Jansen, K. Kapiteyn, T. Trimbos-Kemper, Complications of laparoscopy: a prospective multicenter observational study, Br. J. Obstet. Gynaecol. 104 (1997) 595–600.
[11] E. Diamond, Diagnostic culdoscopy in infertility: a study of 4000 outpatient procedures, J. Reprod. Med. 21 (1978) 23–28.
[12] S. Gordts, et al., Transvaginal hydrolaparoscopy as an outpatient procedure for infertility investigation, Hum. Reprod. 13 (1998) 99–103.
[13] S. Gordts, R. Campo, I. Brosens, Operative transvaginal hydrolaparoscopy of a large ovarian endometrioma, Gynecol. Endosc. 9 (2000) 227–231.
[14] The American Fertility Society, Revised American Fertility Society classification of endometriosis, Fertil. Steril. 43 (1985) 351–352.
[15] I. Brosens, S. Gordts, R. Campo, Transvaginal hydrolaparoscopy but not standard laparoscopy reveals subtle endometriotic adhesions of the ovary, Fertil. Steril. 75 (2001) 1009–1012.
[16] I.A. Brosens, et al., Reconstruction of the ovary containing large endometriomas by an extraovarian endosurgical technique, Fertil. Steril. 66 (1996) 517–521.
[17] I.A. Brosens, P.J. Puttemans, J. Deprest, The endoscopic localization of endometrial implants in the ovarian chocolate cyst, Fertil. Steril. 61 (1994) 1034–1038.

[18] O. Taskin, et al., The effects of duration of $CO_2$ insufflation and irrigation on peritoneal microcirculation assessed by free radical scavengers and total glutathione levels during operative laparoscopy, J. Am. Assoc. Gynecol. Laparosc. 5 (1998) 129–133.
[19] H. Fernandez, et al., Operative transvaginal hydrolaparoscopy for treatment of polycystic ovary syndrome: a new minimally invasive surgery, Fertil. Steril. 75 (2001) 607–611.
[20] S. Gordts, R. Campo, L. Rombauts, Endoscopic visualisation of the process of fimbrial ovum retrieval in the human, Hum. Reprod. 13 (1998) 1425–1428.
[21] S. Gordts, et al., Transvaginal salpingoscopy: an office procedure for infertility investigation, Fertil. Steril. 70 (1998) 523–526.
[22] P.J. Puttemans, I.A. Brosens, P.H. Delattin, Salpingoscopy versus hysterosalpingography in hydrosalpinges, Hum. Reprod. 2 (1987) 535–540.
[23] J.A. Sampson, Peritoneal endometriosis due to the menstrual dissemination of endometrial tissue into the peritoneal cavity, Am. J. Obstet. Gynecol. 14 (1927) 422–469.
[24] P.E. Hughesdon, The structure of endometrial cysts of the ovary, J. Obstet. Gynaecol. Br. Emp. 44 (1957) 481–487.

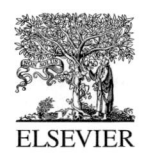

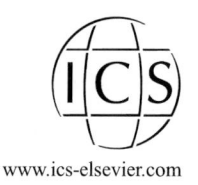

# Ultrasound imaging in human reproduction: what is new?

Sanja Kupesic*

*Department of Obstetrics and Gynecology, Medical School University of Zagreb, Sveti Duh Hospital, Sveti Duh 64, 10000 Zagreb, Croatia*

**Abstract.** Three-dimensional (3D) ultrasound seems to be advantageous in patients scheduled for serial ovarian monitoring, in whom planar reformatted sections allow more accurate and objective volumetric assessment of the leading follicles, which are not always spherical. Ovarian volume measurements by 3D ultrasound may contribute to accurate diagnosis of polycystic ovarian syndrome, prediction of the response to stimulation and estimation of the risk of ovarian hyperstimulation. Transvaginal ultrasound-directed follicular aspiration and embryo transfer under 3D ultrasound guidance improves the operator's spatial evaluation and allows precise follicular and/or catheter tip location during the course of interventional procedures. The use of 3D transvaginal ultrasonography after injection of saline solution and/or echo enhancing contrast medium produces high diagnostic accuracy for visualization of the uterine cavity and fallopian tubes. By providing multiple tomographic sections of the uterine cavity, uterine causes of infertility such as congenital uterine anomalies, submucous leiomyoma and/or intrauterine adhesions become easily visible. Quantification of the endometrial volume by 3D ultrasound, in combination with blood flow studies, contributes to the assessment of endometrial receptivity and has a potential to predict pregnancy rates in assisted reproductive techniques. © 2004 Published by Elsevier B.V.

*Keywords:* Three-dimensional ultrasound; Infertility; Ovarian monitoring and puncture; Hystero-contrast-salpingography; Uterine abnormalities

## 1. Introduction

Recent advances in three-dimensional (3D) ultrasound have made accurate, non-invasive measurements of the follicular, ovarian and endometrial volumes feasible. Storage capacities, reconstruction of the volume images and simultaneous viewing of all three orthogonal planes are the main advantages of this method in the field of infertility. In the not too distant future, this examination may become the method of choice to assess morphology of the uterine cavity and ovaries, as well as to perform ultrasound-directed puncture procedures and evaluate tubal patency. Here I review the

---

* Tel.: +385-1-3712109; fax: +385-1-3745534.
  *E-mail address:* sanja.kupesic@htnet.hr (S. Kupesic).

0531-5131/ © 2004 Published by Elsevier B.V.
doi:10.1016/j.ics.2004.01.065

potential application of this novel technique at each stage of investigation of the infertile patient.

## 2. Ovarian monitoring and ovarian causes of infertility

Monitoring of the ovarian response, essential for safe infertility treatment, can be efficiently performed using 3D ultrasound. Measurement of follicular volume by 3D ultrasound, compared with current standard 2D techniques, produced a more accurate reflection of the true volume estimated by corresponding follicular aspirates [1]. This is because 3D measurement is not affected by the follicular shape, since changing contours are outlined serially to obtain the specific volume measurement. The disparity in accuracy between the 3D assessment of follicular volume and the conventional approach is likely to increase significantly if there is a florid, multifollicular ovarian response, because the conventional formula is less precise with ellipsoid follicles, which predominate in this case.

Feichtinger [2] reported that 3D ultrasound might be useful for distinguishing ovarian cysts from ovarian follicles. 3D ultrasound can be used to search for the presence of cumuli in follicles greater than 15 mm. Follicles without visualization of the cumulus in all three planes were not likely to contain mature fertilizable oocytes. Cumulus visualization by 3D ultrasound appears to be an indicator for mature oocytes and successful fertilization. Follicles in which cumulus cannot be visualized in all three planes are unlikely to contain mature oocytes or oocytes in which fertilization is achieved.

Ovarian volume measurements achieved by 3D ultrasound can predict the ovarian response to stimulation and the risk of ovarian hyperstimulation. Oyesanya et al. [3] measured total ovarian volumes before the administration of human chorionic gonadotropin (HCG) in women undergoing treatment for infertility by IVF-ET, who were considered to have an exaggerated response to stimulation (>20 follicles). The mean total ovarian volume was significantly higher in the group of women who developed moderate or severe OHSS compared with controls ($271.00 \pm 87.00$ vs. $157.30 \pm 54.20$ ml). The 3D scanning can obtain more accurate volume data by outlining the contour of the target organ, which is better than traditional 2D ultrasonographic scanning calculated by the ellipsoid formula.

In patients with polycystic ovary syndrome, the new 3D ultrasound technique enables us to accurately measure ovarian volume. The ovaries of the patients with PCOS are larger in size, area and volume than normal. The stromal areas in PCOS are hypertrophic, and provide yet another subjective ultrasonographic criterion that could differentiate PCOS from the multifollicular ovary. Robert et al. [4] reported that an increased total ovarian stroma of >5.5 cm$^3$ correlated strongly with increased ovarian stroma at a strict longitudinal ovarian section and might contribute to accurate diagnosis of PCOS.

Apart from morphological and volume measurements, assessment of ovarian vessels can be added to the traditional endocrinological and ultrasonographic parameters used clinically for diagnosis of PCOS. Increased ovarian stromal blood flow detected by 3D power Doppler ultrasound may become a new parameter to assist in the ultrasound diagnosis of PCOS. Such a finding seems to explain the excessive response and multifollicular development when PCOS patients are administered gonadotropins during ovulation induction for IVF.

In order to evaluate whether ovarian antral follicle number, ovarian volume, stromal area and ovarian stromal blood flow are predictive of ovarian response and IVF outcome, we constructed a study where pretreatment 3D ultrasound ovarian measurements were compared with subsequent ovulation induction parameters [peak estradiol level (E-2) on HCG administration day and number of the aspirated oocytes] and cycle outcome (fertilization and pregnancy rates) [5]. The total antral follicle number achieved the best predictive value for favorable IVF outcome, followed by ovarian stromal flow index (FI), peak E-2 on HCG administration day, total ovarian volume, total ovarian stromal area and age. Using these six parameters, we were able to predict a favorable IVF outcome in 50% of patients and poor outcome in 85% of patients. 3D ultrasound studies facilitate determination of the antral follicle number, ovarian volume calculation, evaluation of the ovarian stroma and analysis of the intensity of ovarian stromal blood flow in a short time without increasing the patient's discomfort.

In a continuation of the previous study, we monitored the change of 3D ovarian measurements according to patient's age [6]. Pretreatment measurements (number of ovarian antral follicles, ovarian volume, and ovarian stromal flow index determined by 3D and power Doppler ultrasound) were compared with number of recovered oocytes, fertilization rates, and pregnancy rates. As patient age increased, significant trends in ovarian volume, number of follicles, and stromal vascularity decreased. 3D ovarian measurements and fertilization rates differed significantly among age groups. For each age group, a higher number of antral follicles, greater ovarian volume, and favorable ovarian stromal vascularity were associated with higher number of retrieved oocytes and increased pregnancy rates. Increasing patient age is associated with poor ovarian response, as represented by smaller ovarian volume, lower antral follicle count and poor stromal vascularity. Based on our experience, 3D power Doppler ultrasound can help to individualize stimulation protocols in patients undergoing IVF procedures, regardless of age.

## 3. Puncture procedures and 3D hystero-contrast-salpingography

Introduction of the 3D real-time ultrasound technology is the first significant step in obtaining and analyzing dynamic ultrasound images as they happen. By performing up to 25 volume scans per second, real-time 3D ultrasound can allow more precise follicular puncturing. The advantages of this method are: visualization of the organ of interest in all directions, simultaneous multiplanar slice view and volume rendered view and real-time needle visualization. Dynamic multiplanar view enables improved targeting of the object, resulting in a more representative specimen. The needle movement can be assessed within three dimensions, which is especially useful for the puncturing of the static structures such as stimulated ovaries.

Another clinical application of 3D ultrasound in assisted reproductive technology includes evaluation of uterine morphology and tubal patency by 3D hystero-contrast-salpingography (Hy-Co-Sy). The main advantage of this technique is demonstration of the coronal plane and third dimension of the uterine cavity. Demonstration of the coronal plane is mandatory for the diagnosis of uterine pathology, such as septate, arcuate or bicornuate uteri. It also provides the most exact measurement of the endometrial width when transected in a mid-perpendicular manner, since during 3D hysterosonography the typical, triangulated uterine cavity appears in its full shape. Surface or maximal/minimal renderings provide even more information on uterine findings, such as uterine anatomy, uterine cavity, and its content. There are two techniques to accomplish this goal: instillation of the negative contrast medium (normal saline) for demonstration of the entire uterine cavity, its shape, pathology and the frame of the myometrial mantel, and injection of a positive contrast medium for assessment of the permeability of the fallopian tubes.

Hysterosonography is very useful for demonstration of the intracavitary pathologies, such as uterine anomalies, adhesions, submucous leiomyomas and endometrial polyps. Weinraub et al. [7] have demonstrated the feasibility of combined 3D ultrasound and saline contrast hysterosonography. Since volume sampling has a short pick-up time of a few seconds, the examination is over almost immediately after the uterus is reasonably distended. In this uncomfortable examination such an advantage should not be underestimated. Simultaneous display of the three perpendicular planes offers a more comprehensive overview of the examined area and gives access to planes unobtainable by conventional 2D ultrasonographic examination. Surface rendering may confirm the presence of pathological findings in equivocal cases, and characterize their appearance, size, volume and relationship to the surrounding structures. Surface rendering of the polypoid structures shows echogenic masses on a pedicle protruding into the uterine cavity. Submucous leiomyoma appears as a mixed echogenic site bulging into the cavity. Intrauterine synechiae appear as bands of varying thickness traversing the uterine cavity. This can be useful when deciding on treatment options, such as conservative management vs. surgery, and can be a valuable tool in surgical procedures carried out under ultrasonographic guidance. Kyokawa et al. [8] evaluated infertile women using 3D Hy-Co-Sy, with saline as a contrast medium, as a routine outpatient procedure for the assessment of the uterine cavity and tubal patency. The efficacy of the procedure was evaluated with X-ray HSG (hysterosalpingography). The positive predictive value, negative predictive value, sensitivity, and specificity of predicting tubal patency by 3D Hy-Co-Sy were 100%, 33.3%, 84.45, and 100%. The full contour of the uterine cavity was depicted in 96% of cases with 3D Hy-Co-Sy and 64% by X-HSG ($P<0.005$). The uterine cavity area measured on 3D Hy-Co-Sy correlated well with the volume of contrast medium required on X-HSG. 3D Hy-Co-Sy provided advantages of better assessment of the uterine cavity over X-HSG. Compared with conventional X-HSG, the efficacy of 3D Hy-Co-Sy to assess tubal patency was acceptable. The procedure of 3D Hy-Co-Sy appears to be better tolerated, requiring no sedation or anesthesia and a reduced examination time. Therefore, 3D Hy-Co-Sy with saline as a contrast medium is feasible and could comprise a routine outpatient procedure in the initial evaluation of infertile women.

Fallopian tubes can be demonstrated on ultrasound only when they contain fluid (hydrosalpinx, pyosalpinx, bleeding ectopic pregnancy, or a contrast medium). In the case of hydrosalpinx, the fluid-filled Fallopian tube is demonstrated in three multiplanar sections rendered on 3D ultrasound. Instead of visualizing the echo contrast with grayscale ultrasound, it is possible to use 3D power Doppler technology that is sensitive to slow flow. If the tube is patent, Doppler signals should be obtained from flow along the tube and free spill from the fimbrial end should be identified. Sladkevicious et al. [9]

compared the feasibility of 3D power Doppler imaging in the assessment of the patency of the Fallopian tubes during the Hy-Co-Sy procedure with 2D gray-scale scanning. The mean duration of the imaging procedure is less with 3D power Doppler imaging, but the operator time, which includes postprocedure analysis of the stored information, is similar. A lower volume of the contrast medium is required for 3D power Doppler imaging in comparison to that used for conventional 2D Hy-Co-Sy. Sladkevicious et al. [9] reported that color-coded 3D power Doppler imaging with surface rendering allowed visualization of the flow of the contrast through the entire tubal length. Free spill of the contrast from the distal part of the tube was clearly identified in the majority of cases. Furthermore, 3D ultrasound technique allowed better storage of the information for re-analysis and archiving than conventional Hy-Co-Sy. Although examination time for 3D ultrasound is not less than that needed for 2D sonography, some parts of the examination, like measurements, volume assessment, reconstruction of the planes of interest or tomography, and surface rendering can be performed off-line.

## 4. Uterine causes of infertility

Assessment of the uterine morphology and exclusion of the endometrial pathology are essential before commencement of medically assisted reproduction. It is clear that anatomic uterine abnormalities, including submucous leiomyomas, intrauterine adhesions and congenital uterine anomalies interfere with implantation of the developing embryo and may cause recurrent pregnancy loss. Since 3D ultrasound provides images of the uterine cavity in multiple tomographic sections, intracavitary structures become clearly visible.

Congenital uterine malformations are variable in frequency and are usually estimated to represent 3–4%, although less than half have clinical symptoms [10,11]. The respective frequency of symptomatic malformations is dominated by septate uterus. During the first trimester of pregnancy, the risk of spontaneous abortion in this group is between 28% and 45%, while during the second trimester the frequency of late spontaneous abortions is approximately 5%.

Our team attempted to evaluate the combined use of transvaginal ultrasound, transvaginal color and pulsed Doppler sonography, hysterosonography and 3D ultrasound in the preoperative diagnosis of septate uterus [12]. The sensitivity and specificity of 3D ultrasonography were 98.38% and 100%, respectively. A false-negative result in one patient was caused by a fundal leiomyoma distorting the uterine cavity. With 3D ultrasound there was no misinterpretation of the septate uterus for a bicornuate one. 3D ultrasound enables planar reformatted sections through the uterus, which allow precise evaluation of the fundal indentation and the length of the septum. Based on our experience, this technique may give a wrong impression of an arcuate uterus in patients with fundal location of the leiomyoma. In these cases the uterine cavity has a concave shape, while fundal indentation is shallower. Furthermore, shadowing caused by the uterine leiomyomas, irregular endometrial lining and decreased volume of the uterine cavity (in cases of intrauterine adhesions) are obvious limitations of 3D ultrasound. More recently, 3D power Doppler was used to detect vascularization of the uterine septa in a combined angio and gray rendering mode. This approach allows simultaneous analysis of the morphology, texture and vascularization of the uterine septa.

Another study of our group [13] clearly proved that obstetric complications were more frequent among patients with septate uterus than among other women. Furthermore, we demonstrated that ectopic pregnancy occurred at double rate (27.3%) in these patients when compared with controls (13.3%). A possible etiology for this finding is the menstrual reflux, commonly present in patients with uterine anomalies, which sequelae may interfere with passage of the fertilized egg into the uterine cavity. The benefit of removing the intrauterine septum in patients suffering from infertility and recurrent pregnancy wastage has been clearly demonstrated. However, the outcome of hysteroscopic metroplasty depends on patient selection and may be different in the infertile population and women with miscarriages. In the series of Fedele et al. [14], the cumulative live birth rate following hysteroscopic metroplasty at 36 months was 39% in women with infertility, and 62% in women with miscarriages. At present, data obtained from retrospective series suggest that hysteroscopic metroplasty for the septate uterus is associated with a favourable outcome, with a pregnancy rate of approximately 80% and a miscarriage rate of only approximately 15% [15]. It seems that septal incision eliminates an unsuitable site of implantation through revascularization of the connective uterine fundal tissue or elimination of the unfavourable uterine contractions [13]. Since both of these events can be detected by 3D and power Doppler ultrasound, this new modality can be efficiently used for detection of the congenital uterine malformations and follow up of the patients undergoing hysteroscopy.

## 5. Uterine receptivity

The endometrium has been a focus of interest since the beginning of ultrasound diagnosis in gynecology. Although endometrial thickness obtained by 2D ultrasonography is considered the most important parameter of endometrial growth, it does not include the total volume of the endometrium. The ability to quantify the volume of the endometrium using 3D ultrasound may help to resolve the problem presented in the literature where some studies claim that inadequate endometrial thickness is connected to failure of implantation, and others did not find such a correlation. This is because cycle outcome can be correlated with more objective, quantitative parameters rather than endometrial thickness, which is prone to greater subjective variation in measurement.

3D ultrasound has brought the possibility of calculating the volume of endometrium by stepping through the volume in plane mode. The outer limits of endometrium are traced and volume calculations can be performed immediately. To obtain the best results, stepping through the volume should be performed in small units. In each new plane the area tracing has to be corrected to its new extent. According to the experienced sonographers and investigators, 3D ultrasound volume measurements are highly reliable with a small measurement error. Since it is applied in the same manner as 2D vaginal ultrasound, it does not cause additional discomfort.

Turnbull et al. [16] pointed out the reasons why the maximum endometrial thickness is fraught with several problems: first, the uterus may be scanned in an oblique plane thus over- or underestimating the true endometrial thickness; second, a single measurement, usually obtained at the level of the fundus of the uterus is used to represent the entire cross section of the endometrium; third, marked ovarian enlargement may distort the endometrial outline leading to incorrect measurements. Therefore, 3D volumetry may offer a more reliable method to assess the endometrial cavity from the fundal region to the internal cervical os.

In the study of Schild et al. [17] no difference was found between endometrial measurements (thickness and volume) and the pregnancy rates. Interestingly, mean values for endometrial thickness and volume were lower, albeit non-significantly, in the pregnant group. Furthermore, E-2 concentrations were not significantly correlated with endometrial volume. On the contrary, Raga et al. [18] demonstrated that the pregnancy and implantation rates were significantly lower in the group of patients with endometrial volume <2 ml, while no pregnancy was achieved with an endometrial volume <1 ml. Similar results were obtained in our study, indicating that no pregnancy was achieved when endometrial volume was <2 ml, or when it exceeded 8 ml [19]. On the other hand, in the group of patients with endometrial thickness ranging from 2 to 7 ml, no relationship was apparent in terms of pregnancy rate.

Our results indicated that the homogeneous and hyperechogenic endometrial texture on the day of embryo transfer was predictive for implantation. No pregnancy occurred in patients with multilayered endometrial pattern on the day of embryo transfer. The scoring system reported in our study [19] was based on analysis of the endometrial parameters on the day of ET, such as endometrial thickness, volume, echogenicity, and subendometrial blood flow. We demonstrated that measurement of vascular resistance in subendometrial vessels and evaluation of subendometrial vessel density are more indicative than analysis of the presence or absence of the subendometrial blood flow alone. Significantly greater FI values ($13.2 \pm 2.2$), obtained by 3D power Doppler ultrasound, in the pregnant group and the fact that no pregnancy occurred when FI was less than 11.0, enabled us to propose this cutoff value for the 3D US scoring system. A better degree of subendometrial perfusion on the day of embryo transfer indicated a more favorable endometrial milieu for implantation.

Evaluation of endometrial receptivity by 3D power Doppler ultrasound seems to facilitate its routine application in deciding how many embryos or blastocysts will be transferred or cryopreserved. Further studies are needed to evaluate whether such assessment of endometrial receptivity will lead to high pregnancy rates.

## References

[1] A. Kyei-Mensah, J. Zaidi, R. Pittrof, A. Shaker, S. Campbell, S.L. Tan, Transvaginal three-dimensional ultrasound: reproducibility of ovarian and endometrial volume measurements, Fertil. Steril. 66 (1996) 718–722.
[2] W. Feichtinger, Transvaginal three-dimensional imaging for evaluation and treatment of infertility, in: E. Merz (Ed.), 3D Ultrasound in Obstetrics and Gynecology, Lipincott Williams and Wilkins, Philadelphia, 1998, pp. 377–435.
[3] O.A. Oyesanya, J.H. Parsons, W.P. Collins, S. Campbell, Total ovarian volume before human chorionic gonadotropin administration for ovulation induction may predict the hyperstimulation syndrome, Hum. Reprod. 10 (1995) 3211–3212.
[4] Y. Robert, F. Dubrulle, L. Gaillandre, Y. Ardaens, P. Thomas-Desrousseauxe, L. Lemaitre, Ultrasound assessment of ovarian stroma hypertrophy in hyperandrogenism and ovulation disorders: visual analysis versus computerized quantification, Fertil. Steril. 64 (1995) 307–312.
[5] S. Kupesic, A. Kurjak, Predictors of IVF outcome by three-dimensional ultrasound, Hum. Reprod. 17 (2002) 950–955.
[6] S. Kupesic, A. Kurjak, D. Bjelos, S. Vujisic, Three-dimensional ultrasonographic ovarian measurements and in vitro fertilization outcome are related to age, Fertil. Steril. 79 (2003) 190–197.

[7] Z. Weinraub, R. Maymon, A. Shulman, J. Bukovsky, A. Kratochwil, A. Lee, A. Herman, Three-dimensional saline contrast rendering of uterine cavity pathology, Ultrasound Obstet. Gynecol. 8 (1966) 277–282.
[8] K. Kiyokawa, H. Masuda, T. Fuyuki, M. Koseki, N. Uchida, T. Fukuda, K. Anemiya, K. Shouka, K. Suzuki, Three-dimensional hysterosalpingo-contrast sonography (3D HyCoSy) as an outpatient procedure to assess infertile women: a pilot study, Ultrasound Obstet. Gynecol. 6 (2000) 648–654.
[9] P. Sladkeviciuous, K. Ojha, S. Campbell, G. Nargund, Three-dimensional power Doppler imaging in the asssessment of Fallopian tube patency, Ultrasound Obstet. Gynecol. 16 (2000) 644–647.
[10] D. Ashton, H.K. Amin, R.M. Richart, R.S. Neuwirth, The incidence of asmyptomatic uterine anomalies in women undergoing transcervical tubal sterilization, Obstet. Gynecol. 72 (1988) 28–30.
[11] P. Gaucherand, A. Awada, R.C. Rudigoz, D. Dargent, Obstetrical prognosis of septate uterus: a plea for treatment of the septum, Eur. J. Obstet. Gynecol. Reprod. Biol. 54 (1994) 109–112.
[12] S. Kupesic, A. Kurjak, Septate uterus: detection and prediction of obstetrical complications by different forms of ultrasonography, J. Ultrasound Med. 17 (1988) 631–636.
[13] S. Kupesic, A. Kurjak, Diagnosis and treatment outcome of the septate uterus, Croat. Med. J. 39 (1998) 185–190.
[14] L. Fedele, L. Arcaini, F. Parazzini, P. Vercellini, G.D. Nola, Metroplastic hysteroscopy and fertility, Fertil. Steril. 59 (1993) 768–770.
[15] H.A. Homer, T.C. Li, I.D. Cooke, The septate uterus: a review of management and reproductive outcome, Fertil. Steril. 73 (2000) 1–14.
[16] L.W. Turnbull, C.F. Rice, A. Horsmann, J. Robinson, S.R. Killick, Magnetic resonance imaging and transvaginal ultrasound of the uterus prior to embryo transfer, Hum. Reprod. 9 (1994) 2438–2443.
[17] R.L. Schild, D. Indefrei, S. Eschweiler, H. van der Ven, R. Fimmers, M. Hansmann, Three-dimensional endometrial volume calculation and pregnancy rate in an in-vitro fertilization programme, Hum. Reprod. 14 (1999) 1255–1258.
[18] F. Raga, F. Bonilla-Musoles, E.M. Casan, O. Klein, Assessment of endometrial volume by three-dimensional ultrasound prior to embryo transfer: clues to endometrial receptivity, Hum. Reprod. 14 (1999) 2851–2854.
[19] S. Kupesic, I. Bekavac, D. Bjelos, A. Kurjak, Assessment of endometrial receptivity by transvaginal color Doppler and three-dimensional power Doppler ultrasonography in patients undergoing in vitro fertilization procedures, J. Ultrasound Med. 20 (2001) 125–134.

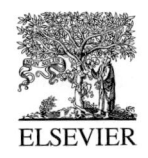

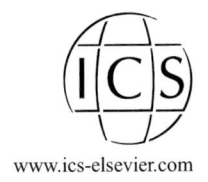

# Pelvic MR imaging in infertility and recurrent pregnancy loss

Caroline Reinhold*

*Diagnostic Radiology, McGill University Health Center, 1650 Cedar Ave., Montreal, Quebec, Canada H3G 1A4*

**Abstract.** Endovaginal sonography and hysterosalpingography (HSG) are the most common imaging modalities used in the evaluation of patients presenting with infertility or recurrent pregnancy loss. In most cases, these modalities adequately address the clinical question. However, magnetic resonance (MR) imaging helps predict the outcome and/or monitor the results of treatment for a number of these clinical entities and may lead to selection of better treatment plans and management. © 2004 Published by Elsevier B.V.

*Keywords:* MR imaging; MRI; Infertility; Pregnancy loss; Uterine anomaly; Endometriosis; Leiomyoma

## 1. Introduction

Endovaginal sonography and hysterosalpingography (HSG) are the most common imaging modalities used in the evaluation of patients presenting with infertility or recurrent pregnancy loss. In the vast majority of patients, these modalities adequately address the clinical question at hand and allow institution of appropriate therapy. Magnetic resonance (MR) imaging in this setting is an important problem solving modality and is usually reserved for cases where endovaginal sonography is suboptimal or inconclusive. However, with reported accuracies of up to 100%, MR imaging is currently the modality of choice in characterizing and evaluating mullerian duct anomalies. At times the distinction between a septate and bicornuate uterus may not be clear on endovaginal sonography, and misclassifications occur not infrequently. In addition, the accuracy of sonography falls further in the setting of complex obstructed anomalies.

MR imaging has only an auxiliary role to HSG in the detection of uterine synechia. The major benefit of MR imaging is to image the uterine cavity above the adhesions, which are not visualized by hysteroscopy. Indeed, determining the presence of endometrial remnants in the fundus is crucial for therapeutic decisions. MR imaging is highly accurate at differentiating leiomyomas from adenomyosis, a critical

---

\* Tel.: +1-514-9341934; fax: +1-514-9348263.
*E-mail address:* caroline.reinhold@synarc.com (C. Reinhold).

diagnostic point in patients for whom uterine conserving therapy is planned. Finally, MR imaging plays an important role in diagnosing endometriomas when the sonographic findings are nonspecific or inconclusive. MR imaging has a greater sensitivity than endovaginal sonography for detecting solid endometriosis or endometriomas measuring less than 1 cm. Although laparoscopy remains the standard of reference for diagnosis endometriosis, MR imaging can assess the extraperitoneal regions for the presence of disease.

HSG remains the standard of reference for assessing tubal patency and evaluating for tubal pathology.

## 2. MR imaging technique

### 2.1. Contraindications

Questions regarding potential pregnancy or late menstrual period are included on the pre-MRI procedure screening form. A possible pregnancy must be identified prior to exposure to the electromagnetic fields of an MR system, so that the referring physician, patient and radiologist may weigh the risks and benefits of the MR procedure. When the referring physician can defend the outcome of the MR examination in a pregnant patient insofar as it has the potential to alter the care or therapy of the mother or fetus, an MR procedure may be performed with informed consent, regardless of the stage of the trimester. However, "elective" MR examinations as a precaution are generally deferred to the second trimester once organogenesis is complete. As stated in the *Policies, Guidelines, and Recommendations for MR Imaging Safety and Patient Management* issued by the Safety Committee of the Society of Magnetic Resonance Imaging in 1991, "MR imaging may be used in pregnant women if other nonionizing forms of diagnostic imaging are inadequate or if the examination provides important information that would otherwise require exposure to ionizing radiation." This information was adopted by the American College of Radiology and is considered to be "standard of care" with respect to the use of MR procedures in pregnant patients [1].

Most absolute contraindications to MR imaging relate to a number of biomedical implants and devices [2]. A detailed discussion of these materials is beyond the scope of this manuscript; however, devices tested in the MRI environment may be reviewed at www.MRIsafety.com. In patients with biomedical implants, the following information should be provided to the MR imaging facility by the referring physician: manufacturer; type (ferromagnetic, weakly ferromagnetic or non-ferromagnetic); material or alloy; lot number; and model and/or serial number. Additional contraindications to MR imaging include patients with metallic ocular foreign bodies. Metallic foreign bodies in other locations need to be evaluated according to metal type, location and size/shape of the object in question.

### 2.2. Patient preparation

To minimize motion artifact produced by bowel peristaltism, patients are asked to fast from 6 to 8 hours before the procedure. Furthermore, patients are administered glucagon (1 mg) or buscopan (40 mg) IM to further reduce bowel peristaltism. When claustrophobia is a consideration, prone scanning or intravenous sedation may be helpful.

## 3. Congenital uterine anomalies

### 3.1. Classification

Buttram and Gibbons proposed a classification system in 1979, which was based on the degree of failure of normal development, while considering similar clinical features, reproductive outcomes, and management [3]. This classification system modified by the American Fertility Society in 1988 (now the American Society of Reproductive Medicine), is the most widely accepted framework of interpreting uterovaginal anomalies [4].

### 3.2. Class I: Mullerian agenesis and hypoplasia

Complete vaginal agenesis, or Mayer-Rokitansky-Kuster-Hauser Syndrome, is the most common presentation. Ninety percent of patients have uterine agenesis, while 10% have a small rudimentary uterus, with or without an obstructed endometrial segment. Ovaries are normal in appearance, however they may be located more cranially outside of the pelvis. Uterine agenesis manifests as lack of a detectable uterus on MRI. Hypoplastic uteri are small, with low signal intensity on T2-weighted images and diminished zonal anatomy even if an endometrial segment is present [5–7]. Vaginal agenesis is best characterized in the transverse plane with no normal vaginal tissue between the urethra and rectum.

### 3.3. Class II: Unicornuate uterus

Unicornuate uteri, without rudimentary horns or those with noncavitary rudimentary horns, are managed expectantly. Unicornuate uteri, with both noncommunicating and communicating rudimentary horns, are usually surgically resected due to dysmenorrhea and hematometra, as well as the potential for pregnancy within the hypoplastic horn. The uterus appears elongated and curved on MRI, presenting as a "banana" shape. Normal zonal anatomy is preserved, although overall uterine volume is decreased. The endometrium may be uniformly narrow or may slightly widen, tapering at the apex in the shape of a bullet. The appearance of the rudimentary horn depends on the presence of endometrial tissue.

### 3.4. Class III: Uterus didelphys

In uterus didelphys, two separate uterine horns (often widely divergent) and two separate cervices are visualized with MR imaging. Normal zonal anatomy is preserved within each hemiuterus, and the two horns stay symmetric in size. Like a unicornuate uterus, the uterine volume of each horn is decreased. A low signal intensity septum may be seen extending to the vagina. Obstructed moieties manifest as varying degrees of dilatation of the vaginal segment and lesser dilatation of the endometrium, with increased signal intensity of blood and debris on T2- and T1-weighted images [8–10].

### 3.5. Class IV: Bicornuate uterus

In the bicornuate uterus, the horns are symmetric in size with a cleft of variable length in the middle extending to the internal cervical os in the "complete" bicornuate uterus, and to a lesser degree in the "incomplete" bicornuate uterus. The cervix may be single (bicornuate unicollis) or duplicated (bicornuate bicollis). Communication of the endometrial segments, most commonly within the lower uterine body, is the hallmark of this anomaly. This characteristic differentiates a complete bicornuate bicollis uterus from a uterus didelphys in which no endometrial communication exists. The fundal cleft on MRI is greater than 1.0 cm, which distinguishes the bicornuate from the septate uterus. Normal zonal anatomy is shown circumferentially within both horns. Communication between the two cavities is essential for the diagnosis, and is demonstrated by confluent, increased signal intensity of the endometrium on T2-weighted images [6–8].

### 3.6. Class V: Septate uterus

In the septate uterus, the external uterine outline can be convex, flat, or mildly concave with the fundal indentation always <1.0 cm [8–11]. In septate anomaly, the size of the uterus is normal on MR imaging with the endometrial cavities appearing smaller than in a normal uterus. The fundal portion of the septum is isointense to myometrium in both partial and complete septa. In complete septa, the inferior segment of the septum is usually of low signal intensity on T2-weighted images, due to a greater fibrous component. This low signal intensity band is frequently absent in partial septa, which are invariably isointense to myometrium [12]. Leiomyomas and adenomyosis arising in the septum confirm the myometrial composition of the septum.

### 3.7. Class VII: DES-exposed uterus

Uterine hypoplasia and the characteristic "T"-shaped contour of the narrowed, irregular endometrial cavity and shortened upper uterine segment are well shown on MR imaging. Constriction bands are seen as focal narrowing of the mid-fundal segment of the endometrium resulting in reduction of the interstitial segments of the fallopian tubes [13]. Cervical hypoplasia and a narrowed, irregular endocervical canal can also be configured. MRI cannot demonstrate fallopian tube abnormalities, unless complicated by hydrosalpinx.

## 4. Endometrial synechiae

The diagnosis is usually offered by hysterography or HSG, and confirmed by hysteroscopy [14].

Hysterography commonly shows the filling defects, typically lacunar defects [15]. On HSG, it is difficult to visualize the synechia unless the endometrial cavity is distended by fluid, when they are seen as traversing bands of tissue within the anechoic cavity. The cavity may be distorted.

MR imaging has only an auxiliary role to HSG in the detection of uterine synechia. T2-weighted MR images show hypointense bands of fibrous tissue representing adhesions of the uterine wall. The major benefit of MR imaging is to image the uterine cavity above the adhesions, which are not visualized by hysteroscopy. Indeed, determining the presence of endometrial remnants in the fundus is crucial for therapeutic decisions [15].

## 5. Leiomyomas

Leiomyomas are best detected on T2-weighted images and appear as well-circumscribed masses of homogeneously decreased signal intensity masses. Orthogonal images allow for accurate localization of leiomyomas as submucosal, intramural or subserosal. Leiomyomas larger than 3 cm are usually heterogeneous due to varying degrees of degeneration. Leiomyomas with hemorrhagic degeneration demonstrate high signal intensity areas on T1-weighted images and do not enhance after contrast administration [16]. Advanced hyaline degeneration may be accompanied by fatty degeneration; however, when macroscopic fat is present in a leiomyoma the diagnosis of benign mixed muellerian tumor or lipoadenofibroma should be a consideration [16,17]. Cellular leiomyomas, a subtype of leiomyomas characterized by densely packed smooth muscle with little intervening collagen, are uniformly high in signal intensity on T2-weighted images [18]. Since they are shown to respond favourably to gonadotropin-releasing hormone (GnRH) analog therapy, prospectively identifying this type of leiomyoma may be advantageous. However, significant overlap in signal characteristics between cellular leiomyomas and degenerated leiomyomas often makes differentiating these lesions difficult.

Enhancement characteristics are becoming increasingly important in predicting which patients may benefit from uterine artery embolization (UAE) and for monitoring patient response post-UAE. Hypervascular leiomyomas show a good response to UAE [19]. In contradistinction, leiomyomas with negligible enhancement and high signal intensity on T1-weighted sequences do not respond to UAE. These imaging features suggest that these leiomyomas have already undergone hemorrhagic infarction. Therefore, patients do not receive any further benefit from embolizing an already infarcted leiomyoma [19]. Pre-UAE MR angiograms are useful for identifying patients with leiomyomas supplied by parasitized ovarian arteries. These may not respond to UAE and/or do not have permanent results as evidenced by re-vascularization and regrowth of their tumour. Such patients may benefit from re-treatment or alternative treatments [20–22].

MR imaging is helpful for distinguishing leiomyomas from other solid pelvic masses, especially in patients with a non-diagnostic or equivocal ultrasound findings [23,16]. Submucosal leiomyomas are usually differentiated from endometrial polyps by identifying their myometrial origin and low signal intensity on T2-weighted images. Lastly, myometrial contractions may mimic both submucosal leiomyomas and adenomyomas [24,25].

## 6. Adenomyosis

Adenomyosis is best shown on T2-weighted sequences that also demonstrate the uterine zonal anatomy. The diagnostic criteria to diagnose adenomyosis includes (1) focal or diffuse widening of the low signal intensity junctional zone, or (2) an ill-defined low signal intensity myometrial mass [26–31]. Based on a retrospective study, we reported that the optimal junctional zone width for diagnosing adenomyosis is ≥12 mm [27]. A junctional zone width of ≤8 mm reliably excludes the disease, whereas a junctional zone width of 9–11 mm is equivocal [27]. In the latter instance, supplementary findings may facilitate the diagnosis. Ancillary findings in adenomyosis include: (1) poorly defined margins; (2) high signal intensity foci on T1- or T2-weighted sequences; and (3) linear, high signal intensity striations radiating out from the endometrial surface [27–29]. These striations probably represent direct invasion of the endometrial zona basalis into the underlying myometrium. The low signal intensity on T2-weighted images seen with adenomyosis is a result of the associated smooth muscle hyperplasia. The high signal intensity foci within a region of adenomyosis occurs in more than 50% of patients and may represent ectopic endometrium, cystically dilated endometrial glands, and/or hemorrhage [27–29].

The differential diagnosis of adenomyosis usually focuses on leiomyomas, although these conditions usually coexist. Differentiating the two entities may be crucial because uterine-conserving therapy is established for leiomyomas, whereas hysterectomy remains the definitive treatment for debilitating adenomyosis. While MRI is extremely accurate in making this distinction, especially in patients with diffuse adenomyosis, the imaging features of focal adenomyosis or adenomyomas can overlap with the imaging findings of leiomyomas [29,30]. Another entity that may mimic focal adenomyosis or an adenomyoma is a myometrial contraction. As mentioned earlier, myometrial contractions are transient and usually change or disappear over the course of the exam. Finally, diffuse muscular hypertrophy may also cause widening of the junctional zone, however the widening tends to be less prominent, uniform and well defined compared with florid diffuse adenomyosis [27]. Cystic adenomyosis should be differentiated from a leiomyoma with central hemorrhagic degeneration or a bicornuate uterus with an obstructed horn.

## 7. Endometriosis

MR imaging can detect extraperitoneal spread of endometriosis, as well as identify lesions hidden by dense adhesions not seen at laparoscopy. MR imaging can also be used to follow up patients with endometriomas and to monitor post-treatment changes. Small implants and adhesions may not be easily visualized on MR.

The most common manifestation of endometriosis on MR imaging is the endometrioma. They appear as large (usually >1 cm), thick-walled, uniformly hyperintense lesions on T1-weighted images, and exhibit a gradient of low signal intensity (shading) on T2-weighted images, which may contain small foci of high signal intensity. Smaller (<1 cm) endometriomas present as multiple, homogeneously hyperintense cysts on T1-weighted images with varying degrees of low signal intensity on T2-weighted images [34]. Based on the above-mentioned findings, the accuracy of MR imaging in detecting endometriomas ranges between 76% and 96% in different studies [34,35]. While variable mural enhancement may happen, contrast-enhanced sequences have not been proven to increase the accuracy of MR imaging in detecting endometriomas. MR imaging demonstrates interval changes in endometriomas in patients with a known diagnosis and can be useful in monitoring response to GnRH analogues [32,33].

Endometrial implants may be predominantly solid in nature, secondary to prominent fibrosis, particularly in implants involving the bladder and bowel walls. These implants are of low signal intensity both on T1- and T2-weighted images, due to fibrosis, with punctate foci of high signal demonstrated on T1-weighted images. Following gadolinium administration, enhancement is demonstrated representing their solid vascularized nature.

## 8. Conclusion

MR imaging plays an important role as a problem solving modality in the infertile patient or patient presenting with recurrent pregnancy loss. In the evaluation of uterine anomalies, MR imaging is the modality of choice.

## References

[1] F.G. Shellock, E. Kanal, Policies, guidelines and recommendations for MR imaging safety and patient management, JMRI 1 (1991) 97–101.
[2] A.M. Sawyer-Glover, F.G. Shellock, Pre-MRI procedure screening: recommendations and safety considerations for biomedical implants and devices, JMRI 12 (2000) 92–106.
[3] V.C. Buttram, W.E. Gibbons, Mullerian anomalies: a proposed classification (an analysis of 144 cases), Fertil. Steril. 32 (1) (1979) 40–46.
[4] The American Fertility Society, The American fertility society classifications of adnexal adhesions, distal tubal obstruction, tubal occlusion secondary to tubal ligation, tubal pregnancies, mullerian anomalies and intrauterine adhesions, Fertil. Steril. 49 (6) (1988) 944–955.
[5] L. Fedele, et al., Magnetic resonance imaging in Mayer-Rokitansky-Kuster-Hauser syndrome, Obstet. Gynecol. 76 (4) (1990) 593–596.
[6] K. Togashi, et al., Vaginal agenesis: classification by MR imaging, Radiology 162 (1987) 675–677.
[7] J.R. Vainright, C.J. Fulp, M.L. Schiebler, MR imaging of vaginal agenesis with hematocolpos, J. Comput. Assist. Tomogr. 12 (5) (1988) 891–893.
[8] B.M. Carrington, et al., Mullerian duct anomalies: MR imaging evaluation, Radiology 176 (1990) 715–720.
[9] J.S. Pellerito, et al., Diagnosis of uterine anomalies: relative accuracy of MR imaging, endovaginal ultrasound, and hysterosalpingography, Radiology 183 (3) (1992) 795–800.
[10] L. Fedele, et al., Magnetic resonance evaluation of double uteri, Obstet. Gynecol. 74 (6) (1989) 844–847.
[11] H.A. Homer, T.C. Li, I.D. Cooke, The septate uterus: a review of management and reproductive outcome, Fertil. Steril. 73 (1) (2000) 1–14.
[12] T.G. Zreik, et al., Myometrial tissue in uterine septa, J. Am. Assoc. Gynecol. Laparosc. 5 (1998) 155–160.
[13] S. Kipersztok, et al., Comparison of magnetic resonance imaging and transvaginal sonography with hysterosonography in the evaluation of women exposed to ddiethylstilbestrol, J. Reprod. Med. 41 (1996) 347–351.
[14] G.S. Letterie, M.F. Haggerty, Magnetic resonance imaging of intrauterine synechiae, Gynecol. Obstet. Invest. 37 (1) (1994) 66–68.
[15] A.C. Bacelar, et al., The value of MRI in the assessment of traumatic intra-uterine adhesions (Asherman's syndrome), Clin. Radiol. 50 (1995) 80–83.
[16] H. Hricak, et al., Uterine leiomyomas: correlation of MR histopathologic findings, and symptoms, Radiology 158 (1986) 385–391.
[17] Y. Horie, et al., Lipoadenofibroma of the uterine corpus: Report of a new variant of adenofibroma (benign mullerian mixed tumor), Arch. Pathol. Lab. Med. 119 (1995) 274–276.
[18] Y. Yamashita, M. Torashima, M. Takahashi, Hyperintense uterine leiomyoma at T2-weighted MR imaging: Differentiation with dynamic enhanced MR imaging and clinical implications, Radiology 189 (1993) 721–725.
[19] R.C. Jha, et al., Symptomatic fibroleiomyomata: MR Imaging of the uterus before and after uterine arterial embolization, Radiology 217 (2000) 228–235.

[20] M. Matson, A. Nicholson, A.M. Belli, Anastomoses of the ovarian and uterine arteries: a potential pitfall and cause of failure of uterine embolization, Cardiovasc. Interv. Radiol. 23 (2000) 393–396.
[21] C.A. Binkert, R.T. Andrews, J.A. Kaufman, Utility of nonselective abdominal aortography in demonstrating ovarian collaterals in patients undergoing uterine artery embolization for fibroids, J. Vasc. Interv. Radiol. 12 (2001) 841–845.
[22] B. Nikolic, et al., Ovarian artery supply of uterine fibroids as a cause of treatment failure after uterine artery embolization: a case report, J. Vasc. Interv. Radiol. 10 (1999) 116–1170.
[23] H.W. Jones, G.S. Jones (Eds.), Gynecology, 3rd ed., Williams and Wilkins, Baltimore, 1982, pp. 245–253.
[24] K. Togashi, et al., Uterine contractions: possible diagnostic pitfall at MR imaging, J. Magn. Reson. Imaging 3 (1993) 889–893.
[25] K. Togashi, et al., Sustained uterine contractions: a cause of hypointense myometrial bulging, Radiology 187 (1993) 707–710.
[26] S.M. Ascher, et al., Adenomyosis: prospective comparison of MR imaging and transvaginal sonography, Radiology 190 (1994) 803–806.
[27] C. Reinhold, et al., Diffuse adenomyosis: comparison of endovaginal US and MR imaging with histopathologic correlation, Radiology 199 (1996) 151–158.
[28] K. Togashi, et al., Adenomyosis: diagnosis with MR imaging, Radiology 166 (1988) 111–114.
[29] K. Togashi, et al., Enlarged uterus: differentiation between adenomyosis and leiomyoma with MR imaging, Radiology 171 (1989) 531–534.
[30] A.S. Mark, et al., Adenomyosis and leiomyoma: differential diagnosis with MR imaging, Radiology 163 (1987) 527–529.
[31] R. Azziz, Adenomyosis: current perspectives, Obstet. Gynecol. Clin. North Am. 16 (1989) 221–235.
[32] D.G. Mitchell, E.K. Outwater, Benign gynecologic disease: applications of magnetic resonance imaging, Top. Magn. Reson. Imaging 7 (1995) 26–43.
[33] K.G. Bis, et al., Pelvic endometriosis: MR imaging spectrum with laparoscopic correlation and diagnostic pitfalls, Radiographics 17 (1997) 639–655.
[34] K. Togashi, et al., Endometrial cysts: diagnosis with MR imaging, Radiology 180 (1991) 73–78.
[35] E. Outwater, et al., Characterization of hemorrhagic adnexal lesions with MR imaging blinded reader study, Radiology 186 (1993) 489–494.

# Author index

Acién, M., 335
Acién, P., 335
Al-Fadhli, R., 197
Andersen, A.N., 32
Anne, D., 303
Apter, D., 81
Arroyo, G., 156

Bahadur, G., 295
Barri, P.N., 156
Bonduelle, M., 343
Boudreaux, M.Y., 233
Boyle, J., 225
Braverman, A.M., 270
Breheny, S., 119
Brugo Olmedo, S., 167

Cacciatore, R., 81
Carp, H.J.A., 328
Chantal, L., 303
Cohlen, B.J., 208
Collins, J.A., 57
Conrads, T.P., 375

Davies, M., 225
Daya, S., 318
Dechaud, H., 96
Demirol, A., 287
Domínguez, F., 177

Englert, Y., 303
Erickson, G.F., 241
Evers, J.L.H., 90

Fabienne, D., 303
Faidherbe, J., 96
Falcone, T., 107
Farquhar, C.M., 191
Foster, W.G., 126

Fujii, S., 183
Fukuhara, K., 183

Gibson, F., 351
Golombok, S., 256
Guérif, F., 170
Gurgan, T., 287

Hamamah, S., 96
Hammer Burns, L., 264
Healy, D.L., 119
Hedon, B., 96
Hermanson, E., 81
Hickey, T., 225
Hochereau de Reviers, M.-T., 170
Hood, B.L., 375
Horcajadas, J.A., 177

Irvine, S., 202

Jensen, T.K., 32

Kanamori, T., 183
Kariya, M., 183
Katabuchi, H., 248
Kovacs, G., 119
Kupesic, S., 393

Laurent-Cadoret, V., 170

MacLachlan, V., 119
Martín, J., 177
Matsumura, N., 183
McLachlan, R.I., 10
McMahon, C., 351
Menkveld, R., 218
Mikkelsen, A.L., 160
Moore, R.K., 241
Moran, L., 225

Neal, M.S., 126
Norman, R.J., 225

Ohba, T., 248
Okamura, H., 248
Otsuka, F., 241

Paavonen, J., 277
Pellicer, A., 177
Pennings, G., 311
Philippe, R., 303

Reinhold, C., 401
Reubinoff, B., 45
Reyftmann, L., 96
Rombauts, L., 119
Royere, D., 170
Rozenbaum, H., 139

Sallam, H.N., 111
Schiff, I., 3
Serena, E., 303
Serour, G.I., 21
Shimasaki, S., 241
Shime, H., 183
Simón, C., 177

Skakkebæk, N.E., 32
Skouby, S.O., 151
Sowter, M.C., 72
Sutcliffe, A.G., 359
Suzuki, A., 183

Takakura, K., 183
Takasaki, A., 248
Talbott, E.O., 233
Tanaka, N., 248
Tapanainen, J.S., 63
Tulandi, T., 197

Utian, W.H., 133

Veenstra, T.D., 375
Veiga, A., 156
Verhoeven, H.C., 381

Wang, J., 225
Weston, G.C., 367

YoungLai, E.V., 126
Yu, S.L., 69

Zborowski, J.V., 233

# Keyword index

Androgens 225
Anonymity 303
Anovulation 57
Antibiotic treatment 218
Apoptosis 170
Assisted reproduction 111, 119, 167, 351
Assisted reproductive therapies 359
Augmented reality 107

Bcl2 170
Bone morphogenetic protein 241
Breast cancer 3

Cardiovascular disease 151
Causality 191
Child 351
Child development 256
Childhood 359
Children 343
Chlamydia trachomatis 277
Conception 295
Condoms 81
Congenital malformation 343
Consent 295
Contraceptive 69
Contraceptive pill 63
Controlled ovarian hyperstimulation–intrauterine insemination 119
Coronary calcium 233
Coronary heart disease 233
Cost-effectiveness 208
Cryopreservation 295
CSF-1 248
Cytokine 183

Definitions 133
Diabetes 233
Diagnosis 225, 318

DNA fragmentation 218
Donor insemination 256
2D PAGE 375

Embryo 295
Embryo quality 156
Embryo selection criteria 156
Embryo transfer 111
Endocrine disrupter 126
Endometrial ablation 72
Endometrial receptivity 177
Endometriosis 57, 90, 381, 401
Estrogen 3
Ethics 303, 311
Ethics-legal 21
Etiology 225
Evidence-based medicine 111, 202, 328

Fas 170
Fecundity 32, 126
Female factors 32
Fertility 32
Fertility, ovary 241
Fertilization 167
Fibroid 183, 197
Fibroids 191
Follicle development 248
Follow-up study 343
Function 270

Gamete 295
Gamete interaction 167
Gender 21
Gender selection 21
Gene expression profile 177
Genomics 367
Gonadotropins 10
Granulosa cell 241

Growth factor 183
Guidelines 202

Habitual abortion 318, 328
Heart disease 3
Heavy menstrual bleeding 69
HERS 139
Histogenesis 183
HLA 311
Hormonal contraception 81
HRT 139
Human embryonic stem cells 45
Human oocytes 160
Hydrosalpinx 96
Hysterectomy 72, 197
Hystero-contrast-salpingography 393
Hysteroscopy 381

ICAT 375
ICSI 111
Infertility 57, 126, 191, 202, 270, 277, 287, 351, 393, 401
Infertility counseling 264
Insemination 295
Intimacy 270
Intracytoplasmatic sperm injection 343
Intrauterine insemination 208
In vitro fertilisation 119, 343
In vitro fertilization 10
IVF 111

Kit 170

Laparoscopy 96
Leiomyoma 183, 197, 401
Leiomyomata 191
Leukocytospermia 218
Levonorgestrel 69
Levonorgestrel intrauterine system 72
Live birth rate per cycle 119
LNG-IUS 69

Macrophage 248
Male factors 32
Male infertility 202

Male subfertility 208
Mass spectrometry 375
Maturation in vitro 160
Menopause 133, 151
Menorrhagia 63, 72
Menstrual disorder 63
Microarray 177
Microarrays 367
Mild ovarian hyperstimulation 208
Mirena 69
Miscarriage 335
MR imaging 401
MRI 401
Multidimensional separation 375
Multiple pregnancy 208
Myolysis 197
Myoma 197
Myomectomy 197

New developments 151

Office endoscopy 381
Oocyte 241, 295
Oocyte donation 303
Outcome 359
Ovarian drilling 381
Ovarian monitoring and puncture 393
Ovarian tissue 295
Ovarian toxicity 126
Ovulation 241
Ovulation enhancement 119
Ovulation induction 119, 248

Paediatric 359
Parenthood 311
Parenting 256, 351
Polycystic ovary syndrome 225, 233
Poor responder 248
Posthumous 295
Predicting factors 208
Pregnancy loss 318, 328, 401
Pregnancy rate 90
Preimplantation genetic diagnosis 311
Prenatal diagnosis 343
Progestogen 69

Prostaglandin inhibitor 63
Proteomics 375
Proximal tubal occlusion 96
Psychosocial 351

Recurrent miscarriage 318, 328
Relationships 270
Reproduction 241, 295, 367
Reproductive health counseling 264
Reproductive staging 133
Review 367
Risk factors 233
Risk groups 151
Risk markers 151
Robotics 107
ROS production 218

SCF 170
Semen 10
Semen parameters 218
Semen quality 32
Sexual health services 81
Sexuality 270
Sexuality education 81
Sexually transmitted infections 277
Single pregnancy 119
Solo mothers 256
Sperm 295
Sperm donation 303
Spermatogenesis 10, 170
STI 81
Subfertility 277

Success rate 119
Surgery 90
Surgical treatment 335

Term gestation 119
Testis 10
Three-dimensional ultrasound 393
Time trends 32
TNF 170
Toxicology 126
Tranexamic acid 63
Transcultural 21
Transplantation 45, 311
Transvaginal endoscopy 381
Treatment 287
Trials 139
Tubal disease 57
Tubal reversal of sterilization 96
Tubal surgery 96
Tuberculosis 287

Unexplained infertility 57
Unexplained subfertility 90
Uterine abnormalities 393
Uterine anomalies 335
Uterine anomaly 401
Uterine artery embolization 197
Uterine fibroid embolization 197

Virtual reality 107

WHI 139